Targeting Oxidative Stress for Disease

Targeting Oxidative Stress for Disease

Guest Editors

Nada Orsolic
Maja Jazvinšćak Jembrek

MDPI

Basel • Beijing • Wuhan • Barcelona • Belgrade • Novi Sad • Cluj • Manchester

Guest Editors
Nada Orsolic
Department of Animal Physiology
Faculty of Science
Zagreb
Croatia

Maja Jazvinšćak Jembrek
Division of Molecular Medicine
Ruđer Bošković Institute
Zagreb
Croatia

Editorial Office
MDPI AG
Grosspeteranlage 5
4052 Basel, Switzerland

This is a reprint of the Special Issue, published open access by the journal *International Journal of Molecular Sciences* (ISSN 1422-0067), freely accessible at: https://www.mdpi.com/journal/ijms/special_issues/B461A9ZK47.

For citation purposes, cite each article independently as indicated on the article page online and as indicated below:

Lastname, A.A.; Lastname, B.B. Article Title. *Journal Name* **Year**, *Volume Number*, Page Range.

ISBN 978-3-7258-4323-7 (Hbk)
ISBN 978-3-7258-4324-4 (PDF)
https://doi.org/10.3390/books978-3-7258-4324-4

Contents

International Journal of *Molecular Sciences*

Editorial

Targeting Oxidative Stress for Disease

Nada Oršolić [1,*] and Maja Jazvinšćak Jembrek [2,3]

[1] Division of Animal Physiology, Faculty of Science, University of Zagreb, Rooseveltov trg 6, HR-10000 Zagreb, Croatia
[2] Croatia Division of Molecular Medicine, Laboratory for Protein Dynamics, Ruđer Bošković Institute, Bijenička Cesta 54, HR-10000 Zagreb, Croatia; maja.jazvinscak.jembrek@irb.hr
[3] School of Medicine, Catholic University of Croatia, Ilica 244, HR-10000 Zagreb, Croatia
* Correspondence: nada.orsolic@biol.pmf.hr; Tel.: +385-1-4877-735; Fax: +385-1-4826-26

Oxidative stress (OS) refers to a metabolic imbalance caused by the excessive production of reactive oxygen species (ROS) and an insufficient antioxidant defense. It plays a key role in the development of numerous diseases, including neurological disorders, type 2 diabetes, cancer, aging, heart and acute renal failure, hypertension, preeclampsia, atherosclerosis, coronary artery disease, asthma, chronic obstructive pulmonary disease, rheumatoid arthritis, glaucoma, osteoporosis, and sexual dysfunction [1–4]. Therefore, this Special Issue, title "Targeting Oxidative Stress for Disease", aimed to provide recent insights into the role of ROS-mediated effects in both physiological and pathological processes underlying disease development.

OS is most commonly associated with neurological disorders. Increasing evidence suggests that OS plays a role in neurodevelopmental disorders, being one of the major environmental factors driving genomic instability and the deregulation of gene expression. Mahmoudi and co-authors [5] analyzed the expression of circular RNAs (circRNAs), a class of non-coding RNAs, and their role in competitive endogenous (ceRNA) networks (including circRNA, miRNA, and mRNA) in differentiating SH-SY5Y neuroblastoma cells that are exposed to OS before and during differentiation. The circRNAs containing miRNA recognition elements are of particular interest, because they act as miRNA sponges. By sequestering miRNAs, circRNAs prevent them from binding to their target mRNAs, thereby influencing various cellular processes, including gene expression [6]. Research on SH-SY5Y cells has shown that circRNAomes' response to OS differs between early neural progenitor cells and cells undergoing neuronal differentiation, with the early stages being the more sensitive to OS exposure. These findings offer valuable insights into the regulatory mechanisms that are induced by OS and other environmental factors that may influence neuronal development [6].

OS and reduced antioxidant capacity have been implicated in the pathogenesis of autism spectrum disorder (ASD), a neurodevelopmental disorder with an increasing global incidence. While the causes of ASD are rather complex and not fully understood, OS biomarkers have been proposed as a potential approach for early diagnosis and the evaluation of pharmacological and nutritional treatments [7]. Moreover, antioxidant supplementation has been considered as a potential strategy for improving metabolic imbalances in ASD [8]. Interestingly, at the molecular level, ASD subtypes may be distinguished based on the ferroptosis score and expression of selected ferroptosis-related genes [9]. Ferroptosis, a form of cell death that is triggered by an Fe^{2+} overload and excessive ROS accumulation, has been linked to the pathophysiology of ASD. In animal models, attenuating ferroptosis has been shown to mitigate autism-like behaviors, further supporting the potential

https://doi.org/10.3390/ijms26062692

clinical application of OS-targeting strategies [10]. ASD is also linked with inflammatory abnormalities, and treatment with anti-inflammatory agents may be beneficial for some individuals. However, further randomized placebo-controlled trials are required to determine the effectiveness of immunoregulatory agents as treatment options for ASD patients [11,12]. The anti-epileptogenic potential of certain compounds may also rely on their ROS scavenging capabilities [13]. Psychiatric disorders are similarly influenced by OS. A better understanding of the role of OS in the development and progression of psychiatric diseases could lead to novel therapeutic approaches aimed at modifying the severity of OS. However, the effects of neuropsychiatric drugs on OS are contradictory: some exhibit protective effects, while others disrupt redox homeostasis [14–16]. Therefore, in order to improve the clinical outcomes, future research should focus on rigorous clinical trials to clarify how different neuropsychiatric drugs modulate OS in distinct patient subgroups.

Antioxidants may also play a beneficial role in bronchopulmonary dysplasia, the most common respiratory complication in premature infants [17]. Although the pathogenesis of this disease is rather complex, it is mainly related to OS due to the limited antioxidant capacity of premature infants, along with inflammatory complications [18]. Emerging evidence suggests that next-generation antioxidants, which combine antioxidant and anti-inflammatory properties, hold promise for preventing and treating this condition [19,20]. The potential of antioxidants has also been explored for the treatment of cardiovascular complications of cirrhosis [21].

The potential of OS has also been studied in the context of cancer treatment. Although further research is needed to fully elucidate the contribution of OS to the development, progression, and treatment outcomes of cancer, an increasing amount of evidence suggests that ROS enhancement correlates with drug resistance, tumor aggressiveness, and poorer survival rates [22,23]. Cancer cells undergo redox reprogramming by simultaneously increasing ROS production and antioxidant defenses, optimizing ROS-driven proliferative signals while minimizing oxidative damage to intracellular targets [24]. Moreover, an ROS increase typically creates an inflammatory environment that promotes tumor growth and metastatic potential [25]. Despite significant advances in cancer treatment, drug resistance remains a major challenge. Therefore, novel chemopreventive agents are urgently needed to improve the overall efficiency of existing treatment options. By their ability to detoxify ROS, increased levels of various antioxidant enzymes may interfere with the efficacy of various anti-cancer therapies that rely on ROS-mediated cytotoxicity. Consequently, inhibitors of antioxidant enzymes and other antioxidant defense mechanisms have emerged as potential strategies for the improvement of anti-cancer therapies and overcoming treatment resistance [26–29].

Dietary approaches may also be effective in cancer prevention and treatment [29,30]. Various phytochemicals and bioactive natural products, such as royal jelly or propolis, show anti-inflammatory and anti-proliferative activities, acting synergistically with anti-cancer drugs to enhance the treatment efficacy and reduce side effects. In addition, these multitarget compounds may regulate the signaling pathways, antioxidant levels, and genetic and epigenetic instability that promote tumor growth [31–33]. However, despite the extensive preclinical evidence supporting the therapeutic potential of natural compounds, future research should prioritize clinical trials to determine their exact role as complementary cancer treatments.

In conclusion, OS contributes to the pathology of numerous diseases. While antioxidants appear to be a rational strategy for preventing and treating OS-related conditions, clinical trial results have been inconsistent. Hopefully, the data presented in this Special Issue should be an incentive for future clinical research that will advance our understanding of the role of OS and the therapeutic potential of OS-targeted therapies for improving human health and well-being.

Conflicts of Interest: The authors declare no conflict of interest.

References

1. Forman, H.J.; Zhang, H. Targeting oxidative stress in disease: Promise and limitations of antioxidant therapy. *Nat. Rev. Drug Discov.* **2021**, *20*, 689–709. [CrossRef] [PubMed]
2. Reddy, V.P. Oxidative Stress in Health and Disease. *Biomedicines* **2023**, *11*, 2925. [CrossRef] [PubMed]
3. Vona, R.; Pallotta, L.; Cappelletti, M.; Severi, C.; Matarrese, P. The Impact of Oxidative Stress in Human Pathology: Focus on Gastrointestinal Disorders. *Antioxidants* **2021**, *10*, 201. [CrossRef] [PubMed]
4. Jomova, K.; Raptova, R.; Alomar, S.Y.; Alwasel, S.H.; Nepovimova, E.; Kuca, K.; Valko, M. Reactive oxygen species, toxicity, oxidative stress, and antioxidants: Chronic diseases and aging. *Arch. Toxicol.* **2023**, *97*, 2499–2574. [CrossRef]
5. Mahmoudi, E.; Khavari, B.; Cairns, M.J. Oxidative Stress-Associated Alteration of circRNA and Their ceRNA Network in Differentiating Neuroblasts. *Int. J. Mol. Sci.* **2024**, *25*, 12459. [CrossRef]
6. Hansen, T.B.; Jensen, T.I.; Clausen, B.H.; Bramsen, J.B.; Finsen, B.; Damgaard, C.K.; Kjems, J. Natural RNA circles function as efficient microRNA sponges. *Nature* **2013**, *495*, 384–388. [CrossRef]
7. Liu, X.; Lin, J.; Zhang, H.; Khan, N.U.; Zhang, J.; Tang, X.; Cao, X.; Shen, L. Oxidative Stress in Autism Spectrum Disorder-Current Progress of Mechanisms and Biomarkers. *Front. Psychiatry* **2022**, *13*, 813304. [CrossRef]
8. Manivasagam, T.; Arunadevi, S.; Essa, M.M.; SaravanaBabu, C.; Borah, A.; Thenmozhi, A.J.; Qoronfleh, M.W. Role of Oxidative Stress and Antioxidants in Autism. *Adv. Neurobiol.* **2020**, *24*, 193–206. [CrossRef] [PubMed]
9. Liu, L.; Lai, Y.; Zhan, Z.; Fu, Q.; Jiang, Y. Identification of Ferroptosis-Related Molecular Clusters and Immune Characterization in Autism Spectrum Disorder. *Front Genet.* **2022**, *13*, 911119. [CrossRef]
10. Wu, H.; Luan, Y.; Wang, H.; Zhang, P.; Liu, S.; Wang, P.; Cao, Y.; Sun, H.; Wu, L. Selenium inhibits ferroptosis and ameliorates autistic-like behaviors of BTBR mice by regulating the Nrf2/GPx4 pathway. *Brain Res. Bull.* **2022**, *183*, 38–48. [CrossRef]
11. Arteaga-Henríquez, G.; Gisbert, L.; Ramos-Quiroga, J.A. Immunoregulatory and/or Anti-inflammatory Agents for the Management of Core and Associated Symptoms in Individuals with Autism Spectrum Disorder: A Narrative Review of Randomized, Placebo-Controlled Trials. *CNS Drugs* **2023**, *37*, 215–229. [CrossRef]
12. Jyonouchi, H. Autism spectrum disorder and a possible role of anti-inflammatory treatments: Experience in the pediatric allergy/immunology clinic. *Front. Psychiatry* **2024**, *15*, 1333717. [CrossRef] [PubMed]
13. Borowicz-Reutt, K.K.; Czuczwar, S.J. Role of oxidative stress in epileptogenesis and potential implications for therapy. *Pharmacol. Rep.* **2020**, *72*, 1218–1226. [CrossRef] [PubMed]
14. Behr, G.A.; Moreira, J.C.; Frey, B.N. Preclinical and clinical evidence of antioxidant effects of antidepressant agents: Implications for the pathophysiology of major depressive disorder. *Oxidative Med. Cell Longev.* **2012**, *2012*, 609421. [CrossRef] [PubMed]
15. Caruso, G.; Grasso, M.; Fidilio, A.; Torrisi, S.A.; Musso, N.; Geraci, F.; Tropea, M.R.; Privitera, A.; Tascedda, F.; Puzzo, D.; et al. Antioxidant Activity of Fluoxetine and Vortioxetine in a Non-Transgenic Animal Model of Alzheimer's Disease. *Front. Pharmacol.* **2021**, *12*, 809541. [CrossRef]
16. Yang, M.; Wang, C.; Zhao, G.; Kong, D.; Liu, L.; Yuan, S.; Chen, W.; Feng, C.; Li, Z. Comparative Analysis of the Pre- and Post-Medication Effects of Antipsychotic Agents on the Blood-Based Oxidative Stress Biomarkers in Patients with Schizophrenia: A Meta-Analysis. *Curr. Neuropharmacol.* **2023**, *21*, 340–352. [CrossRef]
17. Perrone, S.; Tataranno, M.L., Buonocore, G. Oxidative stress and bronchopulmonary dysplasia. *J. Clin. Neonatol.* **2012**, *1*, 109–114. [CrossRef]
18. Saugstad, O.D. Bronchopulmonary dysplasia-oxidative stress and antioxidants. *Semin. Neonatol.* **2003**, *8*, 39–49. [CrossRef]
19. Ferrante, G.; Montante, C.; Notarbartolo, V.; Giuffrè, M. Antioxidants: Role the in prevention and treatment of bronchopulmonary dysplasia. *Paediatr. Respir. Rev.* **2022**, *42*, 53–58. [CrossRef]
20. Teng, M.; Wu, T.-J.; Jing, X.; Day, B.W.; Pritchard, K.A., Jr.; Naylor, S.; Teng, R.-J. Temporal Dynamics of Oxidative Stress and Inflammation in Bronchopulmonary Dysplasia. *Int. J. Mol. Sci.* **2024**, *25*, 10145. [CrossRef]
21. Ferlitsch, A.; Pleiner, J.; Mittermayer, F.; Schaller, G.; Homoncik, M.; Peck-Radosavljevic, M.; Wolzt, M. Vasoconstrictor hyporeactivity can be reversed by antioxidants in patients with advanced alcoholic cirrhosis of the liver and ascites. *Crit. Care Med.* **2005**, *33*, 2028–2033. [CrossRef] [PubMed]
22. Oshi, M.; Gandhi, S.; Yan, L.; Tokumaru, Y.; Wu, R.; Yamada, A.; Matsuyama, R.; Endo, I.; Takabe, K. Abundance of reactive oxygen species (ROS) is associated with tumor aggressiveness, immune response, and worse survival in breast cancer. *Breast Cancer Res. Treat.* **2022**, *194*, 231–241. [CrossRef]
23. Zhou, X.; An, B.; Lin, Y.; Ni, Y.; Zhao, X.; Liang, X. Molecular mechanisms of ROS-modulated cancer chemoresistance and therapeutic strategies. *Biomed. Pharmacother.* **2023**, *165*, 115036. [CrossRef]

24. Gu, X.; Mu, C.; Zheng, R.; Zhang, Z.; Zhang, Q.; Liang, T. The Cancer Antioxidant Regulation System in Therapeutic Resistance. *Antioxidants* **2024**, *13*, 778. [CrossRef]
25. Yu, W.; Tu, Y.; Long, Z.; Liu, J.; Kong, D.; Peng, J.; Wu, H.; Zheng, G.; Zhao, J.; Chen, Y.; et al. Reactive Oxygen Species Bridge the Gap between Chronic Inflammation and Tumor Development. *Oxidative Med. Cell. Longev.* **2022**, *2022*, 2606928. [CrossRef] [PubMed]
26. Yang, H.; Villani, R.M.; Wang, H.; Simpson, M.J.; Roberts, M.S.; Tang, M.; Liang, X. The role of cellular reactive oxygen species in cancer chemotherapy. *J. Exp. Clin. Cancer Res.* **2018**, *37*, 266. [CrossRef] [PubMed]
27. Udomsak, W.; Kucinska, M.; Pospieszna, J.; Dams-Kozlowska, H.; Chatuphonprasert, W.; Murias, M. Antioxidant Enzymes in Cancer Cells: Their Role in Photodynamic Therapy Resistance and Potential as Targets for Improved Treatment Outcomes. *Int. J. Mol. Sci.* **2024**, *25*, 3164. [CrossRef]
28. Kong, Q.; Lillehei, K.O. Antioxidant inhibitors for cancer therapy. *Med. Hypotheses* **1998**, *51*, 405–409. [CrossRef]
29. Sznarkowska, A.; Kostecka, A.; Meller, K.; Bielawski, K.P. Inhibition of cancer antioxidant defense by natural compounds. *Oncotarget* **2017**, *8*, 15996–16016. [CrossRef]
30. Choudhari, A.S.; Mandave, P.C.; Deshpande, M.; Ranjekar, P.; Prakash, O. Phytochemicals in Cancer Treatment: From Preclinical Studies to Clinical Practice. *Front. Pharmacol.* **2020**, *10*, 1614. [CrossRef]
31. Lyubitelev, A.; Studitsky, V. Inhibition of Cancer Development by Natural Plant Polyphenols: Molecular Mechanisms. *Int. J. Mol. Sci.* **2023**, *24*, 10663. [CrossRef] [PubMed]
32. Salama, S.; Shou, Q.; Abd El-Wahed, A.A.; Elias, N.; Xiao, J.; Swillam, A.; Umair, M.; Guo, Z.; Daglia, M.; Wang, K.; et al. Royal Jelly: Beneficial Properties and Synergistic Effects with Chemotherapeutic Drugs with Particular Emphasis in Anticancer Strategies. *Nutrients* **2022**, *14*, 4166. [CrossRef] [PubMed]
33. Oršolić, N.; Jazvinšćak Jembrek, M. Molecular and Cellular Mechanisms of Propolis and Its Polyphenolic Compounds against Cancer. *Int. J. Mol. Sci.* **2022**, *23*, 10479. [CrossRef] [PubMed]

International Journal of *Molecular Sciences*

MDPI

Article

Oxidative Stress-Associated Alteration of circRNA and Their ceRNA Network in Differentiating Neuroblasts

Ebrahim Mahmoudi [1,2,†], Behnaz Khavari [1,2,†] and Murray J. Cairns [1,2,*]

[1] School of Biomedical Sciences and Pharmacy, The University of Newcastle, Newcastle, NSW 2308, Australia
[2] Precision Medicine Research Program, Hunter Medical Research Institute, Newcastle, NSW 2305, Australia
* Correspondence: murray.cairns@newcastle.edu.au
† These authors contributed equally to this work.

Abstract: Oxidative stress from environmental exposures is thought to play a role in neurodevelopmental disorders; therefore, understanding the underlying molecular regulatory network is essential for mitigating its impacts. In this study, we analysed the competitive endogenous RNA (ceRNA) network mediated by circRNAs, a novel class of regulatory molecules, in an SH-SY5Y cell model of oxidative stress, both prior to and during neural differentiation, using RNA sequencing and in silico analysis. We identified 146 differentially expressed circRNAs, including 93 upregulated and 53 downregulated circRNAs, many of which were significantly co-expressed with mRNAs that potentially interact with miRNAs. We constructed a circRNA–miRNA–mRNA network and identified 15 circRNAs serving as hubs within the regulatory axes, with target genes enriched in stress- and neuron-related pathways, such as *signaling by VEGF*, *axon guidance*, *signaling by FGFR*, and the *RAF/MAP kinase cascade*. These findings provide insights into the role of the circRNA-mediated ceRNA network in oxidative stress during neuronal differentiation, which may help explain the regulatory mechanisms underlying neurodevelopmental disorders associated with oxidative stress.

Keywords: circRNAs; ceRNA network; interaction axes; oxidative stress; neuronal differentiation; neurodevelopmental disorders; SH-SY5Y

1. Introduction

Oxidative stress is a common phenomenon induced by an imbalance between the production of reactive oxygen species (ROS) and their clearance by the antioxidant system. This process causes significant molecular and cellular damage to tissues, particularly in the brain, which is highly susceptible to oxidative stress due its elevated level of oxygen consumption and lipid-rich content [1]. A highly oxidative environment affects neuronal structural integrity and disrupts their optimal function, potentially leading to pathological conditions in the human brain [2].

Emerging evidence suggests that oxidative stress may be an important contributor to a host of neurodegenerative and neuropsychiatric disorders, such as Alzheimer's Disease (AD), Parkinson's Disease (PD), schizophrenia, bipolar disorder, and depression, where it impairs critical processes including cognition and neurotransmission [1,3,4]. In psychiatric conditions, these mechanisms may be mediated via the inflammatory response of the brain, which frequently appears in such disorders and may play an important role in their pathophysiology [5]. Perturbation of antioxidant enzymes and elevated levels of free radicals have been observed in bipolar disorder, schizophrenia, and major depression [6–8]. Studies have shown that using antioxidants, such as vitamins C and E, EGb, and ginkgo, improved clinical symptoms in schizophrenia [9], supporting an association between oxidative stress and the disorder's pathophysiology.

Given the potential involvement of oxidative stress in the development of various diseases and its detrimental effects on the genome [10], there has been increasing effort to explore the molecular consequences of oxidative conditions. This includes gene expression studies, which have revealed significant transcriptomic responses to oxidative stress [11–13]. In our recent work, we observed alterations in many genes in response to oxidative stress, particularly in pathways associated with psychiatric disorders and immunity-related clusters [13]. Additionally, associated changes in non-coding RNA (ncRNA), such as microRNA (miRNA) and long non-coding RNA (lncRNA), may mediate the effects of oxidative stress [14,15], and thus play a critical role in its pathophysiological consequences. For example, our lab has demonstrated that oxidative conditions induce dysregulation of numerous miRNAs involved in psychiatric disorders, including 12 miRNAs originating from DLK1-DIO3, a schizophrenia-associated locus [16].

Circular RNAs (circRNAs) are a class of ncRNAs formed through the back-splicing of pre-mRNA transcripts [17]. CircRNAs are evolutionarily conserved and stably expressed in almost all mammalian cells and tissues, and they appear, at least in some cases, to modulate the activity of target nucleic acids, including miRNA and mRNA [18]. These transcripts, primarily present in the cytoplasm, are usually derived from coding genes and in some cases contain open reading frames that support translation [19,20]. CircRNAs are implicated in various cellular processes, including proliferation, differentiation, inflammatory and immune responses, apoptosis, and development [21,22]. Increasing evidence indicates that circRNAs are associated with a range of human diseases, including neuropsychiatric and neurodegenerative disorders such as schizophrenia, AD, autoimmune diseases, cancer, and cardiovascular diseases [23–26]. Mechanistic studies have demonstrated the regulatory function of circRNAs by fine-tuning mRNA at the transcriptional and post-transcriptional levels [17]. These molecules have been shown to act as competitive endogenous RNAs (ceRNAs) that bind miRNAs and attenuate their target gene-silencing activity. For example, a circRNA-associated ceRNA network is known for CDR1as, a brain-enriched circRNA that sponges miR-7, resulting in upregulation of the miRNA gene targets of Fos, Nr4a3, Irs2, and Klf4 [27–29].

Given the association of oxidative stress as a significant risk factor for neurological disorders, a deep understanding of the molecular basis, in particular the regulatory systems that mediate oxidative stress-induced changes, seems essential to uncovering their mechanisms in the pathogenesis of these disorders. This understanding may also aid in developing novel diagnostic agents or therapeutic targets for treating pathological conditions characterised by oxidative features, such as neurodevelopmental diseases. CircRNAs serve as regulatory molecules that have been implicated in oxidative stress-associated pathological processes and disorders. We therefore hypothesised that circRNAs and their ceRNA network may mediate molecular perturbations arising from oxidative stress. To investigate this, we reanalysed our total RNA expression dataset using a circRNA-oriented pipeline and detected thousands of circRNAs, many of which were found to be associated with oxidative stress. Our bioinformatic analysis suggested these circRNAs have the capacity to modulate the expression of target genes through circRNA–miRNA–mRNA interactions.

2. Results

2.1. Oxidative Stress Models and Profiling the circRNAome

In order to explore the circRNA-mediated impacts of oxidative stress and their critical role in neuronal development, we established two models using human SH-SY5Y neuroblast cultures: (i) pre-differentiation oxidative stress (PD-OS), in which oxidative stress was induced prior to neuronal differentiation, and (ii) during-differentiation oxidative stress (DD-OS), where oxidative stress was induced during differentiation. We determined transcriptome-wide profiles of circRNA in the two oxidative stress models by conducting RNA sequencing using total RNA depleted of ribosomal RNA. To predict and quantify the circRNAs, we used CIRIquant, a recent pipeline with high precision and reliability [30]. A total of over 51,000 circRNAs were initially identified in all the samples, but to ensure high confidence in the circRNAs, we applied a cutoff minimum of two junction reads in at least half of the samples in each oxidative stress model. This resulted in detection of 1910 and 1282 circRNAs in PD-OS and DD-OS, respectively (Supplementary Table S2). We used these circRNAs for all the analyses to ensure the reliability of the results. A flowchart of the experimental design and circRNA detection process is illustrated in Figure 1.

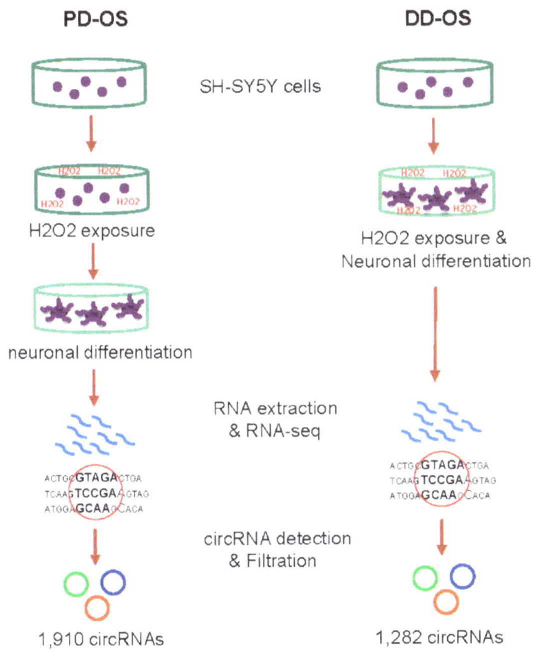

Figure 1. Schematic of the oxidative stress cell models in this study. The two oxidative stress models using SH-SY5Y neuroblastoma cells include: pre-differentiation oxidative stress (PD-OS), in which the oxidative condition was introduced before neuronal differentiation; and during-differentiation oxidative stress (DD-OS), in which the oxidative condition was introduced during differentiation. In the next step, the circRNA profile of each model was identified by RNA sequencing using total RNA depleted of ribosomal RNA, followed by bioinformatic analysis.

2.2. CircRNAs Are Differentially Expressed in Response to Oxidative Stress

To explore the circRNAome response to oxidative stress in neuronal differentiation, we performed differential expression analysis in PD-OS and DD-OS. The results showed that a total of 102 and 45 circRNAs were altered in PD-OS and DD-OS, respectively ($p < 0.05$, FC > 2; Supplementary Table S3). This included circTCONS_12_00000968, circSCARNA10, circCCDC90B, and circC7orf44, which survived multiple testing corrections in PD-OS, and circSIPA1L3 and circCANX in DD-OS. As illustrated in Figure 2a,b, about two thirds of the circRNAs were upregulated following the induction of oxidative stress: 65 circRNAs in PD-OS and 28 circRNAs in DD-OS. To further validate these observations, we examined the expression of the top 11 differentially expressed circRNAs (7 from PD-OS and 4 from DD-OS) using qRT-PCR (Figure 2c), and confirmed that the circRNA expression inferred from sequencing data correlated with qRT-PCR (Spearman's rank, $\rho = 0.74$, $p = 0.013$) (Figure 2d). We also noticed that the circRNA expression response to PD stress was distinct from that of DD stress, as there was only one circRNA, chr4:73956384|73958017 (circANKRD17), common between the two stress conditions. In order to investigate the potential mechanisms of action of the altered circRNAs, we performed Gene Ontology (GO) analysis for their parental genes. We found a significant enrichment of 27 biological processes in PD-OS, including *embryo development*, *brain development*, *neural tube development*, *forebrain development*, *head development*, and *embryonic morphogenesis* (Figure 2e; Supplementary Table S3). In DD-OS, however, there was no significant enrichment observed.

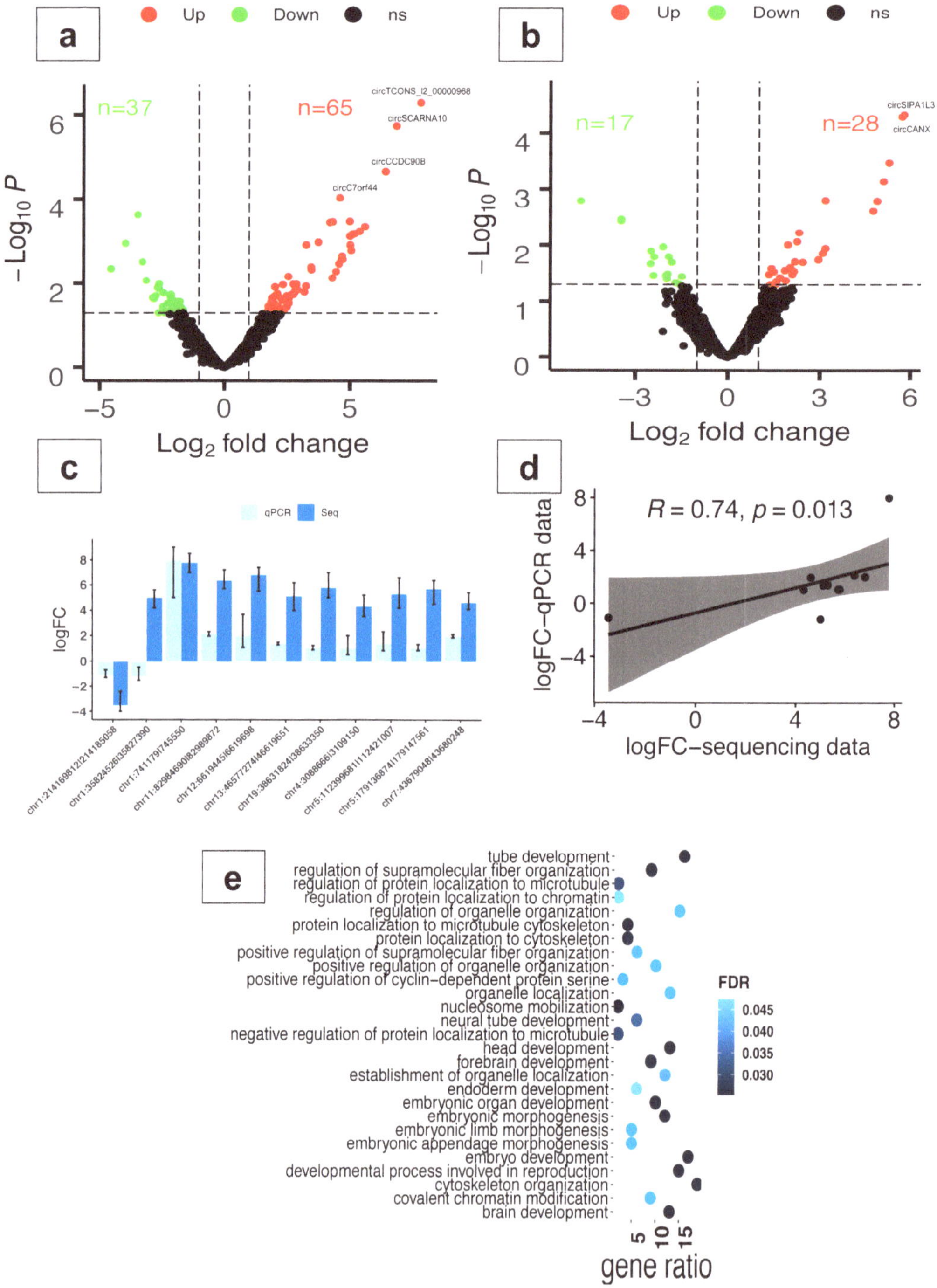

Figure 2. Analysis of circRNA differential expression in oxidative stress. Volcano plot generated using fold change values and *p*-values to illustrate the expression changes of circRNA in oxidative conditions PD-OS (**a**) and DD-OS (**b**). Red and green dots indicate significant upregulation and

downregulation, respectively, with the vertical lines representing a fold change > 2 and the horizontal line representing a $p < 0.05$ cutoff. Differentially expressed circRNAs that survived multiple testing correction are labelled on plots. (**c**) Side-by-side comparison of the expression change from sequencing data and qRT-PCR results for the top 11 differentially expressed circRNAs. All reactions were performed in triplicate. (**d**) Correlation between the expression change from sequencing data and qRT-PCR results (Spearman's rank, $\rho = 0.74$, $p = 0.013$). (**e**) Gene Ontology (GO) enrichment analysis for the altered circRNA parental genes in PD-OS. All the significantly enriched GO terms are shown (FDR < 0.05).

2.3. Identification of circRNA-Mediated ceRNA Network

Recent studies suggest that circRNAs containing MREs can competitively sponge miRNAs and inhibit them from binding to target sites within mRNA transcripts, thereby fine-tuning the expression of mRNA [27–29]. We therefore sought to characterise the circRNA-associated ceRNA regulatory network in oxidative stress. To this end, we integrated the expression profiles of circRNA with mRNA expression obtained from reanalysing our previous dataset [13], as well as miRNA expression results recently published by our lab [16]. As the potential regulatory relationships are reflected in a positive correlation of circRNAs with their mRNA targets, we determined the DE mRNA in oxidative stress (211 in PD-OS and 224 in DD-OS) and then examined their co-expression with the differentially expressed (DE) circRNAs across the samples in each model. This analysis revealed 2301 circRNA–mRNA pairs in PD-OS and 367 pairs in DD-OS that showed a positive expression correlation ($r > 0.90$, adjusted $p < 0.05$; Supplementary Table S4). To construct a ceRNA network of circRNA–miRNA–mRNA, we predicted the miRNA binding sites for each correlated circRNA–mRNA pair. Pairs where both elements shared a common miRNA that was also expressed in the samples were included (Figure 3a). The resulting network identified 454 axes and 245 nodes in PD-OS, which included 301 circRNA–miRNA and 265 miRNA–mRNA interactions, and 122 axes and 103 nodes in DD-OS, including 95 circRNA–miRNA and 84 miRNA–mRNA interactions (Supplementary Table S4). The ceRNA networks of circRNA–miRNA–mRNA are illustrated in Figure 3b for PD-OS and 3c for DD-OS.

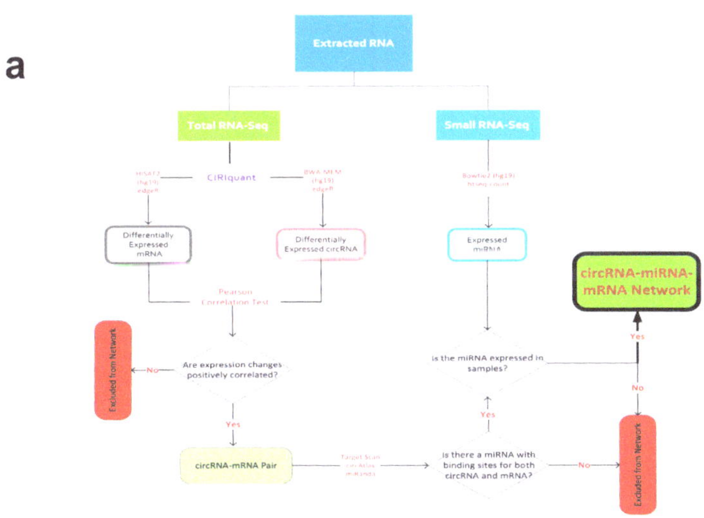

Figure 3. *Cont.*

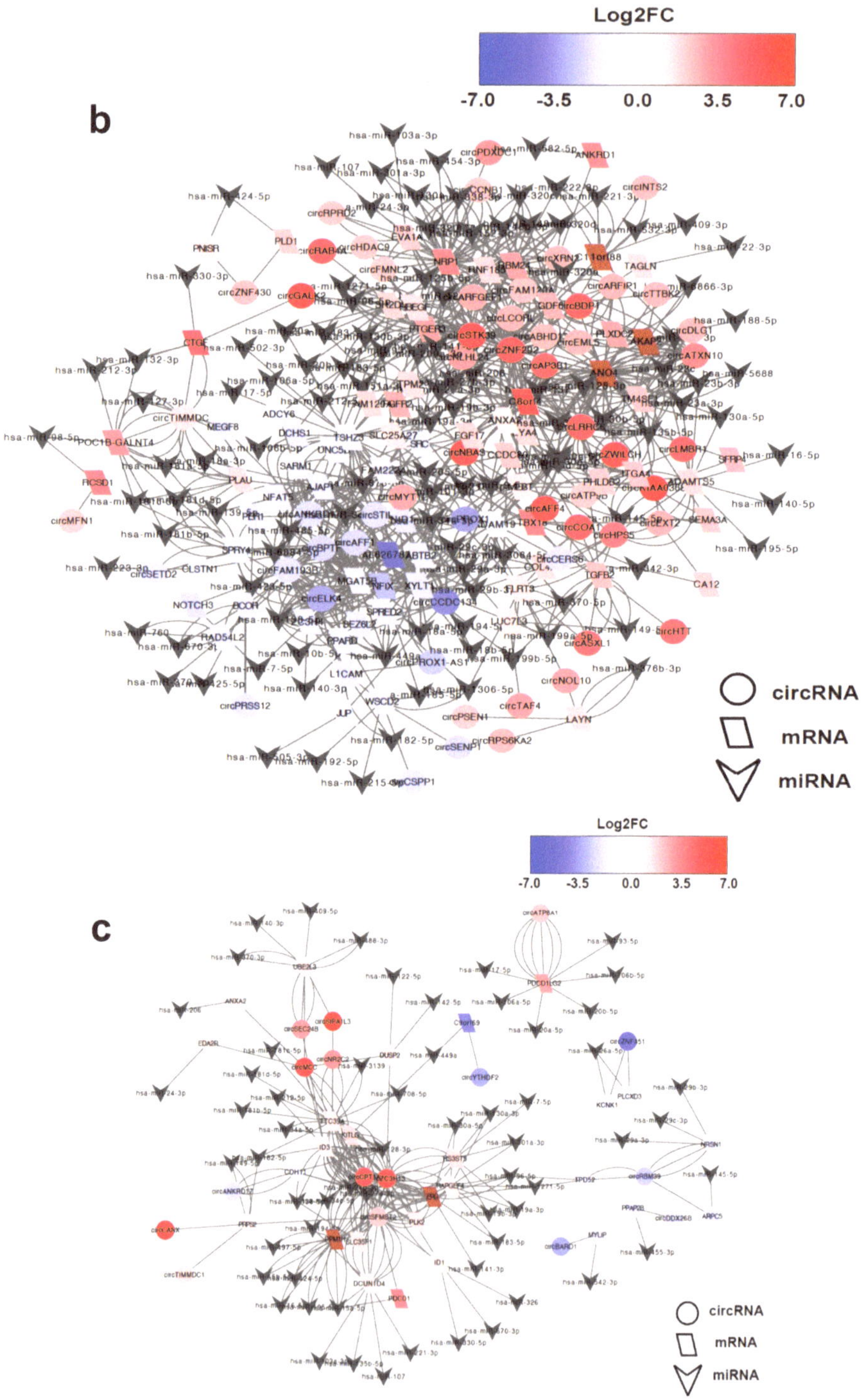

Figure 3. The circRNA-associated ceRNA network in oxidative stress. The potential interaction network of circRNA-miRNA-mRNA. (**a**) The networks are constructed based on the co-expression

between the DE circRNAs and DE mRNAs and the predicted miRNA, with binding sites for each correlated circRNA–mRNA pair. (**b**) The predicted interaction network in PD-OS includes 454 axes and 244 nodes. (**c**) The predicted network in DD-OS includes 122 axes and 103 nodes. The circle and the parallelogram represent DE circRNA and DE mRNA, respectively, with red and blue denoting upregulation and downregulation, respectively. The colour intensity associates with the expression fold change. The gray inverted triangles indicate miRNA.

Intriguingly, we noticed that more than half of the miRNAs predicted to be sponged by differentially expressed circRNAs were previously reported to be dysregulated in the brain and peripheral tissues of psychiatric patients [31]. This included 66/114 miRNAs in PD-OS and 36/60 miRNAs in DD-OS, with 31 miRNAs affected by both conditions (Figure 4a and Supplementary Table S5). A Fisher's exact test revealed a statistically significant enrichment of sponged miRNAs in psychiatric disorders for both conditions (p-value < 0.001) (Figure 4b,c).

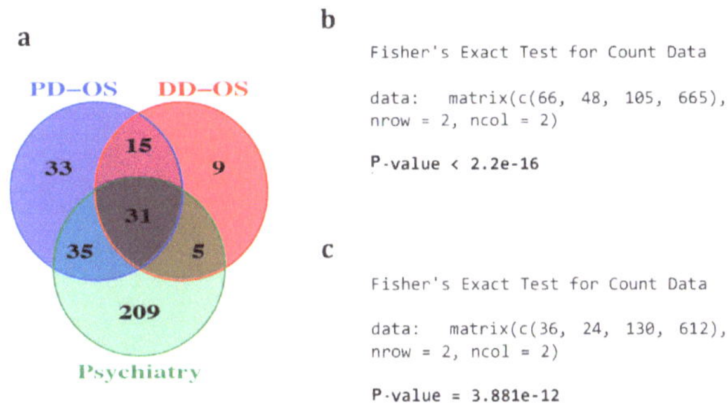

Figure 4. The enrichment of circRNA-sponged miRNAs in psychiatric disorders. (**a**) Of the 114 and 60 miRNAs that were predicted to be sponged by DE circRNA in PD-OS and DD-OS, respectively, more than 50% were dysregulated in psychiatric disorders. We observed significant enrichment of circRNA-sponged miRNAs in these diseases for both PD-OS (**b**) and DD-OS (**c**) conditions, using Fisher's exact test.

2.4. Characterisation of Hub circRNAs in the ceRNA Networks

To determine the central regulatory elements involved in the oxidative stress process, we ranked the circRNA nodes in the network using CytoHubba and found 10 and 5 key circRNAs with highest connectivity in the ceRNA networks of PD-OS and DD-OS, respectively (Supplementary Table S6). A regulatory subnetwork was constructed for each oxidative stress model, as shown in Figure 5. The PD-OS subnetwork was composed of 255 circRNA–miRNA–mRNA interactions where the hub circRNAs potentially regulate 57 mRNAs by sponging 86 miRNAs (Figure 5a; Supplementary Table S6). Similarly, in DD-OS, we detected 97 circRNA–miRNA–mRNA interactions, where the hub circRNAs potentially regulate 20 DE mRNA through binding to 46 miRNAs (Figure 5b; Supplementary Table S6). Three circRNAs, circZNF292, circBPTF, and circFAM193B, were the top regulatory hubs in PD-OS, while circZC3H13, circSFMBT2, and circCPT1A were the top hubs in DD-OS, suggesting potential significant roles for these circRNAs in the biology of stress. Examples of the observed regulatory axes are circZNF292/miR-222-3p/C11orf88, circBPTF/miR-138-5p/AJAP1, and circZC3H13/miR-15a-5p/PPM1H (Figure 5).

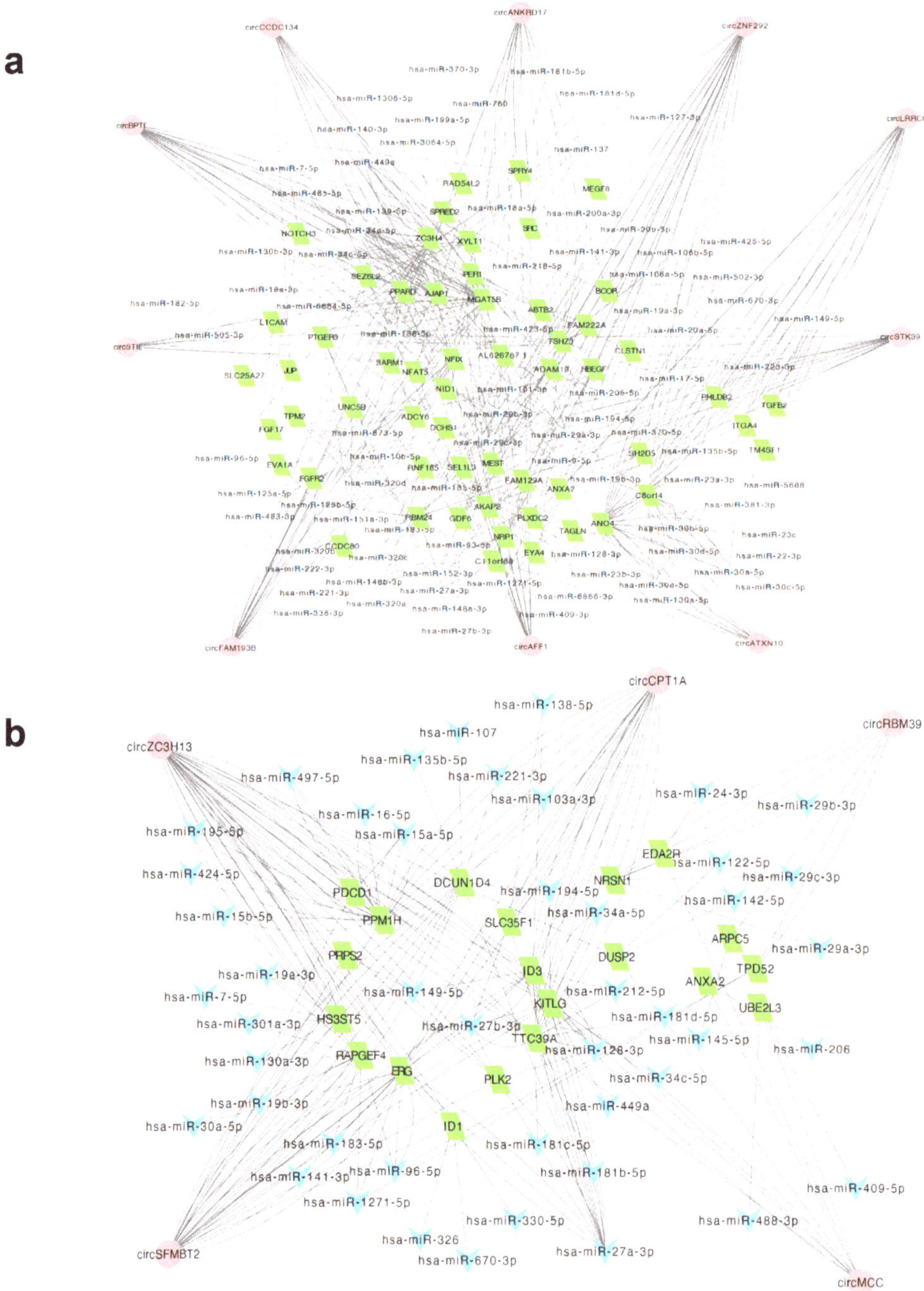

Figure 5. Identification of the ceRNA subnetwork. The interaction subnetwork in (**a**) PD-OS and (**b**) DD-OS. The subnetwork in PD-OS includes 10 hub circRNAs potentially regulating 57 mRNAs through interacting with 86 miRNAs. In the DD-OS subnetwork with 5 circRNA hubs, 20 mRNAs are regulated through 46 miRNAs. The circle represents circRNA, the parallelogram denotes mRNA, and the inverted triangle indicates miRNA.

2.5. Functional Enrichment Analysis of the ceRNA Subnetworks

To glean insight into the biological functions of the key axes of the ceRNA network, we performed GO and pathway enrichment analysis for the target genes. As shown in Figure 6a, the target genes in the PD-OS network were significantly enriched with biological themes related to cell adhesion, development, neuronal processes, and response to stress (FDR< 0.05). We also found significant enrichment of the genes in many pathways, including *signaling by VEGF*, *axon guidance*, *signaling by FGFR*, *Interleukin-2 signaling*, *PI3K/AKT activation*, *negative regulation of PI3K/AKT network*, and *RAF/MAP kinase cascade*, among others, in the PD-OS regulatory network (FDR < 0.05) (Figure 6b). The full list of the enriched GO categories and pathways is provided in Supplementary Table S7. The enrichment analysis for the DD-OS network showed that the *ID signaling pathway* was enriched, while no biological processes reached the statistical significance after multiple testing correction.

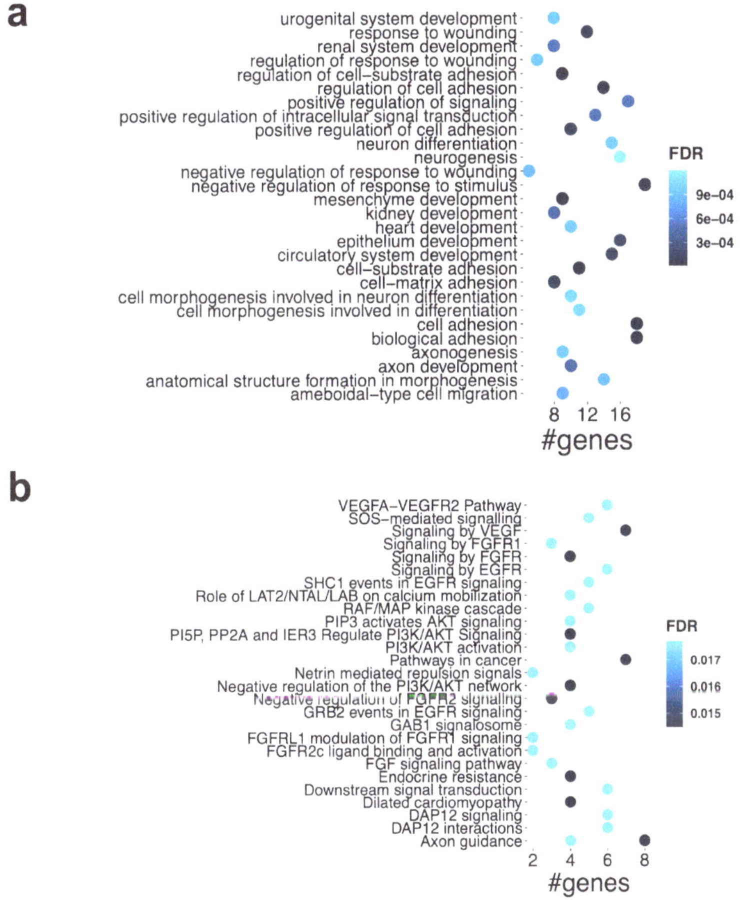

Figure 6. Functional analysis of the ceRNA subnetwork. (**a**) GO enrichment analysis for the target genes in the ceRNA subnetwork in PD-OS, which showed significantly enriched biological processes (FDR < 0.05). (**b**) Pathway enrichment analysis of the target genes in PD-OS, which indicated a significant enrichment of the genes in several pathways (FDR < 0.05). Selected GO terms and pathways are shown.

3. Discussion

Oxidative stress is thought to play a role in the onset of neurodevelopmental disorders and may represent a major environmental factor driving the genomic instability and gene expression deregulation observed in these disorders. In this study, we explored the impact of oxidative stress on circRNA expression and its ceRNA network in differentiating SH-SY5Y neuroblast cells. We observed 102 and 45 differentially expressed circRNAs in cells experiencing stress conditions prior to differentiation (PD-OS) and during differentiation (DD-OS), respectively. Interestingly, eight of these circRNAs were previously found by our group to be differentially expressed in the postmortem cortical grey matter of schizophrenia subjects [23]. These include circXRN2, circKIAA0368, circSTK39, circTTBK2, circDLG1, and circARFGEF1 in PD-OS; and circATP8A1 and circBARD1 in DD-OS.

We observed distinct profiles between the PD-OS and DD-OS conditions, with only one circRNA, circANKRD17, in common, suggesting that the circRNAomes response to oxidative stress in early neural progenitor cells may be different from that in cells undergoing neuronal differentiation. Moreover, alteration of expression was substantially higher in PD-OS, indicating that exposure to stress may be more critical during the early stages of neural development. Our analysis confirmed that the parental genes of the altered circRNAs were significantly enriched in developmental clusters such as *embryo development, brain development, head development,* and *forebrain development* in PD-OS.

Evidence emerging from other studies has demonstrated that circRNA with miRNA recognition elements can function as competing RNA molecules by sponging their target miRNA and inhibiting them from binding to the mRNA targets [27–29]. We performed bioinformatics analysis to explore putative circRNA-related ceRNA regulatory networks, including circRNA, miRNA, and mRNA, in response to oxidative stress. While we integrated our previous miRNA expression results [16] directly into the interaction analyses, we reanalysed the total RNA sequencing using an effective approach, CIRIquant [30], to detect and quantify both linear and circular transcripts. We found that many DE circRNAs were significantly co-expressed with DE mRNA (positive correlation), suggesting a regulatory relationship between these transcripts. Many of these circRNA–mRNA correlation pairs were predicted to interact with common miRNA molecules, which supported the existence of ceRNA networks where circRNA and miRNA compete for the target mRNA. Using in silico interaction analysis, we constructed a ceRNA network including 454 axes in PD-OS and 122 axes in DD-OS (Figure 3).

To further characterise the key regulatory axes implicated in the oxidative stress process, we determined the hub circRNAs in the ceRNA networks and found 15 hub nodes with the highest connectivity in the networks (Figure 4). The top circRNAs include circZNF292, circBPTF, and circFAM193B in PD-OS, and circZC3H13, circSFMBT2, circ-CPT1A in DD-OS, suggesting these circRNAs may have critical regulatory functions in the biology of stress conditions through miRNA sponging, as shown by previous studies. For example, an isoform of circZNF292, hsa_circ_0004058, was recently reported to be significantly reduced following induction of oxidative stress in human lens epithelial HLE-B3 cells. Functional studies showed that circZNF292 overexpression significantly increased cell viability and cell cycle progression but suppressed cell apoptosis in H_2O_2-treated HLE-B3 cells. While H_2O_2 reduced the activity of antioxidant enzymes catalase and superoxide dismutase, and increased the oxidative stress marker malondialdehyde activity, circZNF292 expression significantly reduced these impacts by directly targeting miR-222-3p and regulating E2F3 expression, suggesting a role for circZNF292 in alleviating oxidative stress-induced injury [32]. This circRNA was also responsive to hypoxia in three different cancer cell lines from cervical (HeLa), breast (MCF-7), and lung (A549) cancer [33]. Similarly, it was reported to be hypoxia-induced in cultured human umbilical venous endothelial cells [34]. Another top circRNA, circBPTF (chr17:65941525|65972074), was found to be increased in bladder cancer, with its expression linked to tumour grades associated with poorer prognosis. Mechanistically, circ-BPTF was shown to inhibit miR-31-5p to allow upregulation of the oncogenic molecule RAB27A [35]. A study by Hu et al. demonstrated that circSFMBT2 (chr10:7262373 | 7327916) was upregulated in invasive pituitary adenomas, suggesting that the circRNA could facilitate tumour invasion by targeting an miR-15a/16-Sox-5 axis [36]. These findings are noteworthy given that oxidative stress is known to influence the progression of various cancers [37].

The expression of circFAM193B (chr5:176963359 | 176966148), also differentially expressed in our study, was previously altered in human induced pluripotent stem cell (hiPSC)-derived neurons, six weeks after differentiation, in patients with early-onset schizophrenia, as compared to control samples. Whilst circZC3H13 and circCPT1A have not yet been the subject of functional analysis, they may be involved in molecular mechanisms of stress through their host genes, as previously suggested [38]. This is tantalizing given that ZC3H13 protein is involved in RNA N6-methyladenosine (m6A) methylation writing. RNA m6A modification is thought to play an important role in regulating cellular response to oxidative stress [39]. The CPT1A protein is implicated in mitochondrial oxidation of fatty acids. It enhances oxidative stress and inflammation induced by ROS in liver injury [40], and also increases mitochondrial ROS while promoting antioxidant defences in prostate cancer [41].

To uncover the central regulatory elements involved in oxidative stress, we constructed ceRNA networks (Figure 5) with 255 and 97 circRNA–miRNA–mRNA axes in PD-OS and DD-OS, respectively, where the hub circRNAs associated with the expression of 57 (PD-OS) and 20 (DD-OS) DE mRNA. To further speculate on the biological function of the ceRNA regulatory networks, we conducted functional annotation and pathway analysis for the target genes. Our enrichment analysis for the PD-OS network indicated that the circRNA target genes were significantly associated with *cell adhesion, development, neurogenesis, axon guidance, neuron projection development*, as well as *response to stress* (Figure 6a). There was also a significant enrichment of the genes in various stress- and neuronal- related pathways such as *signaling by VEGF, axon guidance, signaling by FGFR, and RAF/MAP kinase cascade* (Figure 6b). These data provide insight into the molecular regulatory systems that derive critical pathways in oxidative exposure and might explain the mechanism of oxidative stress involvement in neuropathological conditions. In support of this, our previous study indicated that oxidative stress may contribute to the development of psychiatric disorders by disrupting pathways involved in synapsis, neuronal differentiation, and the immune system [13]. This is interesting given that we observed significant enrichment of circRNA-sponged miRNAs in psychiatric diseases, with 31 psychiatry-associated miRNAs common between the two exposure paradigms, including hsa-miR-17-5p, hsa-miR-181b-5p, and hsa-miR-195-5p, all of which have been found by several studies to be dysregulated in different brain regions and peripheral tissues of individuals with psychiatric disorders [31].

Our study has some limitations that warrant further investigation in future studies. Most importantly, the ceRNA networks involved in our observations need to be validated functionally through interventional loss- and/or gain-of-function studies. However, these remain challenging, as our capacity to effectively differentiate between circRNAs and cognate linear mRNAs is limited. Considering that, for many circRNAs, the same exon exists in the cognate mRNA, sequence changes at circRNAs are likely to cause unwanted changes in the expression of cognate linear RNAs, as well [42,43], although techniques such as the CRISPR-Cas13 system have been shown to offer greater efficiency and specificity compared to conventional RNAi-based approaches [43]. Furthermore, RNA pulldown assays may provide support for the interactions underpinning the ceRNA networks involved in our investigation. Proteomics and metabolomics may also provide insight into the downstream molecular changes associated with oxidative stress in the nervous system, particularly when post-transcriptional regulation of mRNA targets alter translation [44,45]. Methodologies coupling liquid chromatography with single-stage mass spectrometry (LC-MS) and nuclear magnetic resonance (NMR) spectroscopy have the potential to provide advantages over other platforms [46], through enhanced sensitivity [47] and resolution [48].

In addition, in this study, we leveraged the SH-SY5Y cell line for its low cost, ease of culture (feasibility), and reproducibility. Using alternative human neuronal models, such as embryonic stem cells, neuronal progenitor cells (NPCs), and induced pluripotent stem cells (iPSCs), offers advantages and could help confirm these results across various biological models. Therefore, repeating this study using these neural cell lines and tissue cultures will enhance our understanding of ceRNA regulation in response to oxidative stress and other environmental factors affecting neuronal development.

In summary, this study provides evidence that circRNA expression is involved in the cellular response to oxidative stress. In addition, bioinformatics analysis suggests that circRNAs emerge as a new layer of regulatory system in the stress process through associating with the ceRNA networks. Discovery of the circRNA-mediated network that responds to oxidative stress would improve our understanding of the basis of this process, and more significantly, could identify novel agents for the diagnosis or targets for therapeutic purposes in disorders with oxidative features, such as neurodevelopmental diseases. Our observation of a more significant response in the ceRNA network of PD-OS compared to the DD-OS model suggests that the most critical impacts of stress may occur before the initiation of neuron differentiation. This may indicate that neuronal progenitor cells in the fetal nervous system may be more vulnerable to stress exposure during the early stages of development. This warrants further studies, such as those conducted with in vivo animal models, to explore the prenatal impacts of oxidative stress and associated regulatory networks on the neuronal phenotypes and development of nervous system disorders.

4. Materials and Methods

4.1. Cell Culture and Differentiation

Human neuroblastoma SH-SY5Y cells were cultured at a density of $2 \times 10^4/cm^2$ in Dulbecco's Modified Eagle's Medium (DMEM, Burlington, VT, USA) complemented with 2 mM L-glutamine ((Hyclone, Logan, USA), 20 mM HEPES (Thermofisher, New York, NY, USA), and 10% foetal bovine serum (FBS, Bovogen Biologicals, Melbourne, Australia). The cells were maintained at 37 °C in a 5% CO_2 with the media replaced every 2–3 days. To obtain neuronal differentiation, the immature neuroblast cells were cultured in 6-well plates, followed by treatment with 10 μM all-trans retinoic acid (ATRA) (Sigma-Aldrich, Burlington, VT, USA) the next day. The ATRA-supplemented media was refreshed after 72 h, and the differentiation protocol was terminated after 7 days of treatment with ATRA. During differentiation, the plates were covered with aluminium foil to protect them from light. The neuronal differentiation was confirmed by observing morphological and molecular changes. The cells demonstrated a neuronal phenotype, with increased growth of neurite projections and stalled cell division. In addition, we detected a significant alteration of neuronal marker genes, including TUBB3, ENO2, MAP2, MAPT, and SV2A in DD-OS (log_2CPM values 9.6, 7.6, 8, 3.9, and 6.7, respectively) and PD-OS (log_2CPM values 9, 7, 8.7, 4, and 6.5, respectively) conditions.

4.2. Inducing Oxidative Stress

As described previously [13], we designed two treatment models for oxidative stress to assess the impact of stress, both before the neuronal differentiation commenced and during the differentiation process, as follows: [1] undifferentiated cells were exposed to H_2O_2 (Sigma-Aldrich, Burlington, VT, USA) throughout the entire 7 days of differentiation using ATRA; we refer to this as "during-differentiation oxidative stress" (DD-OS). This condition highlights the interaction between oxidative stress and differentiation factors [2]. Undifferentiated cells were first exposed to H_2O_2 for 72 h and then, following removal of peroxide, treated with ATRA for 7 days to induce differentiation; we call this "pre-differentiation oxidative stress" (PD-OS). The PD-OS model allows cells sufficient time to activate adaptive mechanisms against the induced oxidative stress, indicating that the observed alterations were not merely due to a rapid increase in the concentration of ROS.

Hydrogen peroxide is commonly used to investigate the impacts of chronic oxidative stress exposure due to its high stability compared to other known reactive oxygen species, such as free radicals, superoxide anion, and hydroxyl radical [49]. To identify a suitable, non-cytotoxic concentration of peroxide that induces oxidative stress without significantly reducing cell viability, we first conducted a literature review of similar studies and then optimised the amount of H_2O_2 used. In a notable study, Brennand et al. treated neural progenitor cells (NPCs) with a 50 μM concentration of H_2O_2, and showed that this dose presented a sub-threshold environmental challenge of oxidative stress [50]. Based on this and other findings, we treated cells with increasing peroxide concentrations of 10, 20, 40, 80, and 100 μM, monitoring cellular morphology over 10 consecutive days through optical microscopy. We observed that 10 μM H_2O_2 had the least adverse effects; therefore, we selected it for our experiments. This choice of optimal dose was based on continuous monitoring of cell health and morphology under the microscope.

Each protocol included six samples: three H_2O_2 treatments and three mock treatment controls that received differentiating culture medium without H_2O_2. This design provided three biological replicates per treatment group for each protocol.

4.3. RNA Extraction and Integrity Check

Cells were lysed by 1 mL Trizol reagent (Sigma-Aldrich, Burlington, VT, USA) and lysate was collected into microcentrifuge tubes to add 200 μL of chloroform (Chem-supply, Gillman, Australia) before centrifugation at 13,000× g at 4 °C for 10 min according to the manufacturer's instructions (ThermoFisher, New York, NY, USA). The resultant aqueous phase was separated from the organic phase and mixed with 80 μg glycogen (Life Technologies, Mulgrave, Australia) and 500 μL isopropanol (Chem-supply, Australia), and incubated at −20 °C overnight. Following centrifugation at 9000× g at 4 °C for 30 min, the supernatant was discarded, and the pellet was washed twice with 75% cold ethanol and then resuspended in nuclease-free water for storage at −80 °C. The concentration and purity of the extracted RNA was analysed by the Agilent small RNA kit and the 2100 Bioanalyzer in accordance with the manufacturer's instructions (Agilent Technologies, Santa Clara, CA, USA). The provided system software was used for automatic calculation of the RNA integrity number (RIN) [51]. All samples had RIN values above 8.5.

4.4. Total RNA-Seq Library Generation and Sequencing

Library generation for total RNA-seq was performed as previously described [13]. Briefly, a total of 350 ng of total RNA was treated with DNase I (1 U/μg RNA, Thermo Scientific, New York, NY, USA), and then depleted of ribosomal RNA using the Ribo-Zero kit (Illumina, San Diego, CA, USA). The sequencing libraries were constructed using the Illumina TruSeq Stranded Total RNA Library Prep Kit according to the manufacturer's protocol. The quality and concentrations of the constructed libraries were assessed by the High Sensitivity DNA Bioanalyzer chip (Agilent Technologies, Santa Clara, CA, USA), followed by pooling the libraries and running in paired-end mode on a NovaSeq 6000 instrument for 100 cycles.

4.5. Small RNA Sequencing

For a separate study [16], small RNA sequencing was performed by the Ramaciotti Centre for Genomics (UNSW, Sydney, Australia), using the QIAseq miRNA Library Kit for small RNA library preparation, and the Illumina NextSeq 500 platform (Illumina, San Diego, CA, USA) for sequencing.

4.6. CircRNA Detection and Expression Analysis

Sequencing reads were demultiplexed based on unique adapter sequences and then converted to FASTQ files using the "bcl2fastq" package from Illumina (https://support.illumina.com/sequencing/sequencing_software/bcl2fastq-conversion-software.html) (accessed on 20 October 2020). The reads were then quality checked using the AfterQC tool (v0.9.7) [52], such that low-quality reads were discarded and sequencing errors were corrected. The resultant clean FASTQ files were analysed by the CIRIquant package (v1.0) [30] to detect and quantify circRNA transcripts. Briefly, the reads were mapped to the reference genome (hg19) using BWA-MEM aligner [53] and unmapped reads were fed into CIRI2 (v2.0) [54] to detect back-spliced junction (BSJ) reads using the ensemble gene annotation GRCh37 (Release 19). The candidate circular reads were then realigned against a constructed reference of pseudo circRNA using HISAT2 (v 2.1.0) [55], and the read pairs mapped concordantly across a 10 bp region of the junction site were considered as circRNA transcripts. Differential expression was conducted using edgeR [56] fed with BSJ reads of circRNA. To identify the DE circRNA we used a p-value (p) of <0.05 and a fold change (FC) of >2.

4.7. cDNA Synthesis and Quantitative PCR

The total RNA was reverse transcribed with random hexamers. Then Real-time PCR was conducted using divergent primers. We used the ΔCt method to normalize the data using GAPDH and HMBS as internal references. Finally, the fold changes were log transformed for visualization. All reactions were performed in triplicate for each biological group. Primer sequences are provided in Supplementary Table S1.

4.8. mRNA and miRNA Expression Analysis

For mRNA expression analysis, the raw reads were demultiplexed, quality checked, and trimmed as explained above. The resulting FASTQ files were subjected to CIRIquant to quantify mRNA expression. In brief, the reads were aligned to the reference genome hg19 using HISAT2, and the mapped reads were fed into StringTie [57] to reassemble the transcriptome and estimate gene expression. Differential expression analysis was conducted by EdgeR, with $FDR < 0.05$ and $FC > 1.5$ set to identify DE mRNA.

Analysis of miRNA expression was performed as part of a separate study [16]. The sequencing reads were quality controlled by FastQC (v0.11.8) (http://www.bioinformatics.babraham.ac.uk/projects/fastqc) (accessed on 23 October 2020), and adaptors were trimmed using Cutadapt (v2.10) (DOI:10.14806/ej.17.1.200) (accessed on 20 October 2020) before aligning to the human reference genome build hg19 using Bowtie2 (v2.4.1) [58]. Then, using the miRBase mature miRNA reference annotation, the reads aligned to the mature miRNAs were counted using htseq-count (v0.7.2).

4.9. Co-Expression Analysis

We used DE circRNAs and DE mRNAs for this analysis. To identify co-expressed pairs, we used the Pearson correlation test (one-sided) and reported pairs with a significant positive correlation by setting an adjusted p-value < 0.05. The circRNA-mRNA pairs were then used to generate the circRNA–miRNA–mRNA network.

4.10. Construction of circRNA–miRNA–mRNA Network

We downloaded the TargetScan Release 7.2 prediction (https://www.targetscan.org/vert_72/) (accessed on 25 October 2020), including conserved mRNA targets of conserved miRNA families [59] and intersected the predictions with the DE mRNA list to find miRNA associating with the DE mRNA and construct miRNA-mRNA interactions. We then determined miRNA binding sites within DE circRNAs using sequences of circRNAs from circAtlas 2.0 [60] and the miRanda prediction algorithm [61], to determine circRNA–miRNA interactions. Finally, the two interaction networks were intersected using the common miRNA; those pairs with a shared miRNA, provided the miRNA was expressed in the samples, were combined to construct the circRNA–miRNA–mRNA regulatory network.

To generate the subnetworks, we first ranked the nodes of the interaction networks using the topological analysis methods provided by CytoHubba [62], and then selected the top nodes as hub nodes to create the subnetworks.

We also applied Fisher's exact test to assess the enrichment of miRNA in the regulatory networks related to psychiatric disorders, using a recent systematic review of differentially expressed miRNA in psychiatric patients compared to healthy controls. Tables 1 and 2 demonstrate the test details for PD-OS and DD-OS, respectively.

Table 1. Fisher's exact test for examining the enrichment of miRNA within the PD-OS regulatory network in psychiatric diseases.

	miRNAs Sponged by circRNAs	miRNAs Not Sponged by circRNAs	Total
miRNAs associated with psychiatry	circRNA-sponged, Psy-associated miRNAs 66	Not sponged, Psy-associated miRNAs 105	Total number of Psy-associated miRNAs 171
miRNAs unassociated with psychiatry	circRNA-sponged, Psy-unassociated miRNAs 48	Not sponged, Psy-unassociated miRNAs 665	Total number of Psy-unassociated miRNAs 713
Total	Total number of circRNA-sponged miRNAs 114	Total number of miRNAs not sponged 770	**Total number of miRNAs expressed in the cell line** 884

fisher.test(matrix(c(66,48,105,665),nrow=2,ncol=2),alternative="greater")

Table 2. Fisher's exact test for examining the enrichment of miRNA within the DD-OS regulatory network in psychiatric diseases.

	miRNAs Sponged by circRNAs	miRNAs Not Sponged by circRNAs	Total
miRNAs associated with psychiatry	circRNA-sponged, Psy-associated miRNAs 36	Not sponged, Psy-associated miRNAs 130	Total number of Psy-associated miRNAs 166
miRNAs unassociated with psychiatry	circRNA-sponged, Psy-unassociated miRNAs 24	Not sponged, Psy-unassociated miRNAs 612	Total number of Psy-unassociated miRNAs 636
Total	Total number of circRNA-sponged miRNAs 60	Total number of miRNAs not sponged 742	**Total number of miRNAs expressed in the cell line** 802

fisher.test(matrix(c(36,24,130,612),nrow=2,ncol=2),alternative="greater")

4.11. Functional Enrichment Analysis

The gene ontology (GO) and pathway enrichment analyses were performed using ToppFun from the ToppGene Suite (https://toppgene.cchmc.org) (accessed on 25 October 2020) [63]. We input either circRNA parental genes or target genes and set all human genes as the reference for the analysis. An FDR < 0.05 was set as the threshold for statistical significance in determining significant terms.

4.12. Visualization

Plots and graphs were constructed using R coding (v3.5). Heatmaps were constructed using the heatmap.2 function from the gplots package (http://CRAN.R-project.org/package=gplots) (accessed on 25 October 2020) (v3.0.1). The volcano plots were constructed using the EnhancedVolcano package (v3.12) [64]. The interaction networks were generated with the Cytoscape tool [65]. The remaining plots and graphs were constructed using the ggplot2 package (v3.2.1) [66].

Supplementary Materials: The following supporting information can be downloaded at: https://www.mdpi.com/article/10.3390/ijms252212459/s1.

Author Contributions: Conceptualization, E.M., B.K. and M.J.C.; data curation, E.M.; formal analysis, E.M.; funding acquisition, M.J.C.; investigation, E.M. and B.K.; methodology, E.M. and B.K.; project administration, M.J.C.; resources, M.J.C.; software, E.M.; supervision, M.J.C.; validation, B.K.; visualization, E.M.; writing—original draft, E.M.; writing—review and editing, B.K., E.M. and M.J.C. All authors have read and agreed to the published version of the manuscript.

Funding: This research was supported by an NHMRC project grant (APP1147894) and an NHMRC ideas grant (1188493). B.K. was supported by the University of Newcastle RHD Scholarship. M.J.C. was supported by an NHMRC Senior Research Fellowship (1121474) and a University of Newcastle Faculty of Health and Medicine Gladys M Brawn Senior Fellowship.

Data Availability Statement: Raw sequencing data for total RNA sequencing is available at the Gene Expression Omnibus (Accession Number: GSE161860). Raw sequencing data for small RNA sequencing is also available at the Gene Expression Omnibus (Accession Number: GSE182627).

Acknowledgments: The authors would like to thank Adam Graham for proofreading the original manuscript.

Conflicts of Interest: The authors declare no conflicts of interest.

References

1. Salim, S. Oxidative Stress and the Central Nervous System. *J. Pharmacol. Exp. Ther.* **2017**, *360*, 201–205. [CrossRef]
2. Castelli, V.; Benedetti, E.; Antonosante, A.; Catanesi, M.; Pitari, G.; Ippoliti, R.; Cimini, A.; d'Angelo, M. Neuronal Cells Rearrangement During Aging and Neurodegenerative Disease: Metabolism, Oxidative Stress and Organelles Dynamic. *Front. Mol. Neurosci.* **2019**, *12*, 132. [CrossRef]
3. Salim, S. Oxidative stress and psychological disorders. *Curr. Neuropharmacol.* **2014**, *12*, 140–147. [CrossRef] [PubMed]
4. Patel, M. Targeting Oxidative Stress in Central Nervous System Disorders. *Trends Pharmacol. Sci.* **2016**, *37*, 768–778. [CrossRef] [PubMed]
5. Popa-Wagner, A.; Mitran, S.; Sivanesan, S.; Chang, E.; Buga, A.M. ROS and brain diseases: The good, the bad, and the ugly. *Oxid. Med. Cell. Longev.* **2013**, *2013*, 963520. [CrossRef] [PubMed]
6. Boskovic, M.; Vovk, T.; Kores Plesnicar, B.; Grabnar, I. Oxidative stress in schizophrenia. *Curr. Neuropharmacol.* **2011**, *9*, 301–312. [PubMed]
7. Andreazza, A.C.; Kauer-Sant'anna, M.; Frey, B.N.; Bond, D.J.; Kapczinski, F.; Young, L.T.; Yatham, L.N. Oxidative stress markers in bipolar disorder: A meta-analysis. *J. Affect. Disord.* **2008**, *111*, 135–144. [CrossRef]
8. Bajpai, A.; Verma, A.K.; Srivastava, M.; Srivastava, R. Oxidative stress and major depression. *J. Clin. Diagn. Res.* **2014**, *8*, CC04–CC07. [CrossRef]
9. Pandya, C.D.; Howell, K.R.; Pillai, A. Antioxidants as potential therapeutics for neuropsychiatric disorders. *Prog. Neuropsychopharmacol. Biol. Psychiatry* **2013**, *46*, 214–223. [CrossRef]
10. Guo, J.D.; Zhao, X.; Li, Y.; Li, G.R.; Liu, X.L. Damage to dopaminergic neurons by oxidative stress in Parkinson's disease (Review). *Int. J. Mol. Med.* **2018**, *41*, 1817–1825. [CrossRef]
11. Kunsch, C.; Medford, R.M. Oxidative stress as a regulator of gene expression in the vasculature. *Circ. Res.* **1999**, *85*, 753–766. [CrossRef] [PubMed]
12. Han, E.S.; Muller, F.L.; Perez, V.I.; Qi, W.; Liang, H.; Xi, L.; Fu, C.; Doyle, E.; Hickey, M.; Cornell, J.; et al. The in vivo gene expression signature of oxidative stress. *Physiol. Genom.* **2008**, *34*, 112–126. [CrossRef]
13. Khavari, B.; Mahmoudi, E.; Geaghan, M.P.; Cairns, M.J. Oxidative Stress Impact on the Transcriptome of Differentiating Neuroblastoma Cells: Implication for Psychiatric Disorders. *Int. J. Mol. Sci.* **2020**, *21*, 9182. [CrossRef] [PubMed]
14. Ghafouri-Fard, S.; Shoorei, H.; Taheri, M. Non-coding RNAs are inolved in the response to oxidative stress. *Biomed. Pharmacother.* **2020**, *127*, 110228. [CrossRef]
15. Wang, W.-T.; Ye, H.; Wei, P.-P.; Han, B.-W.; He, B.; Chen, Z.-H.; Chen, Y.-Q. LncRNAs H19 and HULC, activated by oxidative stress, promote cell migration and invasion in cholangiocarcinoma through a ceRNA manner. *J. Hematol. Oncol.* **2016**, *9*, 117. [CrossRef]
16. Khavari, B.; Michelle, M.B.; Mahmoudi, E.; Geaghan, M.P.; Graham, A.; Cairns, M.J. microRNA and the Post-Transcriptional Response to Oxidative Stress during Neuronal Differentiation: Implications for Neurodevelopmental and Psychiatric Disorders. *Life* **2024**, *14*, 562. [CrossRef]
17. Huang, S.; Yang, B.; Chen, B.J.; Bliim, N.; Ueberham, U.; Arendt, T.; Janitz, M. The emerging role of circular RNAs in transcriptome regulation. *Genomics* **2017**, *109*, 401–407. [CrossRef]
18. Mahmoudi, E.; Cairns, M.J. Circular RNAs are temporospatially regulated throughout development and ageing in the rat. *Sci. Rep.* **2019**, *9*, 2564. [CrossRef]
19. Mahmoudi, E.; Kiltschewskij, D.; Fitzsimmons, C.; Cairns, M.J. Depolarization-Associated CircRNA Regulate Neural Gene Expression and in Some Cases May Function as Templates for Translation. *Cells* **2019**, *9*, 25. [CrossRef]

20. Huang, A.; Zheng, H.; Wu, Z.; Chen, M.; Huang, Y. Circular RNA-protein interactions: Functions, mechanisms, and identification. *Theranostics* **2020**, *10*, 3503–3517. [CrossRef]
21. Yu, C.-Y.; Kuo, H.-C. The emerging roles and functions of circular RNAs and their generation. *J. Biomed. Sci.* **2019**, *26*, 29. [CrossRef]
22. Li, Z.; Cheng, Y.; Wu, F.; Wu, L.; Cao, H.; Wang, Q.; Tang, W. The emerging landscape of circular RNAs in immunity: Breakthroughs and challenges. *Biomark. Res.* **2020**, *8*, 25. [CrossRef]
23. Mahmoudi, E.; Fitzsimmons, C.; Geaghan, M.P.; Shannon Weickert, C.; Atkins, J.R.; Wang, X.; Cairns, M.J. Circular RNA biogenesis is decreased in postmortem cortical gray matter in schizophrenia and may alter the bioavailability of associated miRNA. *Neuropsychopharmacology* **2019**, *44*, 1043–1054. [CrossRef]
24. Li, Z.; Liu, S.; Li, X.; Zhao, W.; Li, J.; Xu, Y. Circular RNA in Schizophrenia and Depression. *Front. Psychiatry* **2020**, *11*, 392. [CrossRef]
25. Qu, S.; Zhong, Y.; Shang, R.; Zhang, X.; Song, W.; Kjems, J.; Li, H. The emerging landscape of circular RNA in life processes. *RNA Biol.* **2017**, *14*, 992–999. [CrossRef]
26. Zhou, Z.; Sun, B.; Huang, S.; Zhao, L. Roles of circular RNAs in immune regulation and autoimmune diseases. *Cell Death Dis.* **2019**, *10*, 503. [CrossRef]
27. Memczak, S.; Jens, M.; Elefsinioti, A.; Torti, F.; Krueger, J.; Rybak, A.; Maier, L.; Mackowiak, S.D.; Gregersen, L.H.; Munschauer, M.; et al. Circular RNAs are a large class of animal RNAs with regulatory potency. *Nature* **2013**, *495*, 333–338. [CrossRef]
28. Hansen, T.B.; Jensen, T.I.; Clausen, B.H.; Bramsen, J.B.; Finsen, B.; Damgaard, C.K.; Kjems, J. Natural RNA circles function as efficient microRNA sponges. *Nature* **2013**, *495*, 384–388. [CrossRef]
29. Piwecka, M.; Glazar, P.; Hernandez-Miranda, L.R.; Memczak, S.; Wolf, S.A.; Rybak-Wolf, A.; Filipchyk, A.; Klironomos, F.; Cerda Jara, C.A.; Fenske, P.; et al. Loss of a mammalian circular RNA locus causes miRNA deregulation and affects brain function. *Science* **2017**, *357*, eaam8526. [CrossRef]
30. Zhang, J.; Chen, S.; Yang, J.; Zhao, F. Accurate quantification of circular RNAs identifies extensive circular isoform switching events. *Nat. Commun.* **2020**, *11*, 90. [CrossRef]
31. Smigielski, L.; Jagannath, V.; Rössler, W.; Walitza, S.; Grünblatt, E. Epigenetic mechanisms in schizophrenia and other psychotic disorders: A systematic review of empirical human findings. *Mol. Psychiatry* **2020**, *25*, 1718–1748. [CrossRef] [PubMed]
32. Xu, X.; Gao, R.; Li, S.; Li, N.; Jiang, K.; Sun, X.; Zhang, J. Circular RNA circZNF292 regulates H2 O2 -induced injury in human lens epithelial HLE-B3 cells depending on the regulation of the miR-222-3p/E2F3 axis. *Cell Biol. Int.* **2021**, *45*, 1757–1767. [CrossRef] [PubMed]
33. Di Liddo, A.; de Oliveira Freitas Machado, C.; Fischer, S.; Ebersberger, S.; Heumüller, A.W.; Weigand, J.E.; Müller-McNicoll, M.; Zarnack, K. A combined computational pipeline to detect circular RNAs in human cancer cells under hypoxic stress. *J. Mol. Cell. Biol.* **2019**, *11*, 829–844. [CrossRef]
34. Boeckel, J.N.; Jaé, N.; Heumüller, A.W.; Chen, W.; Boon, R.A.; Stellos, K.; Zeiher, A.M.; John, D.; Uchida, S.; Dimmeler, S. Identification and Characterization of Hypoxia-Regulated Endothelial Circular RNA. *Circ. Res.* **2015**, *117*, 884–890. [CrossRef]
35. Bi, J.; Liu, H.; Cai, Z.; Dong, W.; Jiang, N.; Yang, M.; Huang, J.; Lin, T. Circ-BPTF promotes bladder cancer progression and recurrence through the miR-31-5p/RAB27A axis. *Aging* **2018**, *10*, 1964–1976. [CrossRef]
36. Hu, Y.; Zhang, N.; Zhang, S.; Zhou, P.; Lv, L.; Richard, S.A.; Ma, W.; Chen, C.; Wang, X.; Huang, S.; et al. Differential circular RNA expression profiles of invasive and non-invasive non-functioning pituitary adenomas: A microarray analysis. *Medicine* **2019**, *98*, e16148. [CrossRef]
37. Saha, S.K.; Lee, S.B.; Won, J.; Choi, H.Y.; Kim, K.; Yang, G.M.; Dayem, A.A.; Cho, S.G. Correlation between Oxidative Stress, Nutrition, and Cancer Initiation. *Int. J. Mol. Sci.* **2017**, *18*, 1544. [CrossRef]
38. You, X.; Vlatkovic, I.; Babic, A.; Will, T.; Epstein, I.; Tushev, G.; Akbalik, G.; Wang, M.; Glock, C.; Quedenau, C.; et al. Neural circular RNAs are derived from synaptic genes and regulated by development and plasticity. *Nat. Neurosci.* **2015**, *18*, 603–610. [CrossRef]
39. Wilkinson, E.; Cui, Y.H.; He, Y.Y. Context-Dependent Roles of RNA Modifications in Stress Responses and Diseases. *Int. J. Mol. Sci.* **2021**, *22*, 1949. [CrossRef]
40. Luo, X.; Sun, D.; Wang, Y.; Zhang, F.; Wang, Y. Cpt1a promoted ROS-induced oxidative stress and inflammation in liver injury via the Nrf2/HO-1 and NLRP3 inflammasome signaling pathway. *Can. J. Physiol. Pharmacol.* **2021**, *99*, 468–477. [CrossRef]
41. Joshi, M.; Kim, J.; D'Alessandro, A.; Monk, E.; Bruce, K.; Elajaili, H.; Nozik-Grayck, E.; Goodspeed, A.; Costello, J.C.; Schlaepfer, I.R. CPT1A Over-Expression Increases Reactive Oxygen Species in the Mitochondria and Promotes Antioxidant Defenses in Prostate Cancer. *Cancers* **2020**, *12*, 3431. [CrossRef]
42. Gao, X.; Ma, X.K.; Li, X.; Li, G.W.; Liu, C.X.; Zhang, J.; Wang, Y.; Wei, J.; Chen, J.; Chen, L.L.; et al. Knockout of circRNAs by base editing back-splice sites of circularized exons. *Genome Biol.* **2022**, *23*, 16. [CrossRef] [PubMed]
43. Pisignano, G.; Michael, D.C.; Visal, T.H.; Pirlog, R.; Ladomery, M.; Calin, G.A. Going circular: History, present, and future of circRNAs in cancer. *Oncogene* **2023**, *42*, 2783–2800. [CrossRef] [PubMed]
44. Di Liegro, C.M.; Schiera, G.; Schirò, G.; Di Liegro, I. RNA-Binding Proteins as Epigenetic Regulators of Brain Functions and Their Involvement in Neurodegeneration. *Int. J. Mol. Sci.* **2022**, *23*, 14622. [CrossRef] [PubMed]
45. Gu, Q.; Liu, H.; Ma, J.; Yuan, J.; Li, X.; Qiao, L. A Narrative Review of Circular RNAs in Brain Development and Diseases of Preterm Infants. *Front. Pediatr.* **2021**, *21*, 706012. [CrossRef]

46. Emwas, A.H.; Roy, R.; McKay, R.T.; Tenori, L.; Saccenti, E.; Gowda, G.A.N.; Raftery, D.; Alahmari, F.; Jaremko, L.; Jaremko, M.; et al. NMR Spectroscopy for Metabolomics Research. *Metabolites* **2019**, *9*, 123. [CrossRef]
47. Chandra, K.; Al-Harthi, S.; Sukumaran, S.; Almulhim, F.; Emwas, A.H.; Atreya, H.S.; Jaremko, Ł.; Jaremko, M. NMR-based metabolomics with enhanced sensitivity. *RSC Adv.* **2021**, *11*, 8694–8700. [CrossRef]
48. Chandra, K.; Al-Harthi, S.; Almulhim, F.; Emwas, A.H.; Jaremko, Ł.; Jaremko, M. The robust NMR toolbox for metabolomics. *Mol. Omics* **2021**, *17*, 719–724. [CrossRef]
49. Hameister, R.; Kaur, C.; Dheen, S.T.; Lohmann, C.H.; Singh, G. Reactive oxygen/nitrogen species (ROS/RNS) and oxidative stress in arthroplasty. *J. Biomed. Mater. Res. B Appl. Biomater.* **2020**, *108*, 2073–2087. [CrossRef]
50. Brennand, K.; Savas, J.N.; Kim, Y.; Tran, N.; Simone, A.; Hashimoto-Torii, K.; Beaumont, K.G.; Kim, H.J.; Topol, A.; Ladran, I.; et al. Phenotypic differences in hiPSC NPCs derived from patients with schizophrenia. *Mol. Psychiatry.* **2015**, *20*, 361–368. [CrossRef]
51. Schroeder, A.; Mueller, O.; Stocker, S.; Pfrieger, F.W. The RIN: An RNA integrity number for the assessment of RNA quality. *Nat. Protoc.* **2006**, *1*, 1044–1050.
52. Chen, S.; Huang, T.; Zhou, Y.; Han, Y.; Xu, M.; Gu, J. AfterQC: Automatic filtering, trimming, error removing and quality control for fastq data. *BMC Bioinform.* **2017**, *18*, 80. [CrossRef] [PubMed]
53. Li, H. Aligning sequence reads, clone sequences and assembly contigs with BWA-MEM. *arXiv* **2013**, arXiv:1303.3997.
54. Gao, Y.; Zhang, J.; Zhao, F. Circular RNA identification based on multiple seed matching. *Brief Bioinform.* **2018**, *19*, 803–810. [CrossRef]
55. Kim, D.; Langmead, B.; Salzberg, S.L. HISAT: A fast spliced aligner with low memory requirements. *Nat. Methods* **2015**, *12*, 357–360. [CrossRef]
56. Robinson, M.D.; McCarthy, D.J.; Smyth, G.K. edgeR: A Bioconductor package for differential expression analysis of digital gene expression data. *Bioinformatics* **2010**, *26*, 139–140. [CrossRef]
57. Pertea, M.; Pertea, G.M.; Antonescu, C.M.; Chang, T.-C.; Mendell, J.T.; Salzberg, S.L. StringTie enables improved reconstruction of a transcriptome from RNA-seq reads. *Nat. Biotechnol.* **2015**, *33*, 290–295. [CrossRef]
58. Langmead, B.; Salzberg, S.L. Fast gapped-read alignment with Bowtie 2. *Nat. Methods* **2012**, *9*, 357–359. [CrossRef] [PubMed]
59. Friedman, R.C.; Farh, K.K.; Burge, C.B.; Bartel, D.P. Most mammalian mRNAs are conserved targets of microRNAs. *Genome Res.* **2009**, *19*, 92–105. [CrossRef]
60. Wu, W.; Ji, P.; Zhao, F. CircAtlas: An integrated resource of one million highly accurate circular RNAs from 1070 vertebrate transcriptomes. *Genome Biol.* **2020**, *21*, 101. [CrossRef]
61. Enright, A.J.; John, B.; Gaul, U.; Tuschl, T.; Sander, C.; Marks, D.S. MicroRNA targets in Drosophila. *Genome Biol.* **2003**, *5*, R1. [CrossRef]
62. Chin, C.-H.; Chen, S.-H.; Wu, H.-H.; Ho, C.-W.; Ko, M.-T.; Lin, C.-Y. cytoHubba: Identifying hub objects and sub-networks from complex interactome. *BMC Syst. Biol.* **2014**, *8*, S11. [CrossRef] [PubMed]
63. Chen, J.; Bardes, E.E.; Aronow, B.J.; Jegga, A.G. ToppGene Suite for gene list enrichment analysis and candidate gene prioritization. *Nucleic Acids Res.* **2009**, *37*, W305–W311. [CrossRef] [PubMed]
64. Blighe, K.; Rana, S.; Lewis, M. EnhancedVolcano: Publication-Ready Volcano Plots with Enhanced Colouring and Labeling. 2018. Available online: https://bioconductor.org/packages/devel/bioc/vignettes/EnhancedVolcano/inst/doc/EnhancedVolcano.html (accessed on 6 November 2024).
65. Shannon, P.; Markiel, A.; Ozier, O.; Baliga, N.S.; Wang, J.T.; Ramage, D.; Amin, N.; Schwikowski, B.; Ideker, T. Cytoscape: A software environment for integrated models of biomolecular interaction networks. *Genome Res.* **2003**, *13*, 2498–2504. [CrossRef] [PubMed]
66. Wickham, H. *Ggplot2: Elegant Graphics for Data Analysis*; Springer: New York, NY, USA, 2016.

International Journal of
Molecular Sciences

MDPI

Communication

Gene Expression and Prognostic Value of NADPH Oxidase Enzymes in Breast Cancer

Andressa de Vasconcelos e Souza †, Caroline Coelho de Faria †, Leonardo Matta Pereira, Andrea Claudia Freitas Ferreira, Pedro Henrique Monteiro Torres and Rodrigo Soares Fortunato *

Instituto de Biofísica Carlos Chagas Filho, Universidade Federal do Rio de Janeiro, Rio de Janeiro 21941-971, Brazil; andvasco.celos@gmail.com (A.d.V.e.S.); carolinefaria@biof.ufrj.br (C.C.d.F.); leonardo.matta@helmholtz-munich.de (L.M.P.); deiaclau@biof.ufrj.br (A.C.F.F.); monteirotorres@biof.ufrj.br (P.H.M.T.)

* Correspondence: rodrigof@biof.ufrj.br

† These authors contributed equally to this work.

Abstract: NADPH oxidase enzymes (NOX) are involved in all stages of carcinogenesis, but their expression levels and prognostic value in breast cancer (BC) remain unclear. Thus, we aimed to assess the expression and prognostic value of NOX enzymes in BC samples using online databases. For this, mRNA expression from 290 normal breast tissue samples and 1904 BC samples obtained from studies on cBioPortal, Kaplan–Meier Plotter, and The Human Protein Atlas were analyzed. We found higher levels of NOX2, NOX4, and Dual oxidase 1 (DUOX1) in normal breast tissue. NOX1, NOX2, and NOX4 exhibited higher expression in BC, except for the basal subtype, where NOX4 expression was lower. DUOX1 mRNA levels were lower in all BC subtypes. NOX2, NOX4, and NOX5 mRNA levels increased with tumor progression stages, while NOX1 and DUOX1 expression decreased in more advanced stages. Moreover, patients with low expression of NOX1, NOX4, and DUOX1 had lower survival rates than those with high expression of these enzymes. In conclusion, our data suggest an overexpression of NOX enzymes in breast cancer, with certain isoforms showing a positive correlation with tumor progression.

Keywords: breast cancer; NADPH oxidases; reactive oxygen species; tumor aggressiveness

1. Introduction

Breast cancer (BC) is the second most commonly diagnosed cancer and the most frequent malignancy in women worldwide. In 2018, an estimated 2.1 million new diagnoses and approximately 626,679 BC-related deaths have occurred [1]. Due to the inherent molecular and clinical heterogeneity, BC is associated with diverse risk factors, etiologies, treatment effectiveness, and prognosis [2–5]. Most studies profiling gene expression signatures have classified BC into five major molecular subtypes: luminal A (estrogen receptor (ER)-positive, progesterone receptor (PR)-positive, human epidermal growth factor receptor 2 (HER2)-negative), luminal B (ER-positive, PR-positive, HER2-positive), HER2-enriched (ER-negative, PR- negative, HER2-positive), basal-like or triple-negative (ER-negative, PR-negative, HER2-negative), and normal breast-like tumors (unclassified) [6,7]. More recently, the claudin-low subtype has been identified and characterized as negative for ER, PR, and HER2 expression, but with low expression of Ki67 and high expression of epithelial–mesenchymal transition (EMT)-related genes, which distinguishes this subtype from the basal-like [8].

The mammalian nicotinamide adenine dinucleotide phosphate (NADPH) oxidases (NOX) are transmembrane proteins that carry electrons across biological membranes, reducing molecular oxygen (O_2) to superoxide anion ($O_2^{\bullet -}$) or hydrogen peroxide (H_2O_2). The NOX enzymes family contains seven members, which are NOX1-5 and Dual oxidases 1 and 2 (DUOX1-2). All isoforms exhibit six highly conserved transmembrane domains, one

NADPH binding site in the C-terminal region, one FAD binding site, and two histidine-linked heme groups in the transmembrane domains III and IV. Additionally, NOX5 and DUOX 1-2 show an intracellular calcium-binding site that is closely related to their activation. Unlike all other sources of reactive oxygen species (ROS), NOX enzymes generate ROS as their main function [9].

Accumulated evidence in recent decades highlights the role of NOX-derived ROS in virtually all steps of carcinogenesis (initiation, promotion, and progression) of different organs/tissues. Furthermore, NOX enzymes have been suggested as a prospective target in novel therapeutic approaches [10,11]. Regarding BC, some studies have shown that NOX might be important players in this disease, although most of them were conducted under in vitro conditions utilizing cell lines, and the expression levels and prognostic value of NOX in patients remain elusive [12–14]. Thus, the aims of this study were first to assess the expression and prognostic value of individual NOX family members in the different BC molecular subtypes using online databases.

2. Results

2.1. Expression of NOX Family Genes in the Breast Tissue

We first compared the mRNA levels of NOX family members in 290 samples of normal breast tissue using the HPA database. As shown in Figure 1, NOX2 mRNA levels were the most expressed, which was followed by NOX4, DUOX1, DUOX2, NOX5, and NOX1. NOX3 mRNA levels were undetectable. Therefore, we did not evaluate NOX3 in the next analysis.

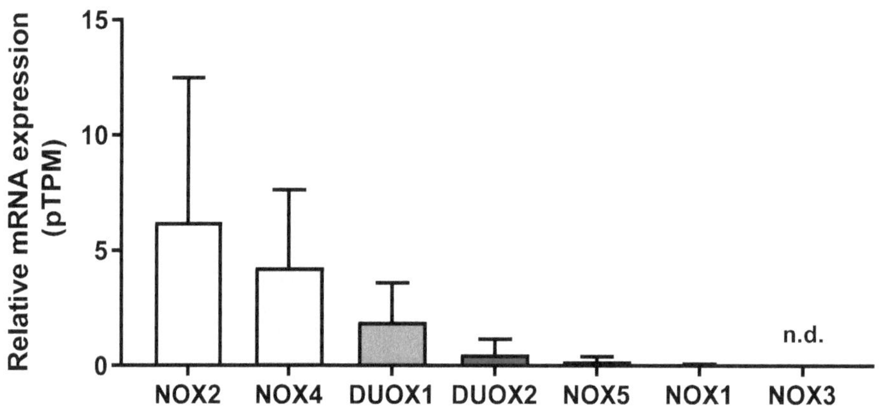

Figure 1. NADPH oxidases mRNA levels in the breast. Differences among NOX family mRNA levels in normal breast tissue. Data were obtained from the online platform Human Protein Atlas (https://www.proteinatlas.org, accessed on 2 July 2022). Results are represented as the mean protein-coding transcripts per million (pTPM) ± standard deviation (N = 290; n.d.: not detectable).

2.2. Comparison of NOX mRNA Levels in Non-Tumoral and Breast Tumor Tissues

We next compared NOX mRNA levels between non-tumoral and breast tumor tissues. No data concerning DUOX2 expression were available, so this isoform was not analyzed. Due to breast cancer heterogeneity, we divided BC samples according to the five major molecular subtypes: luminal A, luminal B, HER2, basal, and claudin-low.

As demonstrated in Table 1, we observed that NOX1 mRNA levels were higher in the HER2 and basal subtypes when compared to the normal group. Similarly, the mRNA levels for NOX2 showed an increase in the HER2 and basal subtypes, in addition to claudin-low. Concerning NOX4 mRNA levels, they were revealed to be high in the luminal A, HER2, and claudin-low subtypes in comparison to normal tissue, while in the basal subtype, NOX4 mRNA levels were decreased. There were no statistically significant differences in NOX5 expression in any of the tumor subtypes when compared to the normal group. In relation to DUOX1, we detected a decrease in the mRNA levels in the luminal A, luminal B, HER2, and claudin-low subtypes when compared to the control.

Table 1. Comparison of NOX1, NOX2, NOX4, and DUOX1 mRNA levels in non-tumoral and different subtypes of breast tumor tissues.

Gene	BC Subtype	Non-Tumor	Tumor	*p* Value
NOX1	Claudin-low	0.03836	−0.02103	0.1291
	Luminal A	−0.02086	0.00429	0.9626
	Luminal B	0.01854	−0.0031	0.2762
	HER2	−0.09212	0.07419	0.0059
	Basal	−0.09197	0.08255	0.011
NOX2	Claudin-low	−2.2	1.576	<0.0001
	Luminal A	0.1081	−0.06415	0.763
	Luminal B	−0.1862	0.05626	0.0888
	HER2	−0.1628	0.2237	0.0483
	Basal	−0.2893	0.24	0.001
NOX4	Claudin-low	−0.3601	0.1767	0.036
	Luminal A	−1.125	0.1626	<0.0001
	Luminal B	−0.3539	0.0578	0.0564
	HER2	−0.9915	0.3326	<0.0001
	Basal	0.2339	−0.2542	0.0298
DUOX1	Claudin-low	0.2405	−0.1769	0.0112
	Luminal A	0.3179	−0.04951	0.0154
	Luminal B	0.1411	−0.00134	0.0104
	HER2	0.3012	−0.1476	0.0329
	Basal	−0.2282	0.1196	0.0686

Data were obtained from the cBioPortal online platform (http://www.cbioportal.org/, accessed on 3 July 2022). Non-tumor (N = 140); claudin-low (N = 199); luminal A (N = 679); luminal B (N = 461); HER2 (N = 220); basal (N = 199). Results are expressed as Log2 median-centered intensity.

As demonstrated in Figure 2, NOX2 mRNA levels were higher in the claudin-low BC subtype in comparison to the luminal A, luminal B, Her2, and basal subtypes. Furthermore, DUOX1 mRNA levels were lower in the luminal B BC subtype when compared to luminal A and Her2, and in luminal A in comparison to the basal subtype.

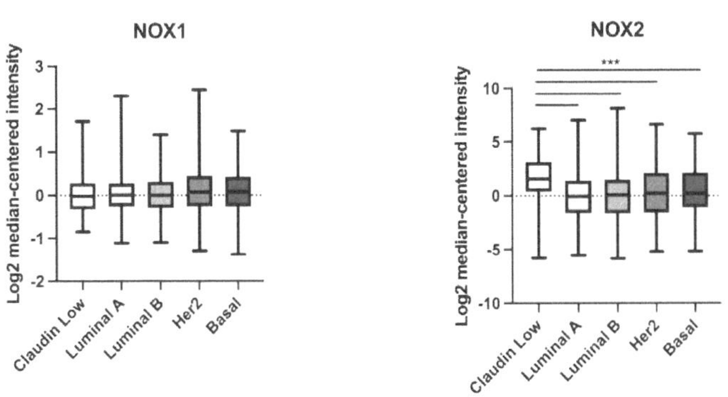

Figure 2. *Cont.*

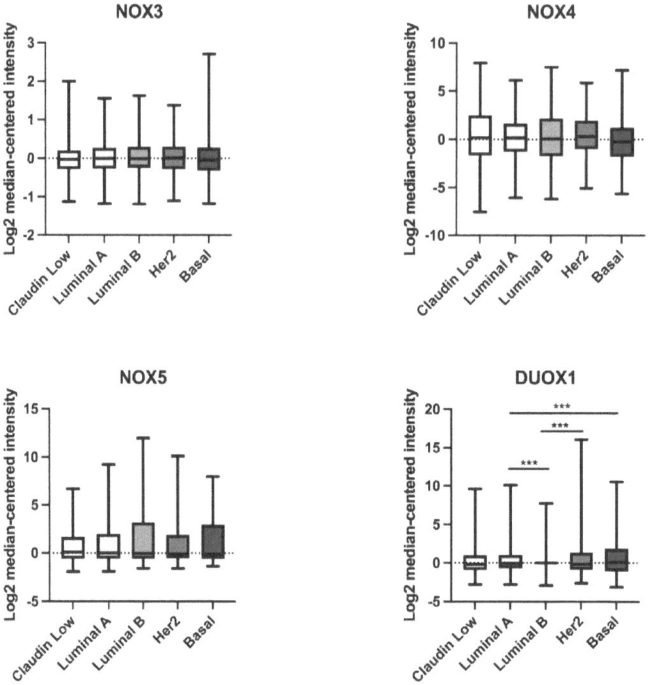

Figure 2. Comparison of NOX1, NOX2, NOX3, NOX4, NOX5, and DUOX1 mRNA levels in different subtypes of breast tumor tissues. Data were obtained from the cBioPortal online platform (http://www.cbioportal.org/, accessed on 3 July 2022) (N = 1904). Claudin-low (N = 199); luminal A (N = 679); luminal B (N = 461); HER2 (N = 220); basal (N = 199). *** $p < 0.001$.

2.3. *mRNA Expression of NOX Genes at Different Stages of Breast Tumor Development*

Another parameter we have taken into consideration is BC staging. The American Joint Committee on Cancer (AJCC) TNM staging system takes into account three primary factors: tumor size (T), regional lymph node status (N), and distant metastases (M). These factors are used to determine an overall stage, which ranges from 0 to 4. Stage 0 is referred to as "carcinoma in situ", indicating that the cancer remains confined to the primary layer of cells where it originated and has not spread. In this context, stage 1 BC is anatomically defined as a tumor smaller than 2 cm in size and shows no involvement of lymph nodes. On the other hand, stage 4 represents a state of advanced disease with distant metastases [4,15].

Based on our analysis, we have not observed any significant variations in the expression of any NOX isoform across the different tumor stages (Figure 3).

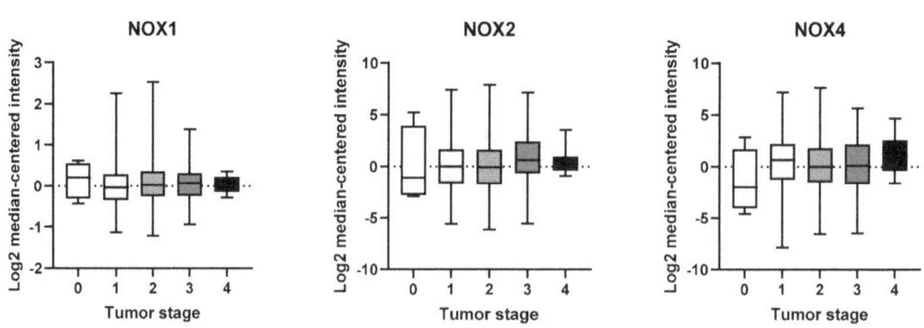

Figure 3. *Cont.*

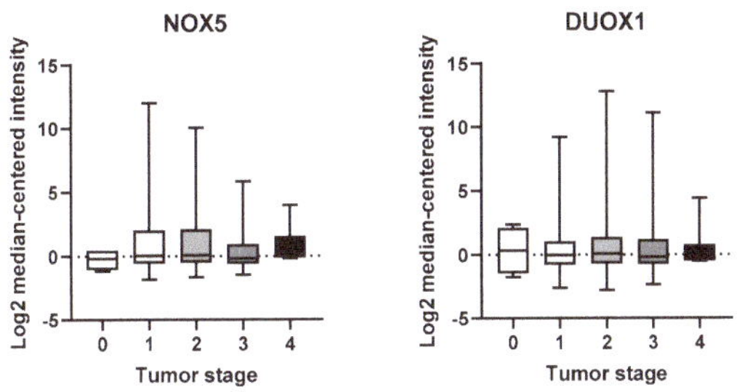

Figure 3. mRNA expression of NOX family at different stages of breast tumor. NOX1, NOX2, NOX4, NOX5, and DUOX1 were evaluated across tumor staging of breast tissues. Data were obtained from the cBioPortal online platform (http://www.cbioportal.org/, accessed on 3 July 2022) (N = 1904).

2.4. Survival Analysis of NOX Members in BC Patients

Afterwards, we examined the potential prognostic values of NOX isoforms in BC. The survival curves are demonstrated in Figure 4. It is important to highlight that there were no patient survival data related to high NOX1 expression after 200 months. We observed that patients with low expression of NOX1, NOX4, and DUOX1 exhibited significantly unfavorable prognoses in BC when compared with patients with high expression of those NOXs (Figure 4A, Figure 4C, and Figure 4E, respectively). Moreover, NOX2, NOX5, and DUOX2 expression were not associated with overall survival in BC (Figure 4B, Figure 4D, and Figure 4F, respectively).

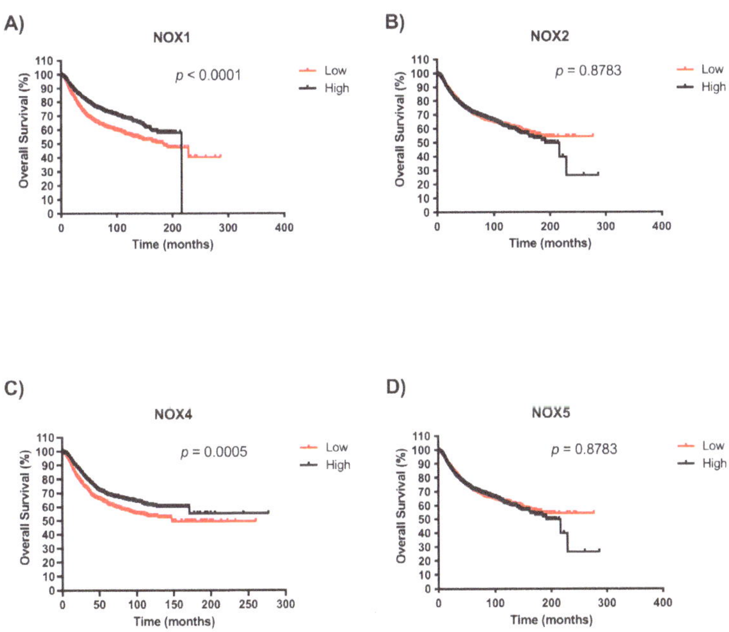

Figure 4. *Cont.*

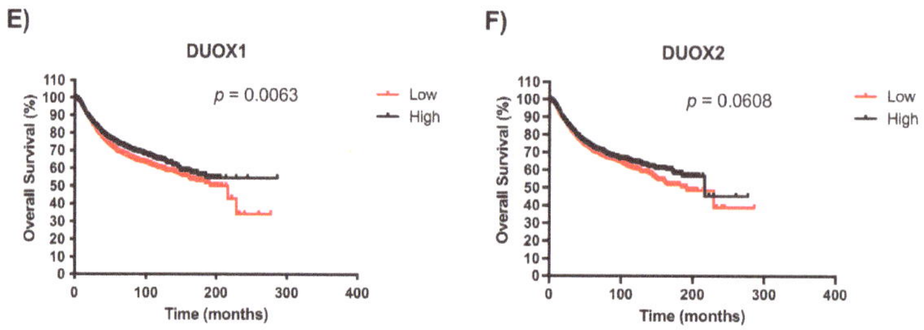

Figure 4. Survival analysis according to NOX family gene expression in BC patients. Comparison between the survival of BC patients with high or low expression of NOX1 (**A**), NOX2 (**B**), NOX4 (**C**), NOX5 (**D**), DUOX1 (**E**), and DUOX2 (**F**) in tumor breast tissues using Kaplan–Meier plotter analysis.

2.5. NOX Gene Expression in Relation to Estrogen Receptor Status in Breast Cancer Samples

We further compared NOX mRNA levels between BC tissues that were positive or negative for the presence of estrogen receptors (ERs). As shown in Figure 5, NOX1 (Figure 5A), NOX2 (Figure 5B), and DUOX1 (Figure 5E) were higher in tissues that were ER-negative when compared to the ER-positive group. On the other hand, NOX4 expression (Figure 5C) was lower in ER-negative tissues in comparison to those with ER-positive status.

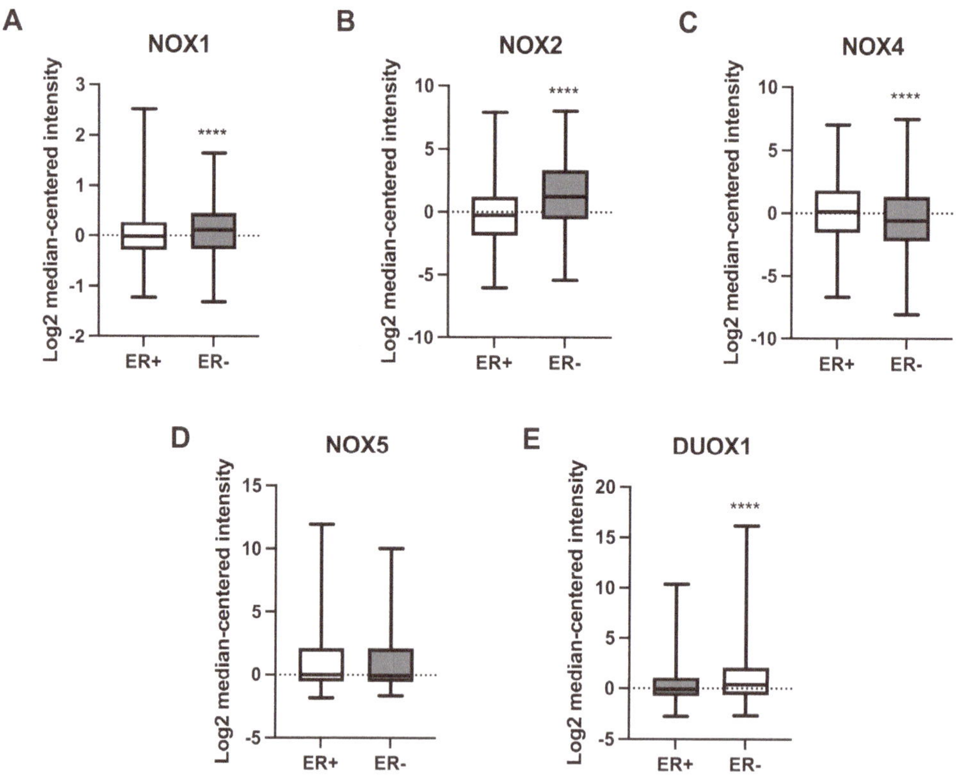

Figure 5. Expression of NOX family genes in relation to estrogen receptor (ER) status in BC samples. mRNA levels of NOX1 (**A**), NOX2 (**B**), NOX4 (**C**), NOX5 (**D**), and DUOX1 (**E**) in relation to the presence (ER+) or absence (ER-) of ER in tumor breast tissues. Data were obtained from the cBioPortal online platform (http://www.cbioportal.org/, accessed on 3 July 2022). N = 1904. **** $p < 0.0001$.

3. Discussion

Here, we show that NOX2 was the most expressed NOX isoform in normal tissue. NOX2 was originally the first identified NOX. It is highly expressed in leukocytes, where it has an essential role in phagocytic oxidative burst and host defense [11]. NOX2 expression was followed by NOX4, the only constitutively active isoform, which has been linked to physiological functions such as differentiation and memory formation [16,17]. Next, we observed DUOX1 and DUOX2 expression, respectively. Although DUOX2 plays an imperative role in hormone synthesis in the thyroid gland, DUOX1 has a diverse tissue distribution, but not a well-established physiological function [18,19]. It seems to be implicated in differentiation, wound responses, and host defense (reviewed in [20]). However, the role of DUOX1 and 2 in mammary tissue physiology is not known. Subsequently, we noticed NOX5, an isoform whose expression is typically found in the endothelium, spermatocytes, and lymphoid organs [21], and, finally, NOX1, which was mainly expressed in the colon and associated with gut immune modulation [22]. NOX3 mRNA levels were undetectable in our analysis, which might be due in part to its restricted distribution, found in high levels, for instance, in the inner ear, participating in ontogenesis [23]. To the best of our knowledge, no other study has evaluated the expression levels of NOX enzymes in normal human breast tissue.

Subsequently, we evaluated the expression levels of each NOX isoform by comparing the normal tissue to the different BC molecular subtypes. In a time in which personalized medicine is moving toward even more individualized treatment, the identification of new biomarkers among the subtypes should facilitate management planning. We found that the luminal A subtype had higher levels of NOX4 mRNA and lower levels of DUOX1. This subtype is low-grade, associated with a better prognosis, and tends to grow slowly [24]. In the luminal B subtype, which is known to grow slightly faster than luminal A cancers and to show worse recurrence-free survival at 5 years and 10 years [25], we observed a significant decrease in DUOX1 expression. In line with these findings, the HER2 subtype presented higher expression levels of NOX1, NOX2, and NOX4, but lower levels of DUOX1. The HER2 BC subtype was characterized as growing faster than luminal cancers and having a worse prognosis. Interestingly, these three subtypes exhibited low levels of DUOX1 expression. Data from our group demonstrated that DUOX1 was downregulated in BC cell lines and tissues. Moreover, non-tumor breast cells silenced for DUOX1 had a higher proliferation rate, as well as less adherence and migratory capacity when compared to control cells, suggesting that DUOX1 may play a tumor-suppressive role [26], which can be disrupted in luminal A, B, and HER2 BC subtypes according to our analysis.

Furthermore, in basal-like, also called triple-negative and considered the most aggressive and resistant BC subtype, NOX1 and NOX2 expression were significantly higher, in contrast to NOX4, which was diminished when compared to non-tumoral tissue. Some studies concerning NOX enzymes and BC have shown an upregulation of NOX1 in tumor tissues compared to normal tissues [27,28]. Desouki et al. (2005) demonstrated that NOX1 is highly expressed in breast tumors (86%). The authors also showed crosstalk between the mitochondria and NOX1 controlling redox signaling, and suggested that a disruption of this pathway could be involved in breast tumorigenesis [27]. Another study has proposed that the activation of the G protein-coupled receptor (GPCR) leukotriene receptor BLT2 promotes cell survival through the induction of NOX1- and NOX4-derived ROS in an ERK- and AKT-dependent mechanism in BC cell lines [29]. In addition, activation of the RAS-Erk1/2-NOX1 pathway was observed in a population of BC stem-like cells exposed to low concentrations of combined carcinogens, with an important function in the maintenance of increased cell proliferation [30].

NOX2 and NOX4 expression levels were higher in the claudin-low BC subtype, which is marked by aggressiveness, resistance to treatment, and poor prognosis [2]. Moreover, we observed higher NOX2 levels in three other BC subtypes (HER2, basal, and claudin-low). NOX2 has been related to angiogenesis, immune suppression, metastasis, and pro-survival signals in tissues such as the lung, as well as in leukemia and melanoma cells [31–35].

NOX2 was found in lipid rafts (LRs) of BC cell lines, whereas the disruption of these structures resulted in downregulation of the enzyme [36]. Mukawera et al. demonstrated that IKKε overexpression in BC cells was dependent on NOX2, leading to increased proliferation. NOX4 expression was also upregulated in three BC subtypes (luminal A, HER2, and claudin-low). Overexpression of NOX4 in non-tumor breast cells has been associated with increased senescence, cellular transformation, and resistance to apoptosis, suggesting an oncogenic role of this enzyme. The same authors also showed that NOX4 was overexpressed in various BC cell lines and primary breast tumors [12]. Additionally, another group has suggested NOX4 as a key player in TGFβ-induced epithelial-to-mesenchymal transition and migration of non-tumor and metastatic human breast cells [13]. In conformity, a subsequent study reported the efficiency of attenuating metastasis in BC cells by targeting NOX4 [37]. Our findings, in conjunction with those exposed in the literature, reinforce the great relevance of NOX4 in BC initiation and development.

Although, herein, we observed no changes in NOX5 expression levels among the BC subtypes, previous reports have identified NOX5 upregulation in BC, but they analyzed a limited number of samples with no molecular subtype distinction [14,38]. More recently, leptin has emerged as a potential activator of NOX5-derived ROS production in human epithelial mammary cells, linking obesity-associated hyperleptinemia with mammary tumorigenesis [39].

Surprisingly, in the present study, we did not identify significant alterations in NOX expression over tumor stages in our analysis. However, we verified the presence of increased expression levels of NOX1, NOX2, and DUOX1 in ER- BC tissues, and significantly low levels of NOX4 in ER+. ER is one of the main prognostic biomarkers in BC. The lack of the receptor is associated with a more aggressive profile of the tumor [40]. There are few studies correlating NOX expression and tumor progression. Liu and colleagues revealed a greater expression of NOX1 according to tumor progression in lung cancer [41]. Moreover, high expression of NOX4 and NOX5 were correlated to poorer overall survival in patients with end-stage gastric cancer [42].

Some studies have proposed that the expression level of NOX enzymes can influence the overall survival of patients. Individuals with hepatocarcinoma seem to have better prognoses when high expression levels of NOX4 mRNA are found, while patients with high levels of NOX2 present poor prognoses [43]. Analysis of gastric tumors has correlated NOX2 overexpression with longer patient survival, in contrast with NOX4 overexpression, which is associated with poorer overall patient survival [44]. It has also been reported that the high expression of DUOXs is related to reduced mortality in thyroid cancer [45]. In our analysis, patients with lower NOX1, NOX4, and DUOX1 expression exhibited shorter survival compared to patients with higher levels. Although we have observed high levels of expression of these proteins in tumor tissues, the survival data suggest that the loss of these NOX may occur in more undifferentiated cells and, consequently, more aggressive tumors, which would explain the lower survival rates of patients.

In conclusion, our data shed light on the role of NOX isoforms in BC. We highlight here that NOX2 is the most expressed NOX isoform in normal breast tissue, whereas, in conjunction with NOX4, it displays high levels in different BC subtypes. In the face of the plurality of BC molecular and histological characteristics, taking NOX expression into account could add significant value to the design and management of new therapies. However, many studies are still needed to elucidate the role of each NOX member in the different types of cancer and their implications.

4. Materials and Methods

4.1. Gene Expression Profiles in Breast Tissue

To analyze the expression of NOX family genes in normal breast tissue, we used the database The Human Protein Atlas (HPA) (https://www.proteinatlas.org, accessed on 2 July 2022). Individual genes (NOX1, CYBB NOX2, NOX3, NOX4, NOX5, DUOX1, and DUOX2) were evaluated. All quantitative transcriptome data (RNA-Seq) were retrieved from the Cancer Genome Atlas (TCGA) portal. A total of 290 normal breast samples were analyzed. The data were downloaded and plotted using the Graphpad Prism 9 software (GraphPad Software, Inc., San Diego, CA, USA).

4.2. Analysis of Gene Expression in Breast Tumor Tissue

The evaluation of NOX mRNA levels in BC patients was achieved through the online analysis tool cBioPortal (http://www.cbioportal.org/, accessed on 3 July 2022). The expression of NOX mRNA levels in human BC and normal tissues was obtained using the METABRIC study [3,45], containing 1904 samples from patients who had their breast tissue samples collected. We compared NOX mRNA levels between the different subtypes of BC and the non-tumoral tissue, as well as the influence of estrogen receptor status.

4.3. Analysis of Patient Survival According to NOX Expression

The significance of the prognosis in BC patients with different levels of NOX isoforms was performed using the Kaplan–Meier database (http://kmplot.com/analysis/, accessed on 15 August 2022). The BC database was established using gene expression data and survival information from 876 patients. Individual genes (NOX1, CYBB NOX2, NOX4, NOX5, DUOX1, and DUOX2) were evaluated on the platform. The patient cases were divided into two groups according to the median expression of the gene (high vs. low expression). The survival of patients in both groups was then analyzed using the Kaplan–Meier survival graph. A p-value less than 0.05 was considered statistically significant. The data were downloaded as text, which was replotted.

4.4. Statistical Analysis

Normality was verified using the D'Agostino and Pearson test. The data were analyzed using ANOVA, except in the results with only 2 groups, in which the t test was applied. Log2 median-centered intensity was calculated by subtracting the median from the values of both groups. The results were expressed as the mean ± standard deviation.

Author Contributions: Conceptualization, R.S.F. and A.d.V.e.S.; methodology, A.d.V.e.S., C.C.d.F., L.M.P. and P.H.M.T.; formal analysis, A.d.V.e.S., C.C.d.F., L.M.P. and P.H.M.T.; data curation, A.d.V.e.S., C.C.d.F., P.H.M.T., A.C.F.F. and R.S.F.; writing—original draft preparation, A.d.V.e.S., C.C.d.F. and R.S.F.; writing—review and editing, L.M.P., P.H.M.T., A.C.F.F. and R.S.F.; supervision, R.S.F.; project administration, R.S.F.; funding acquisition, R.S.F. All authors have read and agreed to the published version of the manuscript.

Funding: This research was funded by Conselho Nacional de Desenvolvimento Científico e Tecnológico (CNPq), Fundação de Amparo à Pesquisa do Estado do Rio de Janeiro (FAPERJ) and Coordenação de Aperfeiçoamento de Pessoal de Nível Superior (CAPES). The APC was funded by Coordenação de Aperfeiçoamento de Pessoal de Nível Superior (CAPES).

Institutional Review Board Statement: Not applicable.

Informed Consent Statement: Not applicable.

Data Availability Statement: Data is contained within the article.

Conflicts of Interest: The authors declare no conflicts of interest.

References

1. Bray, F.; Ferlay, J.; Soerjomataram, I.; Siegel, R.L.; Torre, L.A.; Jemal, A. Global cancer statistics 2018: GLOBOCAN estimates of incidence and mortality worldwide for 36 cancers in 185 countries. *CA Cancer J. Clin.* **2018**, *68*, 394–424. [CrossRef]
2. Turkoz, F.P.; Solak, M.; Petekkaya, I.; Keskin, O.; Kertmen, N.; Sarici, F.; Arik, Z.; Babacan, T.; Ozisik, Y.; Altundag, K. Association between common risk factors and molecular subtypes in breast cancer patients. *Breast* **2013**, *22*, 344–350. [CrossRef]
3. Curtis, C.; Shah, S.P.; Chin, S.F.; Turashvili, G.; Rueda, O.M.; Dunning, M.J.; Speed, D.; Lynch, A.G.; Samarajiwa, S.; Yuan, Y.; et al. The genomic and transcriptomic architecture of 2,000 breast tumours reveals novel subgroups. *Nature* **2012**, *486*, 346–352. [CrossRef]
4. Waks, A.G.; Winer, E.P. Breast Cancer Treatment: A Review. *JAMA—J. Am. Med. Assoc.* **2019**, *321*, 288–300. [CrossRef]

5. Blows, F.M.; Driver, K.E.; Schmidt, M.K.; Broeks, A.; van Leeuwen, F.E.; Wesseling, J.; Cheang, M.C.; Gelmon, K.; Nielsen, T.O.; Blomqvist, C.; et al. Subtyping of breast cancer by immunohistochemistry to investigate a relationship between subtype and short and long term survival: A collaborative analysis of data for 10,159 cases from 12 studies. *PLoS Med.* **2010**, *7*, e1000279. [CrossRef]
6. Cheang, M.C.U.; Martin, M.; Nielsen, T.O.; Prat, A.; Voduc, D.; Rodriguez-Lescure, A.; Ruiz, A.; Chia, S.; Shepherd, L.; Ruiz-Borrego, M.; et al. Defining Breast Cancer Intrinsic Subtypes by Quantitative Receptor Expression. *Oncologist* **2015**, *20*, 474–482. [CrossRef] [PubMed]
7. Harbeck, N.; Penault-Llorca, F.; Cortes, J.; Gnant, M.; Houssami, N.; Poortmans, P.; Ruddy, K.; Tsang, J.; Cardoso, F. Breast cancer. *Nat. Rev. Dis. Primers* **2019**, *5*, 66. [CrossRef] [PubMed]
8. Malhotra, G.K.; Zhao, X.; Band, H.; Band, V. Histological, molecular and functional subtypes of breast cancers. *Cancer Biol. Ther.* **2010**, *10*, 955–960. [CrossRef]
9. Drummond, G.R.; Selemidis, S.; Griendling, K.K.; Sobey, C.G. Combating oxidative stress in vascular disease: NADPH oxidases as therapeutic targets. *Nat. Rev. Drug Discov.* **2011**, *10*, 453–471. [CrossRef] [PubMed]
10. Parascandolo, A.; Laukkanen, M.O. Carcinogenesis and reactive oxygen species signaling: Interaction of the NADPH oxidase NOX1-5 and superoxide dismutase 1-3 signal transduction pathways. *Antioxid. Redox Signal.* **2019**, *30*, 443–486. [CrossRef] [PubMed]
11. Block, K.; Gorin, Y. Aiding and abetting roles of NOX oxidases in cellular transformation. *Nat. Rev. Cancer* **2012**, *12*, 627–637. [CrossRef]
12. Graham, K.A.; Kulawiec, M.; Owens, K.M.; Li, X.; Desouki, M.M.; Chandra, D.; Singh, K.K. NADPH oxidase 4 is an oncoprotein localized to mitochondria. *Cancer Biol. Ther.* **2010**, *10*, 223–231. [CrossRef]
13. Boudreau, H.E.; Casterline, B.W.; Rada, B.; Korzeniowska, A.; Leto, T.L. Nox4 involvement in TGF-beta and SMAD3-driven induction of the epithelial-to-mesenchymal transition and migration of breast epithelial cells. *Free Radic. Biol. Med.* **2012**, *53*, 1489–1499. [CrossRef]
14. Dho, S.H.; Kim, J.Y.; Lee, K.P.; Kwon, E.S.; Lim, J.C.; Kim, C.J.; Jeong, D.; Kwon, K.S. STAT5A-mediated NOX5-L expression promotes the proliferation and metastasis of breast cancer cells. *Exp. Cell Res.* **2017**, *351*, 51–58. [CrossRef]
15. Giuliano, A.E.; Connolly, J.L.; Edge, S.B.; Mittendorf, E.A.; Rugo, H.S.; Solin, L.J.; Weaver, D.L.; Winchester, D.J.; Hortobagyi, G.N. Breast Cancer-Major changes in the American Joint Committee on Cancer eighth edition cancer staging manual. *CA Cancer J. Clin.* **2017**, *67*, 290–303. [CrossRef]
16. Schröder, K.; Wandzioch, K.; Helmcke, I.; Brandes, R.P. Nox4 acts as a switch between differentiation and proliferation in preadipocytes. *Arterioscler. Thromb. Vasc. Biol.* **2009**, *29*, 239–245. [CrossRef]
17. Yoshikawa, Y.; Ago, T.; Kuroda, J.; Wakisaka, Y.; Tachibana, M.; Komori, M.; Shibahara, T.; Nakashima, H.; Nakashima, K.; Kitazono, T. Nox4 Promotes Neural Stem/Precursor Cell Proliferation and Neurogenesis in the Hippocampus and Restores Memory Function Following Trimethyltin-Induced Injury. *Neuroscience* **2019**, *398*, 193–205. [CrossRef] [PubMed]
18. Johnson, K.R.; Marden, C.C.; Ward-Bailey, P.; Gagnon, L.H.; Bronson, R.T.; Donahue, L.R. Congenital hypothyroidism, dwarfism, and hearing impairment caused by a missense mutation in the mouse dual oxidase 2 gene, Duox2. *Mol. Endocrinol.* **2007**, *21*, 1593–1602. [CrossRef] [PubMed]
19. Grasberger, H. Defects of thyroidal hydrogen peroxide generation in congenital hypothyroidism. *Mol. Cell. Endocrinol.* **2010**, *322*, 99–106. [CrossRef]
20. De Faria, C.C.; Fortunato, R.S. The role of dual oxidases in physiology and cancer. *Genet. Mol. Biol.* **2020**, *43*, e20190096. [CrossRef] [PubMed]
21. Jagnandan, D.; Church, J.E.; Banfi, B.; Stuehr, D.J.; Marrero, M.B.; Fulton, D.J.R. Novel mechanism of activation of NADPH oxidase 5: Calcium sensitization via phosphorylation. *J. Biol. Chem.* **2007**, *282*, 6494–6507. [CrossRef]
22. Schwerd, T.; Bryant, R.V.; Pandey, S.; Capitani, M.; Meran, L.; Cazier, J.B.; Jung, J.; Mondal, K.; Parkes, M.; Mathew, C.G.; et al. NOX1 loss-of-function genetic variants in patients with inflammatory bowel disease. *Mucosal Immunol.* **2018**, *11*, 562–574. [CrossRef] [PubMed]
23. Paffenholz, R.; Bergstrom, R.A.; Pasutto, F.; Wabnitz, P.; Munroe, R.J.; Jagla, W.; Heinzmann, U.; Marquardt, A.; Bareiss, A.; Laufs, J.; et al. Vestibular defects in head-tilt mice result from mutations in Nox3, encoding an NADPH oxidase. *Genes Dev.* **2004**, *18*, 486–491. [CrossRef]
24. Dumitrescu, R.G. Interplay between genetic and epigenetic changes in breast cancer subtypes. In *Methods in Molecular Biology*; Humana Press Inc.: Totowa, NJ, USA, 2018; pp. 19–34. [CrossRef]
25. Prat, A.; Pineda, E.; Adamo, B.; Galván, P.; Fernández, A.; Gaba, L.; Díez, M.; Viladot, M.; Arance, A.; Muñoz, M. Clinical implications of the intrinsic molecular subtypes of breast cancer. *Breast* **2015**, *24*, S26–S35. [CrossRef] [PubMed]
26. Fortunato, R.S.; Gomes, L.R.; Munford, V.; Pessoa, C.F.; Quinet, A.; Hecht, F.; Kajitani, G.S.; Milito, C.B.; Carvalho, D.P.; Menck, C.F.M. DUOX1 silencing in mammary cell alters the response to genotoxic stress. *Oxidative Med. Cell. Longev.* **2018**, *2018*, 3570526. [CrossRef]
27. Desouki, M.M.; Kulawiec, M.; Bansal, S.; Das, G.; Singh, K.K. Cross talk between mitochondria and superoxide generating NADPH oxidase in breast and ovarian tumors. *Cancer Biol. Ther.* **2005**, *4*, 1367–1373. [CrossRef] [PubMed]
28. Pervin, S.; Tran, L.; Urman, R.; Braga, M.; Parveen, M.; Li, S.A.; Chaudhuri, G.; Singh, R. Oxidative stress specifically downregulates survivin to promote breast tumour formation. *Br. J. Cancer* **2013**, *108*, 848–858. [CrossRef]

29. Choi, J.A.; Lee, J.W.; Kim, H.; Kim, E.Y.; Seo, J.M.; Ko, J.; Kim, J.H. Pro-survival of estrogen receptor-negative breast cancer cells is regulated by a BLT2-reactive oxygen species-linked signaling pathway. *Carcinogenesis* **2009**, *31*, 543–551. [CrossRef]
30. Pluchino, L.A.; Wang, H.-C.R. Chronic Exposure to Combined Carcinogens Enhances Breast Cell Carcinogenesis with Mesenchymal and Stem-Like Cell Properties. *PLoS ONE* **2014**, *9*, e108698. [CrossRef] [PubMed]
31. Ushio-Fukai, M.; Nakamura, Y. Reactive oxygen species and angiogenesis: NADPH oxidase as target for cancer therapy. *Cancer Lett.* **2008**, *266*, 37–52. [CrossRef]
32. Kusmartsev, S.; Nefedova, Y.; Yoder, D.; Gabrilovich, D.I. Antigen-Specific Inhibition of CD8 + T Cell Response by Immature Myeloid Cells in Cancer Is Mediated by Reactive Oxygen Species. *J. Immunol.* **2004**, *172*, 989–999. [CrossRef]
33. Van Der Weyden, L.; Arends, M.J.; Campbell, A.D.; Bald, T.; Wardle-Jones, H.; Griggs, N.; Velasco-Herrera, M.D.C.; Tüting, T.; Sansom, O.J.; Karp, N.A.; et al. Genome-wide in vivo screen identifies novel host regulators of metastatic colonization. *Nature* **2017**, *541*, 233–236. [CrossRef]
34. Maraldi, T.; Prata, C.; Sega, F.V.D.; Caliceti, C.; Zambonin, L.; Fiorentini, D.; Hakim, G. NAD(P)H oxidase isoform Nox2 plays a prosurvival role in human leukaemia cells. *Free Radic. Res.* **2009**, *43*, 1111–1121. [CrossRef] [PubMed]
35. Brar, S.S.; Kennedy, T.P.; Sturrock, A.B.; Huecksteadt, T.P.; Quinn, M.T.; Whorton, A.R.; Hoidal, J.R. An NAD(P)H oxidase regulates growth and transcription in melanoma cells. *Am. J. Physiol. Cell Physiol.* **2002**, *282*, C1212–C1224. [CrossRef] [PubMed]
36. Malla, R.R.; Raghu, H.; Rao, J.S. Regulation of NADPH oxidase (Nox2) by lipid rafts in breast carcinoma cells. *Int. J. Oncol.* **2010**, *37*, 1483–1493. [CrossRef]
37. Zhang, B.; Liu, Z.; Hu, X. Inhibiting cancer metastasis via targeting NAPDH oxidase 4. *Biochem. Pharmacol.* **2013**, *86*, 253–266. [CrossRef]
38. Juhasz, A.; Ge, Y.; Markel, S.; Chiu, A.; Matsumoto, L.; van Balgooy, J.; Roy, K.; Doroshow, J.H. Expression of NADPH oxidase homologues and accessory genes in human cancer cell lines, tumours and adjacent normal tissues. *Free Radic. Res.* **2009**, *43*, 523–532. [CrossRef] [PubMed]
39. Mahbouli, S.; Der Vartanian, A.; Ortega, S.; Rougé, S.; Vasson, M.P.; Rossary, A. Leptin induces ROS via NOX5 in healthy and neoplastic mammary epithelial cells. *Oncol. Rep.* **2017**, *38*, 3254–3264. [CrossRef] [PubMed]
40. Fragomeni, S.M.; Sciallis, A.; Jeruss, J.S. Molecular Subtypes and Local-Regional Control of Breast Cancer. *Surg. Oncol. Clin. N. Am.* **2018**, *27*, 95–120. [CrossRef] [PubMed]
41. Liu, X.; Pei, C.; Yan, S.; Liu, G.; Liu, G.; Chen, W.; Cui, Y.; Liu, Y. NADPH oxidase 1-dependent ROS is crucial for TLR4 signaling to promote tumor metastasis of non-small cell lung cancer. *Tumor Biol.* **2015**, *36*, 1493–1502. [CrossRef]
42. You, X.; Ma, M.; Hou, G.; Hu, Y.; Shi, X. Gene expression and prognosis of NOX family members in gastric cancer. *OncoTargets Ther.* **2018**, *11*, 3065–3074. [CrossRef] [PubMed]
43. Eun, H.S.; Cho, S.Y.; Joo, J.S.; Kang, S.H.; Moon, H.S.; Lee, E.S.; Kim, S.H.; Lee, B.S. Gene expression of NOX family members and their clinical significance in hepatocellular carcinoma. *Sci. Rep.* **2017**, *7*, 11060. [CrossRef] [PubMed]
44. Pulcrano, M.; Boukheris, H.; Talbot, M.; Caillou, B.; Dupuy, C.; Virion, A.; De Vathaire, F.; Schlumberger, M. Poorly differentiated follicular thyroid carcinoma: Prognostic factors and relevance of histological classification. *Thyroid* **2007**, *17*, 639–646. [CrossRef] [PubMed]
45. Pereira, B.; Chin, S.F.; Rueda, O.M.; Vollan, H.K.M.; Provenzano, E.; Bardwell, H.A.; Pugh, M.; Jones, L.; Russell, R.; Sammut, S.J.; et al. The somatic mutation profiles of 2433 breast cancers refines their genomic and transcriptomic landscapes. *Nat. Commun.* **2016**, *7*, 11479. [CrossRef]

International Journal of
Molecular Sciences

MDPI

Article

Hepatic Alterations in a BTBR T + Itpr3tf/J Mouse Model of Autism and Improvement Using Melatonin via Mitigation Oxidative Stress, Inflammation and Ferroptosis

Rita Rezzani [1,2,3,*], Marzia Gianò [1], Daniela Pinto [4], Fabio Rinaldi [4], Cornelis J. F. van Noorden [5] and Gaia Favero [1,2]

1. Anatomy and Physiopathology Division, Department of Clinical and Experimental Sciences, University of Brescia, 25123 Brescia, Italy; marzia.giano@unibs.it (M.G.); gaia.favero@unibs.it (G.F.)
2. Interdipartimental University Center of Research "Adaption and Regeneration of Tissues and Organs (ARTO)", University of Brescia, 25123 Brescia, Italy
3. Italian Society for the Study of Orofacial Pain (Società Italiana Studio Dolore Orofacciale-SISDO), 25123 Brescia, Italy
4. Human Microbiome Advanced Project Institute, 20129 Milan, Italy; dpinto@giulianipharma.com (D.P.); fabio.rinaldi@studiorinaldi.com (F.R.)
5. Department of Genetic Toxicology and Cancer Biology, National Institute of Biology, 1000 Ljubljana, Slovenia; c.j.vannoorden@nib.si

* Correspondence: rita.rezzani@unibs.it; Tel.: +39-0303717483

Abstract: Autism spectrum disorder (ASD) is a complicated neurodevelopmental disorder, and its etiology is not well understood. It is known that genetic and nongenetic factors determine alterations in several organs, such as the liver, in individuals with this disorder. The aims of the present study were to analyze morphological and biological alterations in the liver of an autistic mouse model, BTBR T + Itpr3tf/J (BTBR) mice, and to identify therapeutic strategies for alleviating hepatic impairments using melatonin administration. We studied hepatic cytoarchitecture, oxidative stress, inflammation and ferroptosis in BTBR mice and used C57BL6/J mice as healthy control subjects. The mice were divided into four groups and then treated and not treated with melatonin, respectively. BTBR mice showed (a) a retarded development of livers and (b) iron accumulation and elevated oxidative stress and inflammation. We demonstrated that the expression of ferroptosis markers, the transcription factor nuclear factor erythroid-related factor 2 (NFR2), was upregulated, and the Kelch-like ECH-associated protein 1 (KEAP1) was downregulated in BTBR mice. Then, we evaluated the effects of melatonin on the hepatic alterations of BTBR mice; melatonin has a positive effect on liver cytoarchitecture and metabolic functions.

Keywords: autism spectrum disorder; liver; oxidative stress; inflammation; ferroptosis

1. Introduction

Autism spectrum disorder (ASD) is a heterogeneous, disabling neurodevelopmental disorder that affects social interactions, limits interests and induces stereotype behavior [1–3]. The prevalence of ASD is increasing and creates a social burden. Currently, psychostimulant and antipsychotic interventions are the only therapeutics available to treat ASD patients [4].

The etiology of ASD is not well understood [2,5], but it is likely that both biological and environmental factors are involved [6]. Biologically, genetic and nongenetic factors play a role, such as immunological and mitochondrial malfunction associated with oxidative stress, neurotrophic dysregulation and inflammation [7–10]. There is increasing evidence that ASD patients show excessive reactive oxygen species (ROS) production [8,11,12]. Environmental factors involve, among others, exposure to both essential and toxic metals [13–15]. Dysregulated iron metabolism, causing an increased availability of free iron, can significantly impact hepatic metabolism [16]. Free iron has been implicated in inducing amyloid-β plaques, contributing to toxicity via oxidative stress in Alzheimer's disease and other neurodegenerative diseases [17].

An autistic mouse model, BTBR T + Itpr3tf/J (BTBR) mice, originally developed to study insulin resistance, diabetes-induced nephropathy and phenylketonuria, has been identified to consistently display autism-like behavior [18]. This animal model is considered a translational tool to evaluate potential therapies for ASD [18,19]. Recently, liver disorders have become a significant health concern and are an issue commonly found in autistic children [9,20]. Moreover, Trinchese et al. [8] showed that inflammation and oxidative stress in these mice induce mitochondrial dysfunction and mitochondrial fission in the liver. Hepatocytes are rich in mitochondria that produce ROS [21], and exposure to ROS induces oxidative stress, which results in lipid peroxidation and reduced antioxidant activity, causing liver damage [22,23] and, subsequently, leading to liver diseases [24,25].

Thus far, the role of the liver in ASD has been poorly investigated. Therefore, we studied the crosstalk between alterations in hepatic functions and ASD. Liver morphology was analyzed with haematoxylin-eosin staining and a common and reliable dye for detecting iron in tissues (Perls staining), and liver functions were analyzed by staining the biological markers of oxidative stress and inflammation, and the master regulators of a recently discovered form of cell death called *ferroptosis* in BTBR mice [16,18,26,27]. Ferroptosis is a recently discovered iron-dependent type of cell death characterized by ROS accumulations in cells, leading to Fe ion deposition and lipid peroxidation that results in cell death [18]. It is a result of redox inequity between the free iron-induced production of lipid hydroperoxides and various antioxidant defense systems, such as glutathione peroxidase 4 (GPX4), which detoxify free radicals and lipid oxidation products [18,28,29]. Moreover, ferroptosis has been implicated in multiple pathologies and is associated with neurodegeneration, nonalcoholic fatty liver diseases and cardiovascular diseases such as atherosclerosis [16]. Disruption of iron metabolism, in relation to the expression of the transcription factor nuclear factor erythroid-related factor 2 (NRF2), may significantly impact the ferroptosis pathway. It has been demonstrated that NRF2 is able to reduce anaerobic glycolysis and ROS levels in glioblastoma stem cells and leukemic stem cells [30]. Under physiological conditions, NRF2 resides in the cytoplasm, where it is attached to Kelch-like ECH-associated protein 1 (KEAP1), which negatively regulates NRF2 and keeps it in the cytoplasm [31]. Under oxidative stress conditions, NRF2 protein is stabilized and initiates a multistep pathway of activation that includes nuclear translocation [32]. After its translocation to the nucleus, NRF2 binds to antioxidant response elements and activates the transcription of cytoplasmic genes. Heme oxygenase-1 (HO-1) and other proteins are strictly under the control of NFR2 [33]. This pathway is considered to have a potential protective role of NFR2 in several types of cells, such as renal proximal tubular epithelial cells, leading to an upregulation of antioxidant enzymes such as superoxide dismutase 3 (SOD3) [33].

On the basis of these considerations, we report that ferroptosis participates in a spectrum of liver diseases, both acute and chronic [19,33], and we hypothesize that ferroptosis is also involved in hepatocyte alterations of BTBR mice. Only after considering the involvement of ferroptosis in the liver of BTBR mice, we evaluated the possible effect of an antioxidant, such as melatonin, in hepatic ASD.

Moreover, BTBR mice were treated with melatonin, a potent antioxidant that has been shown to have many cellular protective effects in neurological and non-neurological disorders [34,35]. Melatonin (N-acetyl-5-methoxytryptamine) is an indoleamine synthesized from the amino acid tryptophan in the pineal gland and other organs, such as the liver [21,36–38]. Studies have extensively demonstrated the effects of melatonin on oxidative stress, lipid peroxidation, and its therapeutic potential in liver injuries and diseases, showing its beneficial effects [35]. A recent study demonstrated that melatonin attenuates hepatocyte ferroptosis induced by lead or lipopolysaccharide exposure through the activation of AMP-activated protein kinase phosphorylation [39]. However, it is crucial to acknowledge that the exploration of the relationship between melatonin and ferroptosis is in a nascent stage, and many uncharted fields require further investigation.

Therefore, the aims of the present study were (a) to analyze morphological and biological alterations in the liver of BTBR mice in combination with markers related to oxidative stress and inflammation and (b) to identify the potential association between ferroptosis-related mechanisms and morphological changes in the liver in the BTBR mice; (c) to evaluate and identify therapeutic strategies for targeting the liver and alleviating metabolic impairments using melatonin administration.

Our research hypothesis is that oxidative stress, inflammation and even ferroptosis may be important tools for ASD evaluation.

2. Results

2.1. Hepatic Histological Features

The BTBR and CTR experimental groups treated with the vehicle were respectively redefined as "BTBR mice" and "CTR mice" for the following morphological, morphometrical and immunohistochemical analyses.

The haematoxylin-eosin staining showed that the cytoarchitecture of BTBR livers was well preserved, except for small signs of inflammation; the hepatocytes presented microvesicular steatosis morphology (hepatocellular ballooning). In addition, increased numbers of Kupffer cells and fat-storing cells were preserved in the parenchyma (Figure 1a). Furthermore, numerous hepatic cells exhibit crenulated nuclei that are irregularly shaped, as well as many nucleoli. Figure 1b shows the cytoarchitecture of the CTR liver for comparison.

In BTBR livers, most nuclei were diploid, either present in mononuclear diploid (MD) hepatocytes or in binuclear diploid (BD) hepatocytes (Figure 1a). Mononuclear tetraploid (MT) hepatocytes were relatively sparse (Figure 1a), whereas in CTR livers, most hepatocytes were MT (Figure 1c). Most hepatocytes in BTBR mice were MD, and only a few of them were identified as MT cells (Figure 1a).

The CTR group showed normal liver morphology (Figure 1b). Hepatocytes display central nuclei with a regular shape and eosinophilic cytoplasm with few lipid droplets (Figure 1b). No clear histopathological changes and no inflammatory cell infiltration were observed in the liver of the CTR group. Several hepatocytes were MT cells, a few of them were BD cells, and a small number were identified as MD cells (Figure 1b).

As mentioned above, numerous BD hepatocytes were found in BTBR mice compared with MD and MT cells in the same animals. This finding was evaluated using quantitative analysis, and the results showed that BTBR mice had three times more BD cells than CTR mice (Figure 1c). After this evaluation, we also observed MD and MT cells in both experimental groups. The quantitative analysis demonstrated a significantly higher number of MD cells in BTBR mice than in CTR mice; instead, the number of MT cells appeared to be significantly lower in BTBR mice compared to CTR mice, as reported in Figure 1c.

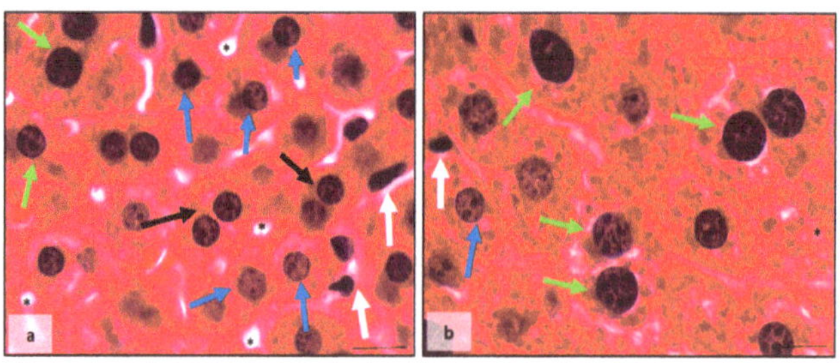

Figure 1. *Cont.*

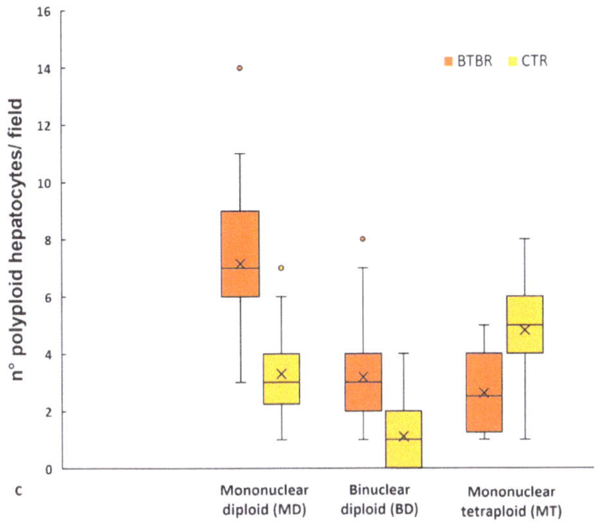

Figure 1. Hepatic histological evaluation. Representative photomicrographs of BTBR (**a**) and CTR (**b**) liver stained with haematoxylin-eosin. Bar: 10 μm. The black and white arrows show binuclear hepatocytes and Kupffer cells, respectively; the asterisks show the vacuoles; the blue and green arrows indicate mononuclear diploid and mononuclear tetraploid cells, respectively. Graph (**c**) reports the symmetrical data distribution of mononuclear diploid, binuclear and mononuclear tetraploid hepatocytes. In the graph, the orange dot indicates the outlier, the (x) indicates the mean value and the line represents the median value for each experimental group subdivided using polyploid hepatocytes.

The Perls staining showed that BTBR mice presented a higher accumulation of iron granules (blue) in the cytoplasm of MD and MT cells. Several blue granules were also observed in Kupffer cells (Figure 2a,b). On the other side, in the liver tissue of CTR mice, we observed no presence of iron either in the cytoplasm of all types of hepatocytes or in Kupffer cells (Figure 2c,d).

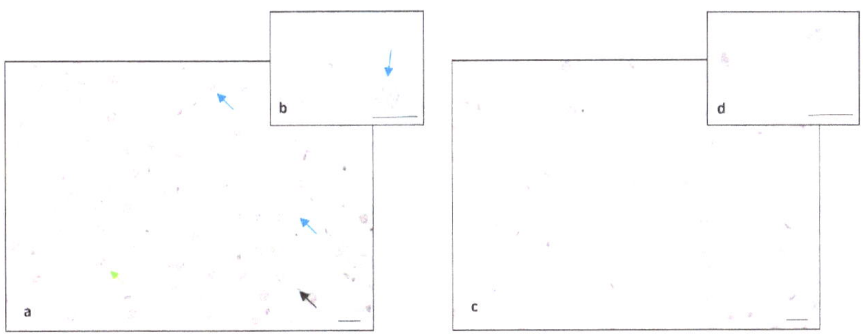

Figure 2. Evaluation of iron accumulation. Representative photomicrographs stained with Perls staining of BTBR (**a**,**b**) and CTR (**c**,**d**) liver. Bar: 10 μm. The black, blue and green arrows showed Kupffer cells, mononuclear diploid and mononuclear tetraploid cells, respectively, positive to Perls staining in BTBR mice.

2.2. Liver Oxidative Stress, Inflammation and the Regulatory Pathways of Ferroptosis

To investigate oxidative stress and inflammation in the liver of BTBR mice, we evaluated the expression of catalase (CAT), superoxide dismutase-1 (SOD-1), GPX4 and interleukin-1 β (IL-1β).

MD, BD and MT cells showed the same expression of the abovementioned proteins in both animal groups; therefore, we identified these cells as hepatocytes.

About CAT expression, in BTBR mice, we observed a weak/moderate immunopositivity in the cytoplasm of all hepatocytes (Figure 3a). Kupffer cells were negative and sometimes very weakly positive. Instead, CTR mice showed moderate/strong cytoplasmic immunopositivity in all the cells of the hepatic parenchyma, including Kupffer cells (Figure 3b).

Regarding SOD-1 expression, we observed a very weak/weak positivity in the hepatic parenchyma of BTBR mice, including Kupffer cells. This positivity was demonstrated in the cytoplasm with a scattered distribution and sometimes in the nuclei (Figure 3d). In CTR mice, SOD-1 showed a moderate/strong immunopositivity in the cytoplasm of all hepatic cells, as shown in Figure 3e. In particular, the expression of SOD-1 was very weak/negative in the nuclei of the hepatic cells of CTR mice.

The negative controls of CAT and SOD-1 immunohistochemistry were similar in both BTBR and CTR hepatic samples, and the inserts in Figure 3c,f showed a control reaction in a representative CTR liver tissue.

Comparing BTBR mice and CTR mice, we observed that in BTBR animals, both CAT and SOD-1 immunopositivity were significantly decreased compared to CTR mice. These data were confirmed through immunomorphometric analysis, as shown in Figure 3g,h.

Regarding the immunopositivity of GPX4, we observed very weak cytoplasmic positivity in BTBR mice compared with CTR mice, which showed moderate/strong positivity in liver parenchyma cells. GPX4 expression was decreased in BTBR mice compared with CTR mice, as summarized in Figure 3i.

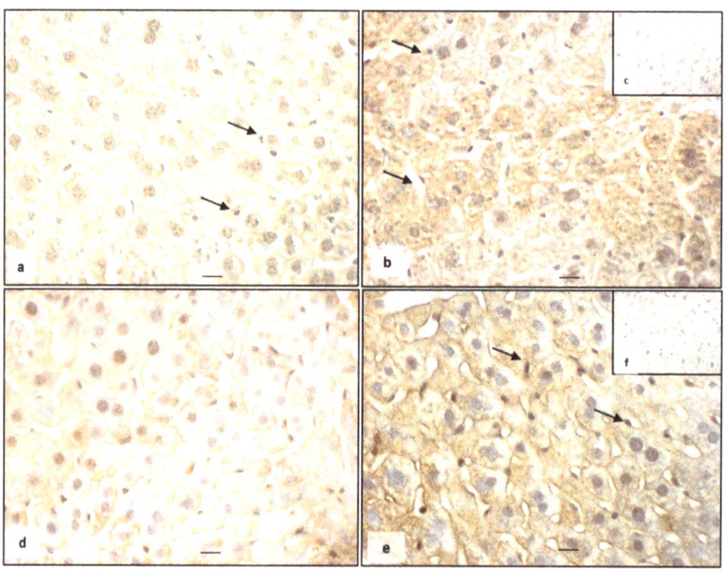

Figure 3. *Cont.*

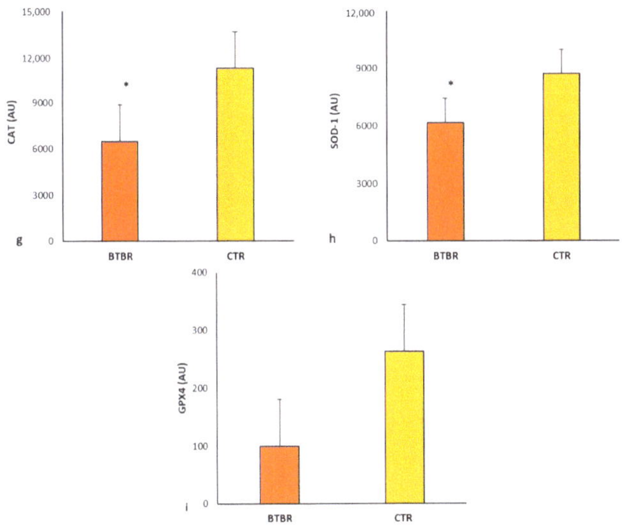

Figure 3. Evaluation of oxidative stress. Representative liver photomicrographs of CAT immunostaining of BTBR (**a**) and CTR (**b**,**c**) mice. Representative liver photomicrographs of SOD-1 immunostaining of BTBR (**d**) and CTR (**e**,**f**) mice. CAT (**c**) and SOD-1 (**f**) representative photomicrographs of the negative control are reported as inserts. The black arrows indicate Kupffer cells. Bars: 10 μm. The graphs summarize liver CAT (**g**), SOD-1 (**h**) and GPX4 (**i**) immunomorphometric measurement. * $p < 0.05$ vs. CTR mice. (AU): arbitrary units.

We also evaluated the expression of IL-1β in both animal groups.

In BTBR mice, the weak/moderate/strong immunopositivity for IL-1β was scattered and diffuse in the cytoplasm of hepatocytes, Kupffer cells and sinusoidal cells (Figure 4a). Only rarely were the nuclei of all hepatic cells positive for IL-1β. The expression of this protein was also observed in the cytoplasm of sinusoidal cells, and it was weak or sometimes moderate (Figure 4a). The hepatocytes of CTR mice showed a very weak cytoplasmic immunopositivity for this interleukin. The nuclei of hepatocytes and Kupffer cells were negative for IL-1β. Very weak or negative positivity of IL-1β was observed in the cytoplasm of sinusoidal cells (Figure 4b).

The negative controls of IL-1β immunohistochemistry were similar in both BTBR and CTR samples, and Figure 4c shows a control reaction in a representative CTR liver tissue.

As summarized in Figure 4d, IL-1β expression was significantly upregulated in BTBR mice compared with CTR mice.

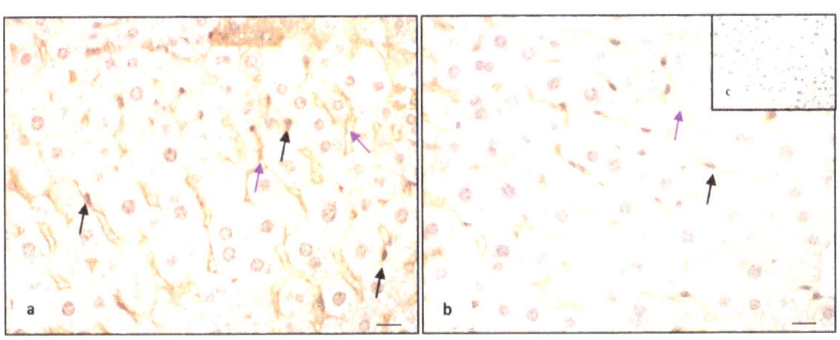

Figure 4. *Cont.*

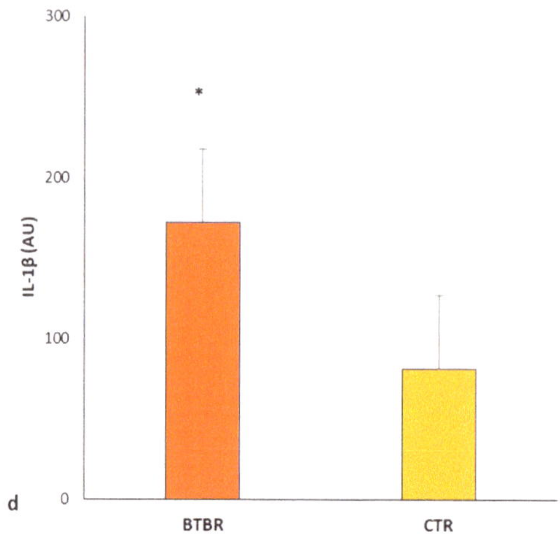

Figure 4. Evaluation of inflammation. Representative liver photomicrographs of IL-1β immunostaining of BTBR (**a**) and CTR (**b**,**c**) mice. IL-1β (**c**) representative photomicrograph of the negative control is reported as an insert. The black and purple arrows indicate Kupffer cells and sinusoids, respectively. Bar: 10 μm. The graph (**d**) summarizes liver IL-1β immunomorphometric measurement. * $p < 0.05$ vs. CTR mice. (AU): arbitrary units.

Then, we studied KEAP1 and NRF2 as the negative regulators of the ferroptosis pathway. Furthermore, to evaluate the effects of NRF2 translocation in the nucleus as a potential trigger of cytoprotective enzyme transcription, we studied the HO-1 enzyme.

It is important to remember that MD, BD and MT cells showed the same expression of the abovementioned proteins in both animal groups; therefore, we identified these cells as hepatocytes.

The KEAP1 immunopositivity in BTBR mice liver was very weak in the hepatocytes cytoplasm compared with CTR animal livers, which showed a strong/moderate expression of this protein. The immunomorphometric analysis confirmed that KEAP1 was weakly expressed in BTBR mice compared with CTR mice, as summarized in Figure 5a.

About NRF2, its cytoplasmic expression was moderate in BTBR mice, but it was very strong in almost all the nuclei of hepatocytes and Kupffer cells (Figure 5b). In fact, a few nuclei were negative for the NFR2 protein. CTR mice showed moderate/weak immunopositivity in the cytoplasm of all hepatocytes, but their nuclei were weakly positive or negative for this protein (Figure 5c). No positivity was observed in the sinusoidal cells in both groups.

The negative controls of NRF2 immunohistochemistry were similar in both BTBR and CTR samples. Figure 5d shows a control reaction in a representative CTR liver tissue.

NRF2 expression was significantly higher in the hepatic parenchyma of BTBR mice compared with the CTR group, as reported in Figure 5e.

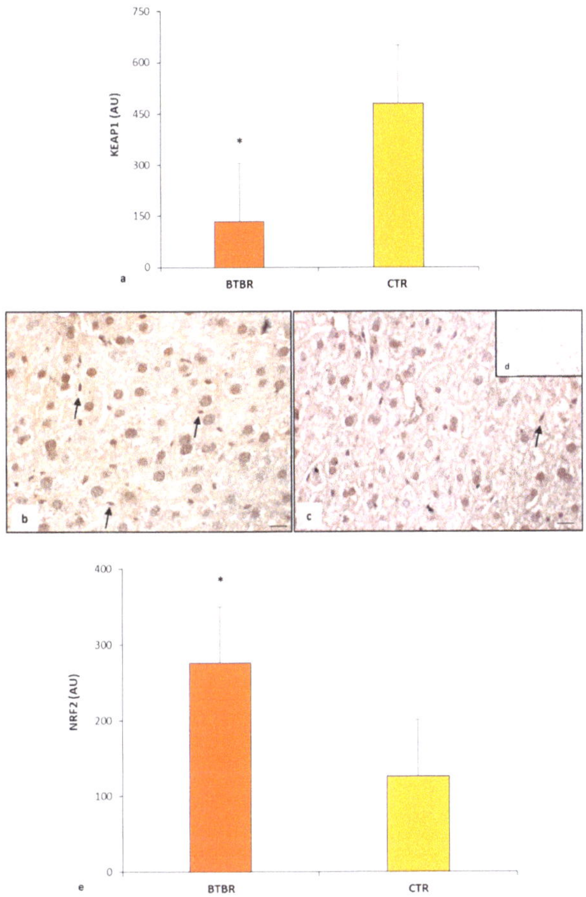

Figure 5. Regulatory pathways of ferroptosis. Graph (**a**) summarizes KEAP1 immunomorphometric measurement in BTBT and CTR mice. Representative photomicrographs of NRF2 immunostaining in liver sample of BTBR (**b**) and CTR (**c**,**d**) mice. NRF2 (**d**) representative photomicrographs of the negative control are reported as an insert. The black arrows indicate Kupffer cells. Bar: 10 μm. Graph (**e**) summarizes liver NRF2 immunohistochemical measurement of BTBR and CTR. * $p < 0.05$ vs. CTR mice. (AU): arbitrary units.

The nuclear presence of NFR2 stimulates the transcription of some genes responsible for inducing the production of proteins with protective effects against the ferroptosis pathway. It is known that one of these proteins is HO-1; therefore, we evaluated this protein through immunohistochemistry and immunomorphometric analyses.

As observed in Figure 6a, the hepatocytes had a moderate/weak/very weak expression of HO-1 together with sinusoidal cells and Kupffer cells. CTR livers presented very weak/negative HO-1 immunopositivity in all hepatic cells, including sinusoidal cells (Figure 6b). No nuclear positivity was observed in hepatic cells in both experimental groups.

The negative controls of HO-1 immunohistochemistry were similar in both BTBR and CTR samples, and Figure 6c shows a control reaction in a representative CTR liver tissue.

The immunomorphometric analysis of HO-1 immunostaining was significantly upregulated in BTBR mice compared with CTR ice (Figure 6d).

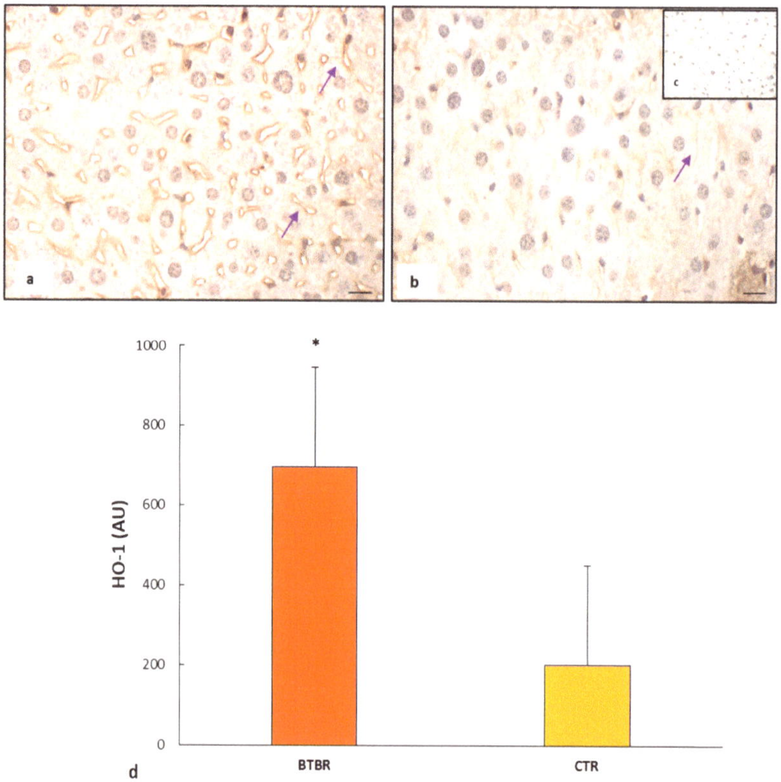

Figure 6. Evaluation of HO-1 in mice liver tissue. Representative photomicrographs of HO-1 immunostaining in the liver sample of BTBR (**a**) and CTR (**b**,**c**) mice. HO-1 (**c**) representative photomicrographs of negative control are reported as insert. The purple arrows indicate sinusoids. Bar: 10 μm. The graph summarizes liver HO-1 (**d**) immunomorphometric measurement comparing BTBR and CTR. * $p < 0.05$ vs. CTR mice. (AU): arbitrary units.

2.3. *Melatonin Effects in the Liver of BTBR and CTR Animals*

After demonstrating morphological and biochemical alterations in the hepatic parenchyma of BTBR compared with the CTR mice of the same age, we continued our study on the liver of BTBR mice treated with melatonin during the same period together with the previously mentioned groups, as reported in the Section 4 Materials and Methods.

2.3.1. Histological Evaluation of Hepatic Tissue in BTBR after Melatonin Treatment

Comparing BTBR animals treated with melatonin to BTBR mice, we observed an improvement in hepatic morphology. The liver had normal hepatocytes, some Kupffer cells and a reduction in vacuolization (Figure 7a). Regarding the number of BD, MD and MT cells, the quantitative analysis and the results demonstrated a significant decrease in BD cells, a nonsignificant decrease in MD cells, and a nonsignificant increase in MT cells compared to BTBR mice (Figure 7b).

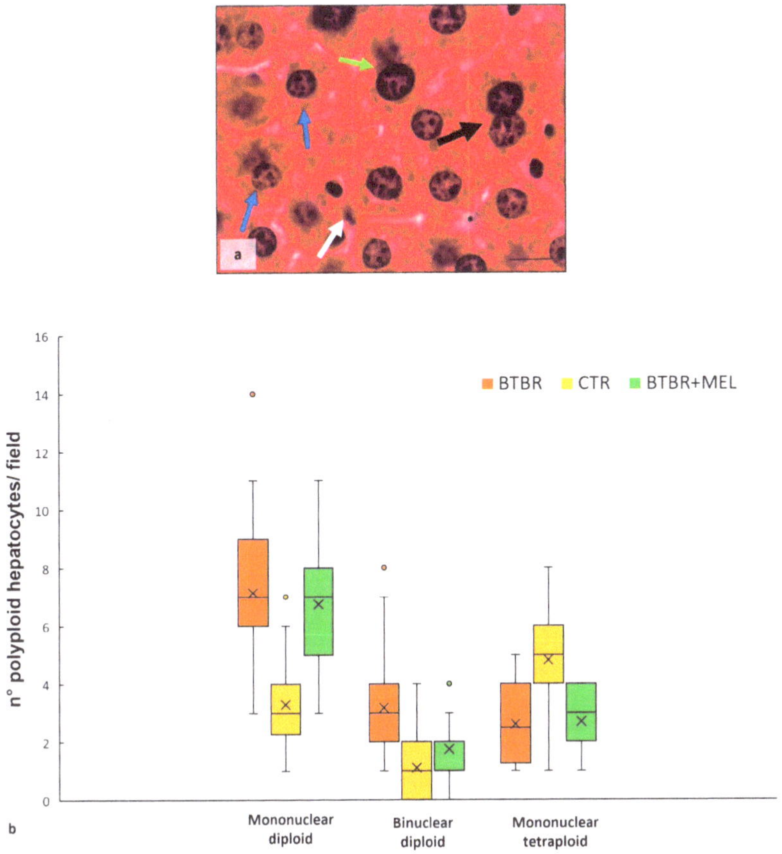

Figure 7. Hepatic histological evaluation. Representative photomicrographs (**a**) of the liver in BTBR mice treated with melatonin and stained with haematoxylin-eosin. Bar: 10 µm. The black and white arrows show binuclear hepatocytes and Kupffer cells respectively; the asterisks show vacuoles; the blue and green arrows indicate mononuclear diploid and mononuclear tetraploid cells, respectively. Graph (**b**) reports the symmetrical data distribution of mononuclear diploid, binuclear and mononuclear tetraploid hepatocytes. In the graph, the orange dot indicates the outlier, the (x) indicates the mean value, and the line represents the median value for each experimental group subdivided using polyploid hepatocytes.

As far as the overaccumulation of iron in the cytoplasm of hepatocytes of BTBR animals, Perls staining showed a reduction in iron in the same mice strain treated with melatonin (Figure 8a,b), resulting in a normalization of the amount of iron similar to the liver tissue of the CTR group (Figure 2). We noted the presence of iron only in Kupffer cells (Figure 8a).

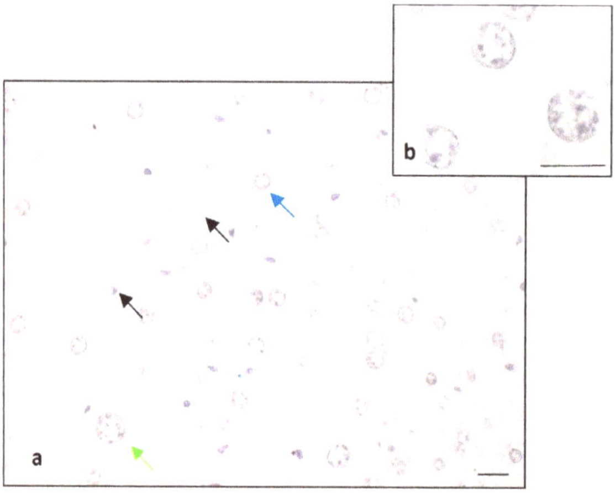

Figure 8. Evaluation of iron accumulation. Representative photomicrographs stained with Perls staining of the liver in BTBR mice treated with melatonin (**a**,**b**). Bar: 10 μm. The blue, green and black arrows showed mononuclear diploid, mononuclear tetraploid and Kupffer cells, respectively.

2.3.2. Oxidative Stress, Inflammation and Regulatory Pathways of Ferroptosis in BTBR Mice after Melatonin Treatment

As previously reported, no difference in the positivity of markers was observed in the types of hepatocytes, so we considered them only as hepatocytes.

BTBR mice treated with melatonin showed moderate cytoplasmic immunopositivity for CAT and SOD-1 in all hepatic cells, including Kupffer cells (Figure 9a,b). The expression of these markers was likely to that observed in the CTR group and reported in Figure 3b,e.

The negative controls of CAT and SOD-1 immunohistochemistry were similar in all the samples and are reported in the inserts (c,f) of Figure 3.

These observations were confirmed using the immunomorphometric analysis, as reported in Figure 9c, even though the increase does not show a significant trend compared to BTBR mice.

Finally, we observed a weak positivity for GPX4 in the hepatocyte cytoplasm of BTBR treated with melatonin, showing an upward trend compared to untreated mice, as reported in Figure 9d.

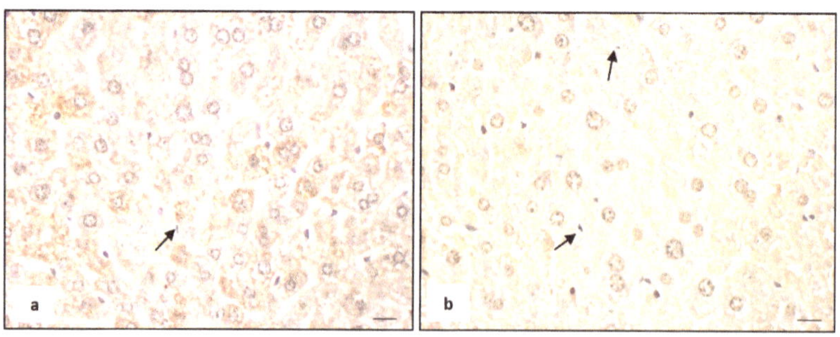

Figure 9. *Cont.*

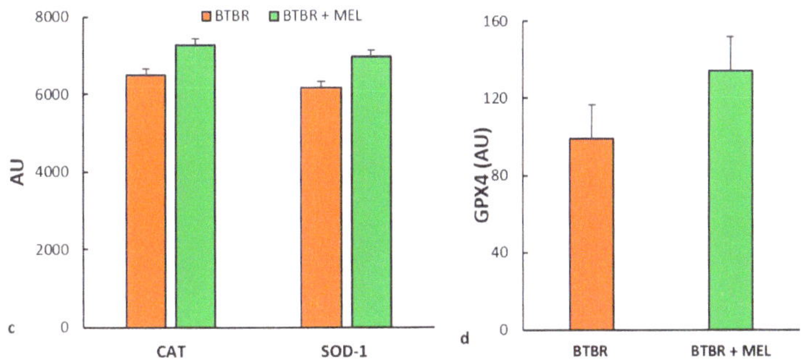

Figure 9. Evaluation of oxidative stress. Representative liver photomicrographs of CAT immunostaining of BTBR mice treated with melatonin (**a**). Representative liver photomicrographs of SOD-1 immunostaining in BTBR mice treated with melatonin (**b**). The black arrows indicate Kupffer cells. Bar: 10 µm. The graphs summarize liver CAT and SOD-1 (**c**) and GPX4 (**d**) immunomorphometric measurements. (AU): arbitrary units.

We also evaluated the expression of IL-1β in BTBR mice treated with melatonin.

We observed weak IL-1β immunopositivity in the cytoplasm of hepatocytes and sinusoidal cells; instead, the hepatocytes nuclei and Kupffer cells were negative for this interleukin (Figure 10a). The negative control of IL-1β immunohistochemistry was reported above as the insert in Figure 4c.

The immunomorphometric analysis, summarized in Figure 10b, confirmed that IL-1β immunopositivity, was significantly decreased in BTBR mice treated with melatonin compared to untreated BTBR mice.

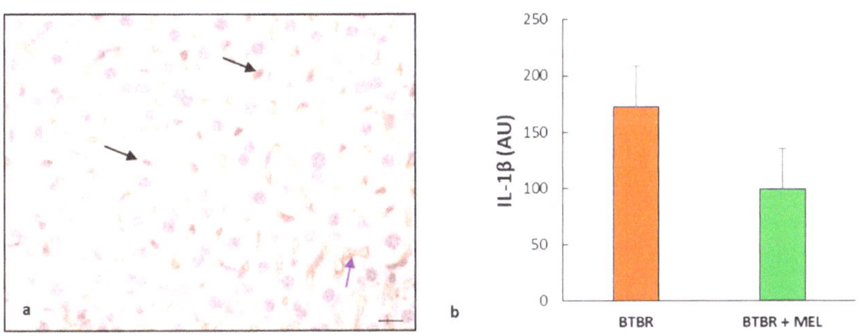

Figure 10. Evaluation of inflammation. Representative liver photomicrographs of IL-1β immunostaining of BTBR mice treated with melatonin (**a**). The black and purple arrows indicate Kupffer cells and sinusoids, respectively. Bar: 10 µm. The graph (**b**) summarizes IL-1β immunomorphometric measurements. (AU): arbitrary units.

The immunohistochemical analysis of BTBR mice treated with melatonin showed a weak cytoplasmic positivity of KEAP1 in all hepatocytes, similar to untreated mice.

The immunomorphometric analysis confirmed that KEAP1 did not differ significantly between BTBR mice treated with melatonin and untreated BTBR mice (Figure 11a).

The nuclei of the cells in the hepatic parenchyma of BTBR mice treated with melatonin are moderately/strongly positive to NFR2; only some nuclei of Kupffer cells were negative (Figure 11b). No positivity was observed in the sinusoidal cells. The negative control of NRF2 immunohistochemistry was reported above as the insert in Figure 5d.

The immunomorphometric analysis showed that NRF2 tended to increase compared to untreated mice (Figure 11c) and significantly improved compared to CTR mice (Figure 5c).

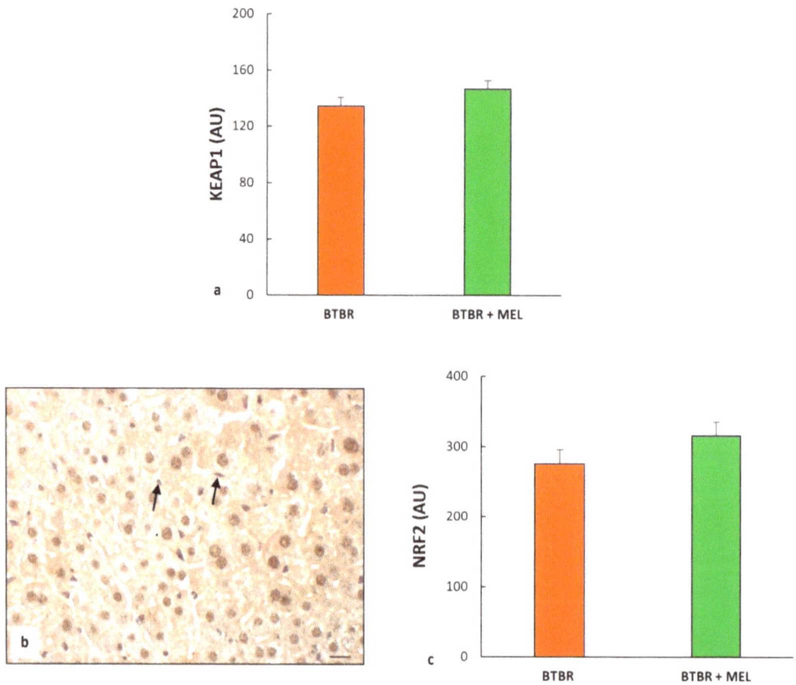

Figure 11. Regulatory pathways of ferroptosis. Plot (**a**) summarizes KEAP1 immunomorphometric measurements in BTBT mice and BTBR animals treated with melatonin. Representative photomicrographs of NRF2 immunostaining in the liver sample of BTBR treated with melatonin (**b**). The black arrows indicate Kupffer cells. Bar: 10 µm. Graph (**c**) summarizes liver NRF2 immunohistochemical measurements of BTBR mice and BTBR animals treated with melatonin. (AU): arbitrary units.

As for the evaluation between BTBR and CTR groups, we studied HO-1 protein to verify the effect of melatonin in ASD mice treated with antioxidants.

The results showed an increase in HO-1 protein in the sinusoidal cells and cytoplasm of hepatocytes (Figure 12a) compared to untreated BTBR and to the CTR group, as reported in Figure 6. This finding was confirmed through immunomorphometrical analysis, showing a significant increase in this protein compared to untreated BTBR mice (Figure 12b).

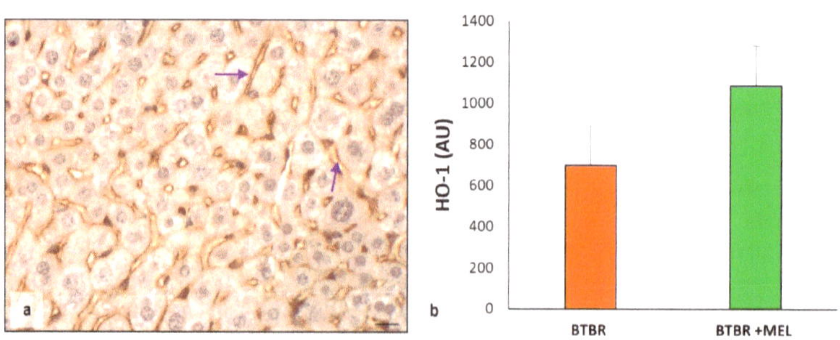

Figure 12. Evaluation of HO-1 in mice liver tissue. Representative photomicrographs of HO-1 immunostaining in liver sample of BTBR mice treated with melatonin (**a**). The purple arrows indicate sinusoids. Bar: 10 µm. The graph summarizes HO-1 (**b**) immunomorphometric measurements, comparing BTBR mice and BTBR animals treated with melatonin. (AU): arbitrary units.

3. Discussion

Our study shows that BTBR mice at the age of 16 weeks have significantly higher numbers of MD and BD cells and fewer MT hepatocytes in their livers compared with CTR mice at the same age. Moreover, we show that oxidative stress and inflammation are involved in the liver pathogenesis of ASD in BTBR mice. A major finding in our study is that ferroptosis, a type of programmed cell death, occurs in the livers of this autistic mouse model, which is similar to defects in the neurological development of ASD [2,40]. Furthermore, we demonstrate that the antioxidant melatonin ameliorates morphological and biochemical alterations in the liver of BTBR mice.

The liver has a remarkable potential to generate new tissue in response to injury due to the proliferative ability of the parenchyma [41]. Hepatocytes are physiologically long-lived cells, similar to neurons and cardiomyocytes [42,43]. Guidotti et al. [44] demonstrated that rat liver consists almost solely of MD hepatocytes during the first postnatal 22 days; thereafter, between the age of 22 and 28 days postnatally, this MD population decreases with a concomitant increase in BD hepatocytes. Moreover, at 30 days postnatally, MT hepatocyte numbers increase, and the MD and BD populations slowly decline. Based on these findings, we propose that there are defects in liver organogenesis in BTBR mice since these mice have large amounts of MD and BD hepatocytes that were inhibited in the formation of MT hepatocytes, as was found in CTR animals at the same age. We consider this defect in the livers of these mice comparable to those observed in hippocampal neurogenesis in various animal ASD models and ASD patients [2,18,26,44–47].

Our study shows that oxidative stress and inflammation are involved in ASD, showing a downregulation of CAT, SOD-1 and GPX4 expression and an upregulation of Il-1β expression. Hepatocellular ballooning and iron accumulation in hepatocytes and sinusoidal cells were found in the livers of BTBR mice but not in CTR mice. Decreased expression of antioxidant proteins has been demonstrated in patients in relationship with ASD and neurodegenerative disorders, including Alzheimer's and Parkinson's diseases. In these patients, the levels of GPX4 and other antioxidant proteins, as well as the expression of their regulatory genes, are usually in dyshomeostasis [48]. Moreover, oxidative stress has been reported in connection with decreased antioxidant enzymes, increased lipid peroxidation and advanced glycation products in peripheral blood [12,49]. In association with these phenomena, we found an accumulation of lipids and iron in the hepatic parenchyma and sinusoidal cells of BTBR mice, as detected in haematoylin-eosin and Perls stained sections, respectively.

Ferroptosis is a recently discovered iron-dependent type of cell death due to ROS accumulation with free iron deposition and lipid accumulation that results in cell death [26,50,51]. The ferroptosis pathway is triggered by the iron-catalyzed accumulation of phospholipid peroxides and reduced glutathione (GSH), which is essential to protect cells in all tissues, particularly in the liver, from ferroptosis [51,52]. We show that GPX-4 expression is remarkably reduced in the livers of BTBR mice, which can induce the ferroptosis pathway.

The transcription factor, NFR2, a master regulator of antioxidant responses and inducible cell defense systems, regulates the activity of the ferroptosis pathway and the expression of lipid peroxidation-related proteins [2,31,32,53]. NFR2 activity as a transcription factor is primarily regulated through KEAP1, which acts as a cytoplasmic anchor and promotes the degradation of NFR2 [32,35,54]. Under conditions of oxidative stress, NFR2 dissociates from KEAP1 and is then translocated into the nucleus [31,54,55]. Our results confirm these findings, showing that NFR2 expression was very strong in all nuclei of hepatocytes and sinusoidal cells, such as Kupffer cells, in BTBR mice. In contrast, CTR mice showed a lower nuclear positivity of NFR2 and a moderate/weak cytoplasmic expression. KEAP1 immunopositivity followed the expression of NFR2 in the cytoplasm of BTBR mice.

In the nucleus, NFR2 dissociated from KEAP1 affects the transcription of specific genes that contain antioxidant response elements (ARE) and cytoprotective genes. In fact, NFR2 regulates a plethora of target genes involved in the regulation of synthesis and conjugation of GSH. HO-1 and both ferritin heavy and light chains are strictly under the control of NFR2 as well [33]. To establish that NFR2 in the liver of BTBR mice induces GSH synthesis, we studied HO-1 expression; we demonstrated that it is moderately expressed in hepatocytes of the autistic mice model and very weakly expressed in CTR mouse hepatocytes.

Inhibition of ferroptosis is a challenge focused on the mitigation of ferroptosis-related diseases. Numerous ferroptosis inhibitors have been identified in recent years, showing potential for the treatment of ferroptosis through various mechanisms [35]. Recent publications showed that the supplementation of antioxidants improves symptoms of ASD related to ferroptosis in the central nervous system [1,18].

As far as we know, only a limited number of studies have considered the role of antioxidants, such as folic acid and selenium, in the brain of BTBR mice [26], but studies on the role of melatonin on the liver parenchyma in BTBR mice have not yet been published.

Therefore, we evaluated the effects of melatonin on the liver of BTBR and CTR mice. The findings suggested improved hepatic cell polyploidy, although not all differences between BTBR and CTR mice and between treatment or no treatment with melatonin were statistically significant. Moreover, markers of oxidative stress, inflammation and ferroptosis showed a clear improvement due to melatonin treatment. We hypothesize that ferroptosis can induce cell death, blocking the evolution of BD hepatocytes into MT hepatocytes.

In conclusion, our study suggests that the liver of the autistic mouse model showed morphological and biochemical alterations, including ferroptosis, as a mechanism that is not well known in hepatic disorders, such as ASD. Moreover, we suggest that melatonin has a positive effect on symptoms and hepatic organization through ferroptosis inhibitions, which may be a potential therapeutic antioxidant for autism intervention.

These initial findings were further investigated on the role of ferroptosis mechanisms in ASD.

4. Materials and Methods

4.1. Experimental Groups

A total of 20 male BTBR T + Itpr3tf/J (BTBR) mice (JAXTM Mice Strain; The Jackson Laboratory, Bar Harbor, ME, USA) as a transgenic animal model of ASD and 20 C57BL6/J (JAXTM Mice Strain; The Jackson Laboratory, Bar Harbor, ME, USA) mice as healthy CTR mice were housed in cages (two/three animals/cage), with food and water ad libitum, starting at post-natal day 21. The animals were kept in an animal house at a constant temperature of 20 °C with a 12 h alternating light–dark cycle to minimize circadian variations. Before the start of the experiment, mice were housed in the animal facility for 1 week. All efforts were made to minimize animal suffering and the number of animals used. All the experimental procedures were approved by the Italian Ministry of Health (n° 446/2018-PR - 20/06/2018) and followed the National Institutes of Health guide for the care and the use of laboratory animals (NIH Publications No. 8023, revised 1978). The animals were randomly subdivided into two subgroups: (a) 10 animals were treated with 10 mg/kg/day per os of melatonin, and (b) 10 animals were treated daily with the melatonin vehicle. The melatonin treatment followed the procedure reported by Borsani et al. [56]. Briefly, melatonin was given in a single daily administration per os through gavage (100 μL). On the last day of the chronic melatonin treatment, all the experimental animals, as reported in our previous study [56], were tested for behavioral tests (marble burying, self-grooming, and reciprocal social interaction tests), confirming that BTRB presented typical ASD behavioral manifestations, such as deficit in social interaction and stereotyped and repetitive behaviors. Five mice from each group were deeply anesthetized (isoflurane 5%) and transcardically perfused with saline, followed by 50 mL of 4% paraformaldehyde in phosphate buffer saline (0.1 M, pH 7.4). The liver of each experimental animal was carefully removed for the subsequent morphological and immunohistochemical evaluations [57,58].

4.2. Sample Processing

After removal, the liver samples were rinsed in a physiological salt solution, dehydrated in graded ethanol, and then embedded in paraffin wax following standard procedure. Serial paraffin sections (5 μm thick) of each sample were cut with a microtome.

4.3. Hepatic Morphological Evaluation

Alternate sections were deparaffinized, rehydrated and stained with haematoxylin-eosin (Bio Optica, Milan, Italy) according to the standard procedure. The sections were then observed using a light optical microscope (Olympus BX50 microscope, Hamburg, Germany). According to Guidotti et al. [44], a blind examiner identified MD, BD and MT hepatocytes using the Olympus BX50 microscope at a final magnification of 1000×. The number of all polyploid hepatocytes was evaluated in 10 random fields in each liver sample.

4.4. Perls Staining: Iron Accumulation

Alternate liver sections stained with the Perls kit (Bio Optica, Milan, Italy) were used to evaluate reactive ferric iron. According to the manufacturer's instructions, liver sections were deparaffinized, rehydrated, and then immersed for 1 h in a solution consisting of potassium ferrocyanide, acid activation buffer and distilled water. Then, the sections were washed in distilled water and stained with Mayer Emallumen for 10 min. Finally, the liver sections were dehydrated, mounted and observed with the Olympus BX50 microscope at a final magnification of 400×. The iron positivity is indicated using blue staining [59–61].

4.5. Immunohistochemical Evaluation

Alternate liver sections were deparaffinized and rehydrated, then subjected to antigen retrieval in 0.01 M sodium citrate buffer (pH 6.0) in a microwave oven for two cycles of 3 min at 600 W [62]. Then, the sections were washed in Tris-buffered saline (TBS) for 5 min and incubated in 3% hydrogen peroxide for 10 min at room temperature. To demonstrate the specificity of antibodies, we used a pre-absorption test (blocking agent): 1% bovine serum albumin in 0.05% Tween 20 for 1 h at room temperature [63]. Subsequently, liver sections were incubated for 1 h and 30 min at room temperature with the following primary antibodies: mouse monoclonal anti-SOD-1 (diluted 1:100; Santa Cruz Biotechnology, Dallas, TX, USA), rabbit polyclonal anti-CAT (diluted 1:200; Abcam, Cambridge, UK), mouse monoclonal anti-IL-1β (diluted 1:100; Santa Cruz Biotechnology, Dallas, TX, USA), mouse monoclonal anti-HO-1 (diluted 1:100; Santa Cruz Biotechnology, Dallas, TX, USA), mouse monoclonal anti-GPX4 (diluted 1:1000; Proteintech, Manchester, UK), rabbit monoclonal anti-NRF2 (diluted 1300; Proteintech, Manchester, UK) and rabbit monoclonal anti-KEAP1 (diluted 1:1000; Proteintech, Manchester, UK). Then, the samples were incubated for 1 h with specific biotinylated secondary antibodies (Vector Laboratories, Newark, CA, USA) and successively conjugated with avidin-biotin peroxidase complex (Vector Laboratories, Newark, CA, USA). The reaction products were visualized using 0.33% hydrogen peroxide and 0.05% 3,3′-diaminobenzidine tetrahydrochloride (DAB) as a chromogen (Sigma, St. Louis, MO, USA). Finally, the liver sections were counterstained with Carazzi's Emallumen (Bio Optica, Milan, Italy), dehydrated, mounted and observed with the Olympus BX50 microscope at a final magnification of 400× [64,65]. Liver sections of BTBR mice treated with melatonin were subjected to immunohistochemical analysis for the following primary antibodies: SOD-1, CAT, GPX4, NRF2 and KEAP1. Immunohistochemical negative controls were performed by omitting the primary antibody and the presence of the isotype-matched IgG.

Five sections of each sample were analyzed by a blinded examiner, and the immunostaining for each primary antibody was evaluated as integrated optical density, expressed in arbitrary units (AU), using an image analyzer [64,65]. In detail, we performed white balancing and background subtraction for all the visual fields evaluated, and then we applied a pixel quantification algorithm to calculate the positive diaminobenzidine tetrahydrocloride-stained pixels area [66,67].

4.6. Statistical Analysis

Results were expressed as the mean ± standard deviation. Data distribution and statistical significance of differences among the experimental groups were analyzed using a one-way analysis of variance (ANOVA one-way test corrected Bonferroni test), with the significance set up at $p \leq 0.05$. The data distribution was symmetrical.

Author Contributions: Conceptualization, R.R., M.G. and G.F.; methodology, M.G. and G.F.; formal analysis, M.G., D.P. and G.F.; investigation, R.R., M.G., D.P., F.R. and G.F.; data curation, M.G. and G.F.; writing—original draft preparation, R.R., F.R. and C.J.F.v.N.; writing—review and editing, R.R., M.G., D.P., F.R., C.J.F.v.N. and G.F.; supervision, R.R. and C.J.F.v.N.; funding acquisition, R.R., F.R. and C.J.F.v.N. All authors have read and agreed to the published version of the manuscript.

Funding: CJF van Noorden was supported by the Slovenian Research Agency (ARRS P1-0245 and J3-2526 research grants).

Institutional Review Board Statement: All the experimental procedures were approved by the Italian Ministry of Health (n° 446/2018-PR - 20/06/2018) and followed the National Institutes of Health guide for the care and the use of laboratory animals (NIH Publications No. 8023, revised 1978).

Informed Consent Statement: Not applicable.

Data Availability Statement: The data underlying this article will be shared upon reasonable request to the corresponding author.

Acknowledgments: The authors sincerely thank Flamma S.p.A. (Chignolo d'Isola, Bergamo, Italy) for courteously providing melatonin (Melapure^{TM}). The authors would like to thank Giuliani S.p.A. (Milan, Italy) and Flamma S.p.A. (Chignolo d'Isola, Bergamo, Italy) for the precious support to research projects of Anatomy and Physiopathology Division (University of Brescia, Italy). Moreover, the authors thank Borsani Elisa and Bonomini Francesca of the Anatomy and Physiopathology Division (University of Brescia, Italy) for the support during the initial part of the project.

Conflicts of Interest: The authors declare no conflicts of interest.

References

1. Jiang, P.; Zhou, L.; Zhao, L.; Fei, X.; Wang, Z.; Liu, T.; Tang, Y.; Li, D.; Gong, H.; Luo, Y.; et al. Puerarin attenuates valproate-induced features of ASD in male mice via regulating Slc7a11-dependent ferroptosis. *Neuropsychopharmacology* **2023**. [CrossRef] [PubMed]
2. Shan, J.; Gu, Y.; Zhang, J.; Hu, X.; Wu, H.; Yuan, T.; Zhao, D. A scoping review of physiological biomarkers in autism. *Front. Neurosci.* **2023**, *17*, 1269880. [CrossRef] [PubMed]
3. Precenzano, F.; Ruberto, M.; Parisi, L.; Salerno, M.; Maltese, A.; Verde, D.; Tripi, G.; Romano, P.; Di Folco, A.; Di Filippo, T.; et al. Sleep habits in children affected by autism spectrum disorders: A preliminary case-control study. *Acta Med. Mediter.* **2017**, *33*, 405–409. [CrossRef]
4. Sharma, A.; Mehan, S. Targeting PI3K-AKT/mTOR signaling in the prevention of autism. *Neurochem. Int.* **2021**, *147*, 105067. [CrossRef] [PubMed]
5. Nestler, E.J.; Hyman, S.E. Animal models of neuropsychiatric disorders. *Nat. Neurosci.* **2010**, *13*, 1161–1169. [CrossRef]
6. Watts, T.J. The pathogenesis of autism. *Clin. Med. Pathol.* **2008**, *1*, 99–103. [CrossRef]
7. Joon, P.; Kumar, A.; Parle, M. What is autism? *Pharmacol. Rep.* **2021**, *73*, 1255–1264. [CrossRef]
8. Trinchese, G.; Cimmino, F.; Cavaliere, G.; Catapano, A.; Fogliano, C.; Lama, A.; Pirozzi, C.; Cristiano, C.; Russo, R.; Petrella, L.; et al. The Hepatic Mitochondrial alterations exacerbate meta-inflammation in autism spectrum disorders. *Antioxidants* **2022**, *11*, 1990. [CrossRef]
9. Mirzavandi, F.; Sabet, N.; Aminzadeh, A.; Heidari, M.; Pouya, F.; Moslemizadeh, A.; Parizi, A.S.; Bashiri, H. Effects of varied-intensity endurance exercise training on oxidative and antioxidant factors in the liver of rats with valproic acid-induced autism. *Acta Neurobiol. Exp.* **2023**, *83*, 25–33. [CrossRef]
10. Singh, R.; Kisku, A.; Kungumaraj, H.; Nagaraj, V.; Pal, A.; Kumar, S.; Sulakhiya, K. Autism spectrum disorders: A recent update on targeting inflammatory pathways with natural anti-inflammatory agents. *Biomedicines* **2023**, *11*, 115. [CrossRef]

11. Messina, A.; Monda, V.; Sessa, F.; Valenzano, A.; Salerno, M.; Bitetti, I.; Precenzano, F.; Marotta, R.; Lavano, F.; Lavano, S.M.; et al. Sympathetic, metabolic adaptations, and oxidative stress in autism spectrum disorders: How far from physiology? *Front. Physiol.* **2018**, *9*, 261. [CrossRef] [PubMed]
12. Usui, N.; Kobayashi, H.; Shimada, S. Neuroinflammation and oxidative stress in the pathogenesis of autism spectrum disorder. *Int. J. Mol. Sci.* **2023**, *24*, 5487. [CrossRef]
13. Braun, J.M.; Kahn, R.S.; Froehlich, T.; Auinger, P.; Lanphear, B.P. Exposures to environmental toxicants and attention deficit hyperactivity disorder in U.S. children. *Environ. Health Perspect.* **2006**, *114*, 1904–1909. [CrossRef] [PubMed]
14. Rossignol, D.A.; Frye, R.E. A review of research trends in physiological abnormalities in autism spectrum disorders: Immune dysregulation, inflammation, oxidative stress, mitochondrial dysfunction and environmental toxicant exposures. *Mol. Psychiatry* **2012**, *17*, 389–401. [CrossRef] [PubMed]
15. Modabbernia, A.; Velthorst, E.; Reichenberg, A. Environmental risk factors for autism: An evidence-based review of systematic reviews and meta-analyses. *Mol. Autism.* **2017**, *8*, 13. [CrossRef]
16. Aschner, M.; Skalny, A.V.; Martins, A.C.; Sinitskii, A.I.; Farina, M.; Lu, R.; Barbosa, F., Jr.; Gluhcheva, Y.G.; Santamaria, A.; Tinkov, A.A. Ferroptosis as a mechanism of non-ferrous metal toxicity. *Arch. Toxicol.* **2022**, *96*, 2391–2417. [CrossRef] [PubMed]
17. Jakaria, M.; Belaidi, A.A.; Bush, A.I.; Ayton, S. Ferroptosis as a mechanism of neurodegeneration in Alzheimer's disease. *J. Neurochem.* **2021**, *159*, 804–825. [CrossRef]
18. Wu, H.; Luan, Y.; Wang, H.; Zhang, P.; Liu, S.; Wang, P.; Cao, Y.; Sun, H.; Wu, L. Selenium inhibits ferroptosis and ameliorates autistic-like behaviors of BTBR mice by regulating the Nrf2/GPx4 pathway. *Brain Res. Bull.* **2022**, *183*, 38–48. [CrossRef]
19. McFarlane, H.G.; Kusek, G.K.; Yang, M.; Phoenix, J.L.; Bolivar, V.J.; Crawley, J.N. Autism-like behavioral phenotypes in BTBR T+tf/J mice. *Genes Brain Behav.* **2008**, *7*, 152–163, Erratum in *Genes Brain Behav.* **2008**, *7*, 163. [CrossRef]
20. Cao, C.; Wang, D.; Zou, M.; Sun, C.; Wu, L. Untargeted metabolomics reveals hepatic metabolic disorder in the BTBR mouse model of autism and the significant role of liver in autism. *Cell Biochem. Funct.* **2023**, *41*, 553–563. [CrossRef]
21. Mortezaee, K.; Khanlarkhani, N. Melatonin application in targeting oxidative-induced liver injuries: A review. *J. Cell Physiol.* **2018**, *233*, 4015–4032. [CrossRef] [PubMed]
22. Rajput, S.A.; Shaukat, A.; Wu, K.; Rajput, I.R.; Baloch, D.M.; Akhtar, R.W.; Raza, M.A.; Najda, A.; Rafał, P.; Albrakati, A.; et al. Luteolin alleviates aflatoxinB1-induced apoptosis and oxidative stress in the liver of mice through activation of Nrf2 signaling pathway. *Antioxidants* **2021**, *10*, 1268. [CrossRef] [PubMed]
23. Rezzani, R.; Franco, C. Liver, oxidative stress and metabolic syndromes. *Nutrients* **2021**, *13*, 301. [CrossRef] [PubMed]
24. Shalaby, A.M.; Shalaby, R.H.; Alabiad, M.A.; Abdelrahman, D.I.; Alorini, M.; Jaber, F.A.; Hassan, S.M.A. Evening primrose oil attenuates oxidative stress, inflammation, fibrosis, apoptosis, and ultrastructural alterations induced by metanil yellow in the liver of rat: A histological, immunohistochemical, and biochemical study. *Ultrastruct. Pathol.* **2023**, *47*, 188–204. [CrossRef] [PubMed]
25. Arumugam, M.K.; Gopal, T.; Kalari Kandy, R.R.; Boopathy, L.K.; Perumal, S.K.; Ganesan, M.; Rasineni, K.; Donohue, T.M., Jr.; Osna, N.A.; Kharbanda, K.K. Mitochondrial Dysfunction-associated mechanisms in the development of chronic liver diseases. *Biology* **2023**, *12*, 1311. [CrossRef]
26. Zhang, Q.; Wu, H.; Zou, M.; Li, L.; Li, Q.; Sun, C.; Xia, W.; Cao, Y.; Wu, L. Folic acid improves abnormal behavior via mitigation of oxidative stress, inflammation, and ferroptosis in the BTBR T+ tf/J mouse model of autism. *J. Nutr. Biochem.* **2019**, *71*, 98–109. [CrossRef]
27. Granata, S.; Votrico, V.; Spadaccino, F.; Catalano, V.; Netti, G.S.; Ranieri, E.; Stallone, G.; Zaza, G. Oxidative stress and ischemia/reperfusion injury in kidney transplantation: Focus on ferroptosis, mitophagy and new antioxidants. *Antioxidants* **2022**, *11*, 769. [CrossRef]
28. Bersuker, K.; Hendricks, J.M.; Li, Z.; Magtanong, L.; Ford, B.; Tang, P.H.; Roberts, M.A.; Tong, B.; Maimone, T.J.; Zoncu, R.; et al. The CoQ oxidoreductase FSP1 acts parallel to GPX4 to inhibit ferroptosis. *Nature* **2019**, *575*, 688–692. [CrossRef]
29. Tak, J.; Kim, S.G. Effects of toxicants on endoplasmic reticulum stress and hepatic cell fate determination. *Toxicol. Res.* **2023**, *39*, 533–547. [CrossRef]
30. van Noorden, C.J.F.; Breznik, B.; Novak, M.; van Dijck, A.J.; Tanan, S.; Vittori, M.; Bogataj, U.; Bakker, N.; Khoury, J.D.; Molenaar, R.J.; et al. Cell biology meets cell metabolism: Energy production is similar in stem cells and in cancer stem cells in brain and bone marrow. *J. Histochem. Cytochem.* **2022**, *70*, 29–51. [CrossRef]
31. Dodson, M.; Castro-Portuguez, R.; Zhang, D.D. NRF2 plays a critical role in mitigating lipid peroxidation and ferroptosis. *Redox Biol.* **2019**, *23*, 101107. [CrossRef] [PubMed]
32. Sun, X.; Ou, Z.; Chen, R.; Niu, X.; Chen, D.; Kang, R.; Tang, D. Activation of the p62-Keap1-NRF2 pathway protects against ferroptosis in hepatocellular carcinoma cells. *Hepatology* **2016**, *63*, 173–184. [CrossRef] [PubMed]
33. Capelletti, M.M.; Manceau, H.; Puy, H.; Peoc'h, K. Ferroptosis in Liver Diseases: An Overview. *Int. J. Mol. Sci.* **2020**, *21*, 4908. [CrossRef] [PubMed]
34. Korczowska-Łącka, I.; Słowikowski, B.; Piekut, T.; Hurła, M.; Banaszek, N.; Szymanowicz, O.; Jagodziński, P.P.; Kozubski, W.; Permoda-Pachuta, A.; Dorszewska, J. Disorders of endogenous and exogenous antioxidants in neurological diseases. *Antioxidants* **2023**, *12*, 1811. [CrossRef] [PubMed]
35. Zhang, D.; Jia, X.; Lin, D.; Ma, J. Melatonin and ferroptosis: Mechanisms and therapeutic implications. *Biochem. Pharmacol.* **2023**, *218*, 115909. [CrossRef]

36. Reiter, R.J.; Mayo, J.C.; Tan, D.X.; Sainz, R.M.; Alatorre-Jimenez, M.; Qin, L. Melatonin as an antioxidant: Under promises but over delivers. *J. Pineal Res.* **2016**, *61*, 253–278. [CrossRef]
37. Kang, J.W.; Hong, J.M.; Lee, S.M. Melatonin enhances mitophagy and mitochondrial biogenesis in rats with carbon tetrachloride-induced liver fibrosis. *J. Pineal Res.* **2016**, *60*, 383–393. [CrossRef]
38. Zhang, J.J.; Meng, X.; Li, Y.; Zhou, Y.; Xu, D.P.; Li, S.; Li, H.B. Effects of melatonin on liver injuries and diseases. *Int. J. Mol. Sci.* **2017**, *18*, 673. [CrossRef]
39. Miao, Z.; Miao, Z.; Teng, X.; Xu, S. Melatonin alleviates lead-induced fatty liver in the common carps (*Cyprinus carpio*) via gut-liver axis. *Environ. Pollut.* **2023**, *317*, 120730. [CrossRef]
40. Gevezova, M.; Sbirkov, Y.; Sarafian, V.; Plaimas, K.; Suratanee, A.; Maes, M. Autistic spectrum disorder (ASD-Gene, molecular and pathway signatures linking systemic inflammation, mitochondrial dysfunction, transsynaptic signalling, and neurodevelopment. *Brain Behav. Immun. Health* **2023**, *30*, 100646. [CrossRef]
41. Heinke, P.; Rost, F.; Rode, J.; Trus, P.; Simonova, I.; Lázár, E.; Feddema, J.; Welsch, T.; Alkass, K.; Salehpour, M.; et al. Diploid hepatocytes drive physiological liver renewal in adult humans. *Cell Syst.* **2022**, *13*, 499–507. [CrossRef] [PubMed]
42. Huttner, H.B.; Bergmann, O.; Salehpour, M.; Rácz, A.; Tatarishvili, J.; Lindgren, E.; Csonka, T.; Csiba, L.; Hortobágyi, T.; Méhes, G.; et al. The age and genomic integrity of neurons after cortical stroke in humans. *Nat. Neurosci.* **2014**, *17*, 801–803. [CrossRef] [PubMed]
43. Bergmann, O.; Zdunek, S.; Felker, A.; Salehpour, M.; Alkass, K.; Bernard, S.; Sjostrom, S.L.; Szewczykowska, M.; Jackowska, T.; Dos Remedios, C.; et al. Dynamics of cell generation and turnover in the human heart. *Cell* **2015**, *161*, 1566–1575. [CrossRef] [PubMed]
44. Guidotti, J.E.; Brégerie, O.; Robert, A.; Debey, P.; Brechot, C.; Desdouets, C. Liver cell polyploidization: A pivotal role for binuclear hepatocytes. *J. Biol. Chem.* **2003**, *278*, 19095–19101. [CrossRef] [PubMed]
45. Wegiel, J.; Kuchna, I.; Nowicki, K.; Imaki, H.; Wegiel, J.; Marchi, E.; Ma, S.Y.; Chauhan, A.; Chauhan, V.; Bobrowicz, T.W.; et al. The neuropathology of autism: Defects of neurogenesis and neuronal migration, and dysplastic changes. *Acta Neuropathol.* **2010**, *119*, 755–770. [CrossRef]
46. Calabrese, V.; Giordano, J.; Ruggieri, M.; Berritta, D.; Trovato, A.; Ontario, M.L.; Bianchini, R.; Calabrese, E.J. Hormesis, cellular stress response, and redox homeostasis in autism spectrum disorders. *J. Neurosci. Res.* **2016**, *94*, 1488–1498. [CrossRef] [PubMed]
47. Grasselli, C.; Carbone, A.; Panelli, P.; Giambra, V.; Bossi, M.; Mazzoccoli, G.; De Filippis, L. Neural stem cells from Shank3-ko mouse model autism spectrum disorders. *Mol. Neurobiol.* **2020**, *57*, 1502–1515. [CrossRef] [PubMed]
48. Bjørklund, G.; Meguid, N.A.; El-Bana, M.A.; Tinkov, A.A.; Saad, K.; Dadar, M.; Hemimi, M.; Skalny, A.V.; Hosnedlová, B.; Kizek, R.; et al. Oxidative stress in autism spectrum disorder. *Mol. Neurobiol.* **2020**, *57*, 2314–2332. [CrossRef]
49. Chauhan, A.; Chauhan, V.; Brown, W.T.; Cohen, I. Oxidative stress in autism: Increased lipid peroxidation and reduced serum levels of ceruloplasmin and transferrin--the antioxidant proteins. *Life Sci.* **2004**, *75*, 2539–2549. [CrossRef]
50. Stockwell, B.R.; Friedmann Angeli, J.P.; Bayir, H.; Bush, A.I.; Conrad, M.; Dixon, S.J.; Fulda, S.; Gascón, S.; Hatzios, S.K.; Kagan, V.E.; et al. Ferroptosis: A regulated cell death nexus linking metabolism, redox biology, and disease. *Cell* **2017**, *171*, 273–285. [CrossRef]
51. Cui, S.; Ghai, A.; Deng, Y.; Li, S.; Zhang, R.; Egbulefu, C.; Liang, G.; Achilefu, S.; Ye, J. Identification of hyperoxidized PRDX3 as a ferroptosis marker reveals ferroptotic damage in chronic liver diseases. *Mol. Cell* **2023**, *83*, 3931–3939.e5. [CrossRef] [PubMed]
52. Jiang, X.; Stockwell, B.R.; Conrad, M. Ferroptosis: Mechanisms, biology and role in disease. *Nat. Rev. Mol. Cell Biol.* **2021**, *22*, 266–282. [CrossRef] [PubMed]
53. Suzuki, T.; Motohashi, H.; Yamamoto, M. Toward clinical application of the Keap1-Nrf2 pathway. *Trends Pharmacol. Sci.* **2013**, *34*, 340–346. [CrossRef] [PubMed]
54. Yang, J.; Fu, X.; Liao, X.; Li, Y. Nrf2 activators as dietary phytochemicals against oxidative stress, inflammation, and mitochondrial dysfunction in autism spectrum disorders: A systematic review. *Front. Psychiatry* **2020**, *11*, 561998. [CrossRef]
55. Silva-Islas, C.A.; Maldonado, P.D. Canonical and non-canonical mechanisms of Nrf2 activation. *Pharmacol. Res.* **2018**, *134*, 92–99. [CrossRef]
56. Borsani, E.; Bonomini, F.; Bonini, S.A.; Premoli, M.; Maccarinelli, G.; Giugno, L.; Mastinu, A.; Aria, F.; Memo, M.; Rezzani, R. Role of melatonin in autism spectrum disorders in a male murine transgenic model: Study in the prefrontal cortex. *J. Neurosci. Res.* **2022**, *100*, 780–797. [CrossRef]
57. Franco, C.; Bonomini, F.; Borsani, E.; Castrezzati, S.; Franceschetti, L.; Rezzani, R. Involvement of intestinal goblet cells and changes in sodium glucose transporters expression: Possible therapeutic targets in autistic BTBR T+Itpr3tf/J mice. *Int. J. Environ. Res. Public Health* **2021**, *18*, 11328. [CrossRef]
58. Rezzani, R.; Franco, C.; Favero, G.; Rodella, L.F. Ghrelin-mediated pathway in Apolipoprotein-E deficient mice: A survival system. *Am. J. Transl. Res.* **2019**, *11*, 4263–4276.
59. Perls, M. Nachweis von Eisenoxyd in geweissen Pigmentation. In *Virchows Archiv für Pathologische Anatomie und Physiologie und für Klinische Medizin*; Springer Publishing: New York, NY, USA, 1867; Volume 39, p. 42.
60. Bancroft, G.J.; Gamble, M. *Theory and Practices of Histological Techniques*; Churchill Livingstone Elsevier: Philadelphia, PA, USA, 2008.
61. Alwahaibi, N.Y.; Alkhatri, A.S.; Kumar, J.S. Hematoxylin and eosin stain shows a high sensitivity but sub-optimal specificity in demonstrating iron pigment in liver biopsies. *Int. J. Appl. Basic Med. Res.* **2015**, *5*, 169–171. [CrossRef]

62. Rezzani, R.; Rodella, L.F.; Bonomini, F.; Tengattini, S.; Bianchi, R.; Reiter, R.J. Beneficial effects of melatonin in protecting against cyclosporine A-induced cardiotoxicity are receptor mediated. *J. Pineal Res.* **2006**, *41*, 288–295. [CrossRef]
63. Franco, C.; Gianò, M.; Favero, G.; Rezzani, R. Impairment in the intestinal morphology and in the immunopositivity of toll-like receptor-4 and other proteins in an autistic mouse model. *Int. J. Mol. Sci.* **2022**, *23*, 8731. [CrossRef] [PubMed]
64. Bonomini, F.; Favero, G.; Rodella, L.F.; Moghadasian, M.H.; Rezzani, R. Melatonin modulation of sirtuin-1 attenuates liver injury in a hypercholesterolemic mouse model. *BioMed Res. Int.* **2018**, *2018*, 7968452. [CrossRef] [PubMed]
65. Stacchiotti, A.; Favero, G.; Lavazza, A.; Golic, I.; Aleksic, M.; Korac, A.; Rodella, L.F.; Rezzani, R. Hepatic macrosteatosis is partially converted to microsteatosis by melatonin supplementation in ob/ob mice non-alcoholic fatty liver disease. *PLoS ONE* **2016**, *11*, e0148115. [CrossRef] [PubMed]
66. Chieco, P.; Jonker, A.; De Boer, B.A.; Ruijter, J.M.; Van Noorden, C.J. Image cytometry: Protocols for 2D and 3D quantification in microscopic images. *Prog. Histochem. Cytochem.* **2013**, *47*, 211–333. [CrossRef]
67. Wiseman, E.J.; Moss, J.I.; Atkinson, J.; Baakza, H.; Hayes, E.; Willis, S.E.; Waring, P.M.; Rodriguez Canales, J.; Jones, G.N. Epitope lability of phosphorylated biomarkers of the DNA Damage response pathway results in increased vulnerability to effects of delayed or incomplete formalin fixation. *J. Histochem. Cytochem.* **2023**, *71*, 237–257. [CrossRef]

International Journal of
Molecular Sciences

MDPI

Article

Comparative Analysis of Anticonvulsant Activity of *Trans* and *Cis* 5,5′-Diphenylhydantoin Schiff Bases

Jana Tchekalarova [1,*], Petar Todorov [2], Tsveta Stoyanova [1] and Milena Atanasova [3]

1 Institute of Neurobiology, Bulgarian Academy of Sciences, 1113 Sofia, Bulgaria; tzafti@abv.bg
2 Department of Organic Chemistry, University of Chemical Technology and Metallurgy, 1756 Sofia, Bulgaria; pepi_37@abv.bg
3 Department of Biology, Medical University of Pleven, 5800 Pleven, Bulgaria; milenaar2001@yahoo.com
* Correspondence: janetchekalarova@gmail.com or jt.chekalarova@inb.bas.bg; Tel.: +359-887267052

Abstract: Recently, the four 5,5′-diphenylhydantoin Schiff bases, possessing different aromatic species (**SB1-Ph, SB2-Ph, SB3-Ph and SB4-Ph**) were synthesized, characterized, and evaluated for anticonvulsant activity in combination with phenytoin. In the present study, the **SB1-Ph** and **SB4-Ph** compounds were selected, based on their anticonvulsant potency, and compared with their *cis* isomers, prepared after a one-hour exposure to the UV source, for their anticonvulsant potency in the maximal electroshock (MES) test and the kainate (KA)-induced status epilepticus (SE) test in mice. In the MES test, the *cis* **SB1-Ph** compound exhibited superior to phenytoin and *trans* isomer activity in the three tested doses, while the *cis* **SB4-Ph** compound entirely suppressed the electroshock-induced seizure spread at the highest dose of 40 mg/kg. Pretreatment with the *cis* **SB1-Ph** compound and the *cis* **SB4-Ph** at the doses of 40 mg/kg, respectively, for seven days, significantly attenuated the severity of KA SE compared to the matched control group pretreated with a vehicle, while phenytoin was ineffective in this test. The *cis* **SB4-Ph** but not the *cis* **SB1-Ph** demonstrated an antioxidant effect against the KA-induced SE in the hippocampus. Our results suggest that *trans–cis* conversion of 5,5′-diphenylhydantoin Schiff bases has potential against seizure spread in the MES test and mitigated the KA-induced SE. The antioxidant potency of *cis* **SB4-Ph** might be associated with its efficacy in mitigating the SE.

Keywords: 5,5′-diphenylhydantoin Schiff bases; *trans–cis*; MES; KA SE; mice

1. Introduction

Epilepsy is a chronic neurological disorder that affects approximately 1% of people worldwide [1]. Spontaneous recurrent seizures represent the main symptom of this disease. Pharmacotherapy with anticonvulsants is the method of choice for epileptic patients. Although there is extensive funding for developing antiepileptic drugs (ASMs), about 30% of patients are resistant to treatment [2]. The first generations of ASMs were characterized by severe side effects, whereas new-generation ASMs have an advantage with good tolerability and low capacity for drug interaction [3].

The first-line ASM phenytoin effectively blocks partial and tonic-clonic seizures [4]. However, this ASM has low solubility and side effects during treatments. Heterocyclic systems and their Schiff bases are an essential class of compounds that have piqued the interest of researchers due to their varied range of biological functions, including anti-inflammatory, anticonvulsant, analgesic, antimicrobial, anticancer, antioxidant, anthelmintic, and antidepressant activities [5–7]. Schiff bases, a universal pharmacophore, are studied in screening investigations [8]. These compounds have an imine or azomethine (-C=N-) functional group. They are condensation products of primary amines with carbonyl compounds, which are gaining importance in medicine and pharmacy due to their ease of synthesis and isolation. A heterocyclic system, such as phenytoin, combined with an azomethine functional group would have a synergistic effect and increase biological activity. Schiff bases tend to isomerize due to the imine group (-C=N-) giving two stereoisomers *cis* and *trans* (E and Z) isomers, and the formation of these stereoisomers can be controlled kinetically or thermodynamically. These compounds have the potential to be photosensitive, undergoing rapid reverse photoisomerization from the more stable *trans* isomer to the less stable *cis* isomer. They can employ this characteristic to control, functionalize, and alter numerous biological functions. As a result, as the Schiff bases' molecular arrangement changes, the compounds' bioactivity also changes [9].

Recently, the four 5,5′-diphenylhydantoin Schiff bases, containing aromatic species (**SB1-Ph, SB2-Ph, SB3-Ph and SB4-Ph**), were synthesized and their structure–property characterization was carried out by X-ray, optical, and electrochemical methods [10]. Furthermore, the four 3-amino-phenytoin Schiff base derivatives were explored alone and in combination with phenytoin against maximal electroshock (MES)-induced seizure spread in mice [11]. Taking into consideration the potential anticonvulsant properties of 3-amino-phenytoin Schiff base derivatives, in the present study, we aimed to compare the anticonvulsant activity of *trans* and *cis* 5,5′-diphenylhydantoin Schiff bases **SB1-Ph** and **SB4-Ph** against the MES-induced seizure spread. Furthermore, the potency to mitigate status epilepticus (SE) induced by kainic acid (KA) and oxidative stress in the hippocampus was evaluated after sub-chronic pretreatment with the more potent *cis* isomers of Schiff bases at the dose of 40 mg/kg, that was effective against tonic-clonic seizures in the MES test.

2. Results

2.1. Grip Strength and Rotarod

No significant effect on the neuromuscular tone, measured in the grip strength apparatus was detected for both the *trans*- and the *cis*-forms of the two Schiff bases (**SB1-Ph** and **SB4-Ph**), administered at doses of 10, 20 or 40 mg/kg [One-way ANOVA: $F(2,23) = 0.543$; $p = 0.621$—*trans* **SB1-Ph**; $F(2,23) = 0.893$; $p = 0.462$—*cis* **SB1-Ph**; $F(2,23) = 1.641$; $p = 0.092$—*trans* **SB4-Ph** $F(2,23) = 1.307$; $p = 0.312$—*cis* **SB4-Ph**] (Table 1). In addition, the tested Schiff bases in *trans*- and *cis*-form, respectively, did not affect the motor coordination of mice, when tested in the three doses mentioned above, suggesting a lack of myorelaxant activity.

Table 1. Effects of *trans* and *cis* 5,5′-diphenylhydantoin Schiff bases—**SB1-Ph** and **SB4-Ph** on neuromuscular tone in the grip strength test and motor coordination in the rotarod test in mice.

Group/Treatment	Dose (mg/kg). i.p.	Neuromuscular Strength (N)	Rotarod Test N/F
Control (saline)	0	2.08 ± 0.48	0/8
trans SB2-Ph	10	1.56 ± 0.28	1/6
	20	1.62 ± 0.39	2/6
	40	1.74 ± 0.29	2/6
cis SB2-Ph	10	2.17 ± 0.36	1/6
	20	1.41 ± 0.21	1/6
	40	1.84 ± 0.36	1/6
trans SB4-Ph	10	2.0 ± 0.41	0/6
	20	1.94 ± 0.4	1/6
	40	1.93 ± 0.32	3/6
cis SB4-Ph	10	2.52 ± 0.14	1/6
	20	1.75 ± 0.35	1/6
	40	2.01 ± 0.13	1/6

Data are presented as mean muscle strength (in Newtons ± S.D. of 3 determinations) in mice subjected to the grip strength test. The Schiff bases were injected i.p. 0.5 h before the tests at different doses (10, 20 and 40 mg/kg) as shown above. One-way ANOVA was used for the grip strength test and Fisher's exact test for statistical analysis of the rotarod test.

2.2. Maximal Electroshock Test

In the MES test, the *cis*-form of **SB1-Ph** but not the *trans* isomer showed protection against the MES-induced hindlimb tonic phase at the three tested doses (10, 20 and 40 mg/kg) (Fisher exact test: $p = 0.003$ compared to the control group) (Figure 1). This effect was comparable to that of the positive control phenytoin ($p = 0.015$ compared to control group). Similarly, the *cis*- but not the *trans*-form of **SB4-Ph** compound exhibited potency to suppress the MES-induced seizure spread (Fisher exact test: $p = 0.003$ **SB4-Ph**, 10 and 20 mg/kg compared to the control group). Notably, the *cis* isomer of **SB4-Ph** demonstrated 100% protection against tonic seizures at the highest dose of 40 mg/kg ($p < 0.001$, 40 mg/kg compared to the control group). No mortality of the *cis*-forms was observed except for **SB4-Ph** at a dose of 20 mg/kg with 16% mortality rate compared to the controls with 87% and 33% mortality rate for most of the *trans* isomers.

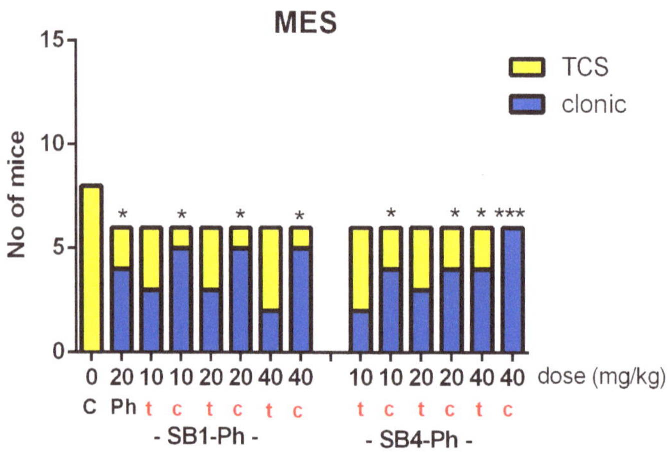

Figure 1. Effect of vehicle (C), phenytoin (Ph) (20 mg/kg), *trans*(t)-form **SB1-Ph** (10, 20 and 40 mg/kg), *cis*(c)-form **SB1-Ph** (10, 20 and 40 mg/kg), *trans*(t)-form **SB4-Ph** (10, 20 and 40 mg/kg), *cis*(c)-form **SB4-Ph** (10, 20, and 40 mg/kg) on seizure activity (tonic-clonic seizures, TCS, and clonic seizures) in mice, injected intraperitoneally (i.p.) 30 min before MES test. $n = 6$–8/group. $p = 0.015$ phenytoin compared to the control group; * $p = 0.003$ *cis*-form **SB1-Ph** (10, 20, 40 mg/kg) and **SB4-Ph** (10 and 20 mg/kg) compared to the controls; *** $p < 0.001$ **SB4-Ph** (40 mg/kg) compared to the controls.

2.3. Kainate-Induced Status Epilepticus

The mice from all groups were pretreated with the positive control phenytoin (Ph group, 20 mg/kg), *cis*-forms of **SB1-Ph** and **SB4-Ph**, respectively (40 mg/kg), i.p. for seven days to assess the efficacy of *cis* isomers of novel phenytoin-related Schiff bases to mitigate seizure intensity during the KA-induced SE as well as its consequences on oxidative stress in the hippocampus. The matched control group was pretreated with a vehicle for a week in the same manner before the KA test. One hour (Ph group) or thirty minutes after the last injection the convulsant KA was i.p. applied at a dose of 30 mg/kg. The intensity of seizures was scored each hour up to 200 min. During the first 20 min of observation, the KA injection induced mild seizure behavior consisting mainly of facial automatisms and head nodding. Furthermore, at about 40th minutes, the seizure intensity progressed to forelimb clonus and rearing with occasional loss of posture (score 3–4). That behavioral reaction was sustainable until 140 min and faded out gradually till 200 min of observation in the control group (Figure 2A). No significant difference in each time interval as well as total seizure intensity was detected between the Ph group and the veh group (Figure 2A,B). Significantly lower seizure scores were demonstrated in the *cis*-form of the **SB1-Ph** compound in the

80th ($p < 0.05$), 120th ($p < 0.001$), 140th ($p < 0.001$) and 160th min ($p < 0.001$), respectively, compared to veh group (Figure 2A). The *cis*-form of **SB4-Ph** compound alleviated SE at the 140th ($p < 0.001$) and 160th minute ($p < 0.01$), respectively, compared to the veh group.

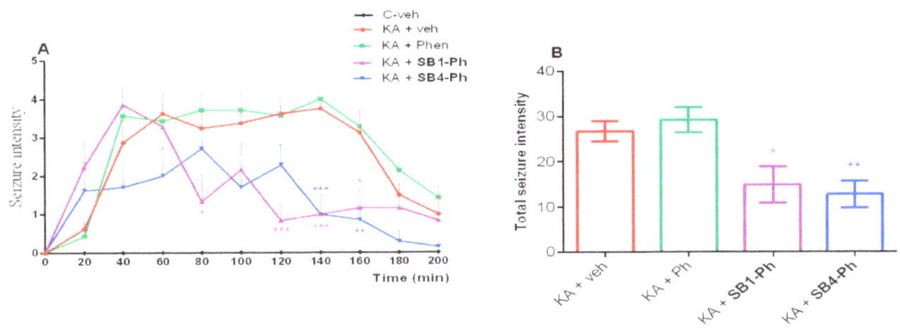

Figure 2. Effect of vehicle (C-veh), kainate (KA) + veh, phenytoin (KA + Ph) (20 mg/kg), *cis*-form **SB1-Ph** (40 mg/kg) and *cis*-form **SB4-Ph** (40 mg/kg) on seizure activity detected for 200 min (**A**) and total seizure intensity (only for KA-treated groups) (**B**) in mice, pretreated i.p. for 7 days with vehicle, phenytoin (20 mg/kg), *cis*-form of **SB1-Ph** (40 mg/kg), and *cis*-form of **SB4-Ph** (40 mg/kg), before the KA injection (30 mg/kg, i.p.). $n = 8$/group. * $p < 0.05$, ** $p < 0.01$, *** $p < 0.001$ compared to KA + veh group.

2.4. Effects of Cis Isomers of SB1-Ph and SB4-Ph Derivates on the KA-Induced Oxidative Stress

The antioxidant capacity of the two *cis* isomers of SB1-Ph and SB4-Ph was assessed by measurement of the level of total glutathione (GSH) and lipid peroxidation in the hippocampus after the KA-induced SE in mice. A significant decrease in the total GSH was detected in the KA-veh group compared to the controls ($p < 0.001$) (Figure 3A). The *cis* isomer of SB4-Ph significantly elevated the level of endogenous antioxidant in the homogenate ($p < 0.001$ compared to the KA + veh group). The antioxidant activity of this derivate was comparable to the effect of phenytoin ($p < 0.001$ compared to the KA-veh group), while the *cis* isomer of SB1-Ph was ineffective ($p > 0.05$).

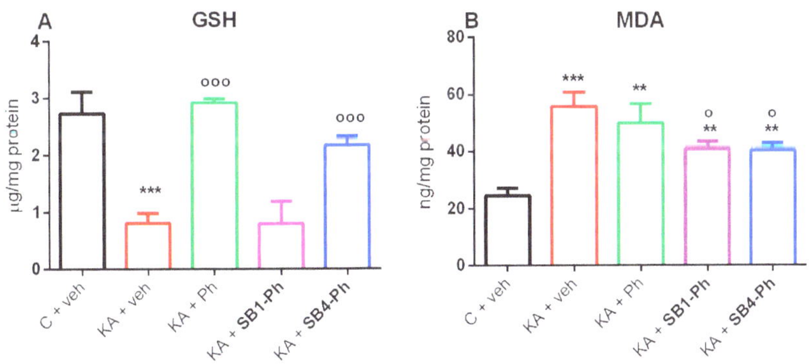

Figure 3. Effect of vehicle (C-veh), kainate (KA) + veh, phenytoin (KA + Ph) (20 mg/kg), *cis*-form SB1-Ph (40 mg/kg) and *cis*-form SB4-Ph (40 mg/kg) on total GSH level (**A**) and MDA (**B**) in the hippocampus of mice. $n = 8$/group. ** $p < 0.01$; *** $p < 0.001$ compared to the veh group; ^{o} $p < 0.05$; ^{ooo} $p < 0.001$ compared to the KA + veh group.

Furthermore, the KA + veh group showed elevated malondialdehyde (MDA) level in the hippocampus ($p < 0.001$ compared to C-veh group) suggesting an enhanced lipid peroxidation as a result of SE (Figure 3B). Neither the phenytoin nor the two *cis* isomers of the new Schiff bases succeeded to suppress the KA-induced lipid peroxidation in the hippocampus though the two phenytoin analogs partly mitigated this process ($p < 0.01$ compared to KA + veh group).

3. Discussion

Our findings revealed that the *trans/cis* conversion of 5,5′-diphenylhydantoin Schiff bases has protective activity against seizure spread in the MES test and mitigated the KA-induced SE. The antioxidant potency of *cis* **SB4-Ph** might be associated with its efficacy in reducing the severity of SE.

Two new 3-amino-5,5′-diphenylhydantoin Schiff Bases (**SB1-Ph** and **SB4-Ph**) were synthesized as described in detail in [10]. The compounds **SB1-Ph**, and **SB4-Ph** were synthesized by a condensation reaction in absolute methanol between 3-amino-5,5′-diphenylimidazolidine-2,4-dione (1) and the corresponding aromatic aldehyde: thiophene-2-carbaldehyde (2) or pyridine-2-carbaldehyde (3) in a 1:1 molar ratio in the presence of catalytic quantities of glacial acetic acid (Scheme 1). Heterocycles thienyl, respectively pyridyl moiety in the **SB1-Ph** and **SB4-Ph** give the electron-donating properties of the molecules.

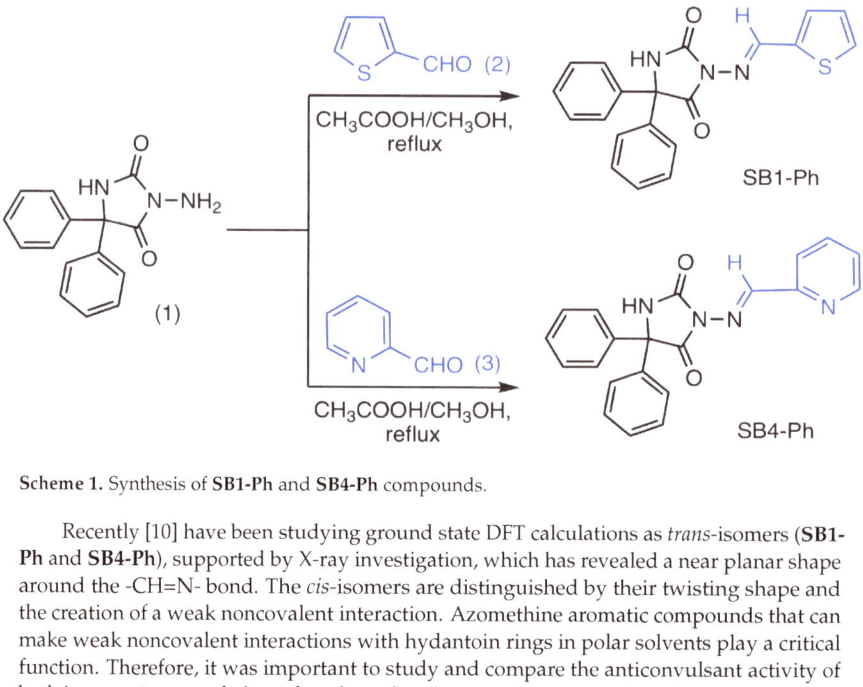

Scheme 1. Synthesis of **SB1-Ph** and **SB4-Ph** compounds.

Recently [10] have been studying ground state DFT calculations as *trans*-isomers (**SB1-Ph** and **SB4-Ph**), supported by X-ray investigation, which has revealed a near planar shape around the -CH=N- bond. The *cis*-isomers are distinguished by their twisting shape and the creation of a weak noncovalent interaction. Azomethine aromatic compounds that can make weak noncovalent interactions with hydantoin rings in polar solvents play a critical function. Therefore, it was important to study and compare the anticonvulsant activity of both isomers *trans*- and *cis*- and to show that the stereoisomeric and conformation states of the molecules play an important role and possess different activity.

We found that compared to the *trans* isomers, the *cis* isomers of the two phenytoin Schiff Bases **SB1-Ph** and **SB4-Ph** exerted higher potency to suppress seizure spread in the MES test, which is consistent with earlier bioactivity investigations [11–14]. Furthermore, unlike phenytoin, the sub-chronic pretreatment with the two *cis* isomers of these Schiff Bases mitigated the severity of the KA-induced SE in mice. The detected potency of the *cis*-form of the **SB4-Ph** analog to elevate the total level of GSH and partly to reduce the lipid peroxidation in the hippocampus, suggest that the potency of this drug to minimize seizure severity during SE is closely related to its antioxidant activity in the hippocampus. However, the seizure-suppressing effect of **SB1-Ph** analog during SE was not accompanied by mitigation of oxidative stress, suggesting a difference from the **SB1-Ph** mechanism of its anticonvulsant effect.

Azomethine aromatic compounds SB1-Ph and SB4-Ph have a donor thiophene/pyridine ring that can give favorable lipophylic interactions with the corresponding receptors. **SB1-Ph** contains the large S atom's sterical hindrance in the molecule's variable ring part, as opposed to **SB4-Ph** which contains an N atom. The enhanced biological activity of the *cis*-form in comparison to the *trans*-form, on the other hand, may also be due to the better conformational states and matches with the target receptors. We hypothesize that the underlying mechanism of the anticonvulsant activity of the two 5,5′-diphenylhydantoin Schiff bases, which are structurally similar to phenytoin, is different [11]. The two heterocyclic substituents, in particular, can be the molecule's key pharmacophore.

4. Materials and Methods

4.1. Chemicals and Instrumentation

Each one of the chemicals and solvents was analytical or HPLC quality, bought from Fluka or Merck, and utilized unpurified. The 3-amino-phenytoin Schiff base derivatives: 5,5-diphenyl-3-((thiophen-2-ylmethylene)amino)-imidazolidine-2,4-dione (SB1-Ph), and 5,5-diphenyl-3-((pyridin-2-ylmethylene)amino)imidazolidine-2,4-dione (SB4-Ph) have been prepared by our recently described procedure [10]. The physicochemical and analytical data of the compounds were identical to those previously described. The *trans/cis* isomerization upon long wavelength UV light at 365 nm and *cis/trans* relaxation at room temperature is demonstrated in Figure 4.

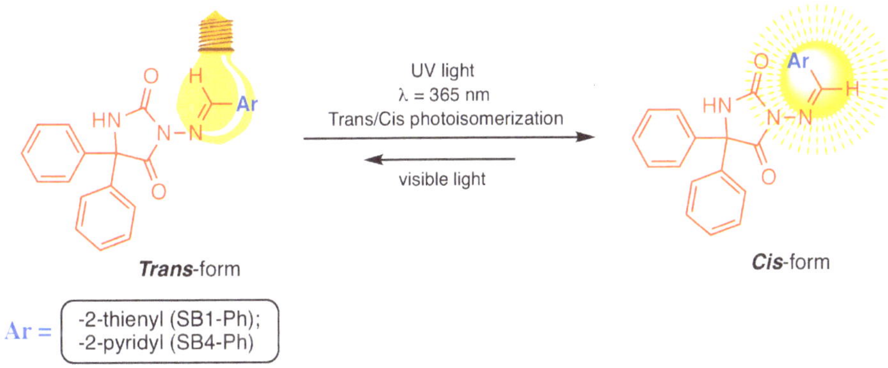

Figure 4. Photochemical conversion of 3-amino-phenytoin Schiff bases: SB1-Ph and SB4 Ph under UV illumination at λ = 365 nm in DMSO.

4.2. Experimental Rodents

Male albino ICR mice (23–26 g), delivered by the vivarium of the Institute of Neurobiology-BAS, were left undisturbed for seven days before experimental procedures. The rodents were kept in transparent cages (10 in groups), with standard pellets and tap water ad libitum and in an artificial light–dark cycle regime (12:12; light on at 07:00 a.m.), T° = 21 ± 1 °C and humidity: 40 ± 5%). The experiments were conducted in the morning (10:00–11:00 p.m.). All performed manipulations were consistent with the Declaration of Helsinki Guiding Principles on Care and Use of Animals (DHEW Publication, NHI 80–23) and with EC Directive 2010/63/EU for animal experiments. The experimental procedures were approved by the Bulgarian Food Safety Agency (License No: 354/2023).

4.3. Experimental Design

A description of experimental groups and consequent procedural steps is described Figure 5. In short, the mice were allocated to two main experimental protocols. In Experiment#1, sixteen groups were used as follows: C group (control group, injected with a vehicle) (n = 16); Ph group (positive control, injected with phenytoin in 20 mg/kg) (n = 12); three groups, injected with *trans*-form of SB1-Ph in doses of 10, 20 and 40 mg/kg, respectively) (12 × 3); three groups, injected with *cis*-form of SB1-Ph in doses of 10, 20 and 40 mg/kg, respectively) (12 × 3); three groups, injected with *trans*-form of SB4-Ph in doses of 10, 20 and 40 mg/kg, respectively) (12 × 3); three groups, injected with *cis*-form of SB4-Ph in doses of 10, 20 and 40 mg/kg, respectively) (12 × 3). In Experiment#2, five groups were used as follows: C-veh group (control group, treated with a vehicle for 7 days) (n = 8); KA + Ph group (positive control, treated with phenytoin at a dose of 20 mg/kg for 7 days) (n = 8); KA + SB1-Ph groups (experimental group treated with *cis*-form of SB1-Ph at a dose of 40 mg/kg) (8); KA + SB4-Ph groups (experimental group treated with *cis*-form of SB4-Ph at a dose of 40 mg/kg) (8).

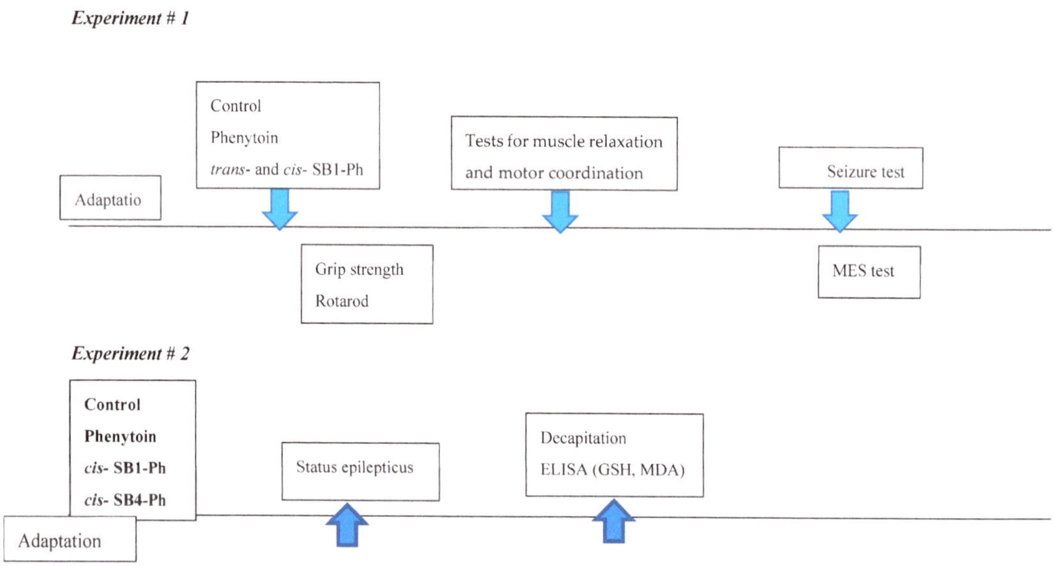

Figure 5. A schematic illustration of Experiment#1 and Experiment#2.

4.4. Drugs and Treatment

The 3-amino-phenytoin Schiff bases: (E)-5,5-diphenyl-3-((thiophen-2-ylmethylene)amino)-imidazolidine-2,4-dione (SB1-Ph) and (E)-5,5-diphenyl-3-((pyridin-2-ylmethylene)amino) imidazolidine-2,4-dione (SB4-Ph) have been prepared as described in our previous study [10]. Their *cis* isomers were freshly prepared before each experiment after UV irradiation exposure at λ = 365 nm to the probe *trans* isomers for 60 min. The compounds and the positive control phenytoin were dissolved in 1% DMSO before each test. Phenytoin was applied intraperitoneally (i.p.) an hour before the grip strength, rotarod, and MES at 30 mg/kg. The two Schiff bases were administered in three doses of 10, 20 and 40 mg/kg 0.5 h before the grip strength, rotarod and MES. The effective dose against tonic-clonic seizures of 40 mg/kg was applied in a sub-chronic regime of 7 days before KA (30 mg/kg., i.p.)-induced SE. The convulsant was administered 0.5 h after the last drug/vehicle injection.

4.5. Rotarod Test

The motor coordination was assessed as previously described [12]. The inability to keep position on a rotating rod (3.2 cm in diameter, at a speed of 10 rpm) for at least of one minute out of three trials was accepted as a criterion for neurotoxicity (>half of mice per group with lost balance).

4.6. Muscle Strength

The grip strength device, attached to the dynamometer (BIOSEB, Chaville, France), was used to determine the muscle strength of each mouse. The animal was pulled backward by the tail after a tough grasp of the steel wire grid (8 cm × 8 cm) via forepaws. The average grasping force, expressed in N (newtons) ± S.E.M., of three trials was assessed for every animal.

4.7. Anticonvulsant Activity

4.7.1. Maximal Electroshock (MES) Test

Corneal electroshock (50 mA, 60 Hz, 0.2 s) via electrodes (Constant Current Shock Generator) was applied to mice in the control group (C), phenytoin group (Ph), three SB1-Ph-treated with *trans* isomer groups as follows: injected with 10 mg/kg (SB1-Ph 10), (SB1-Ph 20) and (SB1-Ph 40), three SB1-Ph-treated with *cis* isomer groups as follows: injected with 10 mg/kg (SB1-Ph 10), (SB1-Ph 20) and (SB1-Ph 40), three SB4-Ph-treated with *trans* isomer groups as follows: injected with 10 mg/kg (SB4-Ph 10), (SB4-Ph 20) and (SB4-Ph 40) and three SB4-Ph-treated with *cis* isomer groups as follows: injected with 10 mg/kg (SB4-Ph 10), (SB4-Ph 20) and (SB4-Ph 40), respectively. Each group consisted of 6–7 mice. The controls exhibited tonic-clonic seizures with 100% of the hind limb tonic extensor component. The lack of an extensor component (forelimb tonic or only clonic seizures) was accepted as an anticonvulsant activity of the treatment.

4.7.2. Kainate-Induced Status Epilepticus

The mice were assigned in groups of 8 mice. On the day of the 7th i.p. injection of the drug/vehicle, each animal was i.p. administered by 30 m/kg KA (FOT, Bulgaria). The convulsant was dissolved in saline (10 mL/kg of body weight). The observation of seizure onset and its intensity was scored according to the scale [15] as follows: stage 1 (facial clonus), stage 2 (nodding), stage 3 (forelimb clonus), stage 4 (forelimb clonus with rearing), and stage 5 (rearing and lost posture). The SE was characterized by continuous clonic seizures of stage 4 or 5. The seizures of the highest score detected during every 20 min up to 200 min were evaluated. Immediately after a 3 h period of observation, the mice were decapitated, brains were dissected rapidly on ice and the two hippocampi were isolated, quickly frozen in liquid nitrogen and stored at −20 °C until ELISA analysis.

4.8. Measurement of Glutathione (GSH) and Malondialdehyde (MDA) in the Hippocampus

The isolated hippocampi were kept on ice, weighed, and preserved at 20 °C until homogenization in cold PBS buffer (pH 7.4) containing 1 mM EGTA, 50 mM NaF, 1 mM 270 EDTA and 1 mM PMSF. After centrifugation of the tissue homogenate at 5000× *g*, 4 °C for 271 10 min, GSH and MDA were measured in duplicates using an ELISA kit (Elabscience cat. 272 No E-EL-0060 and E-EL-0026) according to the manufacturer's instructions. The results (273) were expressed in µg/mg protein (GSH) and ng/mg protein (MDA).

4.9. Data Analysis

The data are expressed as means ± SEM. The results from the MES test and rotarod test 315 were analyzed by Fisher's exact test. Data from the grip strength test, KA test and bio-316 chemistry were assessed by the one-way analysis of variance (ANOVA) followed by the 317 post hoc Bonferroni's test. $p < 0.05$ was considered statistically significant.

5. Conclusions

In conclusion, the *cis* isomers of 3-amino-5,5′-diphenylhydantoin Schiff Bases (SB1-Ph and SB4-Ph) exhibited higher potency than their *trans*-forms to suppress seizure spread and tonic seizures in mice. The anticonvulsant activity of the *cis* isomer SB4-Ph against the neurotoxin KA might be associated with the antioxidant potency in the hippocampus during SE.

Author Contributions: Conceptualization, J.T.; methodology, J.T. and P.T.; formal analysis, J.T., M.A. and T.S.; resources, J.T. and P.T.; data curation, J.T. and P.T.; writing—original draft preparation, J.T.; writing—review and editing, J.T. and P.T.; project administration, J.T. and P.T.; funding acquisition, J.T. and P.T. All authors have read and agreed to the published version of the manuscript.

Funding: This study is funded by the European Union-NextGeneration EU, through the National Recovery and Resilience Plan of the Republic of Bulgaria, project No. BG-RRP-2.004-0002, "BiOrgaMCT".

Institutional Review Board Statement: The procedures with animals were executed according to the Declaration of Helsinki Guiding Principles on Care and Use of Animals (DHEW Publication, NHI 80-23) and the European Communities Council Directives of 24 November 1986 (86/609/EEC). The project was approved by the Bulgarian Food Safety Agency (License No: 354).

Informed Consent Statement: Not applicable.

Data Availability Statement: Data are contained within the article.

Conflicts of Interest: The authors declare no conflict of interest.

References

1. McNamara, J.O. Emerging insights into the genesis of epilepsy. *Nature* **1999**, *399*, 15–22. [CrossRef] [PubMed]
2. Fattorusso, A.; Matricardi, S.; Mencaroni, E.; Dell'Isola, G.B.; Di Cara, G.; Striano, P.; Verrotti, A. The Pharmacoresistant Epilepsy: An Overview on Existant and New Emerging Therapies. *Front. Neurol.* **2021**, *12*, 674483. [CrossRef] [PubMed]
3. Perucca, P.; Gilliam, F.G. Adverse effects of antiepileptic drugs. *Lancet Neurol.* **2012**, *11*, 792–802. [CrossRef] [PubMed]
4. Browne, T.R.; Holmes, G.L. Epilepsy. *N. Engl. J. Med.* **2001**, *344*, 1145–1151. [CrossRef] [PubMed]
5. Wadher, S.J.; Puranik, M.P.; Karande, N.A.; Yeole, P.G. Synthesis and Biological Evaluation of Schiff Base of Dapsone and Their Derivative as Antimicrobial Agents. *Int. J. PharmTech Res.* **2009**, *1*, 22–23.
6. Cates, L.A.; Rasheed, M.S. Phosphorus GABA Analogues as Potential Prodrugs. *Pharm. Res.* **1984**, *1*, 271–273. [CrossRef] [PubMed]
7. Paneersalvam, P.; Raj, T.; Ishar, M.P.; Singh, B.; Sharma, V.; Rather, B.A. Anticonvulsant Activity of Schiff Bases of 3-Amino-6,8-dibromo-2-phenyl-quinazolin-4(3H)-ones. *Indian J. Pharm. Sci.* **2010**, *72*, 375–378. [CrossRef] [PubMed]
8. Kajal, A.; Bala, S.; Kamboj, S.; Sharma, N.; Saini, V. Schiff Bases: A Versatile Pharmacophore. *J. Catal.* **2013**, *14*, 893512. [CrossRef]
9. Huang, Y.; Zhang, G.; Zhao, R.; Zhang, Z. Tetraphenylethene-Based cis/trans Isomers for Targeted Fluorescence Sensing and Biomedical Applications. *Chem.—A Eur. J.* **2023**, *29*, e202300539. [CrossRef] [PubMed]
10. Todorov, P.; Georgieva, S.; Peneva, P.; Rusew, R.; Shivachevc, B.; Georgiev, A. Experimental and theoretical study of bidirectional photoswitching behavior of 5,5′-diphenylhydantoin Schiff bases: Synthesis, crystal structure and kinetic approaches. *New J. Chem.* **2020**, *44*, 15081–15099. [CrossRef]
11. Dugave, C.; Demange, L. Cis–Trans Isomerization of Organic Molecules and Biomolecules: Implications and Applications. *Chem. Rev.* **2003**, *103*, 2475–2532. [CrossRef] [PubMed]
12. Hadidi, S.; Farshad, S.; Mohammadsaleh, N. Conversion mechanism and isomeric preferences of the cis and trans isomers of anti-cancer medicine carmustine; A double hybrid DFT calculation. *Chem. Phys.* **2019**, *522*, 39–43. [CrossRef]
13. Ning, Y.; Liu, Y.-W.; Yang, Z.-S.; Yao, Y.; Kang, L.; Sessler, L.J.; Zhang, J.-L. Split and Use: Structural Isomers for Diagnosis and Therapy. *J. Am. Chem. Soc.* **2020**, *142*, 6761–6768. [CrossRef] [PubMed]
14. Bhurta, D.; Bharate, S.B. Styryl Group, a Friend or Foe in Medicinal Chemistry. *ChemMedChem* **2022**, *17*, 7. [CrossRef] [PubMed]
15. Racine, R.; Rose, P.A.; Burnham, W.M. Afterdischarge thresholds and kindling rates in dorsal and ventral hippocampus and dentate gyrus. *Can. J. Neurol. Sci.* **1977**, *4*, 273–278. [CrossRef] [PubMed]

International Journal of
Molecular Sciences

MDPI

Review

Temporal Dynamics of Oxidative Stress and Inflammation in Bronchopulmonary Dysplasia

Michelle Teng [1,2], Tzong-Jin Wu [1,2], Xigang Jing [1,2], Billy W. Day [3], Kirkwood A. Pritchard, Jr. [2,3,4], Stephen Naylor [3] and Ru-Jeng Teng [1,2,*]

1 Department of Pediatrics, Medical College of Wisconsin, Suite C410, Children Corporate Center, 999N 92nd Street, Milwaukee, WI 53226, USA; mteng@mcw.edu (M.T.); twu@mcw.edu (T.-J.W.); xgjing@mcw.edu (X.J.)
2 Children's Research Institute, Medical College of Wisconsin, 8701 W Watertown Plank Rd., Wauwatosa, WI 53226, USA; kpritch@mcw.edu
3 ReNeuroGen LLC, 2160 San Fernando Dr., Elm Grove, WI 53122, USA; billy.day@rngen.com (B.W.D.); snaylor@rngen.com (S.N.)
4 Department of Surgery, Medical College of Wisconsin, 8701 Watertown Plank Rd., Milwaukee, WI 53226, USA
* Correspondence: rteng@mcw.edu; Tel.: +1-414-266-6820; Fax: +1-414-266-6979

Abstract: Bronchopulmonary dysplasia (BPD) is the most common lung complication of prematurity. Despite extensive research, our understanding of its pathophysiology remains limited, as reflected by the stable prevalence of BPD. Prematurity is the primary risk factor for BPD, with oxidative stress (OS) and inflammation playing significant roles and being closely linked to premature birth. Understanding the interplay and temporal relationship between OS and inflammation is crucial for developing new treatments for BPD. Animal studies suggest that OS and inflammation can exacerbate each other. Clinical trials focusing solely on antioxidants or anti-inflammatory therapies have been unsuccessful. In contrast, vitamin A and caffeine, with antioxidant and anti-inflammatory properties, have shown some efficacy, reducing BPD by about 10%. However, more than one-third of very preterm infants still suffer from BPD. New therapeutic agents are needed. A novel tripeptide, N-acetyl-lysyltyrosylcysteine amide (KYC), is a reversible myeloperoxidase inhibitor and a systems pharmacology agent. It reduces BPD severity by inhibiting MPO, enhancing antioxidative proteins, and alleviating endoplasmic reticulum stress and cellular senescence in a hyperoxia rat model. KYC represents a promising new approach to BPD treatment.

Keywords: bronchopulmonary dysplasia; oxidative stress; inflammation; endoplasmic reticulum stress; senescence; antioxidant; anti-inflammatory; temporal relationship; therapeutic intervention

1. Introduction

Bronchopulmonary dysplasia (BPD) is the most common lung complication in premature infants [1,2], affecting 50–70% of those born before 28 weeks of gestation [3]. The diagnostic criteria for BPD continue to evolve. The diagnosis of BPD is based on clinical metrics such as the need for oxygen at twenty-eight days of age postnatal and radiographic lung abnormalities [4] or, more often, oxygen requirement beyond the postconceptional age of 36 weeks [5]. Roughly one-fourth to one-third of BPD infants develop pulmonary hypertension [6,7], which is associated with 16% mortality before hospital discharge or 48% mortality within two years of the diagnosis [8]. BPD survivors frequently suffer from recurrent respiratory infections [9], growth delays [10], and reactive airway disease or trouble exercising that can persist into adulthood. The impaired lung growth trajectory in BPD survivors also results in their susceptibility to early-onset chronic obstructive pulmonary disease [11,12].

It has been estimated that more than 15,000 new BPD patients are diagnosed each year in the United States alone [13,14]. Notably, the annual number of newly diagnosed premature BPD neonates in the United States has been unchanged for a considerable period [15].

This intractable situation continues despite various new interventions, including gentle ventilation, judicious oxygen therapy [16], aggressive nutritional support [17], intramuscular vitamin A treatment [18], and early caffeine use [19]. This stagnation underscores the urgent need for further research and more effective interventions. Systemic corticosteroid treatment was once commonly prescribed by clinicians to prevent BPD because of its potent anti-inflammatory properties. After realizing that early systemic corticosteroid treatment, especially within the first week of life, is associated with a significant increase in neurodevelopmental deficit [20], its use has been limited to those with established BPD or after one week of life [21]. Stem cell treatment has been considered a promising treatment for BPD. The benefits of stem cell therapy are derived from its anti-inflammatory and antioxidant activity [22]. Clinical studies have shown that premature neonates tolerate stem cell therapy well, but its benefits for BPD remain to be revealed [22]. Still, concerns regarding possible vascular occlusion, potential tumorigenicity, difficulty obtaining the appropriate number of cells, and maintaining the quality are waiting to be resolved [23]. A meager eight clinical trials investigating therapeutic or supplemental intervention for BPD are listed on Clinicaltrials.gov.

This lack of effective therapies and ongoing clinical trials is because BPD is a complex, multifactorial, and poorly understood disease. A thorough understanding of the pathophysiology and mechanisms of onset and progression, including temporal considerations leading to BPD, is required to provide effective BPD treatments. It should be noted that prematurity and low birth weight are the most critical risk factors for BPD and their association with respiratory distress syndrome (RDS) [1]. Premature rupture of the membranes (PROM), preterm labor, intrauterine growth restriction (IUGR), and maternal hypertension are common causes that lead to premature delivery. Regardless of the cause of preterm delivery, oxidative stress has been reported to be a critical factor in human BPD onset and progression [24].

Similarly, inflammation has been detected in human premature births. Histological evidence of chorioamnionitis is commonly seen in the premature placenta and 94% of peri-viable (21–24 weeks of gestation) placentae [25]. Chorioamnionitis increases OS in the sheep model of premature birth [26]. These observations suggest premature neonates have been exposed to an intrauterine environment with OS and inflammation way before their birth. These observations suggest a more thorough understanding of the complex relationship between OS and inflammation in BPD is needed.

Premature human neonates born before the alveolar stage do not produce enough surfactant to keep their lungs open, leading to RDS [27]. Supplemental oxygen, positive pressure respiratory support, and exogenous surfactants are usually required for tissue oxygenation. The primary postnatal risk factors of BPD include exposure to elevated levels of OS from mechanical ventilation [28], supplemental oxygen [29], and inflammation [30]. Premature lungs with immature antioxidative systems face an abrupt oxidative stress (OS) challenge beyond their coping capacity at birth. OS activates alveolar macrophages to recruit neutrophils from the circulation as a form of sterile inflammation [31]. Inflammatory cytokines and chemokines released from the inflammatory cells damage lung cells, inhibit angiogenesis and alveologenesis, and encourage tissue fibrosis resulting in BPD. Many other contributors to BPD in premature human neonates, such as hemodynamically significant patent ductus arteriosus, necrotizing enterocolitis, and nosocomial infection [32], make studying the BPD mechanism in human neonates extremely difficult.

Over the past five decades, research has resulted in a few treatments that reduce BPD. Preventing a premature birth is undoubtedly the most ideal way, which, unfortunately, is unsuccessful [33]. Antenatal corticosteroids given to mothers at risk of preterm delivery can reduce the risk of RDS, but their effects on decreasing BPD remain equivocal. Postnatal systemic corticosteroids were once commonly used by clinicians believing the incidence of BPD could be reduced. Unfortunately, the strong association between its use and severe neurologic deficit [34] led the American Academy of Pediatrics to caution against its routine use [35]. Intramuscular vitamin A injection has been shown to reduce BPD [18], but the route of administration has led to limited acceptance by most practices. An attempt to use enteral vitamin A administration, however, failed to show any decrease in moderate to severe BPD [36]. Early caffeine treatment is the most promising strategy, significantly reducing BPD [19] and yielding better long-term neurological outcomes. We must, however, remember that the reduction in BPD was found in the secondary analysis of that study. Early administration of surfactant, permissive hypercarbia or gentle ventilation, early application of continuous positive airway pressure, and aggressive nutritional intervention are other clinical measures that have been widely implemented to decrease BPD without solid clinical evidence.

In this review, we evaluate the interaction between OS and inflammation during the development of BPD. Initial literature considerations suggest that OS is the primary process in the onset of BPD, but we argue here that this is possibly an overly simplistic interpretation. Understanding the temporal interplay between OS and inflammation is crucial due to this relationship's complex and poorly understood nature in BPD [37]. Determining whether OS or inflammation alone, independent parallel contributions, or synergistic coupled contributions, especially considering intrauterine factors, remains a significant challenge. This knowledge gap hinders the development of effective therapeutic strategies for BPD. The failure of antioxidant and anti-inflammatory treatments in clinical settings underscores the need for a deeper investigation into their temporal dynamics. Unraveling this relationship could reveal better insights for intervention and potentially lead to more targeted and successful therapies. Thus, comprehending the timing and interaction of OS and inflammation is essential for advancing our understanding of BPD pathophysiology and improving patient outcomes [32]. We suggest that pharmacologic drug candidates with both antioxidant and anti-inflammatory properties appear to afford more promising efficacious treatments for BPD.

2. Literature Search

2.1. Eligibility Criteria

We first submitted the outlines to the editorial office and then prepared this review according to the approval outlines. Three authors (M.T., T-J.W., and X.J.) searched PubMed using keywords including premature birth, mechanism, oxidative stress, inflammation, infection, bronchopulmonary dysplasia, or their combination to identify related reports. Both human and animal studies were included. We prioritized our selection criteria to review articles published in journals with high-impact factors. Only articles published in English were eligible for consideration.

2.2. Inclusion Criteria

Two authors (B.W. and K.A.P.J.) first screened the curated articles based on their expertise and article titles. The senior authors (S.N. and R-J.T.) determined which articles should be included after discussion. For treatment effects, only randomized controlled trials were chosen for review. We included human observational studies, human randomized control trials, and animal models for experimental treatments that were important in explaining the crucial mechanisms.

2.3. Exclusion Criteria

We excluded articles that were not written in English.

3. Relationship between OS and Inflammation in General Pathologies

OS and inflammation are closely intertwined biological processes that often co-exist and can mutually exacerbate each other (Figure 1). However, the temporal relationship of these events can vary depending on the specific disease state and underlying causal mechanism of disease onset. Several signaling pathways have also been reported in the literature that link OS and inflammation together, including Nrf2, Ets-1, Sirt1/p66Shc, Sirt1/PPAR/PGC-1α, nitric oxide synthases, NADPH oxidases (NOX), Fe^{2+}, NLRP3/caspase-1/GSDMD,

HMGB1/TLR4/MAPKs/NF-κB, and mTOR/TFEB/NF-κB. This review will focus only on the most commonly discussed ones. As this review is mainly about BPD, a more detailed discussion of mechanisms will be presented in Section 4 (Relationship Between OS and Inflammation in BPD).

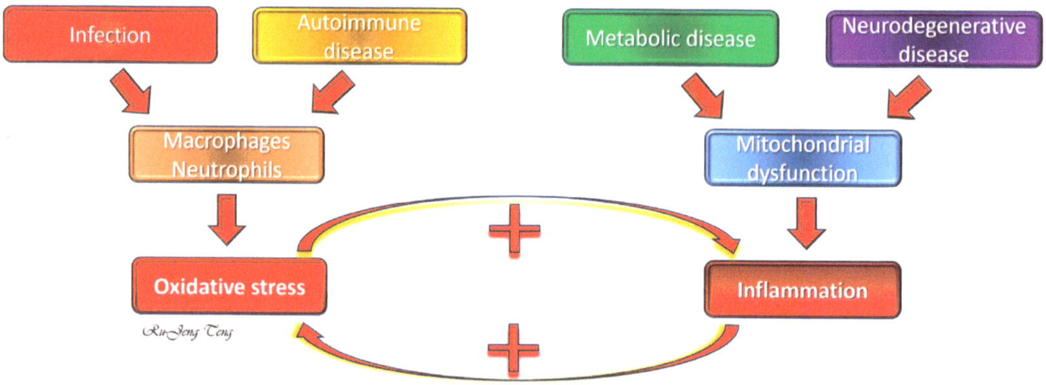

Figure 1. The interaction between oxidative stress (OS) and inflammation in general pathologies. Infection and autoimmune diseases are the most common prototypes that activate macrophages and neutrophils. The reactive oxygen species (ROS) generated by myeloperoxidase (MPO), NADPH oxidase, and uncoupled electron transport chain represent inflammation preceding OS. Metabolic disorders (diabetes mellitus and hyperlipidemia) or neurodegenerative diseases (Parkinson's disease and Alzheimer's disease) have mitochondrial dysfunction with increased OS, which then results in secondary inflammation. However, OS and inflammation frequently form a vicious cycle and reciprocally elicit each other. →: from upstream to downstream; +: positive effect.

3.1. Inflammation Preceding OS

Infection and autoimmune diseases are two typical conditions in this category. During infection, inflammatory cells (neutrophils and macrophages) infiltrate the site to combat pathogens. The inflammatory cells produce reactive oxygen species (ROS) as part of the defense mechanism, leading to OS. The most representative example is viral respiratory infections [38]. The ROS generated by inflammatory cells includes hypochlorous acid (HOCl) from myeloperoxidase (MPO), superoxide (O_2^-) from NOX, xanthine oxidase/dehydrogenase, uncoupled mitochondrial electron transport chains, and uncoupled endothelial nitric oxidase synthase. Superoxide is the primary, most abundant, but not a potent ROS, as it is relatively unreactive with most cell components. Superoxide is converted to other, more potent ROS through several reactions. The presence of free iron (Fe^{2+}) converts superoxide to hydroxyl radical (OH•) through the Fenton reaction. Hydroxyl radical is a highly reactive ROS that quickly penetrates the mitochondrion membrane, peroxidizes lipids, damages DNA/RNA, and kills cells. The three superoxide dismutases (Cu, Zn-SOD, Mn-SOD, extracellular SOD) dismutate superoxide to hydrogen peroxide (H_2O_2). H_2O_2 is a permeable, non-radical ROS that reacts spontaneously with nitrogen or oxygen nucleophiles and π-bonds to damage biomolecules. Another source of hydrogen peroxide generation is monoamine oxidase, mainly found in the central nervous system. Nitric oxide (NO) generated by nitric oxide synthases reacts with superoxide at a diffusion-limited rate ($6.7 \pm 0.9 \times 10^9/\text{mol}^{-1}/\text{s}^{-1}$), which is six times faster than the removal of superoxide by the Cu, Zn-SOD, to form peroxynitrite ($ONOO^-$). HOCl and $ONOO^-$ are potent ROS and reactive nitrogen species (RNS) that react with almost all biomolecules. Tyrosine-containing proteins frequently react with hypochlorous acid and peroxynitrite, yielding chlorotyrosine and nitrotyrosine as stable and characteristic footprints [39].

In autoimmune diseases, chronic inflammation is driven by an overactive immune response, leading to increased ROS production and, hence, OS [40]. The process is more complex than infections, as basal ROS is critical in maintaining the homeostasis of the adaptive immune response, and antioxidant treatments have been shown to increase the mortality rate paradoxically in humans. Initially, it was believed that TNFα released from chronically activated macrophages leads to releasing an oxidoreductase that causes OS. Recent studies suggested ROS may also serve as signaling molecules in many immune cell relationships and functions that prevent the progression of chronic inflammation [41]. This complex relationship between inflammation and OS might explain the antioxidant paradox in humans.

3.2. OS Preceding Inflammation

Metabolic disorders [42] and neurodegenerative diseases [43] are two typical conditions in this category. In diabetes and obesity [44], high glucose and fatty acid levels lead to mitochondrial dysfunction with increased ROS production [45]. The ROS-induced activation of transcription factors (NFκB, AP-1, MAP kinase/Mk2, JAK/STAT, PI3K/AKT/mTOR, and HIF1α) upregulates proinflammatory genes (CAMs, MCP-1, TNFα, IL-1, and TGFβ). It triggers the downstream inflammatory cascades in animal studies [46]. Cells cope with OS through multiple pathways, including the unfolded protein response (UPR) [47], autophagy [48], and cellular senescence [49] in an attempt to survive. The UPR, due to excessive accumulation in the endoplasmic reticulum, can activate neutrophils without infection (sterile inflammation) by upregulating cyclooxygenases and mitochondrial dysgenesis in hyperoxia-exposed rat pup lungs [50]. Autophagy, a mechanism that degrades non-essential biomolecules to obtain raw materials for synthesizing essential biomolecules, can promote and regulate inflammation [51]. Excessive autophagy promotes neutrophil-mediated injury by destructing endothelial cell barriers to facilitate neutrophil invasion, encouraging cytokine and ROS production, and inducing UPR. Senescent cells can consistently release inflammatory cytokines by the senescence-associated secretory phenotype (SASP), which perpetuates inflammatory responses until they are removed by phagocytic cells [49].

There is an extensive interaction between UPR, autophagy, and cellular senescence [50]. When OS becomes unopposed or protracted, it can lead to cell death and release intracellular molecules, including the high mobility group box-B1 (HMGB1). HMGB1 is a non-histone nuclear protein stabilizing DNA when it stays in the nucleus. When HMGB1 leaks out from the nuclei to the extracellular compartment, it becomes the most potent damage-associated molecular patterns (DMAP) or pathogen-associated molecular patterns (PMAP) molecule (Table 1) that binds the pattern recognition receptors (PRR) (Table 2), triggering more inflammatory reactions. HMGB1 is also seen in SASP [49]. The receptor for advanced glycation end-products (RAGE), Toll-like receptors (TLRs), CXC chemokine receptor type 4 (CXCR4), macrophage antigen-1, syndecan-3, T cell Ig mucin-3, and CD24-Siglec-10 are the main PRRs for HMGB1 [52]. Once HMGB1 binds the PRR, a cascade of signaling pathways is activated to augment (sterile) inflammation. In Alzheimer's [53] and Parkinson's diseases [54], OS from mitochondrial dysfunction or accumulation of damaged proteins (UPR) often occurs first, leading to chronic neuronal inflammation.

3.3. Reciprocal Influence between Inflammation and OS

In many diseases, inflammation and OS form a damaging, synergistic cycle [46]. For instance, in chronic inflammatory diseases, persistent ROS production causes tissue damage and perpetuates the inflammatory state. Conversely, ongoing OS can perpetuate inflammation mainly through modulating NFκB signaling [55], leading to the expression of pro-inflammatory cytokines. The temporal relationship between inflammation and OS depends on the nature of the disease and the developmental stage of the animal. One example is neonatal lungs preferentially activate the NFκB pathway upon exposure to hyperoxia compared to adult lungs [56]. These process-specific sequences and interplay can provide insights into disease mechanisms and potential therapeutic targets for any disease state where OS and inflammation are involved in causal onset and progression.

Table 1. The damage-associated molecular patterns (DAMPs) molecules. The table is reproduced from [52] under the CC 4.0 license.

Origin	Subcellular Compartment	Molecule
Intracellular	Nuclear	DNA Histones HMGB1 HMGN1 IL1a IL33 RNA SAP130
	Cytosol	Aβ ATP Cyclophilin A F-actin HSPs S100s Urate
	Endoplasmic reticulum	Calreticulin
	Mitochondrion	Formyl peptide mROS mtDNA TFAM
	Granule	Defensins Cathelicidin
Extracellular matrix		Biglycan Decorin Fibronectin Fibrinogen Heparan sulfate LMW hyaluronan Tenascin C Versican

Aβ: amyloid beta; F-actin: filamentous actin; HSP: heat shock protein; HMGB1: high mobility group box 1; HMGN1: high mobility group nucleosome binding domain 1; LMW: low molecular weight; mROS: mitochondrial reactive oxygen species; SAP130: spliceosome-associated protein 130; TFAM: mitochondrial transcription factor A.

Table 2. Pattern recognition receptors. The table is reproduced from [52] under the CC 4.0 license.

Family	CDCs	CLRs	FPRs	NLRs	RLRs	TLRs	Scavenger Receptor
Members	AIM2-like receptor	DC-SIGN DEC-2-5 Dectin-1 Dectin-2 DNGR-1 Mincle MMR	FPR1–3	NOD1 NOD2 NLRPs	LGP2 MDA5 RIG-1	TLR1–9	CD36 CD44 CD68 CD91 CXCL16 RAGE

Table 2. *Cont.*

Family	CDCs	CLRs	FPRs	NLRs	RLRs	TLRs	Scavenger Receptor
Ligands	DNA	F-actin SAP130	Formyl peptide Cathelicidin	Aβ Biglycan Histones LMW hyaluronan mtROS Uric acid	RNA	Biglycan Decorin DNA Fibrinogen Glypicans Heparan sulfate Histones HMGB1 HSPs LMW hyaluronan mtDNA RNA S100s Syndecans Tenascin C Versican	Calreticulin HMGB1 HSPs S100s Versican

AIM2: absent in melanoma 2; CDCs: cytosolic DNA sensor; CLR: C-type lectin receptor; FPR: formyl peptide receptor; LGP2: laboratory of genetics and physiology 2; MDA5: melanoma differentiation-associated protein 5; MMR: mismatch repair; NLR: NOD-like receptor; RIG-I: retinoic acid-inducible gene I.

4. Relationship between OS and Inflammation in BPD

Premature human neonates, especially those born as extremely premature before 28 weeks of gestation, are often subject to mechanical ventilation and supplemental oxygen shortly after birth to maintain metabolic homeostasis. The treatment readily leads to conditions favoring OS onset [50] and a mistaken belief that OS is the dominant factor in BPD causality. However, the situation is somewhat more complicated, as outlined here (Figure 2). Human observational studies demonstrate a strong association between increased OS, inflammation, and premature births. Evidence from animal studies suggests these intrauterine changes contribute to BPD development [57]. The underdeveloped antioxidant system and RDS make premature neonates more susceptible to injury caused by OS and infection. The postnatal OS from respiratory treatment and infection undoubtedly aggravates the injury. Inflammation and OS are the most critical postnatal contributors to BPD, and they inhibit vascular endothelial growth factor A signaling with impaired angiogenesis and alveolar formation and, hence, the BPD phenotype [58].

4.1. Antenatal Temporal Phase and BPD

Compared to other complex disease conditions, BPD has several unique features, including the probable involvement of antenatal conditions and events. Considering this, the temporal phase is essential to understanding the role of inflammation and OS in BPD onset and progression. In addition, this temporal phase is heavily influenced by the balance between survival and morbidity, early postnatal fluid management, and nutritional management. Lungs also differ from other organs by directly facing the highest oxygen content and mechanical damage from ventilator support. The high expression of RAGE by type I alveolar epithelial cells, a PRR that binds HMGB1 [59], may also explain why lungs are frequently involved in systemic inflammatory response syndrome.

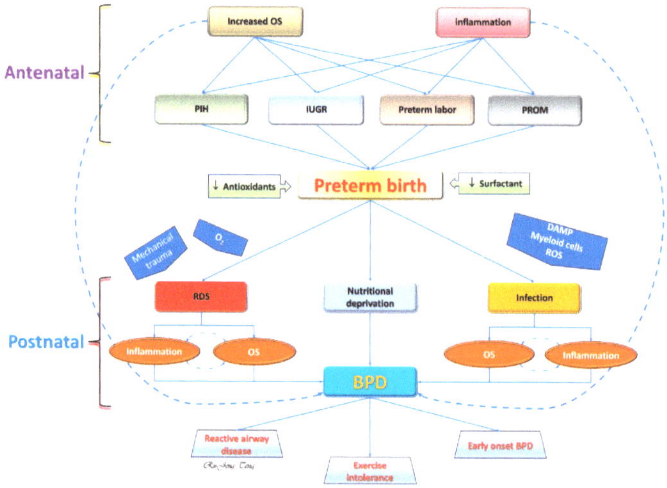

Figure 2. The contributing role of OS and inflammation in developing bronchopulmonary dysplasia (BPD). Increased OS and inflammation are seen antenatally for preterm birth. The surfactant deficiency after preterm birth results in respiratory distress, and antioxidant deficiency leads to sensitivity to OS-induced injury. Postnatal oxygen support, mechanical ventilation, and infection further aggravate OS and inflammation in the premature lung that culminates into BPD. Nutritional deprivation, which weakens the regenerative process, also contributes to BPD. DAMP: damage-associated molecular pattern; IUGR: intrauterine growth restriction; PIH: pregnancy-induced hypertension (pre-eclampsia, eclampsia, and chronic hypertension); PROM: premature rupture of the membranes; ROS: reactive oxygen species. Solid blue arrow: direct relationship; Dashed blue arrow: distant relationship; Broken blue arrow: positive reinforcement.

Approximately one-half of all premature births are considered to have no etiology (idiopathic), which is considered by some researchers as genetically mediated [33]. Other premature births can be the result of preterm labor, PROM, IUGR, or maternal hypertensive disorders. Despite the etiology, ample evidence from human studies suggests that inflammation and OS are highly associated with these antenatal causes of premature delivery through measuring markers for inflammation or OS. The combination of OS and inflammation can result in complex and damaging consequences.

4.1.1. Intrauterine Inflammation

An ample amount of evidence came from human studies. Peripheral neutrophilia [60] and increased OS [61] in pregnant human women are common occurrences during the third trimester. The intrauterine immune milieu is pro-inflammatory during the first trimester and right before labor but anti-inflammatory between these two periods in human studies [62]. The anti-inflammatory status allows the fetus to develop inside the womb without being rejected by the maternal immune system. The pro-inflammatory status during the first trimester is thought to assist implantation and placentation. The pro-inflammatory status right before labor may help the labor process, protect pregnant women against infections, and even facilitate postpartum recovery. The immune profiling of human cord blood, however, showed inconsistent changes in pro-inflammatory mediators with decreased levels of IL-1β, IL-6, IL-17A, IL-8, eotaxin, MIP-1α, and MIP-1β but increased levels of IL-15 and MCP-1 in premature neonates as compared to term neonates. These findings suggest a reduced capacity for pro-inflammatory immune responses in premature infants in response to maternal inflammation [63].

Chorioamnionitis is an acute inflammation of the chorion and membranes of the placenta [64]. We must remember that physiological parturition is an inflammatory process (sterile inflammation) [65] with neutrophil infiltration into the placenta and membranes [66]. This neutrophil infiltration into the maternal–fetal interface during parturition is exaggerated during human preterm birth [67]. The exact role of neutrophils in the onset of labor remains an enigma, as their infiltration is not required for preterm birth in the mouse model of infection-induced preterm labor [68,69]. Unfortunately, obtaining placenta tissue for histology before delivery for studies is impossible, preventing us from studying the temporal changes in human placentas.

Overall, 1–4% of all human births are complicated by chorioamnionitis [70]. The prevalence varies by diagnostic criteria, risk factors, and gestational age. Around 40% of spontaneous human premature births are considered to be infection-related with inflammatory cell infiltration [71]. It results from ascending infection, often polymicrobial [72], and can occur even with intact membranes. IUGR is a frequent cause of elective preterm delivery. Pregnant women with IUGR also have increased TNFα levels in their blood, indicating an inflammatory status [73]. Sustained maternal inflammation is also known to cause IUGR in sheep [74] and human fetuses [75] and sensitizes the neonate to inflammatory disorders, including BPD [76].

Most obstetricians use clinical findings and laboratory tests to diagnose chorioamnionitis without pursuing microbiology or histology. The clinical findings include a fever of at least 102.2 °F (39 °C), increased white blood cell count, uterine tenderness, abdominal pain, foul-smelling vaginal discharge, fetal and maternal tachycardia, and purulent fluid coming from the cervical os [77]. Occasionally, bacterial culture from amniotic fluid, vaginal discharge, amniotic fluid, or urogenital discharge will be ordered to support the diagnosis. Although histological and clinical chorioamnionitis significantly increases the odds of early onset (<72 h of birth) neonatal sepsis, less than 8% of neonates develop culture-positive early onset neonatal septicemia. However, it is essential to point out that more than 20% of neonates born to mothers with chorioamnionitis develop late-onset (≥72 h of birth) or nosocomial neonatal sepsis, indicating maternal chorioamnionitis increases the susceptibility to infections [78]. An extensive meta-analysis out of 158 human studies (including a total of 244,096 premature infants) showed chorioamnionitis is associated with an increased risk of BPD as defined by oxygen-dependence at 28 days (odds ratio 2.32) or postconceptional age of 36 weeks (odds ratio 1.29). Interestingly, the association between chorioamnionitis and BPD is not a consequence of RDS, as the odds of having RDS do not increase with chorioamnionitis (odds ratio 1.1) [79]. In fact, in an animal study, perinatal maternal antibiotic exposure augments the severity of BPD [80].

4.1.2. OS during Pregnancy

The levels of OS in pregnant women vary during their gestation and reach the highest level in the last trimester [61]. The increased OS may be necessary to stimulate cell proliferation, assist the differentiation and invasion of trophoblasts, and promote placentation [81]. It is hypothesized that increased OS may be required to initiate labor-inducing pathways [82]. Although the exact mechanism by which OS initiates labor remains unclear, increased OS levels have been demonstrated in human preterm labor [24]. One piece of evidence came from a study showing maternal blood levels of malondialdehyde (MDA) were higher in those who delivered premature neonates than those who delivered at term. The same study also showed that maternal blood MDA levels were positively correlated with the corresponding cord blood levels at birth [83]. The evidence suggests that an increased OS may promote premature cellular senescence, with senescence-associated (sterile) inflammation and proteolysis predisposing to the PROM [84].

At birth, human premature neonates have higher levels of OS markers than their full-term counterparts [85], such as plasma F2-isoprostane [86], total and hemoglobin-bound MDA [87,88], erythrocyte membrane hydroperoxides [89], 8-hydroxy-2-deoxyguanosine (8-OHdG) [90], and chelatable iron [86]. Some of these markers are negatively correlated with gestational age [85]. Although there is no difference in maternal blood levels of protein carbonyl between term and premature delivery, the cord blood levels are significantly higher in premature neonates than in term neonates [91]. These findings prove that premature human neonates are born with higher endogenous OS. One common cause that results in premature birth is IUGR, which accounts for over 40% of all induced preterm births before 34 weeks of gestation [92]. It can be idiopathic or, more commonly, secondary to maternal hypertension. Regardless of the etiology, they all result in placental insufficiency with prenatal hypoxia and increased generation of ROS [93]. Irrespective of the etiology, increased OS is consistently seen in premature human neonates.

4.2. Postnatal Temporal Phase and BPD

Neonates born prematurely, especially those born before 32 weeks postconceptional age, frequently require respiratory support, including supplemental oxygen and mechanical ventilation. Both relative hyperoxia from supplemental oxygen and mechanical injury from the ventilator generate OS in the immature lungs. Invasive lines are commonly needed to provide adequate fluid and nutritional support or blood work, offering an opportunity for nosocomial infections. Supplemental oxygen, mechanical ventilation, and infection are well-known risk factors for BPD [50]. Necrotizing enterocolitis has recently been identified to increase the odds of BPD through increased inflammation [94].

4.2.1. Postnatally Increased OS

Preterm infants are susceptible to OS due to an imbalance between the oxidant and antioxidant systems [95]. This imbalance results from insufficient antioxidant capacity due to prematurity and increased OS due to respiratory treatment or infections.

- Decreased Antioxidant Capacity

Premature human neonates are born with a deficient antioxidant system, including superoxide dismutase (SOD) [96] and catalase [97] activities in the blood, and SOD and cytosolic glutathione peroxidase activities in red blood cells [89]. The levels of non-enzymatic antioxidants are also decreased in premature neonates, such as vitamin E in blood [81] and red blood cells [89], blood vitamin C [98], reduced glutathione in red blood cells [83], blood transferrin [99], and decreased glutathione in tracheal aspirates [100]. These culminate in lower antioxidant capacity and susceptibility to OS-induced injury in premature neonates.

- Supplemental oxygen

The uterus is a relatively hypoxic environment. This relative hypoxia is believed to encourage stabilizing the hypoxia-inducible factors that encourage placentation and fetal lung development [101]. The abrupt transition from an intrauterine oxygen tension of 40–50 torr to an ambient oxygen tension above 140 torr (21% O_2, room air) is challenging for neonatal lungs. Clinicians face the dilemma of choosing between mortality and morbidity when deciding the optimal oxygen concentration to support neonatal tissue oxygenation. High fractional inspired oxygen (FiO_2) for neonatal resuscitation is known to be associated with increased OS damage in neonates, especially premature neonates [102]. In neonatal animal studies, both high oxygen concentration and mechanical ventilation decrease hypoxia-inducible factors [99], AMP-activated protein kinase [103], mitochondrial function [104], endothelial nitric oxidase synthase activity [105], matrix metalloproteinase-9 expression [106], and vascular endothelial growth factor abundance [107], which result in arrested alveolarization.

- Mechanical ventilation

Although mechanical ventilation is often life-saving for premature neonates, neonatal animal studies have shown that barotrauma and volutrauma from mechanical ventilation can damage premature lungs and contribute to BPD development by causing OS, inflammation, scarring, and tissue destruction [108,109]. Mechanical ventilation can also cause the downregulation of the vascular endothelial growth factor and its receptor, along with the upregulation of endoglin, which contributes to impaired angiogenesis and alveologenesis [110]. The release of inflammatory mediators also contributes to impaired alveolar formation [111].

- Infection

Macrophages and neutrophils activated by infections generate ROS and RNS through NADPH-oxidase (NOX), inducible nitric oxide synthase (iNOS), and MPO. $ONOO^-$ from inducible nitric oxide synthase [112] and HOCl, from MPO [113], are the two most potent free radicals generated by myeloid cells in the lungs that contribute to the increased OS (see detailed description in Section 3.1).

- Consequence of OS to neonatal lungs

Increased OS in human BPD lungs is evidenced by the increased levels of 8-OHdG, a specific biomarker for OS-induced DNA damage, in histology [114]. Animal studies have shown that hyperoxia-induced OS leads to endoplasmic reticulum stress, mitochondrial dysfunction, activation of myeloid activity [115], sterile inflammation [116], autophagy, apoptosis, and cellular senescence [114]. These sequential events form a self-perpetuated destructive cycle, suppressing alveolar formation (Figure 3).

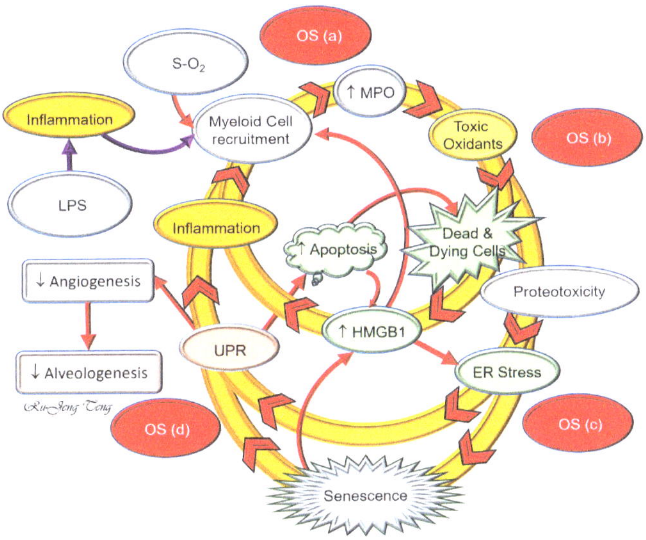

Figure 3. The BPD destructive cycle. The destructive cycle is constructed according to the results of the rat BPD model. OS from hyperoxia or inflammation caused by lipopolysaccharide (LPS) causes myeloid cell infiltration. Myeloperoxidase (MPO) released by macrophages and neutrophils will generate hypochlorous acid (HOCl) from the surrounding chloride anion and H_2O_2 released by activated myeloid cells. As one of the most potent free radicals, HOCl can kill or injure nearby cells by releasing high mobility group box 1 (HMGB1), eliciting endoplasmic reticulum (ER) stress, apoptosis, and cellular senescence. HMGB1 is the most potent DAMP, which binds to Toll-like receptor 4 (TLR4) or the receptor for advanced glycation end product (RAGE). ER stress can generate ROS to regain its ability to fold protein and glycosylate nascent proteins. ER stress will activate sterile inflammation and promote cellular senescence. The senescence-associate secretory phenotype (SASP) can lead to chronic inflammation by releasing pro-inflammatory cytokines (IL6, TNFα, HMGB1). The hypermetabolic state of senescent cells and proliferation arrest of the stem/progenitor cells contribute to impaired alveolar formation. These changes form a complex interaction network and self-perpetuate the destructive cycle. The figure is reproduced from [50] under the Creative Commons CC BY 4.0 license). Solid red and purple arrows: direct relationship; Arrowhead: direction of the destructive cycle.

4.2.2. Postnatal Inflammation

- Infection

Multiple studies show a strong association between postnatal infection and human BPD [117,118]. New knowledge has recently emerged from animal studies showing how pattern recognition receptors and DAMP, or PAMP, are involved in the infection-mediated disruption of neonatal lung developmental processes such as angiogenesis, extracellular matrix deposition, and alveolar formation [52] (see detailed description in Section 3.2). Activating the endothelial cell TLR by endotoxin or HMGB1 during infection will lead to deviant vascular formation, epithelial cell injury and reprogramming, disruption of extracellular matrix organization, and pro-inflammatory polarization of the myeloid cells in animal studies. These changes are similar to acute lung injury in adults and can be expected to impact the neonatal lung during the first wave of alveolar formation [117,118].

- Sterile inflammation

Animal studies show that an excessive or unopposed OS can elicit sterile inflammation without microorganisms; this type of inflammation results from sterile cell death or injury caused by the OS. Several endogenous molecules released during cellular injury are considered DAMPs [52,119] (Table 1) that initiate sterile inflammation by interacting with PRRs (Table 2). HMGB1 is the most extensively studied DAMP, binding mainly to TLR2, TLR4, and RAGE when released extracellularly. After HMGB1 binds to TLR4 and RAGE, inflammatory cytokines' transcription, translation, and secretion increase through NFκB signaling [120]. Other interesting facts are that HMGB1–RAGE binding will promote TLR4 translocation to the cell surface, and the HMGB1–TLR4 binding will result in increased transcription and translation of RAGE, forming a self-perpetuating vicious cycle [120].

ER stress caused by excessive OS will also amplify cytokine-mediated inflammation without pathogens [121] and contribute to cellular senescence [122]. DNA damage by excessive OS will activate a cascade of tumor suppressors that arrest the cell cycle so that DNA repair will succeed [123]. Tumor suppressor TP53 is the master regulator for DNA damage response. TP53 upregulation can result in apoptosis or cellular senescence, which is context-related [124]. Senescent cells can cause chronic inflammation through their characteristic SASP [125]. Inflammatory mediators in SASP, especially HMGB1, can cause chronic sterile inflammation unless phagocytic cells can effectively remove senescent cells.

4.3. *OS and Inflammation Mutually Affect Each Other in BPD*

OS and inflammation are closely related biological processes that can mutually elicit each other [45]. Their complex interdependence might be the root cause of the antioxidant paradox, in which antioxidants fail to protect against OS-mediated human disorders, including BPD [126]. Existing data from human studies show that both OS and inflammation are involved in premature births and BPD. Animal models have not examined the temporal relationship between OS and inflammation in BPD onset and progression. Evidence shows, however, that both HOX and LPS can lead to HMGB1 release, endoplasmic reticulum stress, and cellular senescence in the lungs [50] (Figure 3). There are rare conditions of BPD in which inflammation might precede OS. These conditions are early neonatal pneumonia, necrotizing enterocolitis in late premature or full-term neonates, or postsurgical infections. These rare conditions start from systemic inflammatory response syndrome or neonatal acute lung injury, resulting in BPD after prolonged respiratory support.

Although our extensive literature review and animal experiments cannot reveal the exact temporal relationship between OS and inflammation in BPD, we summarize that they exert a complex interactive role in the onset and progression of BPD. We suggest that additional studies are needed to understand the intrauterine OS and inflammation relationship and that more well-designed animal studies are needed to further clarify this critical temporal relationship.

5. Strategies for BPD Treatment

Our current understanding and best practices for BPD can be summarized as follows. It is believed that BPD development starts from RDS due to premature birth. Clinicians might be capable of postponing preterm delivery, but maintaining the pregnancy until term is almost impossible. The antenatal steroid has been proven to decrease the severity of RDS and should be given to women with preterm labor [127]. As mechanical trauma and oxygen-related injury start right after birth, early surfactant replacement therapy, judicious oxygen use, and gentle ventilation strategy should be implemented. Aggressive nutritional support and adequate fluid management will facilitate the healing of injured premature lungs, which must start as early as possible. Stringent hygienic practice that decreases nosocomial infections is also crucial in reducing BPD. Early administration of caffeine and intramuscular vitamin A injection should be prescribed. These best practices have evolved slowly with time in treating BPD, and further cautious developments continue to occur.

5.1. *Early Surfactant Replacement*

Preventing prematurity and antenatal corticosteroids are the most effective ways to reduce RDS, but obstetricians manage them, and this is beyond the scope of this review. Since premature neonates with RDS require supplemental oxygen and mechanical ventilation, it is hypothesized that early surfactant administration might avoid high oxygen concentrations and prolonged mechanical ventilation and result in reduced BPD. Several new methods of early surfactant administration have been studied. So far, only less invasive surfactant administration (LISA) has shown a significant reduction in BPD for survivors [128]. Currently, two ongoing clinical trials (NCT05711966 and NCT04984057) evaluate the further use of surfactants in BPD treatment (ClinicalTrials.Gov). Results from these two studies may provide helpful information about optimal surfactant treatment strategies for decreasing BPD.

5.2. *Judicious Use of Oxygen*

5.2.1. During Resuscitation

Randomized studies and meta-analysis in term neonates comparing 100% FiO_2 and 21% FiO_2 during resuscitation revealed an unexpectedly decreased survival rate in the FiO_2 21% group [129]. The results spurred changes in practice to use lower FiO_2 in the resuscitation of premature neonates [130]. The most recent network meta-analysis showed, however, that higher FiO_2 (60–90%) for resuscitation results in significant survival in premature neonates born under 32 weeks of gestation [131]. The new finding will undoubtedly stir up a debate about the optimal FiO_2 for premature neonates.

5.2.2. After Initial Stabilization

Unlike most term neonates, who frequently recover from initial respiratory distress within days with their fully developed antioxidant system, premature neonates require more extended oxygen support to maintain tissue oxygenation and, hence, cause excessive OS. The appropriate oxygen treatment strategy after initial resuscitation and stabilization that offers the best survival rate with the lowest OS-induced morbidities has been studied for decades. The optimal FiO_2 for premature neonates after initial resuscitation is challenging to study due to their limited blood amount. The noninvasive tissue oxygen saturation (SpO2) measurement through a pulse oximeter has been adopted as the most practical tool for clinical studies. Results from the "Supplemental Therapeutic Oxygen for Prethreshold Retinopathy Of Prematurity" (STOP-ROP) study clearly showed that maintaining SpO2 above 96% increased BPD without improving the neurodevelopmental outcome [132]. The most recent systemic review showed no difference in either survival rate or neurodevelopmental outcome at 18 to 24 months between those who maintained SpO2 between 85–89% and 91–95% [133]. Maintaining SpO2 91–95% during early postnatal life is thus recommended by most neonatal units [134].

5.2.3. After BPD Is Established

When the diagnosis of BPD is established, oxygen use becomes more liberalized for a very different purpose. Experts suggest maintaining SpO2 at 92–95% to promote growth and prevent pulmonary hypertension development [135].

5.3. Gentle Ventilation

The trauma inflicted by mechanical ventilation is considered a significant contributor to BPD. Noninvasive respiratory support is slowly being accepted by neonatologists worldwide as the best way to support premature neonates [136]. The so-called noninvasive ventilation includes nasal high-frequency ventilation [137], noninvasive neurally adjusted ventilatory assistance [138], nasal intermittent positive pressure ventilation [139], and nasal continuous positive pressure ventilation [140], which have all been reported. Although nasal continuous positive pressure is the most cost-effective gentile ventilation, we must recognize its 30–80% failure rate and the need for endotracheal intubation [141]. After five large multicenter randomized controlled trials including over 3000 infants born at 24–29 weeks gestation, nearly 50% of surviving infants continue to develop BPD [16]. Although no evidence supports the efficacy, the noninvasive ventilation strategy has become routine for most neonatologists [136]. It is not which ventilatory support is more protective but how aggressive clinicians are willing to de-escalate the aggressive mode of positive airway pressure support that can reduce mechanical trauma to the lungs.

5.4. Antioxidant Treatment for BPD

5.4.1. Selenium

Selenium is an essential trace element required for the formation of selenoproteins. It also has antioxidant, anti-inflammatory, and anti-aging properties [142]. Although meta-analysis suggested low plasma selenium was associated with increased complications in premature human infants, selenium supplementation did not reduce BPD [143].

5.4.2. Superoxide Dismutase (SOD)

There are three types of SODs, including Cu, Zn-SOD (SOD1), Mn-SOD (SOD2), and extracellular SOD (ec-SOD, SOD3). Animal studies revealed that ec-SOD deficiency aggravates hyperoxia lung injury. At the same time, Mn-SOD overexpression in type II alveolar cells enhances the tolerance to hyperoxia leading to the assumption that SOD treatment might decrease BPD [144]. There are three randomized controlled trials (RCTs) concerning SOD in premature neonates available for meta-analysis. Unfortunately, there is no evidence that SOD reduces BPD [145].

5.4.3. Vitamin C

The encouraging study showing vitamin C treatment in pregnant smokers led to improved lung function in their offspring [146], offering hope for BPD prevention as maternal smoking was considered a risk factor for BPD [50]. Unfortunately, there has been no vitamin C study on premature human infants. High doses of vitamin C and E treatments in premature baboons exposed to prolonged hyperoxia did increase the level of vitamin C and E in blood and tracheal aspirates. Still, they failed to improve lung histology [147].

5.4.4. Vitamin E

Vitamin E is a fat-soluble essential vitamin with eight isoforms [148]. Both α- and γ-tocopherols have anti-inflammatory properties. Maternal α-tocopherol intake during pregnancy is an important growth factor for fetal lung development [149]. The literature has seven randomized controlled trials of high-dose α-tocopherol to prevent BPD. Although one study reported a significant reduction in BPD, the meta-analysis did not show efficacy [150].

5.4.5. N-Acetylcysteine

Glutathione is the largest antioxidant pool in the body. As the precursor of glutathione, *N*-acetylcysteine has been studied in extreme low-birth-weight neonates requiring positive airway pressure support. The multicenter RCT showed no difference in the severity and incidence of BPD by a six-day course of *N*-acetylcysteine started within 36 h of life [151]. However, a recent single-center study showed an encouraging result for antenatal *N*-acetylcysteine treatment in pregnant women showing signs of preterm labor or inflammation that decreased BPD by 90%. This is the only clinical study showing that exogenous antioxidants prevent premature neonates from developing BPD. It deserves our attention that the treatment did not increase the maternal blood glutathione levels. The authors hypothesized that the effect might be epigenetic instead of related to antioxidant activity [152].

5.4.6. Lactoferrin

Lactoferrin is an endogenous protein that has antioxidant activity by binding non-protein-bound iron. Premature neonates who later develop BPD have a more rapid drop of lactoferrin levels in the tracheal fluid within three days [153]. There are three randomized controlled studies using enteral lactoferrin to prevent prematurity-associated morbidities, including BPD. Meta-analysis showed no reduction in BPD by enteral lactoferrin [154].

5.5. Anti-Inflammatory Treatment for BPD

System corticosteroids are the only anti-inflammatory agents that have been well-studied in BPD. Although initial human studies showed a reduction in BPD if administered within the first week of life, the early treatment strategy was disappointing. The systemic administration of corticosteroids in the first eight days of life led to a significant increase in long-term neurodevelopmental impairment [34] and other short-term complications such as high blood pressure, high blood sugar, bowel perforation, and bleeding from the stomach or bowel [155]. Systemic corticosteroid treatment after the eighth day might reduce the composite outcome of BPD/death without affecting the neurodevelopmental outcome [156]. When focused on extremely premature neonates, late systemic corticosteroid treatment is beneficial to those with a high risk of death or moderate-to-severe BPD. Still, it may harm those at low risk [21]. It is apparent that clinical experience suggests systemic corticosteroid treatment does decrease BPD but will be associated with an increased risk of neurodevelopmental impairment if started at the onset stage of BPD.

Non-steroid anti-inflammatory drugs (NSAIDs) have been studied for other purposes. The trial of indomethacin prophylaxis in preterms (TIPP) showed no reduction in BPD [157]. A retrospective cohort study comparing indomethacin prophylaxis within 24 h of birth in extremely premature neonates (<29 weeks or 401–1000 g birth weight) registered in the NICHD Neonatal Research Network database showed no difference in BPD [158]. Another NSAID that is commonly used in premature neonates is ibuprofen. A retrospective study in extremely premature infants (<28 weeks) showed that ibuprofen effectively closed hemodynamically significant patent ductus arteriosus but increased the odds (odds ratio 2.3) of having BPD [159]. Acetaminophen has become a popular NSAID in treating patent ductus arteriosus, but its impact on BPD is presently unknown [160].

Although neonatal infection is an independent risk factor for BPD, prophylactic antimicrobial treatment is not recommended due to the high probability of cultivating multi-resistant bacteria. Both early exposure to broad-spectrum antibiotics and prolonged antibiotic treatment in human premature neonates have been shown to increase the odds of moderate to severe BPD [161]. One recent animal study showed that perinatal maternal antibiotic exposure augments the severity of BPD [80]. These findings have been explained by changing the microbiomes in premature neonates, leading to dysbiosis that increases the susceptibility to BPD [162]. Unlike broad-spectrum antibiotics, macrolides are used more specifically to treat Ureaplasma or Mycoplasma infections with anti-inflammatory properties [163]. Among all studied macrolides, only prophylactic azithromycin treatment significantly reduced BPD [164]. There is, however, a lack of pharmacokinetic data and information about the potential side effects of their use in premature neonates.

5.6. Pharmacology Agents with Anti-Inflammatory and Antioxidative Properties for BPD

5.6.1. Vitamin A

The efficacy of intramuscular vitamin A injection has been shown to decrease BPD in premature infants [18]. Vitamin A has antioxidative properties due to its hydrophobic chain of polyene units, which can quench singlet oxygen, neutralize thiyl radicals, and stabilize peroxyl radicals [165]. However, we must remember that this antioxidative property is effective only in low-oxygen tension environments. When oxygen tension is high, such as in the lungs under a hyperoxic condition, vitamin A will auto-oxidize. Multiple randomized controlled trials have shown its anti-inflammatory activity [166]. Although systemic analysis demonstrated its efficacy in decreasing BPD [167], clinicians do not commonly use it because it needs to be administered by intramuscular injection [168]. Enteral low-dose vitamin A has been studied in four trials (800 neonates <1500 g birth weight or <32 weeks) but did not show any decrease in BPD by meta-analysis [169]. Inhaled vitamin A offered better protection against BPD than intramuscular injections in the rat hyperoxia model [170]. An NIH-funded Phase-IIB study was recently granted to study the efficacy of inhaled vitamin A on BPD after a successful rat study [171].

5.6.2. Caffeine

Caffeine is a commonly used drug to treat the apnea of prematurity. The successful reduction in BPD in premature neonates from the CAP trial as the secondary outcome analysis [19] prompted us to investigate the mechanisms. We first showed in the rat hyperoxia BPD model that hyperoxia caused endoplasmic reticulum stress, mitochondrial fission, inflammation, and OS-mediated lung injury. Early administration of caffeine effectively reversed these hyperoxia-mediated changes [172]. Our group further showed in the same animal model that caffeine reversed endothelial nitric oxidase synthase uncoupling, at least in part, by preserving the tetrahydrobiopterin levels [112]. The antioxidative effect of caffeine was further demonstrated by Endesfelder et al. by showing decreased H_2O_2, malondialdehyde, and 8-OHdG with increased expression of SODs in the hyperoxia rat BPD model [173]. Using an intra-amniotic lipopolysaccharide injection BPD model in rats, Köroğlu et al. demonstrated the anti-inflammatory effect of caffeine with a reduction in the inflammatory response and improved lung morphometry and the measured resistance of the respiratory system [174]. Endesfelder et al. further showed that caffeine achieves its anti-inflammatory effect by decreasing NFkB expression in hyperoxia-exposed neonatal rat lungs [175]. These animal studies show that caffeine attenuates BPD through antioxidative and anti-inflammatory effects.

5.6.3. Stem Cell Therapy

Stem cell treatment has been considered a promising treatment for BPD. Mesenchymal stem cells (MSC) have attracted the most attention for their ease of isolation, low immune reaction, anti-inflammatory and antioxidative activities [176,177], and reparative properties, mainly in animal studies [22,178]. Studies have shown that MSC therapy reduces inflammation, mitochondrial dysfunction, and fibrosis of neonatal lungs. MSC secretome [179] or exosome [180] are new stem cell therapy modalities that may avoid some of the side effects of MSC therapy. Still, concerns regarding possible vascular occlusion, potential tumorigenicity, and difficulty obtaining the appropriate number of cells and maintaining the quality are waiting to be resolved [23]. A clinical study has shown that human premature neonates tolerate stem cell therapy well, but its benefits for BPD remain to be revealed [22].

5.6.4. N-Acetyl-Lysyltyrosylcysteine Amide (KYC)

KYC is a novel N- and C-capped tripeptide that reversibly inhibits MPO activity to decrease HOCl production [181]. This MPO-inhibiting activity is not seen in vitamin A and caffeine [114]. All reported KYC studies were conducted in animal studies. It has been shown that KYC decreases vascular stress and increases vasorelaxation in sickle cell disease mice [182,183], attenuates experimental autoimmune encephalomyelitis in mice [184], reduces stroke in mice [185], mitigates inflammatory response to rat peritonitis [186], and ameliorates plaque psoriasis in mice [187]. Since neutrophil infiltration is commonly seen in BPD rat lungs shortly after hyperoxia exposure [172], it was hypothesized that KYC might be able to attenuate the severity of BPD by reducing MPO activity. In hyperoxia rat BPD lungs, KYC decreases neutrophil infiltration and MPO expression, indicating anti-inflammatory activity [114]. In that study, the reduced expressions of cyclooxygenases, TLR4, RAGE, and extracellular HMGB1 in BPD lungs further support the presence of an anti-inflammatory property of KYC. It is crucial to know that the anti-inflammatory activity of KYC requires the presence of MPO. MPO transforms KYC into a thiylating species that oxidizes HMGB1 and inhibits HMGB1 binding to TLR4 and RAGE [114]. Reducing ER stress [113], autophagy, and cellular senescence [112] provides more mechanisms by which KYC decreases inflammation in BPD lungs.

The increased protein tyrosine chlorination in BPD rat lungs is significantly decreased by KYC treatment, indicating a reduction in HOCl formation. KYC's reduced 8-OHdG in BPD rat lungs under immunofluorescent staining agrees with the finding above [114]. KYC facilitates the expression of Nrf2-induced antioxidative enzymes through thiylation and glutathionylation of the Keap1, followed by stabilizing Nrf2, which offers one more mechanism for its antioxidative activity [114]. KYC further reduces ROS formation during the UPR by stabilizing the endoplasmic reticulum [112]. KYC thus has multiple mechanisms to achieve its antioxidative activity.

Compared to vitamin A and caffeine, KYC offers more protection mechanisms against hyperoxia-induced BPD, such as its impact on Nrf2 and HMGB1 signalings. By maintaining a higher count of type 2 alveolar cells for the presumptive resident progenitor cells in neonatal lungs [188] under hyperoxia, KYC might support better lung growth potential. We thus coined the term systems pharmacological agent for KYC to describe its multi-layer protection against BPD. Transcriptomic studies show increased leukocyte (macrophage, neutrophil, and lymphocyte) migration, chemotaxis, degranulation, differentiation, proliferation, and NETosis, with decreased WNT-catenin and Notch signalings in hyperoxia BPD rat lungs. KYC can reverse all these transcriptomic changes in BPD rat lungs. From the transcriptomic results, it is clear that KYC offers more mechanisms to reduce BPD. KYC is currently being studied in an NIH-funded preclinical study for BPD.

6. Conclusions

BPD is a common complication of prematurity [1,2]. BPD's most critical risk factors include supplemental oxygen, mechanical ventilation, and infection [1]. As evidence of increased OS [84] and inflammation [62] are consistently detected in human preterm birth, we believe both prenatal mechanisms play crucial roles in BPD onset. Unfortunately, the clinical reports do not allow us to interpret the temporal relationship between OS and inflammation confidently. The limited clinical studies showing the benefit of antenatal *N*-acetylcysteine in reducing BPD [152] and maternal antibiotic exposure increasing BPD [79] suggest OS is the more critical antenatal mechanism for BPD onset. Postnatal respiratory support and infections undoubtedly add more OS and inflammation to premature lungs and contribute to BPD progression.

Most neonatologists have already adopted early surfactant replacement and gentle respiratory support in managing premature neonates [189]. However, meta-analysis has yet to confirm the efficacy of gentle respiratory support for BPD. Animal studies have revealed that postnatal OS and inflammation mutually affect each other during BPD development [54], but the available evidence does not allow us to detail the temporal relationship between them. Prolonged use and prophylactic broad-spectrum antibiotics are not recommended for their strong association with the emergence of multi-resistant bacteria and dysbiosis in premature neonates, and surprisingly, a strong association with moderate to severe BPD was reported [161].

Early caffeine treatment and intramuscular vitamin A injection are proven therapeutic strategies that decrease BPD [18,19]. Both reagents have dual antioxidative and anti-inflammatory activities. The original intramuscular vitamin A study improved the survival rate without BPD by 7% compared to the control group [190]. Unfortunately, the three times weekly intramuscular injection to small premature neonates has made it unpopular to most neonatologists [170]. The original CAP trial shows caffeine decreased BPD by 9% [19]. Meta-analysis of five cohort studies showed that early caffeine treatment (<three days) reduces the BPD compared to late (>three days) caffeine treatment but increases the death rate [191]. Another meta-analysis of 15 cohorts shows that high-dose caffeine (>10 mg/kg/d) offers better BPD reduction than low-dose caffeine (<10 mg/kg/d) but with worse weight gain [192]. More studies are thus needed to determine the best starting time and dose of caffeine treatment.

Although early caffeine and vitamin A treatment reduce BPD by ~10%, more than 35% of premature infants will still develop BPD. There remains room for improvement. As OS and inflammation mutually elicit each other [46], we hypothesize that therapeutic agents with antioxidant and anti-inflammatory properties are needed for BPD treatment. Knowing whether combining intramuscular vitamin A with early caffeine treatment will decrease BPD in premature infants will be essential. The newly developed systems pharmacology agent KYC also holds promise as it involves many layers of protection against BPD. As so many mechanisms are involved in BPD development, a systems pharmacology approach will be required for its treatment.

Author Contributions: Conceptualization, writing, and visualization: T.-J.W., X.J., M.T., S.N. and R.-J.T.; organization and supervision: K.A.P.J., B.W.D., S.N. and R.-J.T.; funding acquisition: R.-J.T., B.W.D., K.A.P.J. and S.N. All authors have read and agreed to the published version of the manuscript.

Funding: This work was supported by NHLBI R44HL166018 (X.J., B.W.D., K.A.P.J., S.N. and R.-J.T.) and NHLBI R01HL128371 (R.-J.T. and K.A.P.J.).

Institutional Review Board Statement: Not applicable.

Informed Consent Statement: Not applicable.

Data Availability Statement: The original contributions presented in the study are included in the article; further inquiries can be directed to the corresponding author.

Conflicts of Interest: K.A.P.J., B.W.D. and S.N. own ReNeuroGen LLC, which is developing the drug candidate KYC as a potential therapeutic intervention in BPD. At present, KYC is in the preclinical phase of development. All other authors report no conflicts of interest.

References

1. Thébaud, B.; Goss, K.N.; Laughon, M.; Whitsett, J.A.; Abman, S.H.; Steinhorn, R.H.; Aschner, J.L.; Davis, P.G.; McGrath-Morrow, S.A.; Soll, R.F.; et al. Bronchopulmonary dysplasia. *Nat. Rev. Dis. Primers* **2019**, *5*, 78. [CrossRef] [PubMed]
2. Nuthakki, S.; Ahmad, K.; Johnson, G.; Cuevas Guaman, M. Bronchopulmonary Dysplasia: Ongoing Challenges from Definitions to Clinical Care. *J. Clin. Med.* **2023**, *12*, 3864. [CrossRef] [PubMed]
3. Stoll, B.J.; Hansen, N.I.; Bell, E.F.; Shankaran, S.; Laptook, A.R.; Walsh, M.C.; Hale, E.C.; Newman, N.S.; Schibler, K.; Carlo, W.A.; et al. Neonatal outcomes of extremely preterm infants from the NICHD Neonatal Research Network. *Pediatrics* **2010**, *126*, 443–456. [CrossRef] [PubMed]
4. Bancalari, E.; Jain, D. Bronchopulmonary Dysplasia: 50 Years after the Original Description. *Neonatology* **2019**, *115*, 384–391. [CrossRef] [PubMed]
5. Shennan, A.T.; Dunn, M.S.; Ohlsson, A.; Lennox, K.; Hoskins, E.M. Abnormal pulmonary outcomes in premature infants: Prediction from oxygen requirement in the neonatal period. *Pediatrics* **1988**, *82*, 527–532. [CrossRef]
6. Hansmann, G.; Sallmon, H.; Roehr, C.C.; Kourembanas, S.; Austin, E.D.; Koestenberger, M.; European Pediatric Pulmonary Vascular Disease Network (EPPVDN). Pulmonary hypertension in bronchopulmonary dysplasia. *Pediatr. Res.* **2021**, *89*, 446–455. [CrossRef]
7. Berkelhamer, S.K.; Mestan, K.K.; Steinhorn, R.H. Pulmonary hypertension in bronchopulmonary dysplasia. *Semin. Perinatol.* **2013**, *37*, 124–131. [CrossRef]

8. Chan, S.; Brugha, R.; Quyam, S.; Moledina, S. Diagnosis and management of pulmonary hypertension in infants with bronchopulmonary dysplasia: A guide for paediatric respiratory specialists. *Breathe* **2022**, *18*, 220209. [CrossRef]
9. Doyle, L.W.; Anderson, P.J. Long-term outcomes of bronchopulmonary dysplasia. *Semin. Fetal Neonatal Med.* **2009**, *14*, 391–395. [CrossRef]
10. Homan, T.D.; Nayak, R.P. Short- and Long-Term Complications of Bronchopulmonary Dysplasia. *Respir. Care* **2021**, *66*, 1618–1629. [CrossRef]
11. Islam, J.Y.; Keller, R.L.; Aschner, J.L.; Hartert, T.V.; Moore, P.E. Understanding the Short- and Long-Term Respiratory Outcomes of Prematurity and Bronchopulmonary Dysplasia. *Am. J. Respir. Crit. Care Med.* **2015**, *192*, 134–156. [CrossRef] [PubMed]
12. McGrath-Morrow, S.A.; Collaco, J.M. Bronchopulmonary dysplasia: What are its links to COPD? *Ther. Adv. Respir. Dis.* **2019**, *13*, 1753466619892492. [CrossRef] [PubMed]
13. McEvoy, C.T.; Jain, L.; Schmidt, B.; Abman, S.; Bancalari, E.; Aschner, J.L. Bronchopulmonary dysplasia: NHLBI Workshop on the Primary Prevention of Chronic Lung Diseases. *Ann. Am. Thorac. Soc.* **2014**, *11* (Suppl. 3), S146–S153. [CrossRef] [PubMed]
14. Davidson, L.M.; Berkelhamer, S.K. Bronchopulmonary Dysplasia: Chronic Lung Disease of Infancy and Long-Term Pulmonary Outcomes. *J. Clin. Med.* **2017**, *6*, 4. [CrossRef] [PubMed]
15. Lee, H.C.; Liu, J.; Profit, J.; Hintz, S.R.; Gould, J.B. Survival without Major Morbidity among Very Low Birth Weight Infants in California. *Pediatrics* **2020**, *146*, e20193865. [CrossRef]
16. Hysinger, E.B.; Ahlfeld, S.K. Respiratory support strategies in the prevention and treatment of bronchopulmonary dysplasia. *Front. Pediatr.* **2023**, *11*, 1087857. [CrossRef]
17. Panagiotounakou, P.; Sokou, R.; Gounari, E.; Konstantinidi, A.; Antonogeorgos, G.; Grivea, I.N.; Daniil, Z.; Gourgouliannis, K.I. Very preterm neonates receiving "aggressive" nutrition and early nCPAP had similar long-term respiratory outcomes as term neonates. *Pediatr. Res.* **2019**, *86*, 742–748. [CrossRef]
18. Tyson, J.E.; Wright, L.L.; Oh, W.; Kennedy, K.A.; Mele, L.; Ehrenkranz, R.A.; Stoll, B.J.; Lemons, J.A.; Stevenson, D.K.; Bauer, C.R.; et al. Vitamin A supplementation for extremely-low-birth-weight infants. National Institute of Child Health and Human Development Neonatal Research Network. *N. Engl. J. Med.* **1999**, *340*, 1962–1968. [CrossRef]
19. Schmidt, B.; Roberts, R.S.; Davis, P.; Doyle, L.W.; Barrington, K.J.; Ohlsson, A.; Solimano, A.; Tin, W.; Caffeine for Apnea of Prematurity Trial Group. Caffeine therapy for apnea of prematurity. *N. Engl. J. Med.* **2006**, *354*, 2112–2121. [CrossRef]
20. Yeh, T.F.; Lin, Y.J.; Huang, C.C.; Chen, Y.J.; Lin, C.H.; Lin, H.C.; Hsieh, W.S.; Lien, Y.J. Early dexamethasone therapy in preterm infants: A follow-up study. *Pediatrics* **1998**, *101*, E7. [CrossRef]
21. Jensen, E.A.; Wiener, L.E.; Rysavy, M.A.; Dysart, K.C.; Gantz, M.G.; Eichenwald, E.C.; Greenberg, R.G.; Harmon, H.M.; Laughon, M.M.; Watterberg, K.L.; et al. Assessment of Corticosteroid Therapy and Death or Disability according to Pretreatment Risk of Death or Bronchopulmonary Dysplasia in Extremely Preterm Infants. *JAMA Netw. Open* **2023**, *6*, e2312277. [CrossRef] [PubMed]
22. Omar, S.A.; Abdul-Hafez, A.; Ibrahim, S.; Pillai, N.; Abdulmageed, M.; Thiruvenkataramani, R.P.; Mohamed, T.; Madhukar, B.V.; Uhal, B.D. Stem-Cell Therapy for Bronchopulmonary Dysplasia (BPD) in Newborns. *Cells* **2022**, *11*, 1275. [CrossRef] [PubMed]
23. Simones, A.A.; Beisang, D.J.; Panoskaltsis-Mortari, A.; Roberts, K.D. Mesenchymal stem cells in the pathogenesis and treatment of bronchopulmonary dysplasia: A clinical review. *Pediatr. Res.* **2018**, *83*, 308–317. [CrossRef]
24. Eick, S.M.; Geiger, S.D.; Alshawabkeh, A.; Aung, M.; Barrett, E.S.; Bush, N.; Carroll, K.N.; Cordero, J.F.; Goin, D.E.; Ferguson, K.K.; et al. Urinary oxidative stress biomarkers are associated with preterm birth: An Environmental Influences on Child Health Outcomes program study. *Am. J. Obstet. Gynecol.* **2023**, *228*, 576.e1–576.e22. [CrossRef]
25. Kim, C.J.; Romero, R.; Chaemsaithong, P.; Chaiyasit, N.; Yoon, B.H.; Kim, Y.M. Acute chorioamnionitis and funisitis: Definition, pathologic features, and clinical significance. *Am. J. Obstet. Gynecol.* **2015**, *213* (Suppl. 4), S29–S52. [CrossRef]
26. Cheah, F.C.; Jobe, A.H.; Moss, T.J.; Newnham, J.P.; Kallapur, S.G. Oxidative stress in fetal lambs exposed to intra-amniotic endotoxin in a chorioamnionitis model. *Pediatr. Res.* **2008**, *63*, 274–279. [CrossRef]
27. Rubarth, L.B.; Quinn, J. Respiratory Development and Respiratory Distress Syndrome. *Neonatal Netw.* **2015**, *34*, 231–238. [CrossRef]
28. Zergeroglu, M.A.; McKenzie, M.J.; Shanely, R.A.; Van Gammeren, D.; DeRuisseau, K.C.; Powers, S.K. Mechanical ventilation-induced oxidative stress in the diaphragm. *J. Appl. Physiol.* **2003**, *95*, 1116–1124. [CrossRef] [PubMed]
29. Perveen, S.; Chen, C.M.; Sobajima, H.; Zhou, X.; Chen, J.Y. Editorial: Bronchopulmonary dysplasia: Latest advances. *Front. Pediatr.* **2023**, *11*, 1303761. [CrossRef]
30. Speer, C.P. Inflammation and bronchopulmonary dysplasia: A continuing story. *Semin. Fetal Neonatal Med.* **2006**, *11*, 354–362. [CrossRef]
31. Murch, S.H.; Costeloe, K.; Klein, N.J.; MacDonald, T.T. Early production of macrophage inflammatory protein-1 alpha occurs in respiratory distress syndrome and is associated with poor outcome. *Pediatr. Res.* **1996**, *40*, 490–497. [CrossRef] [PubMed]
32. Balany, J.; Bhandari, V. Understanding the Impact of Infection, Inflammation, and Their Persistence in the Pathogenesis of Bronchopulmonary Dysplasia. *Front. Med.* **2015**, *2*, 90. [CrossRef] [PubMed]
33. Ratajczak, C.K.; Fay, J.C.; Muglia, L.J. Preventing preterm birth: The past limitations and new potential of animal models. *Dis. Model. Mech.* **2010**, *3*, 407–414. [CrossRef] [PubMed]
34. Yeh, T.F.; Lin, Y.J.; Lin, H.C.; Huang, C.C.; Hsieh, W.S.; Lin, C.H.; Tsai, C.H. Outcomes at school age after postnatal dexamethasone therapy for lung disease of prematurity. *N. Engl. J. Med.* **2004**, *350*, 1304–1313. [CrossRef] [PubMed]

35. Cummings, J.J.; Pramanik, A.K.; Committee on Fetus and Newborn. Postnatal Corticosteroids to Prevent or Treat Chronic Lung Disease Following Preterm Birth. *Pediatrics* **2022**, *149*, e2022057530. [CrossRef]
36. Meyer, S.; Bay, J.; Franz, A.R.; Erhardt, H.; Klein, L.; Petzinger, J.; Binder, C.; Kirschenhofer, S.; Stein, A.; Hüning, B.; et al. Early postnatal high-dose fat-soluble enteral vitamin A supplementation for moderate or severe bronchopulmonary dysplasia or death in extremely low birthweight infants (NeoVitaA): A multicentre, randomised, parallel-group, double-blind, placebo-controlled, investigator-initiated phase 3 trial. *Lancet Respir. Med.* **2024**, *12*, 544–555.
37. Stone, W.L.; Bharti, D.; Shah, D.S.; Hollinger, S. The Redoxomics of Bronchopulmonary Dysplasia. In *Oxidative Stress in Lung Diseases*; Chakraborti, S., Chakraborti, T., Das, S., Chattopadhyay, D., Eds.; Springer: Singapore, 2019. [CrossRef]
38. Gambadauro, A.; Galletta, F.; Li Pomi, A.; Manti, S.; Piedimonte, G. Immune Response to Respiratory Viral Infections. *Int. J. Mol. Sci.* **2024**, *25*, 6178. [CrossRef]
39. Mittal, M.; Siddiqui, M.R.; Tran, K.; Reddy, S.P.; Malik, A.B. Reactive oxygen species in inflammation and tissue injury. *Antioxid. Redox Signal.* **2014**, *20*, 1126–1167. [CrossRef]
40. Furman, D.; Campisi, J.; Verdin, E.; Carrera-Bastos, P.; Targ, S.; Franceschi, C.; Ferrucci, L.; Gilroy, D.W.; Fasano, A.; Miller, G.W.; et al. Chronic inflammation in the etiology of disease across the life span. *Nat. Med.* **2019**, *25*, 1822–1832. [CrossRef]
41. Di Dalmazi, G.; Hirshberg, J.; Lyle, D.; Freij, J.B.; Caturegli, P. Reactive oxygen species in organ-specific autoimmunity. *Auto. Immun. Highlights* **2016**, *7*, 11. [CrossRef]
42. Masenga, S.K.; Kabwe, L.S.; Chakulya, M.; Kirabo, A. Mechanisms of Oxidative Stress in Metabolic Syndrome. *Int. J. Mol. Sci.* **2023**, *24*, 7898. [CrossRef] [PubMed]
43. Olufunmilayo, E.O.; Gerke-Duncan, M.B.; Holsinger, R.M.D. Oxidative Stress and Antioxidants in Neurodegenerative Disorders. *Antioxidants* **2023**, *12*, 517. [CrossRef]
44. Marseglia, L.; Manti, S.; D'Angelo, G.; Nicotera, A.; Parisi, E.; Di Rosa, G.; Gitto, E.; Arrigo, T. Oxidative Stress in Obesity: A Critical Component in Human Diseases. *Int. J. Mol. Sci.* **2015**, *16*, 378–400. [CrossRef]
45. Rovira-Llopis, S.; Bañuls, C.; Diaz-Morales, N.; Hernandez-Mijares, A.; Rocha, M.; Victor, V.M. Mitochondrial dynamics in type 2 diabetes: Pathophysiological implications. *Redox Biol.* **2017**, *11*, 637–645. [CrossRef]
46. Biswas, S.K. Does the Interdependence between Oxidative Stress and Inflammation Explain the Antioxidant Paradox? *Oxid. Med. Cell. Longev.* **2016**, *2016*, 5698931. [CrossRef] [PubMed]
47. Cao, S.S.; Kaufman, R.J. Endoplasmic reticulum stress and oxidative stress in cell fate decision and human disease. *Antioxid. Redox Signal.* **2014**, *21*, 396–413. [CrossRef] [PubMed]
48. Filomeni, G.; De Zio, D.; Cecconi, F. Oxidative stress and autophagy: The clash between damage and metabolic needs. *Cell Death Differ.* **2015**, *22*, 377–388. [CrossRef] [PubMed]
49. Faraonio, R. Oxidative Stress and Cell Senescence Process. *Antioxidants* **2022**, *11*, 1718. [CrossRef]
50. Wu, T.-J.; Jing, X.; Teng, M.; Pritchard, K.A., Jr.; Day, B.W.; Naylor, S.; Teng, R.-J. Role of Myeloperoxidase, Oxidative Stress, and Inflammation in Bronchopulmonary Dysplasia. *Antioxidants* **2024**, *13*, 889. [CrossRef]
51. Roh, J.S.; Sohn, D.H. Damage-Associated Molecular Patterns in Inflammatory Diseases. *Immune Netw.* **2018**, *18*, e27. [CrossRef]
52. Qian, M.; Fang, X.; Wang, X. Autophagy and inflammation. *Clin. Transl. Med.* **2017**, *6*, 24. [CrossRef] [PubMed]
53. Bhatia, S.; Rawal, R.; Sharma, P.; Singh, T.; Singh, M.; Singh, V. Mitochondrial Dysfunction in Alzheimer's Disease: Opportunities for Drug Development. *Curr. Neuropharmacol.* **2022**, *20*, 675–692. [CrossRef] [PubMed]
54. Moon, H.E.; Paek, S.H. Mitochondrial Dysfunction in Parkinson's Disease. *Exp. Neurobiol.* **2015**, *24*, 103–116. [CrossRef] [PubMed]
55. Lingappan, K. NF-κB in Oxidative Stress. *Curr. Opin. Toxicol.* **2018**, *7*, 81–86. [CrossRef] [PubMed]
56. Savani, R.C. Modulators of inflammation in Bronchopulmonary Dysplasia. *Semin. Perinatol.* **2018**, *42*, 459–470. [CrossRef]
57. Yang, G.; Abate, A.; George, A.G.; Weng, Y.-H.; Dennery, P.A. Maturational differences in lung NF-kappaB activation and their role in tolerance to hyperoxia. *J. Clin. Invest.* **2004**, *114*, 669–678. [CrossRef]
58. Perrone, S.; Manti, S.; Buttarelli, L.; Petrolini, C.; Boscarino, G.; Filonzi, L.; Gitto, E.; Esposito, S.M.R.; Nonnis Marzano, F. Vascular Endothelial Growth Factor as Molecular Target for Bronchopulmonary Dysplasia Prevention in Very Low Birth Weight Infants. *Int. J. Mol. Sci.* **2023**, *24*, 2729. [CrossRef]
59. Dahlin, K.; Mager, E.M.; Allen, L.; Tigue, Z.; Goodglick, L.; Wadehra, M.; Dobbs, L. Identification of genes differentially expressed in rat alveolar type I cells. *Am. J. Respir. Cell Mol. Biol.* **2004**, *31*, 309–316. [CrossRef]
60. Griffin, J.F.T.; Beck, I. A Longitudinal Study of Leucocyte Numbers and Mitogenesis during the Last Ten Weeks of Human Pregnancy. *J. Reprod. Immunol.* **1983**, *5*, 239–247. [CrossRef]
61. Hung, T.H.; Lo, L.M.; Chiu, T.H.; Li, M.J.; Yeh, Y.L.; Chen, S.F.; Hsieh, T.T. A longitudinal study of oxidative stress and antioxidant status in women with uncomplicated pregnancies throughout gestation. *Reprod. Sci.* **2010**, *17*, 401–409. [CrossRef]
62. Aghaeepour, N.; Ganio, E.A.; Mcilwain, D.; Tsai, A.S.; Tingle, M.; Van Gassen, S.; Gaudilliere, D.K.; Baca, Q.; McNeil, L.; Okada, R.; et al. An Immune Clock of Human Pregnancy. *Sci. Immunol.* **2017**, *2*, eaan2946. [CrossRef] [PubMed]
63. Anderson, J.; Thang, C.M.; Thanh, L.Q.; Dai, V.T.T.; Phan, V.T.; Nhu, B.T.H.; Trang, D.N.X.; Trinh, P.T.P.; Nguyen, T.V.; Toan, N.T.; et al. Immune Profiling of Cord Blood From Preterm and Term Infants Reveals Distinct Differences in Pro-inflammatory Responses. *Front. Immunol.* **2021**, *12*, 777927. [CrossRef] [PubMed]
64. Tita, A.T.; Andrews, W.W. Diagnosis and management of clinical chorioamnionitis. *Clin. Perinatol.* **2010**, *37*, 339–354. [CrossRef] [PubMed]

65. Gimeno-Molina, B.; Muller, I.; Kropf, P.; Sykes, L. The Role of Neutrophils in Pregnancy, Term and Preterm Labour. *Life* **2022**, *12*, 1512. [CrossRef] [PubMed]
66. Rinaldi, S.F.; Hutchinson, J.L.; Rossi, A.G.; Norman, J.E. Anti-inflammatory mediators as physiological and pharmacological regulators of parturition. *Expert. Rev. Clin. Immunol.* **2011**, *7*, 675–696. [CrossRef]
67. Tong, M.; Abrahams, V.M. Neutrophils in preterm birth: Friend or foe? *Placenta* **2020**, *102*, 17–20. [CrossRef]
68. Rinaldi, S.F.; Catalano, R.D.; Wade, J.; Rossi, A.G.; Norman, J.E. Decidual Neutrophil Infiltration Is Not Required for Preterm Birth in a Mouse Model of Infection-Induced Preterm Labor. *J. Immunol.* **2014**, *192*, 2315–2325. [CrossRef]
69. Timmons BC and Mahendroo MS, Timing of neutrophil activation and expression of pro-inflammatory markers do not support a role for neutrophils in cervical ripening in the mouse. *Biol. Reprod.* **2006**, *74*, 236–245. [CrossRef]
70. Gibbs, R.S.; Duff, P. Progress in pathogenesis and management of clinical intraamniotic infection. *Am. J. Obstet. Gynecol.* **1991**, *164*, 1317. [CrossRef]
71. Agrawal, V.; Hirsch, E. Intrauterine infection and preterm labor. *Semin. Fetal Neonatal Med.* **2012**, *17*, 12–19. [CrossRef]
72. Lukanović, D.; Batkoska, M.; Kavšek, G.; Druškovič, M. Clinical chorioamnionitis: Where do we stand now? *Front. Med.* **2023**, *10*, 1191254. [CrossRef] [PubMed]
73. Bartha, J.L.; Romero-Carmona, R.; Comino-Delgado, R. Inflammatory cytokines in intrauterine growth retardation. *Acta Obstet. Gynecol. Scand.* **2003**, *82*, 1099–1102. [CrossRef] [PubMed]
74. Cadaret, C.N.; Merrick, E.M.; Barnes, T.L.; Beede, K.A.; Posont, R.J.; Petersen, J.L.; Yates, D.T. Sustained maternal inflammation during the early third-trimester yields intrauterine growth restriction, impaired skeletal muscle glucose metabolism, and diminished β-cell function in fetal sheep1,2. *J. Anim. Sci.* **2019**, *97*, 4822–4833. [CrossRef]
75. White, M.R.; Yates, D.T. Dousing the flame: Reviewing the mechanisms of inflammatory programming during stress-induced intrauterine growth restriction and the potential for ω-3 polyunsaturated fatty acid intervention. *Front. Physiol.* **2023**, *14*, 1250134. [CrossRef] [PubMed]
76. Goldstein, J.A.; Gallagher, K.; Beck, C.; Kumar, R.; Gernand, A.D. Maternal-Fetal Inflammation in the Placenta and the Developmental Origins of Health and Disease. *Front. Immunol.* **2020**, *11*, 531543. [CrossRef]
77. Gibbs, R.S.; Blanco, J.D.; St Clair, P.J.; Castaneda, Y.S. Quantitative bacteriology of amniotic fluid from women with clinical intraamniotic infection at term. *J. Infect. Dis.* **1982**, *145*, 1–8. [CrossRef]
78. Beck, C.; Gallagher, K.; Taylor, L.A.; Goldstein, J.A.; Mithal, L.B.; Gernand, A.D. Chorioamnionitis and Risk for Maternal and Neonatal Sepsis: A Systematic Review and Meta-analysis. *Obstet. Gynecol.* **2021**, *137*, 1007–1022. [CrossRef]
79. Villamor-Martinez, E.; Álvarez-Fuente, M.; Ghazi, A.M.T.; Degraeuwe, P.; Zimmermann, L.J.I.; Kramer, B.W.; Villamor, E. Association of Chorioamnionitis with Bronchopulmonary Dysplasia Among Preterm Infants: A Systematic Review, Meta-analysis, and Metaregression. *JAMA Netw. Open* **2019**, *2*, e1914611. [CrossRef] [PubMed]
80. Willis, K.A.; Siefker, D.T.; Aziz, M.M.; White, C.T.; Mussarat, N.; Gomes, C.K.; Bajwa, A.; Pierre, J.F.; Cormier, S.A.; Talati, A.J. Perinatal maternal antibiotic exposure augments lung injury in offspring in experimental bronchopulmonary dysplasia. *Am. J. Physiol. Lung Cell. Mol. Physiol.* **2020**, *318*, L407–L418. [CrossRef]
81. Wu, F.; Tian, F.-J.; Lin, Y. Oxidative stress in placenta: Health and diseases. *BioMed Res. Int.* **2015**, *2015*, e293271. [CrossRef]
82. Menon, R. Oxidative stress damage as a detrimental factor in preterm birth pathology. *Front. Immunol.* **2014**, *5*, 567. [CrossRef] [PubMed]
83. Chakravartya, S.; Sontakkeb, A.N. A correlation of antioxidants and lipid peroxidation between maternal and cord blood in full term and preterm deliveries. *Curr. Pediatr. Res.* **2012**, *16*, 167–174.
84. Dutta, E.H.; Behnia, F.; Boldogh, I.; George; Saade, R.; Brandie; Taylor, D.; Kacerovský, M.; Menon, R. Oxidative stress damage-associated molecular signaling pathways differentiate spontaneous preterm birth and preterm premature rupture of the membranes. *Mol. Hum. Reprod.* **2016**, *22*, 143–157. [CrossRef] [PubMed]
85. Martin, A.; Faes, C.; Debevec, T.; Rytz, C.; Millet, G.; Pialoux, V. Preterm birth and oxidative stress: Effects of acute physical exercise and hypoxia physiological responses. *Redox Biol.* **2018**, *17*, 315–322. [CrossRef]
86. Comporti, M.; Signorini, C.; Signorini, C.; Leoncini, S.; Buonocore, G.; Rossi, V.; Ciccoli, L. Plasma F2-isoprostanes are elevated in newborns and inversely correlated to gestational age. Free Radic. *Biol. Med.* **2004**, *37*, 724–732.
87. Negi, R.; Pande, D.; Kumar, A.; Khanna, R.S.; Khanna, H.D. Evaluation of biomarkers of oxidative stress and antioxidant capacity in the cord blood of preterm low birth weight neonates. *J. Matern. Fetal Neonatal Med.* **2012**, *25*, 1338–1341. [CrossRef]
88. Cipierre, C.; Haÿs, S.; Maucort-Boulch, D.; Steghens, J.P.; Picaud, J.C. Malondialdehyde adduct to hemoglobin: A new marker of oxidative stress suitable for full-term and preterm neonates. *Oxid. Med. Cell. Longev.* **2013**, *2013*, e694014. [CrossRef]
89. Ochoa, J.J.; Ramirez-Tortosa, M.C.; Quiles, J.L.; Palomino, N.; Robles, R.; Mataix, J.; Huertas, J.R. Oxidative stress in erythrocytes from premature and full-term infants during their first 72 h of life. *Free Radic. Res.* **2003**, *37*, 317–322. [CrossRef]
90. Negi, R.; Pande, D.; Kumar, A.; Khanna, R.S.; Khanna, H.D. In vivo oxidative DNA damage and lipid peroxidation as a biomarker of oxidative stress in preterm low-birthweight infants. *J. Trop. Pediatr.* **2012**, *58*, 326–328. [CrossRef]
91. Weber, D.; Stuetz, W.; Bernhard, W.; Franz, A.; Raith, M.; Grune, T.; Breusing, N. Oxidative stress markers and micronutrients in maternal and cord blood in relation to neonatal outcome. *Eur. J. Clin. Nutr.* **2014**, *68*, 215–222. [CrossRef]
92. Zeitlin, J.; Ancel, P.Y.; Saurel-Cubizolles, M.J.; Papiernik, E. The relationship between intrauterine growth restriction and preterm delivery: An empirical approach using data from a European case-control study. *BJOG* **2000**, *107*, 750–758. [CrossRef] [PubMed]

93. Silvestro, S.; Calcaterra, V.; Pelizzo, G.; Bramanti, P.; Mazzon, E. Prenatal Hypoxia and Placental Oxidative Stress: Insights from Animal Models to Clinical Evidences. *Antioxidants* **2020**, *9*, 414. [CrossRef] [PubMed]
94. Willis, K.A.; Ambalavanan, N. Necrotizing enterocolitis and the gut-lung axis. *Semin. Perinatol.* **2021**, *45*, 151454. [CrossRef]
95. Lembo, C.; Buonocore, G.; Perrone, S. Oxidative Stress in Preterm Newborns. *Antioxidants* **2021**, *10*, 1672. [CrossRef]
96. Norishadkam, M.; Andishmand, S.; Zavar Reza, J.; Zare Sakhvidi, M.J.; Hachesoo, V.R. Oxidative stress and DNA damage in the cord blood of preterm infants. *Mutat. Res.* **2017**, *824*, 20–24. [CrossRef]
97. Abdel Ghany, E.A.; Alsharany, W.; Ali, A.A.; Youness, E.R.; Hussein, J.S. Antioxidant profiles and markers of oxidative stress in preterm neonates. *Paediatr. Int. Child. Health* **2016**, *36*, 134–140. [CrossRef] [PubMed]
98. Chahin, N.; Yitayew, M.S.; Richards, A.; Forsthoffer, B.; Xu, J.; Hendricks-Muñoz, K.D. Ascorbic Acid and the Premature Infant. *Nutrients* **2022**, *14*, 2189. [CrossRef]
99. Moison, R.M.W.; Palinckx, J.J.S.; Roest, M.; Houdkamp, E.; Berger, H.M. Induction of lipid peroxidation of pulmonary surfactant by plasma of preterm babies. *Lancet* **1993**, *341*, 79–82. [CrossRef]
100. Lavoie, J.-C.; Chessex, P. Gender and maturation affect glutathione status in human neonatal tissues. *Free Radic. Biol. Med.* **1997**, *23*, 648–657. [CrossRef]
101. Shimoda, L.A.; Semenza, G.L. HIF and the lung: Role of hypoxia-inducible factors in pulmonary development and disease. *Am. J. Respir. Crit. Care Med.* **2011**, *183*, 152–156. [CrossRef]
102. Saugstad, O.D.; Oei, J.L.; Lakshminrusimha, S.; Vento, M. Oxygen therapy of the newborn from molecular understanding to clinical practice. *Pediatr. Res.* **2019**, *85*, 20–29. [CrossRef] [PubMed]
103. Yadav, A.; Rana, U.; Michalkiewicz, T.; Teng, R.J.; Konduri, G.G. Decreased AMP-activated protein kinase (AMPK) function and protective effect of metformin in neonatal rat pups exposed to hyperoxia lung injury. *Physiol. Rep.* **2020**, *8*, e14587. [CrossRef] [PubMed]
104. Yu, X.; Zhao, X.; Cai, Q.; Zhang, D.; Liu, Z.; Zheng, H.; Xue, X.; Fu, J. Effects of Hyperoxia on Mitochondrial Homeostasis: Are Mitochondria the Hub for Bronchopulmonary Dysplasia? *Front. Cell Dev. Biol.* **2021**, *9*, 642717.
105. Jing, X.; Huang, Y.W.; Jarzembowski, J.; Shi, Y.; Konduri, G.G.; Teng, R.J. Caffeine ameliorates hyperoxia-induced lung injury by protecting GCH1 function in neonatal rat pups. *Pediatr. Res.* **2017**, *82*, 483–489. [CrossRef]
106. Hosford, G.E.; Fang, X.; Olson, D.M. Hyperoxia decreases matrix metalloproteinase-9 and increases tissue inhibitor of matrix metalloproteinase-1 protein in the newborn rat lung: Association with arrested alveolarization. *Pediatr. Res.* **2004**, *56*, 26–34. [CrossRef] [PubMed]
107. Thébaud, B.; Ladha, F.; Michelakis, E.D.; Sawicka, M.; Thurston, G.; Eaton, F.; Hashimoto, K.; Harry, G.; Haromy, A.; Korbutt, G.; et al. Vascular endothelial growth factor gene therapy increases survival, promotes lung angiogenesis, and prevents alveolar damage in hyperoxia-induced lung injury: Evidence that angiogenesis participates in alveolarization. *Circulation* **2005**, *112*, 2477–2486. [CrossRef]
108. Carvalho, C.G.; Procianoy, R.S.; Neto, E.C.; Silveira, R.C. Preterm Neonates with Respiratory Distress Syndrome: Ventilator-Induced Lung Injury and Oxidative Stress. *J. Immunol. Res.* **2018**, *2018*, 6963754. [CrossRef]
109. Joelsson, J.P.; Asbjarnarson, A.; Sigurdsson, S.; Kricker, J.; Valdimarsdottir, B.; Thorarinsdottir, H.; Starradottir, E.; Gudjonsson, T.; Ingthorsson, S.; Karason, S. Ventilator-induced lung injury results in oxidative stress response and mitochondrial swelling in a mouse model. *Lab. Anim. Res.* **2022**, *38*, 23. [CrossRef]
110. Mohamed, T.; Abdul-Hafez, A.; Gewolb, I.H.; Uhal, B.D. Oxygen injury in neonates: Which is worse? hyperoxia, hypoxia, or alternating hyperoxia/hypoxia. *J. Lung Pulm. Respir. Res.* **2020**, *7*, 4–13.
111. Jónsson, B.; Tullus, K.; Brauner, A.; Lu, Y.; Noack, G. Early increase of TNF alpha and IL-6 in tracheobronchial aspirate fluid indicator of subsequent chronic lung disease in preterm infants. *Arch. Dis. Child. Fetal Neonatal Ed.* **1997**, *77*, F198–F201. [CrossRef]
112. Beckman, J.S.; Viera, L.; Estévez, A.G.; Teng, R. Nitric oxide and peroxynitrite in the perinatal period. *Semin. Perinatol.* **2000**, *24*, 37–41. [CrossRef] [PubMed]
113. Pattison, D.I.; Davies, M.J.; Hawkins, C.L. Reactions and reactivity of myeloperoxidase-derived oxidants: Differential biological effects of hypochlorous and hypothiocyanous acids. *Free Radic. Res.* **2012**, *46*, 975–995. [CrossRef] [PubMed]
114. Jing, X.; Jia, S.; Teng, M.; Day, B.W.; Afolayan, A.J.; Jarzembowski, J.A.; Lin, C.W.; Hessner, M.J.; Pritchard, K.A., Jr.; Naylor, S.; et al. Cellular Senescence Contributes to the Progression of Hyperoxic Bronchopulmonary Dysplasia. *Am. J. Respir. Cell Mol. Biol.* **2024**, *70*, 94–109. [CrossRef] [PubMed]
115. Pritchard, K.A., Jr.; Jing, X.; Teng, M.; Wells, C.; Jia, S.; Afolayan, A.J.; Jarzembowski, J.; Day, B.W.; Naylor, S.; Hessner, M.J.; et al. Role of endoplasmic reticulum stress in impaired neonatal lung growth and bronchopulmonary dysplasia. *PLoS ONE* **2022**, *17*, e0269564. [CrossRef]
116. Teng, R.J.; Jing, X.; Martin, D.P.; Hogg, N.; Haefke, A.; Konduri, G.G.; Day, B.W.; Naylor, S.; Pritchard, K.A., Jr. N-acetyl-lysyltyrosylcysteine amide, a novel systems pharmacology agent, reduces bronchopulmonary dysplasia in hyperoxic neonatal rat pups. *Free Radic. Biol. Med.* **2021**, *166*, 73–89. [CrossRef]
117. Pryhuber, G.S. Postnatal Infections and Immunology Affecting Chronic Lung Disease of Prematurity. *Clin. Perinatol.* **2015**, *42*, 697–718. [CrossRef] [PubMed]
118. Salimi, U.; Dummula, K.; Tucker, M.H.; Dela Cruz, C.S.; Sampath, V. Postnatal Sepsis and Bronchopulmonary Dysplasia in Premature Infants: Mechanistic Insights into "New BPD". *Am. J. Respir. Cell Mol. Biol.* **2022**, *66*, 137–145. [CrossRef]
119. Chen, G.Y.; Nuñez, G. Sterile inflammation: Sensing and reacting to damage. *Nat. Rev. Immunol.* **2010**, *10*, 826–837. [CrossRef]

120. Zhong, H.; Li, X.; Zhou, S.; Jiang, P.; Liu, X.; Ouyang, M.; Nie, Y.; Chen, X.; Zhang, L.; Liu, Y.; et al. Interplay between RAGE and TLR4 Regulates HMGB1-Induced Inflammation by Promoting Cell Surface Expression of RAGE and TLR4. *J. Immunol.* **2020**, *205*, 767–775. [CrossRef]
121. Chipurupalli, S.; Samavedam, U.; Robinson, N. Crosstalk Between ER Stress, Autophagy and Inflammation. *Front. Med.* **2021**, *8*, 758311. [CrossRef]
122. Pluquet, O.; Pourtier, A.; Abbadie, C. The unfolded protein response and cellular senescence. A review in the theme: Cellular mechanisms of endoplasmic reticulum stress signaling in health and disease. *Am. J. Physiol. Cell Physiol.* **2015**, *308*, C415–C425. [CrossRef] [PubMed]
123. Zhou, B.B.; Mattern, M.R.; Khanna, K.K. Role of tumor suppressors in DNA damage response. *Methods Mol. Biol.* **2003**, *223*, 39–50. [PubMed]
124. Bourgeois, B.; Madl, T. Regulation of cellular senescence via the FOXO4-p53 axis. *FEBS Lett.* **2018**, *592*, 2083–2097. [CrossRef]
125. Ohtani, N. The roles and mechanisms of senescence-associated secretory phenotype (SASP): Can it be controlled by senolysis? *Inflamm. Regen.* **2022**, *42*, 11. [CrossRef] [PubMed]
126. Halliwell, B. The antioxidant paradox. *Lancet* **2000**, *355*, 1179–1180. [CrossRef]
127. Jobe, A.H.; Goldenberg, R.L.; Kemp, M.W. Antenatal corticosteroids: An updated assessment of anticipated benefits and potential risks. *Am. J. Obstet. Gynecol.* **2024**, *230*, 330–339. [CrossRef]
128. Kribs, A.; Roberts, K.D.; Trevisanuto, D.; O'Donnell, C.; Dargaville, P.A. Surfactant delivery strategies to prevent bronchopulmonary dysplasia. *Semin. Perinatol.* **2023**, *47*, 151813. [CrossRef]
129. Saugstad, O.D.; Ramji, S.; Soll, R.F.; Vento, M. Resuscitation of newborn infants with 21% or 100% oxygen: An updated systematic review and meta-analysis. *Neonatology* **2008**, *94*, 176–182. [CrossRef] [PubMed]
130. Perlman, J.M.; Wyllie, J.; Kattwinkel, J.; Atkins, D.L.; Chameides, L.; Goldsmith, J.P.; Guinsburg, R.; Hazinski, M.F.; Morley, C.; Richmond, S.; et al. Neonatal resuscitation: 2010 International Consensus on Cardiopulmonary Resuscitation and Emergency Cardiovascular Care Science with Treatment Recommendations. *Pediatrics* **2010**, *126*, e1319–e1344. [CrossRef]
131. Sotiropoulos, J.X.; Oei, J.L.; Schmölzer, G.M.; Libesman, S.; Hunter, K.E.; Williams, J.G.; Webster, A.C.; Vento, M.; Kapadia, V.; Rabi, Y.; et al. Initial Oxygen Concentration for the Resuscitation of Infants Born at Less than 32 Weeks' Gestation: A Systematic Review and Individual Participant Data Network Meta-Analysis. *JAMA Pediatr.* **2024**, *178*, 774–783. [CrossRef]
132. STOP-ROP Multicenter Study Group. Supplemental Therapeutic Oxygen for Prethreshold Retinopathy of Prematurity (STOP-ROP), a randomized, controlled trial. I: Primary outcomes. *Pediatrics* **2000**, *105*, 295–310. [CrossRef] [PubMed]
133. Manja, V.; Saugstad, O.D.; Lakshminrusimha, S. Oxygen Saturation Targets in Preterm Infants and Outcomes at 18-24 Months: A Systematic Review. *Pediatrics* **2017**, *139*, e20161609. [CrossRef]
134. Stenson, B.J. Achieved Oxygenation Saturations and Outcome in Extremely Preterm Infants. *Clin. Perinatol.* **2019**, *46*, 601–610. [CrossRef]
135. Abman, S.H.; Hansmann, G.; Archer, S.L.; Ivy, D.D.; Adatia, I.; Chung, W.K.; Hanna, B.D.; Rosenzweig, E.B.; Raj, J.U.; Cornfield, D.; et al. Pediatric Pulmonary Hypertension: Guidelines From the American Heart Association and American Thoracic Society. *Circulation* **2015**, *132*, 2037–2099. [CrossRef] [PubMed]
136. Dumpa, V.; Bhandari, V. Noninvasive Ventilatory Strategies to Decrease Bronchopulmonary Dysplasia-Where Are We in 2021? *Children* **2021**, *8*, 132. [CrossRef]
137. Ackermann, B.W.; Klotz, D.; Hentschel, R.; Thome, U.H.; van Kaam, A.H. High-frequency ventilation in preterm infants and neonates. *Pediatr. Res.* **2023**, *93*, 1810–1818. [CrossRef] [PubMed]
138. Yagui, A.C.; Meneses, J.; Zólio, B.A.; Brito, G.M.G.; da Silva, R.J.; Rebello, C.M. Nasal continuous positive airway pressure (NCPAP) or noninvasive neurally adjusted ventilatory assist (NIV-NAVA) for preterm infants with respiratory distress after birth: A randomized controlled trial. *Pediatr. Pulmonol.* **2019**, *54*, 1704–1711. [CrossRef]
139. Jasani, B.; Ismail, A.; Rao, S.; Patole, S. Effectiveness and safety of nasal mask versus binasal prongs for providing continuous positive airway pressure in preterm infants-A systematic review and meta-analysis. *Pediatr. Pulmonol.* **2018**, *53*, 987–992. [CrossRef] [PubMed]
140. Subramaniam, P.; Ho, J.J.; Davis, P.G. Prophylactic nasal continuous positive airway pressure for preventing morbidity and mortality in very preterm infants. *Cochrane Database Syst. Rev.* **2016**, *6*, CD001243. [CrossRef]
141. Fischer, H.S.; Bührer, C. Avoiding endotracheal ventilation to prevent bronchopulmonary dysplasia: A meta-analysis. *Pediatrics* **2013**, *132*, e1351–e1360. [CrossRef]
142. Bjørklund, G.; Shanaida, M.; Lysiuk, R.; Antonyak, H.; Klishch, I.; Shanaida, V.; Peana, M. Selenium: An Antioxidant with a Critical Role in Anti-Aging. *Molecules* **2022**, *27*, 6613. [CrossRef] [PubMed]
143. Darlow, B.A.; Austin, N.C. Selenium supplementation to prevent short-term morbidity in preterm neonates. *Cochrane Database Syst. Rev.* **2003**, *2003*, CD003312. [CrossRef] [PubMed]
144. Davis, J.M. Superoxide dismutase: A role in the prevention of chronic lung disease. *Biol. Neonate* **1998**, *74* (Suppl. 1), 29–34. [CrossRef] [PubMed]
145. Albertella, M.; Gentyala, R.R.; Paraskevas, T.; Ehret, D.; Bruschettini, M.; Soll, R. Superoxide dismutase for bronchopulmonary dysplasia in preterm infants. *Cochrane Database Syst. Rev.* **2023**, *10*, CD013232. [PubMed]

146. McEvoy, C.T.; Shorey-Kendrick, L.E.; Milner, K.; Schilling, D.; Tiller, C.; Vuylsteke, B.; Scherman, A.; Jackson, K.; Haas, D.M.; Harris, J.; et al. Oral Vitamin C (500 mg/d) to Pregnant Smokers Improves Infant Airway Function at 3 Months (VCSIP). A Randomized Trial. *Am. J. Respir. Crit. Care Med.* **2019**, *199*, 1139–1147. [CrossRef]
147. Berger, T.M.; Frei, B.; Rifai, N.; Avery, M.E.; Suh, J.; Yoder, B.A.; Coalson, J.J. Early high dose antioxidant vitamins do not prevent bronchopulmonary dysplasia in premature baboons exposed to prolonged hyperoxia: A pilot study. *Pediatr. Res.* **1998**, *43*, 719–726. [CrossRef]
148. Stone, C.A., Jr.; McEvoy, C.T.; Aschner, J.L.; Kirk, A.; Rosas-Salazar, C.; Cook-Mills, J.M.; Moore, P.E.; Walsh, W.F.; Hartert, T.V. Update on Vitamin E and Its Potential Role in Preventing or Treating Bronchopulmonary Dysplasia. *Neonatology* **2018**, *113*, 366–378. [CrossRef]
149. Turner, S.W.; Campbell, D.; Smith, N.; Craig, L.C.A.; McNeill, G.; Forbes, S.H.; Harbour, P.J.; Seaton, A.; Helms, P.J.; Devereux, G.S. Associations between fetal size, maternal alpha-tocopherol and childhood asthma. *Thorax* **2010**, *65*, 391–397. [CrossRef]
150. Brion, L.; Bell, E.; Raghuveer, T. Vitamin E supplementation for prevention of morbidity and mortality in preterm infants. *Cochrane Database Syst. Rev.* **2003**, *2003*, CD003665. [CrossRef]
151. Ahola, T.; Lapatto, R.; Raivio, K.O.; Selander, B.; Stigson, L.; Jonsson, B.; Jonsbo, F.; Esberg, G.; Stövring, S.; Kjartansson, S.; et al. N-acetylcysteine does not prevent bronchopulmonary dysplasia in immature infants: A randomized controlled trial. *J. Pediatr.* **2003**, *143*, 713–719. [CrossRef]
152. Buhimschi, C.S.; Bahtiyar, M.O.; Zhao, G.; Abdelghany, O.; Schneider, L.; Razeq, S.A.; Dulay, A.T.; Lipkind, H.S.; Mieth, S.; Rogers, L.; et al. Antenatal N-acetylcysteine to improve outcomes of premature infants with intra-amniotic infection and inflammation (Triple I): Randomized clinical trial. *Pediatr. Res.* **2021**, *89*, 175–184. [CrossRef] [PubMed]
153. Revenis, M.E.; Kaliner, M.A. Lactoferrin and lysozyme deficiency in airway secretions: Association with the development of bronchopulmonary dysplasia. *J. Pediatr.* **1992**, *121*, 262–270. [CrossRef] [PubMed]
154. Gao, Y.; Hou, L.; Lu, C.; Wang, Q.; Pan, B.; Wang, Q.; Tian, J.; Ge, L. Enteral Lactoferrin Supplementation for Preventing Sepsis and Necrotizing Enterocolitis in Preterm Infants: A Meta-Analysis with Trial Sequential Analysis of Randomized Controlled Trials. *Front. Pharmacol.* **2020**, *11*, 1186. [CrossRef] [PubMed]
155. Doyle, L.W.; Cheong, J.L.; Ehrenkranz, R.A.; Halliday, H.L. Early (<8 days) systemic postnatal corticosteroids for prevention of bronchopulmonary dysplasia in preterm infants. *Cochrane Database Syst. Rev.* **2017**, *10*, CD001146. [PubMed]
156. Doyle, L.W.; Cheong, J.L.; Hay, S.; Manley, B.J.; Halliday, H.L. Late (≥7 days) systemic postnatal corticosteroids for prevention of bronchopulmonary dysplasia in preterm infants. *Cochrane Database Syst. Rev.* **2021**, *11*, CD001145. [CrossRef]
157. Schmidt, B.; Roberts, R.S.; Fanaroff, A.; Davis, P.; Kirpalani, H.M.; Nwaesei, C.; Vincer, M.; TIPP Investigators. Indomethacin prophylaxis, patent ductus arteriosus, and the risk of bronchopulmonary dysplasia: Further analyses from the Trial of Indomethacin Prophylaxis in Preterms (TIPP). *J. Pediatr.* **2006**, *148*, 730–734. [CrossRef]
158. Jensen, E.A.; Dysart, K.C.; Gantz, M.G.; Carper, B.; Higgins, R.D.; Keszler, M.; Laughon, M.M.; Poindexter, B.B.; Stoll, B.J.; Walsh, M.C.; et al. Association between Use of Prophylactic Indomethacin and the Risk for Bronchopulmonary Dysplasia in Extremely Preterm Infants. *J. Pediatr.* **2017**, *186*, 34–40.e2. [CrossRef]
159. Chen, X.; Qiu, X.; Sun, P.; Lin, Y.; Huang, Z.; Yang, C.; Walther, F.J. Neonatal ibuprofen exposure and bronchopulmonary dysplasia in extremely premature infants. *J. Perinatol.* **2020**, *40*, 124–129. [CrossRef]
160. Mitra, S.; Florez, I.D.; Tamayo, M.E.; Mbuagbaw, L.; Vanniyasingam, T.; Veroniki, A.A.; Zea, A.M.; Zhang, Y.; Sadeghirad, B.; Thabane, L. Association of Placebo, Indomethacin, Ibuprofen, and Acetaminophen with Closure of Hemodynamically Significant Patent Ductus Arteriosus in Preterm Infants: A Systematic Review and Meta-analysis. *JAMA* **2018**, *319*, 1221–1238. [CrossRef]
161. Shi, W.; Chen, Z.; Shi, L.; Jiang, S.; Zhou, J.; Gu, X.; Lei, X.; Xiao, T.; Zhu, Y.; Qian, A.; et al. Early Antibiotic Exposure and Bronchopulmonary Dysplasia in Very Preterm Infants at Low Risk of Early-Onset Sepsis. *JAMA Netw. Open* **2024**, *7*, e2418831. [CrossRef]
162. Lal, C.V.; Ambalavanan, N. Maternal antibiotics augment hyperoxia-induced lung injury in neonatal mice. *Am. J. Physiol. Lung Cell Mol. Physiol.* **2020**, *318*, L405–L406. [CrossRef] [PubMed]
163. Aghai, Z.H.; Kode, A.; Saslow, J.G.; Nakhla, T.; Farhath, S.; Stahl, G.E.; Eydelman, R.; Strande, L.; Leone, P.; Rahman, I. Azithromycin suppresses activation of nuclear factor-kappa B and synthesis of pro-inflammatory cytokines in tracheal aspirate cells from premature infants. *Pediatr. Res.* **2007**, *62*, 483–488. [CrossRef]
164. Nair, V.; Loganathan, P.; Soraisham, A.S. Azithromycin and other macrolides for prevention of bronchopulmonary dysplasia: A systematic review and meta-analysis. *Neonatology* **2014**, *106*, 337–347. [CrossRef]
165. Palace, V.P.; Khaper, N.; Qin, Q.; Singal, P.K. Antioxidant potentials of vitamin A and carotenoids and their relevance to heart disease. *Free Radic. Biol. Med.* **1999**, *26*, 746–761. [CrossRef] [PubMed]
166. Gholizadeh, M.; Basafa Roodi, P.; Abaj, F.; Shab-Bidar, S.; Saedisomeolia, A.; Asbaghi, O.; Lak, M. Influence of Vitamin A supplementation on inflammatory biomarkers in adults: A systematic review and meta-analysis of randomized clinical trials. *Sci. Rep.* **2022**, *12*, 21384. [CrossRef]
167. Huang, L.; Zhu, D.; Pang, G. The effects of early vitamin A supplementation on the prevention and treatment of bronchopulmonary dysplasia in premature infants: A systematic review and meta-analysis. *Transl. Pediatr.* **2021**, *10*, 3218–3229. [CrossRef]
168. Rakshasbhuvankar, A.; Pillow, J.J. Vitamin A and bronchopulmonary dysplasia: The next steps. *Lancet Respir. Med.* **2024**, *12*, 503–505. [CrossRef] [PubMed]

169. Manapurath, R.M.; Kumar, M.; Pathak, B.G.; Chowdhury, R.; Sinha, B.; Choudhary, T.; Chandola, N.; Mazumdar, S.; Taneja, S.; Bhandari, N.; et al. Enteral Low-Dose Vitamin A Supplementation in Preterm or Low Birth Weight Infants to Prevent Morbidity and Mortality: A Systematic Review and Meta-analysis. *Pediatrics* **2022**, *150* (Suppl. 1), e2022057092L. [CrossRef]
170. Gelfand, C.A.; Sakurai, R.; Wang, Y.; Liu, Y.; Segal, R.; Rehan, V.K. Inhaled vitamin A is more effective than intramuscular dosing in mitigating hyperoxia-induced lung injury in a neonatal rat model of bronchopulmonary dysplasia. *Am. J. Physiol. Lung Cell Mol. Physiol.* **2020**, *319*, L576–L584. [CrossRef]
171. Available online: https://grantome.com/grant/NIH/R43-HL142353-01A1 (accessed on 1 July 2024).
172. Teng, R.J.; Jing, X.; Michalkiewicz, T.; Afolayan, A.J.; Wu, T.J.; Konduri, G.G. Attenuation of endoplasmic reticulum stress by caffeine ameliorates hyperoxia-induced lung injury. *Am. J. Physiol. Lung Cell Mol. Physiol.* **2017**, *312*, L586–L598. [CrossRef]
173. Endesfelder, S.; Strauß, E.; Scheuer, T.; Schmitz, T.; Bührer, C. Antioxidative effects of caffeine in a hyperoxia-based rat model of bronchopulmonary dysplasia. *Respir. Res.* **2019**, *20*, 88. [CrossRef] [PubMed]
174. Köroğlu, O.A.; MacFarlane, P.M.; Balan, K.V.; Zenebe, W.J.; Jafri, A.; Martin, R.J.; Kc, P. Anti-inflammatory effect of caffeine is associated with improved lung function after lipopolysaccharide-induced amnionitis. *Neonatology* **2014**, *106*, 235–240. [CrossRef] [PubMed]
175. Endesfelder, S.; Strauß, E.; Bendix, I.; Schmitz, T.; Bührer, C. Prevention of Oxygen-Induced Inflammatory Lung Injury by Caffeine in Neonatal Rats. *Oxid. Med. Cell Longev.* **2020**, *2020*, 3840124. [CrossRef] [PubMed]
176. Luo, Q.; Xian, P.; Wang, T.; Wu, S.; Sun, T.; Wang, W.; Wang, B.; Yang, H.; Yang, Y.; Wang, H.; et al. Antioxidant activity of mesenchymal stem cell-derived extracellular vesicles restores hippocampal neurons following seizure damage. *Theranostics* **2021**, *11*, 5986–6005. [CrossRef] [PubMed]
177. Stavely, R.; Nurgali, K. The emerging antioxidant paradigm of mesenchymal stem cell therapy. *Stem Cells Transl. Med.* **2020**, *9*, 985–1006. [CrossRef] [PubMed]
178. Zhang, S.; Mulder, C.; Riddle, S.; Song, R.; Yue, D. Mesenchymal stromal/stem cells and bronchopulmonary dysplasia. *Front. Cell Dev. Biol.* **2023**, *11*, 1247339. [CrossRef]
179. Kumar, P.; Kandoi, S.; Misra, R.; Vijayalakshmi, S.; Rajagopal, K.; Verma, R.S. The mesenchymal stem cell secretome: A new paradigm towards cell-free therapeutic mode in regenerative medicine. *Cytokine Growth Factor. Rev.* **2019**, *46*, 1–9.
180. Mendt, M.; Rezvani, K.; Shpall, E. Mesenchymal stem cell-derived exosomes for clinical use. *Bone Marrow Transplant.* **2019**, *54* (Suppl. 2), 789–792. [CrossRef]
181. Zhang, H.; Jing, X.; Shi, Y.; Xu, H.; Du, J.; Guan, T.; Weihrauch, D.; Jones, D.W.; Wang, W.; Gourlay, D.; et al. N-acetyl lysyltyrosylcysteine amide inhibits myeloperoxidase, a novel tripeptide inhibitor. *J. Lipid Res.* **2013**, *54*, 3016–3029. [CrossRef]
182. Zhang, H.; Xu, H.; Weihrauch, D.; Jones, D.W.; Jing, X.; Shi, Y.; Gourlay, D.; Oldham, K.T.; Hillery, C.A.; Pritchard, K.A., Jr. Inhibition of myeloperoxidase decreases vascular oxidative stress and increases vasodilatation in sickle cell disease mice. *J. Lipid Res.* **2013**, *54*, 3009–3015. [CrossRef]
183. Rarick, K.R.; Li, K.; Teng, R.J.; Jing, X.; Martin, D.P.; Xu, H.; Jones, D.W.; Hogg, N.; Hillery, C.A.; Garcia, G.; et al. Sterile inflammation induces vasculopathy and chronic lung injury in murine sickle cell disease. *Free Radic. Biol. Med.* **2024**, *215*, 112–126. [CrossRef] [PubMed]
184. Zhang, H.; Ray, A.; Miller, N.M.; Hartwig, D.; Pritchard, K.A.; Dittel, B.N. Inhibition of myeloperoxidase at the peak of experimental autoimmune encephalomyelitis restores blood-brain barrier integrity and ameliorates disease severity. *J. Neurochem.* **2016**, *136*, 826–836. [CrossRef] [PubMed]
185. Yu, G.; Liang, Y.; Huang, Z.; Jones, D.W.; Pritchard, K.A., Jr.; Zhang, H. Inhibition of myeloperoxidase oxidant production by N-acetyl lysyltyrosylcysteine amide reduces brain damage in a murine model of stroke. *J. Neuroinflamm.* **2016**, *13*, 119. [CrossRef]
186. Yu, H., Liu, Y.; Wang, M.; Restrepo, R.J.; Wang, D.; Kalogeris, T.J.; Neumann, W.L.; Ford, D.A.; Korthuis, R.J. Myeloperoxidase instigates pro-inflammatory responses in a cecal ligation and puncture rat model of sepsis. *Am. J. Physiol. Heart Circ. Physiol.* **2020**, *319*, H705–H721. [CrossRef]
187. Neu, S.D.; Strzepa, A.; Martin, D.; Sorci-Thomas, M.G.; Pritchard, K.A., Jr.; Dittel, B.N. Myeloperoxidase Inhibition Ameliorates Plaque Psoriasis in Mice. *Antioxidants* **2021**, *10*, 1338. [CrossRef]
188. Vaughan, A.E.; Chapman, H.A. Failure of Alveolar Type 2 Cell Maintenance Links Neonatal Distress with Adult Lung Disease. *Am. J. Respir. Cell Mol. Biol.* **2017**, *56*, 415–416. [CrossRef]
189. van Kaam, A.H. Optimal Strategies of Mechanical Ventilation: Can We Avoid or Reduce Lung Injury? *Neonatology* **2024**, *121*, 570–575. [CrossRef]
190. Araki, S.; Kato, S.; Namba, F.; Ota, E. Vitamin A to prevent bronchopulmonary dysplasia in extremely low birth weight infants: A systematic review and meta-analysis. *PLoS ONE* **2018**, *13*, e0207730. [CrossRef] [PubMed]
191. Kua, K.P.; Lee, S.W. Systematic review and meta-analysis of clinical outcomes of early caffeine therapy in preterm neonates. *Br. J. Clin. Pharmacol.* **2017**, *83*, 180–191. [CrossRef]
192. Oliphant, E.A.; Hanning, S.M.; McKinlay, C.J.D.; Alsweiler, J.M. Caffeine for apnea and prevention of neurodevelopmental impairment in preterm infants: Systematic review and meta-analysis. *J. Perinatol.* **2024**, *44*, 785–801. [CrossRef]

International Journal of
Molecular Sciences

MDPI

Review

The Effect of Neuropsychiatric Drugs on the Oxidation-Reduction Balance in Therapy

Karina Sommerfeld-Klatta [1,*], Wiktoria Jiers [1], Szymon Rzepczyk [2], Filip Nowicki [2], Magdalena Łukasik-Głębocka [3], Paweł Świderski [2], Barbara Zielińska-Psuja [1], Zbigniew Żaba [3] and Czesław Żaba [2]

1 Department of Toxicology, Poznań University of Medical Sciences, 3 Rokietnicka Street, 60-806 Poznań, Poland
2 Department of Forensic Medicine, Poznań University of Medical Sciences, 10 Rokietnicka Street, 60-806 Poznań, Poland
3 Department of Emergency Medicine, Poznań University of Medical Sciences, 7 Rokietnicka Street, 60-806 Poznań, Poland
* Correspondence: ksommerfeld@ump.edu.pl

Abstract: The effectiveness of available neuropsychiatric drugs in the era of an increasing number of patients is not sufficient, and the complexity of neuropsychiatric disease entities that are difficult to diagnose and therapeutically is increasing. Also, discoveries about the pathophysiology of neuropsychiatric diseases are promising, including those initiating a new round of innovations in the role of oxidative stress in the etiology of neuropsychiatric diseases. Oxidative stress is highly related to mental disorders, in the treatment of which the most frequently used are first- and second-generation antipsychotics, mood stabilizers, and antidepressants. Literature reports on the effect of neuropsychiatric drugs on oxidative stress are divergent. They are starting with those proving their protective effect and ending with those confirming disturbances in the oxidation–reduction balance. The presented publication reviews the state of knowledge on the role of oxidative stress in the most frequently used therapies for neuropsychiatric diseases using first- and second-generation antipsychotic drugs, i.e., haloperidol, clozapine, risperidone, olanzapine, quetiapine, or aripiprazole, mood stabilizers: lithium, carbamazepine, valproic acid, oxcarbazepine, and antidepressants: citalopram, sertraline, and venlafaxine, along with a brief pharmacological characteristic, preclinical and clinical studies effects.

Keywords: neuropsychiatric drugs; oxidative stress; first- and second-generation antipsychotics; mood stabilizers; antidepressants

1. Introduction

Mental disorders have constituted a burden on society for many years. The situation has deteriorated significantly as a result of the pandemic, as well as the risks associated with the increasing stress and direct neuropsychiatric effects of the SARS-CoV-2 virus. Unfortunately, the efficacy of available neuropsychiatric drugs is not sufficient in an era of increasing numbers of patients, and the involvement of both diagnostically and therapeutically complex diseases is rising. Psychiatric disorders are a range of various conditions associated with abnormal functioning of the nervous system, which are common in patients with nervous system disorders [1]. As a result of these abnormalities, in response to a stressful situation, the body activates maladaptive behavioral patterns that impede daily functioning [2]. The most common mental disorders include mood swings, neurotic disorders, dementia disorders, schizoaffective disorders, eating and personality disorders, sleep disorders, or addictions (Table 1) [3–23]. According to the World Health Report, mental disorders affect approximately 25% of people at some point during their lifetime. The co-occurrence of neurological diseases with mood disorders and anxiety syndromes is common in patients with neurodegenerative diseases (Parkinson's, Alzheimer's, and

Huntington's), stroke, epilepsy, and demyelinating diseases. The choice of treatment for neurological patients with co-occurring mood and anxiety disorders is often difficult, as it has to take into account the symptoms of the underlying disease and poorer drug tolerance [1]. According to the International Neuropsychiatry Association, discoveries in the pathophysiology of neuropsychiatric diseases are promising, including those initiating a new round of innovation within the contribution of oxidative stress to the etiology of neuropsychiatric diseases [2,24,25]. Oxidative stress is a significant risk factor for many psychiatric disorders, for the treatment of which first- and second-generation antipsychotics, mood stabilizers, and antidepressants are most commonly used (Table 2) [2].

Table 1. Mental and behavioural disorders in selected categories with clinical details [3–23].

Mental and Behavioural Disorders	Selected Categories	Clinical Details	Publications
Organic, including symptomatic, mental disorders	Dementia in Alzheimer's disease	Progressive, neurodegenerative disease Loss of cognitive function	[3,4]
	Vascular dementia	Result of infraction of the brain due to vascular disease	
	Delirium, not induced by alcohol and other psychoactive substances	Non-specific organic cerebral syndrome Including: disturbances of consciousness, attention, perception and emotional disturbances	
	Unspecified organic or symptomatic mental disorder	Brain disorder, injury, or toxicity Mental and behavioural disorders	
Mental and behavioural disorders due to psychoactive substance use	Mental and behavioural disorders due to use of alcohol	Wide variety of disorders resulting from abuse or misuse of alcohol/psychoactive substances	[5–8]
	Mental and behavioural disorders due to use of sedatives or hypnotics		
	Mental and behavioural disorders due to use of other stimulants, including caffeine		
	Mental and behavioural disorders due to multiple drug use and use of other psychoactive substances		
Schizophrenia, schizotypal, and delusional disorders	Schizophrenia	Multifactorial, combination of genetic and environmental factors Abnormalities in the perception or expression of reality	[9–11]
	Schizotypal disorder	Eccentric thoughts, inappropriate affect and behaviour, extreme social anxiety, and limited interpersonal interaction	
Mood (affective) disorders	Manic episode	Extreme changes in behaviour, and mood that drastically affect their functioning	[12,13]
	Bipolar affective disorder	Severe mood swings (mania and depression)	
Neurotic, stress-related and somatoform disorders	Phobic anxiety disorders	Strong, irrational fear, anxiety	[14,15]
	Obsessive-compulsive disorder	Intrusive ideas, thoughts and images	
Behavioural syndromes associated with physiological disturbances and physical factors	Eating disorders	Physiological and psychological disturbances in appetite or food intake	[16–18]
	Nonorganic sleep disorders	Disturbance of normal sleep patterns	
	Abuse of non-dependence-producing substances	The use of non-addictive drugs, particularly those purchased without a prescription (antacids, herbal, folk remedies, steroids, hormones and vitamins)	

Table 1. *Cont.*

Mental and Behavioural Disorders	Selected Categories	Clinical Details	Publications
Disorders of adult personality and behaviour	Specific personality disorders	Disorders characterized by disturbances in the personality	[19–21]
	Gender identity disorders	Incongruence between experienced or expressed gender and the one assigned at birth	
	Disorders of sexual preference	Intense sexually arousing fantasies, urges, or behaviours	
Behavioural and emotional disorders with onset usually occurring in childhood and adolescence	Hyperkinetic disorders	Difficulty sustaining cognitive engagement in activities	[22,23]
	Tic disorders	Recurrent tics (involuntary, rapid, nonrhythmic motor movement or vocal)	

Table 2. Antipsychotic, mood stabilizers and antidepressants drugs (SSRI, selective serotonin reuptake inhibitor) and (SNRI, serotonin and norepinephrine reuptake inhibitors)—generations and applications [1,3,9,24,25].

Antipsychotic Drugs					Mood Stabilizers				Antidepressants		
Schizophrenia					Bipolar Disorder				Depression		
I	II	III	First-Line Drugs	Second-Line Drugs	I	II	First-Line Drugs	Add-on Therapy	SSRI	SNRI	First-Line Drugs
Haloperidol	Clozapine Quetiapine Risperidone Olanzapine	Aripiprazole	Risperidone Olanzapine Quetiapine Aripiprazole	Clozapine	Lithium Valproate Carbamazepine	Oxcarbazepine	Lithium Valproate Carbamazepine	Oxcarbazepine	Sertraline Citalopram	Venlafaxine	Sertraline Citalopram Venlafaxine

Oxidative stress is a state of imbalance between antioxidants and free radicals in the body. Both oxidants and antioxidants, essential for vital processes, should remain in quantitative balance for the safety of the entire system. However, there are known factors under the influence of which one overpowers the other, resulting in changes, i.e., DNA damage, disruption of protein, lipid, or carbohydrate function and structure. In addition, oxidative stress may be involved in the etiology of many conditions, i.e., hypertension, obesity, atherosclerosis, or diabetes. Also, in terms of many neuropsychiatric diseases, despite advances in neurobiological research, the pathophysiology of many of these diseases has yet to be more extensively described. Advances in the understanding of the pathomechanism of many psychiatric disorders, as well as neuropsychiatric diseases, may help to discover effective therapies and indicators for their early diagnosis. Oxidative stress, which damages biomolecules and causes dysfunctions of, among others, cellular systems at the level of, e.g., mitochondria or dopamine receptors, is also referred to as a critical phenomenon in patients with mental disorders [2,26–29] (Figure 1).

Under conditions of homeostasis, and thus at safe concentrations, the presence of reactive oxygen species (ROS) is not harmful to the organism and acts as a regulator and mediator of physiological processes. ROS play an essential role in the ordinary course of inflammatory reactions, regulation of immune processes, or T-lymphocyte activation, with concomitant adhesion of leukocyte cells to the endothelium [27–30]. Currently, the diagnostic market makes available numerous analytical tools and biomarkers that can be used to assess oxidative stress. Examples of oxidative markers include myeloperoxidase (MPO), 4-hydroxynonenal (HNE), F2-isoprostanes (IsoP), 8-hydroxy-2-deoxyguanosine (8-OHdG), malondialdehyde (MDA), allantoin, and thiobarbituric acid reactive substances (TBARS). They are used to monitor tissue damage resulting from a loss of balance between antioxidants and free radicals [31–33]. Table 3 brings together the oxidative stress markers according to the adverse changes they are used to assess.

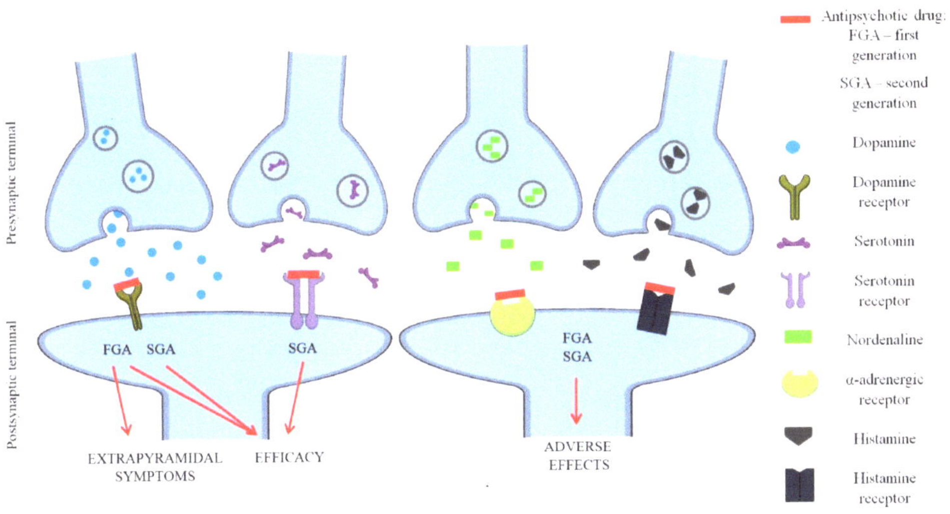

Figure 1. First (FGA) and second-generation (SGA) antipsychotics and extrapyramidal adverse effects—receptor scheme and mechanism [24–26].

Table 3. Biological markers of oxidative stress [31,33,34].

Destructive Changes	Markers of Oxidative Stress
Lipid peroxidation	Malondialdehyde F2-isoprostanes Oxidized low density lipoproteins Oxidized LDL (low-density lipoprotein) antibodies 4-hydroxynonenal Acrolein
Oxidation of nucleic acids	8-hydroxy-2-deoxyguanosine Reactive aldehydes Reduced sugars, e.g., ribose
Carbohydrate oxidation	3-nitrotyrosine
Protein oxidation	Substances that react with thiobarbituric acid Glycation end products Oxidized thiol groups

Knowledge of the biotransformation of drugs used to treat psychiatric disorders involving enzymatic systems may support the hypothesis of oxidative disorders generated by, among other things, reactive metabolites or radicals. However, the link between the effects of many drugs and oxidative stress is still the subject of few scientific publications aiming to confirm their antioxidant or pro-oxidant effects in groups of treated patients [35,36].

The presented publication reviews the state of knowledge on the share of oxidative stress in the most commonly used therapies for neuropsychiatric diseases using first- and second-generation antipsychotics, i.e., haloperidol (HLP), clozapine (CLO), risperidone (RIS), olanzapine (OLZ), quetiapine (QT) or aripiprazole (ARP), mood stabilizers: lithium (Li), carbamazepine (CBZ), valproic acid (VPA), oxcarbazepine (OXC), and antidepressants: citalopram (CIT), sertraline (SER), venlafaxine (VEN), along with an explanation of the obtained results and their comparison. The data provided and discussed come from the US National Library of Medicine (PubMed) bibliographic sources, selecting publications from the last ten years and older for analysis in order to discuss the results of more recent preclinical and clinical studies. The key search terms for the literature search were oxidative stress and neuropsychiatric drugs.

2. First and Second-Generations of Antipsychotic Drugs

2.1. Haloperidol (HLP)

2.1.1. Pharmacological HLP Data

Haloperidol (HLP), synthesized in 1958, belongs to the butyrophenone derivatives. Its discovery came during research into new derivatives of pethidine and methadone, both of which were claimed to have analgesic activity. However, it has been proven that this drug has significant efficacy in the treatment of psychiatric disorders, including schizophrenia, especially hallucinations and delusions [37–39]. The antipsychotic effect of the drug is due to the blockade of dopamine D_2 receptors. Its high affinity for the receptor, together with a low cholinolytic effect, minimizes the occurrence of symptoms such as constipation, dry mouth, and visual disturbances [38,40–43].

2.1.2. Preclinical HLP Studies

Oxidative stress occurring with a first-generation antipsychotic drug such as haloperidol is not a fully understood issue. The use of the drug has been shown to increase oxidative stress, which has an impact on the pathophysiology of schizophrenia. On the one hand, oxidative imbalance may be part of the pathogenesis of the disease, but on the other hand, it can lead to patients experiencing extrapyramidal symptoms (EPS). Preclinical and in vitro (cell) studies conducted on HLP have revealed that the use of the drug is associated with a decrease in antioxidant enzyme activity and an increase in reactive oxygen species (ROS) levels [44–51]. Perera et al. demonstrated that biochemical changes in the rat brain after haloperidol administration are accompanied by histopathological changes such as necrosis and fibrosis. Although the exact pathophysiology of EPS is not known, the authors here point to an important role for ROS in inducing oxidative stress, representing one mechanism of haloperidol-induced long-term neurotoxicity [44]. When HLP is used, dopamine is increased, which deaminates and generates significant amounts of free radicals and hydrogen peroxide, among other things. Reactive metabolites leading to multicellular damage and lipid peroxidation contribute to the cytotoxic effects of the drug. Raudenska et al. showed that long-term haloperidol administration to rats leads to changes in sigma-1R receptor and inositol triphosphate receptor (IP3R) expression, modifying myocardial contractility. This may underlie cardiac arrhythmias and QT interval prolongation in patients using haloperidol [45]. Haloperidol can also lead to changes in brain tissue, as evidenced by the study by El-Awadan et al. After 14 days of administering the drug to rats at a dose of 1 mg/kg, the concentrations of GSH, malondialdehyde (MDA), and nitric oxide (NO) in the brain and liver were determined. Levels of the former were significantly reduced in both tissues. In contrast, there was an increase in NO and MDA levels in brain tissue [47]. The adverse effects of the drug on antioxidant enzymes in the brain were also confirmed by measuring the expression of the enzyme peroxiredoxin-6. After a 28-day administration of haloperidol (1 mg/kg) to rats, significantly increased levels of the test protein were observed in the grey matter of the brain, with a concomitant increase in lipid peroxidation. However, peroxiredoxin-6 concentrations were unchanged in the white matter of the brain and liver of rats [48].

Subsequent studies in human cell lines confirmed that, under prooxidant conditions, therapeutic concentrations of haloperidol increase TBARS levels. However, a significant correlation between the used drug and lipid peroxidation was not observed for cells not treated with hydrogen peroxide. In addition, the combination of lithium and haloperidol significantly reduced cell survival. Despite the lack of statistical significance of the results obtained, they indicate the need for particular caution when combining drugs used in the treatment of psychiatric disorders [50,51].

2.1.3. Clinial HLP Studies

Available clinical data on the relationship between HLP and oxidative stress points to the use of biomarkers such as superoxide dismutase (SOD), catalase (CAT), and glutathione (GSH). The use of haloperidol results in a decrease in the activity of the above antioxidant enzymes, as confirmed by a study by Bošković et al. conducted on a group of patients treated with haloperidol for a minimum of six months. In addition, they observed significantly lower concentrations of the biomarkers determined in patients with extrapyramidal symptoms [46]. In contrast, Singh et al. further assessed markers of lipid peroxidation by determining serum thiobarbituric acid reactive substances (TBARS). TBARS levels were significantly elevated in patients treated with haloperidol (for at least six weeks) compared with patients taking the second-generation antipsychotic drug olanzapine. SOD has also been shown to be negatively correlated with serum TBARS [49].

2.2. Clozapine (CLO)

2.2.1. Pharmacological CLO Data

Clozapine (CLO), which belongs to the atypical antipsychotics, has structural similarities to tricyclic antidepressants. Its synthesis took place in the early 1960s. A clear advantage of clozapine appeared to be the absence of extrapyramidal side effects. Nonetheless, the drug was initially skeptically assessed and withdrawn from use, a factor contributed to by the significant risk of agranulocytosis during its use. However, continued research has confirmed significant effectiveness in the treatment of symptoms of psychosis, especially drug-resistant schizophrenia [52,53]. Regular blood tests of patients have also been shown to control the risk of agranulocytosis. Consequently, the drug was reintroduced to the pharmaceutical market in 1989 in Europe—and a year later in the USA. However, its use is limited, and it is not a first-line drug. The inclusion of CLO in pharmacotherapy occurs primarily when treatment with other antipsychotics is unsuccessful. In addition, its use is associated with adverse effects that are troublesome for patients, e.g., weight gain, constipation, metabolic disorders, and the development of diabetes [52,54,55]. The antipsychotic effect of clozapine is due to its diverse pharmacological profile. This is because it shows affinity for dopamine D_1, D_4, and D_2 receptors. In the case of the D_2 receptor, dissociation occurs very rapidly, thus reducing the risk of hyperprolactinemia and extrapyramidal symptoms. Clozapine also has an affinity for serotonin, adrenergic, histamine, and muscarinic receptors [52,54,55].

2.2.2. Preclinical CLO Studies

There are numerous attempts to link oxidative stress to adverse effects, including metabolic disorders occurring during clozapine use, in preclinical studies. This points to the involvement of free radicals leading to the oxidation of proteins, which results in their disruption or loss of function [56–61]. In the study by Walss-Bass et al., human neuroblastoma cells were used to identify changes in proteins under oxidative stress after administration of CLO (in three concentrations of 1, 10, or 20 μM). The level of reactive oxygen species increased with dose until reaching a maximum value at a drug concentration of 10 μM. Among others, malate dehydrogenase, calumenin, or the muscle isoenzyme of keratin kinase were found to be particularly susceptible to oxidation. Irreversible changes in enzymes involved in key metabolic processes can lead to the occurrence of multiple disorders in the body [57].

A study by Abdel-Wahab et al. in rats further revealed an association between oxidative stress and myocardial ischemia. Clozapine causes an increased release of catecholamines, which in turn increases the production of free radicals. As a consequence, cell damage occurs with the infiltration of neutrophils, which release cytokines, among others, TNF-α. Rats treated with CLO for 21 days showed a significant increase in MDA and 8-hydroxy-2-deoxyguanosine (8-OHdG), which was observed at doses of 15 and 25 mg/kg/day. This indicates lipid peroxidation and oxidative damage to DNA. The cardiotoxic effect was further confirmed by an increase in the activity of the biomarkers of cardiac damage—lactate dehydrogenase (LDH) and cardiac creatine kinase isoenzyme (CK-MB). At the same time, GSH levels decreased significantly [58]. Similar results were obtained during clozapine cardiotoxicity studies using striped danios. After a three-day exposure of embryos to the drug (concentration range 12.5–100 μM), cardiac morphological abnormalities and bradycardia were detected. In addition, levels of ROS, MDA, and pro-inflammatory cytokines increased. In contrast, CAT and SOD activity decreased. These results confirmed that CLO contributes to both oxidative stress and inflammation, thus leading to cardiotoxicity in preclinical studies [59].

2.2.3. Clinial CLO Studies

Clozapine-induced oxidative stress also affects blood cells in patients with agranulocytosis and in patients without agranulocytosis. A clinical study by Fehsel et al. suggests that the use of the drug is associated with an increase in ROS production in neutrophils, which may contribute to the induction of their apoptosis. In addition, increased expression of the proapoptotic gene p53 was observed, and this also occurred in patients treated with other antipsychotics, including olanzapine [60].

However, the results of a study comparing oxidative stress parameters in patients treated with perphenazine, risperidone, and clozapine led the authors to a completely different conclusion. Indeed, it has been shown that in patients treated with clozapine for at least three months, serum GSH and SOD levels increased, and MDA levels were significantly lower compared to patients treated with perphenazine and risperidone [61].

2.3. *Risperidone (RIS)*

2.3.1. Pharmacological RIS Data

During studies conducted in the 1960s and 1970s, it was observed that the administration of lysergic acid diethylamide (LSD) to rats produced symptoms similar to the negative symptoms of schizophrenia. This phenomenon has been linked to 5-HT_2 receptor agonism and serotonin overactivation. A new target in the field of treatment of psychotic disorders has, therefore, become the development of compounds that block D_2 and 5-HT_2 receptors simultaneously. In the early 1980s, a benzoxazole derivative was obtained, which was classified as an atypical antipsychotic drug in the form of risperidone (RIS). The drug was approved by the US Food and Drug Administration in a relatively short time, as early as 1993, for the treatment of schizophrenia [62–64]. The drug also binds to $\alpha_1$adrenergic receptors and α_2 and histamine H_1 receptors. A particular advantage of the drug is its lack of affinity for muscarinic receptors; thus, there is little likelihood of anticholinergic symptoms developing. Although it is not without side effects and can lead to weight gain, hyperprolactinemia, hyperlipidemia, and diabetes, among others, it has a limited side effect profile compared to its predecessors [64–68].

2.3.2. Preclinical RIS Studies

With risperidone, the incidence of serious side effects such as extrapyramidal symptoms is limited, which is attributed to lower levels of oxidative stress [69–72]. Stojkovic et al. demonstrated that the drug affects parameters such as MDA, GSH, and SOD in the brain structures of rats. An increase in previously reduced GSH levels was observed in the brains of rats administered phencyclidine (PCP) initially for redox imbalance, followed by RIS for nine weeks. PCP led to oxidative damage in the brain and lipid peroxidation, but long-term administration of risperidone resulted in reduced levels of MDA and SOD [69].

However, some researchers indicate that risperidone has a cytotoxic effect by increasing the production of reactive oxygen species, thus inducing oxidative stress. In isolated hepatocytes of lab rats incubated with risperidone, a significant decrease in GSH levels was observed compared to the control group, as well as signs of cell damage, including, among others, a decrease in mitochondrial membrane potential and lipid peroxidation [72].

2.3.3. Clinial CLO Studies

Similar results were observed in a group of patients treated with RIS for 12 weeks at a dose of 6 mg/day. The concentration of SOD in the blood decreased significantly. However, the effect of the drug on NO levels remains inconclusive. The above study did not show a decrease in elevated NO levels in patients' blood [70]. Different results were obtained in the blood of patients undergoing six weeks of pharmacotherapy with risperidone at individually selected doses in the range of 3–11 mg/day, as there was an increase in the levels of NO and its metabolites. At the same time, NO levels in the blood of patients with schizophrenia have also been shown to be significantly lower than in healthy individuals [71]. The aforementioned study by Hendouei et al. also assessed the effect of risperidone on oxidative stress parameters. Although clozapine showed a significant advantage in antioxidant activity, the total antioxidant capacity of plasma (FRAP, ferric reducing antioxidant power) reached the highest value compared to the patient group treated with risperidone [61].

2.4. Olanzapine (OLZ)

2.4.1. Pharmacological OLZ Data

In 1996, olanzapine (OLZ) was approved by the FDA for the treatment of schizophrenia, and in 2004, it was also approved for the treatment of bipolar disorder [73,74]. Due to its structural similarity to clozapine, olanzapine has a similar receptor profile. It shows high affinity for both dopamine receptors (e.g., D_2, D_4), serotonin (among others, 5-HT_{2A}, 5H-T_{2C}), adrenergic, histamine, as well as muscarinic. It has been shown that this drug also affects the glutamatergic system by interacting with NMDA receptors. However, the exact mechanism is not known [74,75]. The use of OLZ is associated with a limited risk of extrapyramidal symptoms and small increases in prolactin levels. Despite the above-mentioned advantages, the drug, especially during long-term therapy, significantly interferes with the body's metabolic processes, leading to numerous disorders such as hyperlipidemia, diabetes, and weight gain. The latter is more common with olanzapine compared to other antipsychotics. Drowsiness, dry mouth, dizziness, and fatigue, as well as other symptoms, may also occur [73–75]. Olanzapine is classified as a second-choice drug due to its significant impact on metabolism. Nevertheless, due to its considerable efficacy, it continues to be one of the most commonly used second-generation antipsychotics, along with quetiapine, risperidone, and aripiprazole [41,68,76].

2.4.2. Preclinical OLZ Studies

There are numerous findings to compare oxidative stress with OLZ toxicity, including preclinical and clinical studies [77–81]. In numerous projects, olanzapine is compared with other antipsychotics, both first- and second-generation. In the animal study by Reinke et al., it was combined with haloperidol and clozapine. The obtained results indicate a significant advantage of atypical drugs over classical ones. Unlike haloperidol, they did not cause oxidative brain damage in the studied rats. A 28-day treatment with olanzapine administered intravenously at doses of 2.5, 5, and 10 mg/kg resulted in lower TBARS and carbonyl levels. Two-month treatment of rats with schizophrenia (doses of 10–20 mg/day) also resulted in improvements in oxidative stress parameters. Lipid peroxidation was assessed by analyzing MDA concentrations. Compared to pre-treatment values, biomarker levels decreased significantly [79].

Research from recent years also indicates an important role of the prefrontal cortex in the treatment of schizophrenia. Olanzapine-induced inflammation of this area and activation of the immune response are most likely linked to the pathogenesis of schizophrenia. Administration of the drug to rats for 1, 8, and 36 days (dose 3 mg/kg/day) resulted in activation of IKKβ/NF-κB inflammatory signaling pathways, increased expression of the pro-inflammatory cytokines TNF-α, IL-6, and IL-1β, and immune system proteins including iNOS, TLR4, and CD14 in the prefrontal cortex [81].

OLZ also shows effects on hypothalamic cells, with dose- and time-dependent effects suggested. During in vitro studies on cell lines, a significant decrease in cell survival was observed at concentrations ≥100 μM after 24 h of incubation. Quantification of live hypothalamic cells confirmed the neurotoxicity of OLZ after both 24 and 48 h of incubation, which was for concentrations of 100 μM. No significant changes in cell survival were observed at a concentration of 25 μM. Based on the results, it can be concluded that olanzapine leads to dose-dependent neurotoxicity, where low concentrations of olanzapine (<100 μM) show beneficial antioxidant properties, but high doses (≥100 μM) result in cell damage [78].

2.4.3. Clinial OLZ Studies

Schizophrenic patients have been shown to have elevated levels of free radicals, with reduced levels of antioxidants. However, a significant number of studies show improvements in oxidative stress parameters in the blood of patients treated with OLZ. In the group of patients receiving the drug for 3 months at a dose of 5–20 mg/day, there was a decrease in the elevated MDA levels. The improvement was also noticeable for GSH, the concentration of which decreased significantly. In addition, the initially reduced levels of α-tocopheryl and ascorbic acid increased significantly. In this study, similar effects were obtained for risperidone, but better results in improving levels of oxidative stress biomarkers were obtained in the group of patients treated with olanzapine [77].

Total antioxidant status (TAS) was measured in schizophrenic patients. As a result of treatment, the blood levels of patients increased significantly. On the basis of the obtained data, researchers concluded that olanzapine showed a partial ability to regulate elevated levels of oxidative stress in patients with schizophrenia [80].

2.5. *Quetiapine (QT)*

2.5.1. Pharmacological QT Data

Quetiapine (QT), like clozapine and olanzapine, belongs to the dibenzoazepine derivatives. In 1997, it was approved by the FDA for the treatment of schizophrenia. In 2004, the registration indication was expanded to include the treatment of bipolar disorder and, a few years later, also the treatment of depression, with quetiapine being recognized as an adjunctive therapy drug [73,82,83]. It is characterized by strong antagonism to the 5-HT_{2A} receptor. It binds to a small extent to the D_2 receptor. Its sedative effect is most likely related to its very strong affinity for histamine H_1 receptors. In turn, the occurrence of orthostatic hypotonia is explained by its affinity for α_1-adrenergic receptors. Although the mechanisms of action of quetiapine are not fully understood, it is indicated that its metabolite—norquetiapine—influences antidepressant efficacy. This compound not only acts agonistically at 5-HT_{1A} receptors but also inhibits norepinephrine transport factor (NET). Side effects include drowsiness, dry mouth, dyslipidemia, and weight gain. However, compared to olanzapine and clozapine, the intensity of metabolic disturbances occurring during quetiapine use is lower [41,68,73,83–85].

2.5.2. Preclinical QT Studies

Studies have shown that quetiapine presents different directions of action from the damaging effects of oxidative stress [86–91]. Han et al. induced free radical production by a seven-day intra-peritoneal administration of 20% ethanol (2 g/kg/day) to rats. An increase in total antioxidant capacity (TAC), SOD, and CAT activity was observed in brain areas of animals receiving the drug at a dose of 10 mg/kg/day. This effect was not observed in the liver, where there was an increase in MDA and ROS concentrations despite drug administration [86]. Similar results were also obtained with fourteen days of quetiapine therapy (20 mg/kg), which produced a significant increase in SOD activity and a decrease in TBARS levels in the rat brain areas studied (hippocampus, amygdala, and prefrontal cortex). This indicates a reduction in lipid peroxidation and protein damage, thereby reducing oxidative stress [87]. Due to the significant effectiveness of quetiapine in the treatment of cognitive deficits, studies were also conducted to assess its impact on behavioral changes resulting from anticancer treatment with doxorubicin. The results of the 30-day study revealed that oxidative stress and inflammation parameters were improved in the brain tissue of the rats. Quetiapine administration reduced high concentrations of MDA and GSH in the brains of rats [91].

2.5.3. Clinical QT Studies

In contrast to preclinical data, determination of myeloperoxidase (MPO) and C-reactive protein (CRP) activity in patients after QT overdose revealed oxidative dysfunction and the development of inflammation. Levels of both biomarkers increased significantly, which was further related to serum drug concentration and the patient's clinical condition. Quetiapine concentrations above 1 μg/mL in blood correlated with both increased MPO and CRP levels [88]. However, in other studies conducted with quetiapine-treated patients, the antioxidant effect of the drug has been observed. After four weeks of therapy, a decrease in baseline-elevated plasma TBARS and urinary F2-isoprostane concentrations was noted. Initial levels of the lipid peroxidation marker 4-hydroxynonenal (4-HNE) in the schizophrenia group were not significantly different from the control group, and these levels did not change after quetiapine treatment. This study also allowed a comparison of the antioxidant properties of selected atypical antipsychotics. Quetiapine, together with clozapine and olanzapine, showed the most beneficial effect on oxidative stress parameters [89].

This effect was also confirmed during in vitro studies using blood drawn from healthy volunteers. Significant reductions in lipid peroxidation in the form of reduced TBARS levels occurred after both 1 and 24 h of plasma incubation with the drug [90].

2.6. Aripiprazole (ARP)

2.6.1. Pharmacological ARP Data

In 2002, the FDA approved the new drug aripiprazole (ARP) for the treatment of schizophrenia. As a quinoline derivative, it exhibits a unique mechanism of action, making it classed as a third-generation antipsychotic. Like quetiapine, aripiprazole has received approval for the treatment of bipolar affective disorder and depression as adjunctive therapy. This occurred in 2004 and 2007 [73]. It is called a dopamine system stabilizer. When the activity of the dopaminergic system is reduced, it acts as an agonist for D_2 receptors by stimulating them. In contrast, when dopamine concentrations are too high, aripiprazole acts as an antagonist. This allows for antipsychotic effects while reducing the risk of EPS. This drug also has an affinity for 5-HT_{1A}, 5-HT_{2A}, 5-HT_7, and D_3 receptors and moderate activity at D_4, H_1, and α_1-adrenergic receptors. A particular advantage of aripiprazole is its beneficial effect on prolactin. This is because it does not increase serum concentrations of the hormone. In addition, it can lead to the normalization of prolactin levels in patients whose levels were initially elevated. The most common side effects include drowsiness, akathisia, anxiety, nausea, vomiting, and headache [56,68,73,92–96].

2.6.2. Preclinical ARP Studies

Preclinical, in vitro, and clinical studies have shown that ARP can generate or reduce oxidative stress [97–101]. It was observed that in both isolated mouse liver mitochondria and in isolated blood cells from healthy patients, mitochondrial respiration was disrupted by aripiprazole administration. This drug led to the induction of reactive oxygen species production and lipid peroxidation, as indicated by increased levels of modified HNE proteins [97].

In contrast, some studies confirm the induction of an antioxidant response by ARP. In view of its potential antidepressant effect, an analysis was made of the drug's effect on oxidative stress parameters that also play an important role in the pathogenesis of depression. Lipid peroxidation levels in the cerebral cortex of rats receiving aripiprazole (2.5 mg/kg) for four weeks did not differ from those of the control group. However, glutathione peroxidase activity, GSH, and vitamin C concentrations increased significantly [99].

Recent studies also indicate a potential antioxidant effect on neurons. Administration of aripiprazole to rats for 30 days at doses of 1 and 2 mg/kg resulted in reduced levels of the oxidative stress marker MDA and the inflammatory marker COX-2 for both drug concentrations. In addition, the antioxidant activities of GSH and CAT increased. According to the researchers, the results obtained demonstrate the neuroprotective mechanism of action of aripiprazole [100].

Equally beneficial effects of the drug on antioxidant protection and cell viability were observed in relation to rat hepatocytes. Under oxidative conditions, after eight weeks of treatment, there was an increase in the activity of the antioxidant enzymes, SOD and CAT, which applied to both 2.23 and 6 μM ARP concentrations. At the same time, the dose-dependent effect of the drug was shown, and the largest increase in enzymes occurred after the drug was administered at a higher concentration [101].

2.6.3. Clinical ARP Studies

In contrast, the results of a clinical study conducted to assess the effect of therapeutic doses of antipsychotics on oxidative stress parameters suggest that aripiprazole has a dose-dependent effect. Plasma samples from healthy volunteers were incubated with the drug for 24 h. For both drug concentrations of 163 and 242 ng/mL, no significant effect was observed on plasma TBARS levels. However, at lower concentrations, there was a slight induction of lipid peroxidation, indicating possible prooxidant properties [98].

3. Mood Stabilizers

3.1. Lithium (Li)

3.1.1. Pharmacological Li Data

The origins of the use of lithium (Li) date back to the 19th century, but the first publications demonstrating its effectiveness were published in the mid-20th century [102,103]. It is currently used mainly in the treatment of schizoaffective disorders, including bipolar mood disorders, as a mood stabilizer [104]. It is also suggested for use in the treatment of schizophrenia as a next-line treatment and in severe forms of depression due to its anti-suicidal properties [105,106]. Its use in neurodegenerative diseases has also been postulated [107–109]. Despite its long history of use, the mechanism of action of lithium is not yet fully understood. However, two main mechanisms of action have been postulated: by blocking inositol phosphatases involved in intracellular signal transduction and by inhibiting glycogen synthase kinase 3 [110,111]. In addition, it increases GABA-based inhibitory neurotransmission, which is of particular importance in the treatment of mania [112]. Side effects associated, particularly with long-term use, include kidney damage and endocrine disruption in the form of deterioration of thyroid functions [113,114].

3.1.2. Preclinical Li Studies

Preclinical, clinical, and in vitro studies have shown that lithium enhances or inhibits oxidative stress [115–123]. In preclinical studies conducted on rats induced into a state of mania by methamphetamine, it was shown that the oxidative effect of lithium is influenced by the dose of the substance inducing the manic state in the model and the site of action in the nervous tissue [118]. Results confirming the antioxidant properties of lithium were also shown in a study by Jornad et al., which was also conducted on rats introduced into a model of mania. SOD activity was statistically significantly reduced with lithium treatment compared to the group introduced into mania without lithium treatment in both the prefrontal and hippocampus. In the case of CAT, increased activity was also observed in both brain regions. In addition, a significant reduction in TBARS was also observed after lithium therapy in neural tissue. In contrast, in non-manic animals, the use of lithium did not affect oxidative stress parameters in any case [119]. Another study in rats showed a significant increase in SOD levels only in the group treated with higher concentrations of lithium, suggesting a dose-dependent increase in oxidative damage [121].

Additionally, in an in vitro model study, lithium was shown to inhibit oxidative stress-induced senescence in nerve cells [120]. In a study conducted on rat liver cells in vitro, lithium cytotoxicity associated with its participation in the formation of oxygen-free radicals was demonstrated. Moreover, cytotoxicity increased with increasing ion concentrations. In addition, the role of the CYP2E1 isoenzyme in oxidative stress associated with the intake of lithium was postulated [123].

3.1.3. Clinical Li Studies

A clinical study conducted on a group of bipolar disorder patients treated with lithium showed a statistically significant reduction in TBARS level, an exponent of increased lipid peroxidation, after starting therapy. Similar observations have been shown for superoxide dismutase (SOD). CAT and GPx levels did not change statistically significantly after lithium treatment but were significantly higher compared to the control group, which is explained by the pathophysiology of the disease. In addition, changes in oxidative stress parameters have been linked to the response to lithium therapy [115,116]. A study by Banerjee et al., also conducted on a group of bipolar disorder patients, showed significantly reduced lipid peroxidation exponents in lithium-treated patients compared to lithium-naive patients. Moreover, an increase in Na^+-K^+-ATPase activity associated with lithium treatment and affecting the reduction of oxidative stress was demonstrated [117]. In contrast, a study in healthy volunteers showed a statistically significant reduction in SOD after Li therapy, with no significant effect on CAT or TBARS levels [122].

3.2. *Valproic Acid (VPA)*

3.2.1. Pharmacological VPA Data

The action of valproic acid (VPA) is based on blocking voltage-gated ion channels and modulating GABA-nergic and monoamine-based transmission within neural tissue. Through the induction of glutamic acid decarboxylase, VPA increases levels of GABA, which is an inhibitory neurotransmitter. In addition, VPA inhibits the enzymes that break down GABA, which further contributes to its levels. This reduces impulse conduction, which translates into a reduction in the occurrence of convulsions. The effect on NMDA receptor-based conduction is also not insignificant. This is carried out by weakening the action of glutamate, which is a stimulating neurotransmitter. In addition, VPA reduces glucose utilization within the brain, which results in reduced ATP production and indirectly translates into a slower metabolism in the neural tissue. Common side effects associated with the use of VPA include weakness, lethargy, nausea, weight gain, and hair condition deterioration. In addition, hematological disorders and hepatotoxicity associated with VPA intake are observed. In addition, valproic acid has shown significant teratogenic properties [124–136].

3.2.2. Preclinical VPA Studies

The use of valproic acid affects the redox balance in the body [137–145]. Studies in rats have shown VPA-associated significant reductions in GTx, SOD, and CAT activity in neural tissue. In addition, oxidative stress exponents such as TBARS and carbonyls have been shown to be elevated [137]. However, this effect can be inhibited by selenium and L-carnitine supplementation, which has also been confirmed in studies conducted on rats [138,139]. In turn, work carried out on the same animal model showed neuroprotective properties of VPA against nerve cells after the occurrence of mechanical trauma in the mechanism of inhibiting oxidative stress [140]. VPA also has a similar effect in the case of nerve tissue damage as a result of stroke, which has been demonstrated in studies on the same animal model [141].

Studies conducted on human neuroblastoma cells in an in vitro model showed a reduction in hydrogen peroxide levels in cells subjected to stimulated excitotoxicity in the case of incubation with VPA. In addition, an increase in SOD and a slight increase in CAT were also observed in samples incubated with VPA. However, when excitotoxicity was induced, the relationships were not statistically significant [142]. Also, a study conducted on a mouse embryo model showed an increase in reactive oxygen species associated with VPA administration and a negative impact on the embryo. In addition, administration of exogenous CAT showed potential embryonic protective properties, which could not be demonstrated for SOD [144]. Elevated markers of oxidative stress associated with the use of VPA have also been demonstrated in work on glioma cell lines. VPA-related reactive oxygen species caused damage within mitochondria, affected cell–cell communication pathways, and regulated VPA-induced apoptosis [145].

3.2.3. Clinical VPA Studies

A clinical study conducted on a group of VPA-treated patients showed a significant reduction in antioxidant potential (FRAP) between the VPA-treated and the control group. Importantly, no such relationship was shown for reduced to oxidized glutathione (GSH/GSSG ratio) [143].

3.3. *Carbamazepine (CBZ)*

3.3.1. Pharmacological CBZ Data

The origins of the use of carbamazepine (CBZ) date back to the mid-20th century. Its mechanism is based on the modulation and blocking of potential-gated sodium channels. Its effects on serotonin- and catecholamine-based conductance have also been postulated. Among its other uses are the treatment of seizures, neuropathic pain, and manic episodes in the course of bipolar disorder. Side effects associated with its use include feelings of fatigue, headaches, blurred vision, and ataxia. Cases of Stevens–Johnson syndrome, severe hematological disorders, and toxic epidermal necrolysis associated with carbamazepine use have also been described [146–152].

3.3.2. Preclinical CBZ Studies

The studies of the effect of CBZ on the condition of oxidative stress are varied [153–160]. In vitro studies on erythrocytes showed no significant effect of the drug on oxidative stress in the cell [155]. In contrast, a study conducted on a plant cell model showed an increase in lipid peroxidation and levels of hydroperoxide and carbonyl proteins. In addition, a statistically non-significant increase in CAT levels was observed [160].

Studies of CBZ nephrotoxicity in rats suggest an association of renal cell damage with increased rates of oxidative stress [156]. In another study conducted on rats, no significant changes in malondialdehyde, glutathione, and SOD levels were observed in neural tissue during CBZ treatment. A significant decrease in GSH and SOD levels and an increase in MDA levels were only visible in the group with induced epilepsy [157]. A study in another animal model showed an increase in lipid peroxidation and hydroperoxide levels after exposure to CBZ. At the same time, a reduction in SOD, CAT, and GPx activity was confirmed [158]. Similar conclusions were reached in a similar study on the same animal model. A reduction in SOD, CAT, and GPx activity was shown with a concomitant increase in TBARS and carbonyl protein [159].

3.3.3. Clinical CBZ Studies

A study conducted on a pediatric population showed a significant reduction in antioxidant capacity and an increase in the oxidative stress index among epilepsy patients treated with carbamazepine compared to a healthy control group. In addition, an association was found between the use of CBZ and increased total oxidative status [160]. Similarly, a study by Varoglu et al. found a significant reduction in some antioxidative markers, with an increase in selected oxidative markers during carbamazepine monotherapy [154].

3.4. Oxcarbazepine (OXC)

3.4.1. Pharmacological OXC Data

The origins of the use of oxcarbazepine (OXC) in therapy date back to the 1990s. It is a structural derivative of carbamazepine, which is a pro-drug that is activated in the body as an active metabolite. It is postulated to act mainly by blocking and influencing voltage-gated sodium channels. The primary uses of the drug include the treatment of epilepsy and affective disorders. Compared to carbamazepine, OXC is characterized by greater safety and fewer side effects and interactions. Common side effects associated with OXC use include dizziness, headaches, and nausea [161–166].

3.4.2. Preclinical OXC Studies

The studies of the effect of OXC on the status of oxidative stress are not very numerous and clear [167–171]. Studies in mice have shown no significant effect of OXC use on levels of oxidative stress exponents such as MDA, GSH, CAT, and SOD determined in brain tissue. Elevated MDA levels and reduced glutathione levels were only observed with OXC use in individuals with pharmacologically induced epilepsy [168]. In turn, studies conducted in rats showed a significant protective effect of the use of OXC on nerve cells after hypoxia induced by cardiac arrest. It is postulated that these protective properties result from the attenuation of oxidative stress by increasing the presence of SOD [169]. The neuroprotective properties of OXC through its effect on redox balance are also confirmed by a rodent study by Park et al., which showed a reduction in the production of superoxide anions.

In addition, elevated levels of SOD, CAT, and GPx were observed in nerve cells [170]. An increase in the formation of ROS as a result of epileptic seizures has been demonstrated [171].

3.4.3. Clinical OXC Studies

A meta-analysis by Rezaei et al. found no significant statistical difference between OXC-treated and healthy individuals in blood-assessed homocysteine levels, which are directly related to redox balance regulation [167]. Similar observations have also been made regarding folic acid and cobalamin's indirect involvement in the regulation of oxidative stress [168].

4. Antidepressants

4.1. Citalopram (CIT)

4.1.1. Pharmacological CIT Data

Citalopram (CIT) is a selective serotonin reuptake inhibitor (SSRI), authorized in 1998. In addition, it has a low affinity for dopaminergic D_2 receptors, 5-HT_{1A} and 5-HT_{2A} receptors, α-adrenergic and β-adrenergic, muscarinic, and histamine H_1 receptors [172]. It is used in the treatment of depressive disorders, anxiety disorders with or without anxiety attacks with agoraphobia, as well as obsessive-compulsive disorders. Common side effects include sleep disturbances, nausea, decreased sex drive, excessive sweating, and dry mouth [173].

4.1.2. Preclinical CIT Studies

The research results provide a lot of data on the impact of CIT on oxidative stress [174–181]. Hepatotoxicity of CIT, resulting from free radical effects, has been observed in rat studies. Treatment took place in vitro and in vivo. In the in vitro group, hepatocyte death was noted at 500 μM, as well as increased ROS formation, breakdown of mitochondrial potential, lysosomal membrane leakage, GSH depletion, and lipid peroxidation. The in vivo tests at a dose of citalopram (20 mg/kg), confirmed the above damage [174].

In addition, other studies conducted on male rats have shown that CIT causes testicular damage to the mechanisms of oxidative stress as well as hormonal changes. The drug was used at doses of 5, 10, and 20 mg/kg. Sperm showed abnormal morphology and DNA damage, while their concentration decreased. In addition, histopathological changes in the testicles were observed. Luteinizing hormone concentrations increased with each dose of citalopram, while testosterone concentrations increased with doses of 5 and 10 mg/kg. Reduced glutathione levels signaled increased oxidative stress in the male rats given citalopram at doses of 10 and 20 mg/kg [175]. Studies conducted on Daphnia magna have shown that citalopram causes oxidative damage. The microorganisms were exposed to citalopram in the water at a concentration of 1.03 mg/L. In Daphnia, an increase in the concentration of the antioxidant molecule glutathione S-transferase (GST) was observed, as well as an increase in the activity of SOD, CAT, and GPx. In addition, MDA, protein carbonyl, and 8-OHdG concentrations increased. CIT has been shown to cause oxidative damage [176].

Antitumor effects of citalopram on hepatocellular carcinoma cells have also been observed. The cytotoxic effect of the drug on HepG2 cells was manifested by decreased cell viability and increased ROS formation. An increase in mitochondrial Bax and a decrease in Bcl2, as well as cytochrome C release, were observed. It has been suggested that citalopram may exhibit apoptotic effects against a hepatocellular carcinoma cell line via induction of cell death via a cytochrome C release mechanism and ROS-dependent activation of NFκB [177].

In addition, studies on the effect of citalopram on the processing of amyloid-β precursor protein (AβPP) have suggested that the drug may increase AβPP processing and also reduce oxidative stress. The study was conducted on induced pluripotent stem cells (iPSCs). Citalopram was administered for 45 days at concentrations of 0.8, 5, and 10 μM. In cells with the *PSEN1* gene mutation, O_2 concentrations were significantly reduced after each dose of citalopram. In contrast, no change in the formation of terminal oxidative stress markers was observed after treatment [180].

In addition, in studies conducted in rats, it was observed that co-administration of citalopram combined with rosuvastatin intensifies oxidative stress. The concomitant medications were used for 14 days. The results showed an increase in peroxidase and glutathione reductase activity, with no effect on antioxidant concentrations [178]. On the other hand, in studies conducted in Wistar rats, a neuroprotective effect of citalopram was observed, induced by the alleviation of oxidative stress, inflammation, apoptosis, and an altered metabolic profile. Treatment with CIT at 4 mg/kg significantly altered 17 metabolites with attenuation of malondialdehyde, reduced glutathione, matrix metalloproteinases, and apoptosis markers [179].

4.1.3. Clinical CIT Studies

A limited number of studies examine oxidative stress measured in patient groups. There was a significant increase in serum SOD, serum MDA, and decrease in plasma ascorbic acid levels in patients treated with CIT for major depression as compared to control subjects [181].

4.2. Sertraline (SER)

4.2.1. Pharmacological SER Data

Sertraline (SER) was introduced in 1991. It is a naphthaleneamine derivative. The mechanism of action of the drug is to inhibit the presynaptic reuptake of serotonin from the synaptic cleft (SSRI). Norepinephrine and dopamine transport are also blocked to a small extent. Sertraline slightly binds to adrenergic, histamine, muscarinic, dopaminergic, serotonergic, benzodiazepine, and GABA receptors. It is used to treat depressive disorders, obsessive-compulsive disorder, post-traumatic stress disorder, and seizure disorders. Common side effects include insomnia, drowsiness, anorexia, tremors, dizziness and headaches, diarrhea, nausea, or sexual dysfunction. In addition, movement disorders, paresthesias, visual disturbances, or increased sweating have been noted. In addition, sertraline-induced hepatotoxicity has also been described [182–184].

4.2.2. Preclinical SER Studies

The effects of SER on lipoperoxidation and antioxidant enzyme activity in plasma and brain tissues were studied in Wistar albino rats. Animals were administered the drug at doses of 10, 40, and 80 mg/kg. Lipid peroxidation (MDA) levels in plasma and brain tissue increased in all rats treated with sertraline. SOD activity in brain tissue decreased, while plasma concentrations increased compared to the control group. In contrast, plasma and brain tissue CAT concentrations and plasma paraoxonase (PON) concentrations decreased compared to the control group. Administration of higher doses of sertraline has been found to increase oxidative stress [185]. Studies in Drosophila melanogaster have shown sertraline-induced DNA damage and cell toxicity. Antidepressant-treated larvae manifested delayed development and reduced survival. It was observed that, through the action of sertraline, mitotically active tissues had DNA breaks and underwent apoptosis with increased frequency. Interestingly, the toxicity of the drug was partially mitigated by the administration of ascorbic acid. It has been suggested that sertraline induces oxidative DNA damage [186]. Sertraline-induced hepatotoxicity is probably due to mitochondrial dysfunction. The study was conducted on male Sprague Dawley rats. It has been observed that at doses of 75 and 100 μM, sertraline inhibits mitochondrial function by uncoupling oxidative phosphorylation and inhibiting the activity of complexes I and V. This process is further mediated by the loss of ATP and the induction of microsomal TG transport protein (MPT) [184].

The effects of sertraline (also in combination with haloperidol) on oxidative stress in mice were also compared. SER was administered at doses of 10–20 mg/kg. In antidepressant monotherapy, brain concentrations of GSH, MDA, TAC, and nitrite remained unchanged, while catalase and PON1 activity decreased. It has been found that sertraline, through its effects, can expose the brain to further oxidative damage [187]. Importantly, some studies suggest using the oxidative properties of sertraline to treat certain diseases. Sertraline can be used in the treatment of prostate cancer. Antidepressant-induced apoptosis and autophagy by activating free radical production, hydrogen peroxide (H_2O_2) formation, lipid peroxidation, and decreasing GSH concentration. Furthermore, sertraline significantly reduced the expression of aldehyde dehydrogenase 1 (ALDH1) and the stem cell marker CD44 [188].

Other studies have investigated the oxidative properties of sertraline against the Leishmania infantum parasite. The drug-induced uncoupling of respiration, a significant decrease in intracellular ATP concentration, and oxidative stress in the promastigote *L. infantum*. In addition, prolonged metabolic dysfunction was demonstrated. Sertraline killed *Leishmania* through a multidirectional mechanism of action, eliminating the parasite's primary metabolic pathways. The use of sertraline to treat visceral leishmaniasis in an off-label regimen has been suggested [189].

4.2.3. Clinical SER Studies

In contrast, a pilot study comparing the effects of sertraline on markers of oxidative stress (MDA) revealed a different effect on oxidative properties. People with depression, also diagnosed with heart failure, were divided into two groups: those receiving sertraline and those not receiving any antidepressant. After three months of treatment, patients treated with sertraline showed a significant reduction in MDA. It has been suggested that SER treatment reduces plasma markers of oxidative stress in depressed patients with additionally diagnosed heart failure [190].

4.3. *Venlafaxine (VEN)*

4.3.1. Pharmacological VEN Data

Venlafaxine (VEN) was launched in 1994 [191]. This substance, together with its metabolite—O-desmethylvenlafaxine—acts as a serotonin and norepinephrine reuptake inhibitor (SNRI). In addition, venlafaxine shows weak properties as a dopamine reuptake inhibitor. Its serotonergic effect contributes to sedative, drowsiness-increasing, and neutralizing effects, while its noradrenergic action can result in the opposite effects, i.e., agitation, deterioration of sleep quality, and sometimes even induce feelings of anxiety. The drug is approved for a variety of uses, such as the treatment of episodes of major depression, prevention of recurrent episodes of major depression, treatment of generalized anxiety disorder, treatment of social phobia, and treatment of paroxysmal anxiety [192]. Most patients tolerate VEN well, although symptoms such as dizziness and headache, nausea, dry mouth, and night sweats are most commonly seen in clinical practice. An increase in blood pressure is also observed, especially at the beginning of therapy or with high daily doses (300 mg/day) [193]. Other potential side effects mentioned in the literature include tinnitus, palpitations, sleep disturbances, vomiting, diarrhea, constipation, decreased appetite, and nervousness [194].

4.3.2. Preclinical VEN Studies

A study in male mice assessed venlafaxine's ability to damage DNA in the brain and liver and its oxidative effects on DNA, lipids, and proteins. An intermediate dose of the drug (50 mg/kg) caused significant DNA damage at 2 and 6 h after exposure, while a high dose (250 mg/kg) caused even more pronounced oxidative damage over the same time interval. Damage was observed in both the brain and liver, with the liver being, however, more severe. Lipoperoxidation effects in the brain and liver were evident after 6 and 12 h at doses of 50 and 250 mg/kg. In contrast, liver nitrite content induced 2 h after exposure to venlafaxine (250 mg/kg) was elevated [195].

Similar observations were made on the effect of VEN on hepatocyte cytotoxicity—in this study, the drug was administered to male rats, and then liver cells were isolated from them. Venlafaxine has been observed to cause hepatotoxicity through the induction of oxidative stress and subsequent toxic effects, including GSH depletion, lipid peroxidation, breakdown of mitochondrial potential, and lysosomal membrane leakage in hepatocytes. In addition, functional mitochondrial damage was observed through inhibition of mitochondrial respiratory complexes II and IV. Lysosomes and mitochondria have been shown to be the earliest target structures for venlafaxine-induced hepatotoxicity [196].

In addition, chronic VEN administration affects the methylation of promoters of genes involved in oxidative and nitrosative stress. This includes mRNA expression of SOD1, SOD2, and NOS1 in peripheral blood mononuclear cells (PBMC) and in the brain, as well as gene expression of CAT, Gpx1, and Gpx4 only in the brain [197]. In a study in mice, co-administration of VEN (40 mg/kg) with morphine showed inhibition of naloxone-induced withdrawal symptoms. In addition, the drug reduces the expression of TNF-α, IL-1β, IL-6, NO, and the concentration of MDA in brain tissue. Repeated administration of venlafaxine inhibits the decline in brain-derived neurotrophic factor (BDNF), thiol, and GPx [198]. Studies evaluating the effects of venlafaxine on glucose homeostasis and oxidative stress showed that the drug's effects were associated with a TBARS decrease and an increase in GSH levels in the brain. Mice with diabetes were studied; VEN was administered at doses of 8 and 16 mg/kg/day for 21 days. Glucose levels did not change significantly after administration [199]. No clinical VEN study results were found in the literature.

5. Discussion

Understanding the mechanisms and role of oxidative stress in the possible etiopathogenesis of psychiatric diseases makes it possible to develop new therapeutic approaches based on its modulation. Such research has been conducted in the case of bipolar disorder, where oxidative stress has been shown to affect molecule damage at the neurobiological level. This observation makes it possible to try to use drugs that affect the balance between antioxidative and oxidative processes to induce remission of the disease [1].

A compilation of the many publications on in vitro and animal experiments and the few findings from studies conducted in patient groups indicates considerable interest in the topic of the involvement of oxidative stress in the mechanism of many neurodegenerative diseases treated with older and newer generation drugs.

The findings indicate that significant differences can be observed in clinical practice regarding the prescribing of the classic drug haloperidol. Although second-generation drugs are preferred in most cases, haloperidol still stands out among the classic antipsychotics, as its prescription frequency has not changed significantly over the past decade [41–43]. Despite this, the contribution of oxidative stress during HLP use is still not fully understood. A substantial body of research allows the authors to conclude that haloperidol increases oxidative stress in brain tissue, showing a tendency to increase neuronal damage [47]. Hence, one of the main directions of recent research is the study of the interaction of antipsychotic drugs, including haloperidol, with other substances. This is because they can exhibit both adverse and beneficial joint effects on oxidative stress parameters [44,47,51].

Continued research among neuropsychiatric drugs has confirmed the significant efficacy of clozapine in the treatment of symptoms of psychosis, particularly drug-resistant schizophrenia [52,53]. Studies on the involvement of clozapine in oxidative stress further revealed the cardiotoxic effects of the drug, confirmed by elevated activities of biomarkers of cardiac damage, i.e., LDH and cardiac creatine kinase isoenzyme, CK-MB, with a concomitant decrease in GSH levels, such an important antioxidant in the body [58]. However, the results of a study comparing oxidative stress parameters in patients treated with perphenazine, risperidone, and clozapine led the authors to a completely different conclusion. Indeed, it was shown that in the group of patients treated with clozapine for at least three months, serum GSH and SOD levels increased, and MDA levels were significantly lower compared to patients treated with perphenazine and risperidone. It has, therefore, been suggested that clozapine, contributes to a significant alleviation of the negative symptoms of schizophrenia by exhibiting antioxidant effects [61].

The results suggest that atypical antipsychotics (clozapine, risperidone) have a more favorable effect on levels of oxidative stress biomarkers compared to classical drugs (perphenazine), which may be important in the context of both schizophrenia treatment and symptom relief [61]. The success of clozapine led to a search for its chemical analog, which would not be associated with such a high risk of developing agranulocytosis. This research allowed the synthesis of olanzapine, a new tricyclic dibenzoazepine derivative belonging to the second generation of antipsychotics. The drug quickly gained popularity after its approval and, along with risperidone, became one of the most widely used antipsychotics. Its prescribing frequency declined slightly in the 2000s, most likely driven by patient concerns about side effects [41,68,76].

Numerous studies have been conducted to clarify the relationship between OLZ treatment and changes in antioxidant and oxidant levels in the body [77]. Given the lack of oxidative damage induced by olanzapine, researchers point to a possible neuroprotective mechanism of action of the drug [79]. The results suggest that the use of olanzapine in the short term, unfortunately, leads to the development of inflammation in both the central and peripheral nervous system, which induces the occurrence of altered immunological responses in patients with schizophrenia. These changes may be related to the therapeutic effects of olanzapine, but their association with adverse side effects, e.g., weight gain, is also not excluded [81].

QT shows a complex effect on oxidative stress. As with the other second-generation drugs, research results indicate their antioxidant properties [86,87]. The authors pointed to the potential use of quetiapine to improve cognition and reduce oxidative damage to the brain, drawing additional attention to the drug's neuroprotective properties. Indeed, a reduction in Bax and caspase-3 protein levels provides protection against neuronal apoptosis [91,96]. The favorable side-effect profile makes aripiprazole one of the drugs preferred by patients. Along with risperidone, quetiapine, and olanzapine, it is the most commonly prescribed atypical antipsychotic drug [56,68,96]. Given the unique mechanism of action of aripiprazole and its favorable side-effect profile, it is expected to have an equally favorable effect on oxidative stress parameters. However, the studies conducted do not provide a clear answer regarding the potential pro- or antioxidant effect of the drug [97]. Recent studies also indicate a potential antioxidant effect on neurons. According to the researchers, the results obtained demonstrate the neuroprotective mechanism of action of aripiprazole [100]. Based on the results, it was inferred that aripiprazole provides potential protection for liver cells under oxidative conditions found in people with schizophrenia [101].

The effect of lithium on oxidative status is still not fully understood. A number of factors have now been postulated to influence the effect of lithium on oxidative stress. Among them, factors related to the conduct of therapy should be distinguished, such as the doses used, the time of taking, or interactions with other drugs used. The type of tissue affected by lithium also has an impact. Furthermore, when assessing the effect of lithium on oxidative stress, the pre-existing redox balance disturbances, which form the pathophysiological basis of diseases, must also be taken into account [114,115]. A study in healthy volunteers showed a statistically significant reduction in SOD after lithium therapy, with no significant effect on CAT or TBARS levels [122]. In a study conducted on rat liver cells in vitro, Li cytotoxicity was demonstrated to be associated with participation in the formation of oxygen-free radicals. Moreover, cytotoxicity increased with increasing blood lithium concentrations. In addition, the role of the CYP2E1 isoenzyme in oxidative stress associated with the intake of lithium was postulated [123].

Valproic acid and carbamazepine were among the first drugs to be used in the treatment of epilepsy. Toxicity related to the oxidative stress effects of VPA is also seen in rat hepatocyte cells, which is related to the intensive and multi-step hepatic metabolism of the drug [139].

Capacity and increased oxidative stress index among epilepsy patients treated with carbamazepine compared to a healthy control group. In addition, a correlation was found between the use of carbamazepine and increased total oxidative status [153].

The effect of oxcarbazepine on oxidative stress remains a subject of research [166]. Also, in the case of epilepsy, the role of oxidative stress as one of the components in epileptogenesis has been demonstrated [171].

The effect of citalopram on the development of oxidative stress is important. Studies on Daphnia magna have shown that citalopram causes oxidative damage [176]. Antitumor effects of citalopram on hepatocellular carcinoma cells have also been observed. It has been suggested that citalopram may exhibit apoptotic effects against a hepatocellular carcinoma cell line via induction of cell death via a cytochrome C release mechanism and ROS-dependent activation of NFκB [177].

The topic of sertraline-induced oxidative stress is frequently addressed in research. Studies in Drosophila melanogaster have shown sertraline-induced DNA damage and cell toxicity. Sertraline-induced hepatotoxicity is probably due to mitochondrial dysfunction [184]. Significantly, some studies suggest using the oxidative properties of sertraline to treat certain diseases. Sertraline can be used in the treatment of prostate cancer [188]. In contrast, a pilot study comparing the effects of sertraline on markers of oxidative stress (MDA) revealed different effects on oxidative properties [190].

The relationship between venlafaxine and oxidative stress is a topic addressed in the literature. Studies evaluating the effects of venlafaxine on glucose homeostasis and oxidative stress showed that the drug's effects were associated with a decrease in TBARS and an increase in brain GSH levels [198].

6. Conclusions

In conclusion, oxidative stress is an important risk factor for many psychiatric disorders in the treatment of which first- and second-generation antipsychotics are most commonly used, mood stabilizers, and antidepressants, and this publication reviews the state of the art of the contribution of oxidative stress to the most commonly used treatments of neuropsychiatric diseases, with first- and second-generation antipsychotics as important in treatment success as discoveries in the pathophysiology of neuropsychiatric diseases, including those initiating a new round of innovations in the contribution of oxidative stress to the etiology of neuropsychiatric diseases. For neurological patients, it is important to identify the cause of the oxidation–reduction disturbances, which can be led by pharmacological drug properties, mechanism of action, drug–drug interaction, dose, and nutritional status [2,6,8,77,99,138,139,167,168,181,200]. All changes should be taken into account in oxidative stress generation because it is necessary to understand the characteristics and scope of each neuropsychiatric drug used in therapy.

Author Contributions: Conceptualization, K.S.-K.; methodology, W.J.; software, S.R. and F.N.; formal analysis, K.S.-K., W.J., S.R. and F.N.; resources, M.Ł.-G. and P.Ś.; writing—original draft preparation, K.S.-K.; writing—review and editing, K.S.-K., W.J., S.R. and F.N.; visualization, K.S.-K.; supervision, B.Z.-P.; project administration, C.Ż.; funding acquisition, Z.Ż. All authors have read and agreed to the published version of the manuscript.

Funding: This research received no external funding.

Conflicts of Interest: The authors declare no conflicts of interest.

References

1. Sachdev, P.S. Whither Neuropsychiatry? *J. Neuropsychiatry Clin. Neurosci.* **2005**, *17*, 140–144. [CrossRef] [PubMed]
2. Salim, S. Oxidative Stress and Psychological Disorders. *Curr. Neuropharmacol.* **2014**, *12*, 140–147. [CrossRef] [PubMed]
3. Morandi, A.; Davis, D.; Bellelli, G.; Arora, R.C.; Caplan, G.A.; Kamholz, B.; Kolanowski, A.; Fick, D.M.; Kreisel, S.; MacLullich, A.; et al. The Diagnosis of Delirium Superimposed on Dementia: An Emerging Challenge. *J. Am. Med. Dir. Assoc.* **2017**, *18*, 12–18. [CrossRef] [PubMed]
4. Adamis, D.; Van Munster, B.C.; Macdonald, A.J.D. The Genetics of Deliria. *Int. Rev. Psychiatry* **2009**, *21*, 20–29. [CrossRef] [PubMed]
5. Lees, B.; Meredith, L.R.; Kirkland, A.E.; Bryant, B.E.; Squeglia, L.M. Effect of Alcohol Use on the Adolescent Brain and Behavior. *Pharmacol. Biochem. Behav.* **2020**, *192*, 172906. [CrossRef]
6. Jee, H.J.; Lee, S.G.; Bormate, K.J.; Jung, Y.-S. Effect of Caffeine Consumption on the Risk for Neurological and Psychiatric Disorders: Sex Differences in Human. *Nutrients* **2020**, *12*, 3080. [CrossRef] [PubMed]
7. Cappelletti, S.; Piacentino, D.; Sani, G.; Aromatario, M. Caffeine: Cognitive and Physical Performance Enhancer or Psychoactive Drug? *Curr. Neuropharmacol.* **2015**, *13*, 71–88. [CrossRef]
8. Urits, I.; Gress, K.; Charipova, K.; Li, N.; Berger, A.A.; Cornett, E.M.; Hasoon, J.; Kassem, H.; Kaye, A.D.; Viswanath, O. Cannabis Use and Its Association with Psychological Disorders. *Psychopharmacol. Bull* **2020**, *50*, 56–67. [PubMed]
9. McCutcheon, R.A.; Reis Marques, T.; Howes, O.D. Schizophrenia-An Overview. *JAMA Psychiatry* **2020**, *77*, 201–210. [CrossRef]
10. Rosell, D.R.; Futterman, S.E.; McMaster, A.; Siever, L.J. Schizotypal Personality Disorder: A Current Review. *Curr. Psychiatry Rep.* **2014**, *16*, 452. [CrossRef]
11. Joseph, S.M.; Siddiqui, W. Delusional Disorder. In *StatPearls*; StatPearls Publishing: Treasure Island, FL, USA, 2024.
12. Dailey, M.W.; Saadabadi, A. Mania. In *StatPearls*; StatPearls Publishing: Treasure Island, FL, USA, 2024.
13. Phillips, M.L.; Kupfer, D.J. Bipolar Disorder Diagnosis: Challenges and Future Directions. *Lancet* **2013**, *381*, 1663–1671. [CrossRef]
14. Klein, R.G. Anxiety Disorders. *J. Child Psychol. Psychiatry* **2009**, *50*, 153–162. [CrossRef]
15. Goodman, W.K.; Grice, D.E.; Lapidus, K.A.B.; Coffey, B.J. Obsessive-Compulsive Disorder. *Psychiatr. Clin. North Am.* **2014**, *37*, 257–267. [CrossRef]
16. Treasure, J.; Duarte, T.A.; Schmidt, U. Eating Disorders. *Lancet* **2020**, *395*, 899–911. [CrossRef]
17. Szelenberger, W.; Soldatos, C. Sleep Disorders in Psychiatric Practice. *World Psychiatry* **2005**, *4*, 186–190. [PubMed]
18. Cooper, R.J. Over-the-Counter Medicine Abuse—A Review of the Literature. *J. Subst. Use* **2013**, *18*, 82–107. [CrossRef]
19. Schulte Holthausen, B.; Habel, U. Sex Differences in Personality Disorders. *Curr. Psychiatry Rep.* **2018**, *20*, 107. [CrossRef] [PubMed]
20. Garg, G.; Elshimy, G.; Marwaha, R. Gender Dysphoria. In *StatPearls*; StatPearls Publishing: Treasure Island, FL, USA, 2024.
21. Sharma, B.R. Disorders of Sexual Preference and Medicolegal Issues Thereof. *Am. J. Forensic. Med. Pathol.* **2003**, *24*, 277–282. [CrossRef]
22. Mahone, E.M.; Denckla, M.B. Attention-Deficit/Hyperactivity Disorder: A Historical Neuropsychological Perspective. *J. Int. Neuropsychol. Soc.* **2017**, *23*, 916–929. [CrossRef] [PubMed]
23. Martino, D.; Mink, J.W. Tic Disorders. *Contin. (Minneap Minn)* **2013**, *19*, 1287–1311. [CrossRef]
24. Divac, N.; Prostran, M.; Jakovcevski, I.; Cerovac, N. Second-Generation Antipsychotics and Extrapyramidal Adverse Effects. *Biomed. Res. Int.* **2014**, *2014*, 656370. [CrossRef] [PubMed]
25. Lehman, A.F.; Lieberman, J.A.; Dixon, L.B.; McGlashan, T.H.; Miller, A.L.; Perkins, D.O.; Kreyenbuhl, J.; American Psychiatric Association; Steering Committee on Practice Guidelines. Practice Guideline for the Treatment of Patients with Schizophrenia, Second Edition. *Am. J. Psychiatry* **2004**, *161* (Suppl. 2), 1–56.
26. Klier, C.M.; Mossaheb, N.; Saria, A.; Schloegelhofer, M.; Zernig, G. Pharmacokinetics and Elimination of Quetiapine, Venlafaxine, and Trazodone during Pregnancy and Postpartum. *J. Clin. Psychopharmacol.* **2007**, *27*, 720–722. [CrossRef]
27. Yoshikawa, T.; Naito, Y. What Is Oxidative Stress? *Jpn. Med. Assoc. J.* **2002**, *45*, 271–276.

28. Teleanu, D.M.; Niculescu, A.-G.; Lungu, I.I.; Radu, C.I.; Vladâcenco, O.; Roza, E.; Costăchescu, B.; Grumezescu, A.M.; Teleanu, R.I. An Overview of Oxidative Stress, Neuroinflammation, and Neurodegenerative Diseases. *Int. J. Mol. Sci.* **2022**, *23*, 5938. [CrossRef]
29. Pizzino, G.; Irrera, N.; Cucinotta, M.; Pallio, G.; Mannino, F.; Arcoraci, V.; Squadrito, F.; Altavilla, D.; Bitto, A. Oxidative Stress: Harms and Benefits for Human Health. *Oxid. Med. Cell. Longev.* **2017**, *2017*, 8416763. [CrossRef]
30. Nishimura, Y.; Kanda, Y.; Sone, H.; Aoyama, H. Oxidative Stress as a Common Key Event in Developmental Neurotoxicity. *Oxid. Med. Cell. Longev.* **2021**, *2021*, 6685204. [CrossRef]
31. Gonçalves, R.V.; Costa, A.M.A.; Grzeskowiak, L. Oxidative Stress and Tissue Repair: Mechanism, Biomarkers, and Therapeutics. *Oxid. Med. Cell. Longev.* **2021**, *2021*, 6204096. [CrossRef] [PubMed]
32. Liguori, I.; Russo, G.; Curcio, F.; Bulli, G.; Aran, L.; Della-Morte, D.; Gargiulo, G.; Testa, G.; Cacciatore, F.; Bonaduce, D.; et al. Oxidative Stress, Aging, and Diseases. *Clin. Interv. Aging* **2018**, *13*, 757–772. [CrossRef]
33. Gyurászová, M.; Kovalčíková, A.; Janšáková, K.; Šebeková, K.; Celec, P.; Tóthová, Ľ. Markers of Oxidative Stress and Antioxidant Status in the Plasma, Urine and Saliva of Healthy Mice. *Physiol. Res.* **2018**, *67*, 921–934. [CrossRef]
34. Marrocco, I.; Altieri, F.; Peluso, I. Measurement and Clinical Significance of Biomarkers of Oxidative Stress in Humans. *Oxid. Med. Cell. Longev.* **2017**, *2017*, 6501046. [CrossRef] [PubMed]
35. Li, X.; Cameron, M.D. Potential Role of a Quetiapine Metabolite in Quetiapine-Induced Neutropenia and Agranulocytosis. *Chem. Res. Toxicol.* **2012**, *25*, 1004–1011. [CrossRef] [PubMed]
36. Soeiro-DE-Souza, M.G.; Dias, V.V.; Missio, G.; Balanzá-Martinez, V.; Valiengo, L.; Carvalho, A.F.; Moreno, R.A. Role of Quetiapine beyond Its Clinical Efficacy in Bipolar Disorder: From Neuroprotection to the Treatment of Psychiatric Disorders (Review). *Exp. Ther. Med.* **2015**, *9*, 643–652. [CrossRef] [PubMed]
37. Granger, B.; Albu, S. The Haloperidol Story. *Ann. Clin. Psychiatry* **2005**, *17*, 137–140. [CrossRef] [PubMed]
38. Tyler, M.W.; Zaldivar-Diez, J.; Haggarty, S.J. Classics in Chemical Neuroscience: Haloperidol. *ACS Chem. Neurosci.* **2017**, *8*, 444–453. [CrossRef] [PubMed]
39. López-Muñoz, F.; Alamo, C. The Consolidation of Neuroleptic Therapy: Janssen, the Discovery of Haloperidol and Its Introduction into Clinical Practice. *Brain Res. Bull* **2009**, *79*, 130–141. [CrossRef]
40. Joy, C.B.; Adams, C.E.; Lawrie, S.M. Haloperidol versus Placebo for Schizophrenia. *Cochrane Database Syst. Rev.* **2006**, *4*, CD003082.
41. Radojčić, M.R.; Pierce, M.; Hope, H.; Senior, M.; Taxiarchi, V.P.; Trefan, L.; Swift, E.; Abel, K.M. Trends in Antipsychotic Prescribing to Children and Adolescents in England: Cohort Study Using 2000-19 Primary Care Data. *Lancet Psychiatry* **2023**, *10*, 119–128. [CrossRef] [PubMed]
42. Anczewska, M.; Balicki, M.; Droździkowska, A.; Gorczyca, P.; Janus, J.; Paciorek, S.; Plisko, R.; Zięba, M. Practice of Prescribing Antipsychotics in Schizophrenia during 2013-2018 Based on Data from the National Health Fund. *Psychiatr. Pol.* **2022**, *56*, 751–766. [CrossRef]
43. Haloperidol—Drug Usage Statistics, ClinCalc DrugStats Database. Available online: https://clincalc.com/DrugStats/Drugs/Haloperidol (accessed on 26 January 2024).
44. Perera, J.; Tan, J.H.; Jeevathayaparan, S.; Chakravarthi, S.; Haleagrahara, N. Neuroprotective Effects of Alpha Lipoic Acid on Haloperidol-Induced Oxidative Stress in the Rat Brain. *Cell Biosci.* **2011**, *1*, 12. [CrossRef]
45. Raudenska, M.; Gumulec, J.; Babula, P.; Stracina, T.; Sztalmachova, M.; Polanska, H.; Adam, V.; Kizek, R.; Novakova, M.; Masarik, M. Haloperidol Cytotoxicity and Its Relation to Oxidative Stress. *Mini Rev. Med. Chem.* **2013**, *13*, 1993–1998. [CrossRef] [PubMed]
46. Bošković, M.; Grabnar, I.; Terzič, T.; Kores Plesničar, B.; Vovk, T. Oxidative Stress in Schizophrenia Patients Treated with Long-Acting Haloperidol Decanoate. *Psychiatry Res.* **2013**, *210*, 761–768. [CrossRef] [PubMed]
47. El-Awdan, S.A.; Abdel Jaleel, G.A.; Saleh, D.O. Alleviation of Haloperidol Induced Oxidative Stress in Rats: Effects of Sucrose vs Grape Seed Extract. *Bull. Fac. Pharm. Cairo Univ.* **2015**, *53*, 29–35. [CrossRef]
48. Andreazza, A.C.; Barakauskas, V.E.; Fazeli, S.; Feresten, A.; Shao, L.; Wei, V.; Wu, C.H.; Barr, A.M.; Beasley, C.L. Effects of Haloperidol and Clozapine Administration on Oxidative Stress in Rat Brain, Liver and Serum. *Neurosci. Lett.* **2015**, *591*, 36–40. [CrossRef] [PubMed]
49. Singh, O.P.; Chakraborty, I.; Dasgupta, A.; Datta, S. A Comparative Study of Oxidative Stress and Interrelationship of Important Antioxidants in Haloperidol and Olanzapine Treated Patients Suffering from Schizophrenia. *Indian J. Psychiatry* **2008**, *50*, 171–176. [CrossRef]
50. Gawlik-Kotelnicka, O.; Mielicki, W.; Rabe-Jabłońska, J.; Strzelecki, D. Impact of Lithium Alone or in Combination with Haloperidol on Selected Oxidative Stress Parameters in Human Plasma in Vitro. *Redox Rep.* **2016**, *21*, 45–49. [CrossRef]
51. Kajero, J.A.; Seedat, S.; Ohaeri, J.U.; Akindele, A.; Aina, O. The Effects of Cannabidiol on Behavioural and Oxidative Stress Parameters Induced by Prolonged Haloperidol Administration. *Acta Neuropsychiatr.* **2022**, *4*, 1–11. [CrossRef]
52. Khokhar, J.Y.; Henricks, A.M.; Sullivan, E.D.K.; Green, A.I. Unique Effects of Clozapine: A Pharmacological Perspective. *Adv. Pharmacol.* **2018**, *82*, 137–162.
53. Crilly, J. The History of Clozapine and Its Emergence in the US Market: A Review and Analysis. *Hist. Psychiatry* **2007**, *18*, 39–60. [CrossRef]
54. Seeman, P. Clozapine, a Fast-off-D2 Antipsychotic. *ACS Chem. Neurosci.* **2014**, *5*, 24–29. [CrossRef]

55. Masdrakis, V.G.; Baldwin, D.S. Prevention of Suicide by Clozapine in Mental Disorders: Systematic Review. *Eur. Neuropsychopharmacol.* **2023**, *69*, 4–23. [CrossRef]
56. Griffiths, K.; Martínez-Gutiérrez, A.D.; Rentería, M.E.; Patel, R. Antipsychotic Prescribing Trends in Schizophrenia between 2011 and 2021: Real-World Data from a US Electronic Health Record Database. *Neurosci. Appl.* **2022**, *1*, 269. [CrossRef]
57. Walss-Bass, C.; Weintraub, S.T.; Hatch, J.; Mintz, J.; Chaudhuri, A.R. Clozapine Causes Oxidation of Proteins Involved in Energy Metabolism: A Possible Mechanism for Antipsychotic-Induced Metabolic Alterations. *Int. J. Neuropsychopharmacol.* **2008**, *11*, 1097–1104. [CrossRef] [PubMed]
58. Abdel-Wahab, B.; Abdalla, M.; El-Khawanky, M. Does Clozapine Induce Myocarditis, Myocardial Oxidative Stress and DNA Damage in Rats. *Egypt. J. Forensic Sci.* **2014**, *4*, 75–82. [CrossRef]
59. Zhang, F.; Han, L.; Wang, J.; Shu, M.; Liu, K.; Zhang, Y.; Hsiao, C.; Tian, Q.; He, Q. Clozapine Induced Developmental and Cardiac Toxicity on Zebrafish Embryos by Elevating Oxidative Stress. *Cardiovasc. Toxicol.* **2021**, *21*, 399–409. [CrossRef] [PubMed]
60. Fehsel, K.; Loeffler, S.; Krieger, K.; Henning, U.; Agelink, M.; Kolb-Bachofen, V.; Klimke, A. Clozapine Induces Oxidative Stress and Proapoptotic Gene Expression in Neutrophils of Schizophrenic Patients. *J. Clin. Psychopharmacol.* **2005**, *25*, 419–426. [CrossRef]
61. Hendouei, N.; Farnia, S.; Mohseni, F.; Salehi, A.; Bagheri, M.; Shadfar, F.; Barzegar, F.; Hoseini, S.D.; Charati, J.Y.; Shaki, F. Alterations in Oxidative Stress Markers and Its Correlation with Clinical Findings in Schizophrenic Patients Consuming Perphenazine, Clozapine and Risperidone. *Biomed. Pharmacother.* **2018**, *103*, 965–972. [CrossRef] [PubMed]
62. Awouters, F.H.L.; Lewi, P.J. Forty Years of Antipsychotic Drug Research--from Haloperidol to Paliperidone—with Dr. Paul Janssen. *Arzneimittelforschung* **2007**, *57*, 625–632. [CrossRef]
63. Colpaert, F.C. Discovering Risperidone: The LSD Model of Psychopathology. *Nat. Rev. Drug Discov.* **2003**, *2*, 315–320. [CrossRef]
64. Chopko, T.C.; Lindsley, C.W. Classics in Chemical Neuroscience: Risperidone. *ACS Chem. Neurosci.* **2018**, *9*, 1520–1529. [CrossRef]
65. Pajonk, F.-G. Risperidone in Acute and Long-Term Therapy of Schizophrenia—A Clinical Profile. *Prog Neuropsychopharmacol. Biol. Psychiatry* **2004**, *28*, 15–23. [CrossRef]
66. Taurines, R.; Fekete, S.; Preuss-Wiedenhoff, A.; Warnke, A.; Wewetzer, C.; Plener, P.; Burger, R.; Gerlach, M.; Romanos, M.; Egberts, K.M. Therapeutic Drug Monitoring in Children and Adolescents with Schizophrenia and Other Psychotic Disorders Using Risperidone. *J. Neural. Transm.* **2022**, *129*, 689–701. [CrossRef] [PubMed]
67. Yunusa, I.; El Helou, M.L. The Use of Risperidone in Behavioral and Psychological Symptoms of Dementia: A Review of Pharmacology, Clinical Evidence, Regulatory Approvals, and Off-Label Use. *Front. Pharmacol.* **2020**, *11*, 596. [CrossRef]
68. Atypical Antipsychotics—Drug Usage Statistics, ClinCalc DrugStats Database. Available online: https://clincalc.com/DrugStats/TC/AtypicalAntipsychotics (accessed on 26 January 2024).
69. Stojkovic, M.; Radmanovic, B.; Jovanovic, M.; Janjic, V.; Muric, N.; Ristic, D.I. Risperidone Induced Hyperprolactinemia: From Basic to Clinical Studies. *Front. Psychiatry* **2022**, *13*, 874705. [CrossRef]
70. Zhang, X.Y.; Zhou, D.F.; Shen, Y.C.; Zhang, P.Y.; Zhang, W.F.; Liang, J.; Chen, D.C.; Xiu, M.H.; Kosten, T.A.; Kosten, T.R. Effects of Risperidone and Haloperidol on Superoxide Dismutase and Nitric Oxide in Schizophrenia. *Neuropharmacology* **2012**, *62*, 1928–1934. [CrossRef]
71. Lee, B.-H.; Kim, Y.-K. Reduced Plasma Nitric Oxide Metabolites before and after Antipsychotic Treatment in Patients with Schizophrenia Compared to Controls. *Schizophr. Res.* **2008**, *104*, 36–43. [CrossRef] [PubMed]
72. Eftekhari, A.; Ahmadian, E.; Azarmi, Y.; Parvizpur, A.; Hamishehkar, H.; Eghbal, M.A. In Vitro/Vivo Studies towards Mechanisms of Risperidone-Induced Oxidative Stress and the Protective Role of Coenzyme Q10 and N-Acetylcysteine. *Toxicol. Mech. Methods* **2016**, *26*, 520–528. [CrossRef] [PubMed]
73. Pryor, K.; Storer, K. Chapter 11—Drugs for Neuropsychiatric Disorders. In *Pharmacology and Physiology for Anesthesia: Foundations and Clinical Application*; Elsevier: Amsterdam, The Netherlands, 2013; pp. 180–207.
74. Citrome, L.; McEvoy, J.P.; Todtenkopf, M.S.; McDonnell, D.; Weiden, P.J. A Commentary on the Efficacy of Olanzapine for the Treatment of Schizophrenia: The Past, Present, and Future. *Neuropsychiatr. Dis. Treat.* **2019**, *15*, 2559–2569. [CrossRef] [PubMed]
75. McCormack, P.L.; Wiseman, L.R. Olanzapine: A Review of Its Use in the Management of Bipolar I Disorder. *Drugs* **2004**, *64*, 2709–2726. [CrossRef]
76. Meftah, A.M.; Deckler, E.; Citrome, L.; Kantrowitz, J.T. New Discoveries for an Old Drug: A Review of Recent Olanzapine Research. *Postgrad. Med.* **2020**, *132*, 80–90. [CrossRef]
77. Zerin Khan, F.; Sultana, S.P.; Akhter, N.; Mosaddek, A.S.M. Effect of Olanzapine and Risperidone on Oxidative Stress in Schizophrenia Patients. *Int. Biol. Biomed. J.* **2018**, *4*, 89–97.
78. Boz, Z.; Hu, M.; Yu, Y.; Huang, X.-F. N-Acetylcysteine Prevents Olanzapine-Induced Oxidative Stress in mHypoA-59 Hypothalamic Neurons. *Sci. Rep.* **2020**, *10*, 19185. [CrossRef] [PubMed]
79. Reinke, A.; Martins, M.R.; Lima, M.S.; Moreira, J.C.; Dal-Pizzol, F.; Quevedo, J. Haloperidol and Clozapine, but Not Olanzapine, Induces Oxidative Stress in Rat Brain. *Neurosci. Lett.* **2004**, *372*, 157–160. [CrossRef] [PubMed]
80. Al-Chalabi, B.M.; Thanoon, I.A.J.; Ahmed, F.A. Potential Effect of Olanzapine on Total Antioxidant Status and Lipid Peroxidation in Schizophrenic Patients. *Neuropsychobiology* **2009**, *59*, 8–11. [CrossRef] [PubMed]
81. Li, W.-T.; Huang, X.-F.; Deng, C.; Zhang, B.-H.; Qian, K.; He, M.; Sun, T.-L. Olanzapine Induces Inflammation and Immune Response via Activating ER Stress in the Rat Prefrontal Cortex. *Curr. Med. Sci.* **2021**, *41*, 788–802. [CrossRef] [PubMed]
82. Wang, P.; Si, T. Use of Antipsychotics in the Treatment of Depressive Disorders. *Shanghai Arch. Psychiatry* **2013**, *25*, 134–140.

83. Ignácio, Z.M.; Calixto, A.V.; da Silva, R.H.; Quevedo, J.; Réus, G.Z. The Use of Quetiapine in the Treatment of Major Depressive Disorder: Evidence from Clinical and Experimental Studies. *Neurosci. Biobehav. Rev.* **2018**, *86*, 36–50. [CrossRef]
84. El-Khalili, N. Update on Extended Release Quetiapine Fumarate in Schizophrenia and Bipolar Disorders. *Neuropsychiatr. Dis. Treat.* **2012**, *8*, 523–536. [CrossRef]
85. Brett, J. Concerns about Quetiapine. *Aust. Prescr.* **2015**, *38*, 95–97. [CrossRef]
86. Han, J.-H.; Tian, H.-Z.; Lian, Y.-Y.; Yu, Y.; Lu, C.-B.; Li, X.-M.; Zhang, R.-L.; Xu, H. Quetiapine Mitigates the Ethanol-Induced Oxidative Stress in Brain Tissue, but Not in the Liver, of the Rat. *Neuropsychiatr. Dis. Treat.* **2015**, *11*, 1473–1482.
87. Ignácio, Z.M.; Réus, G.Z.; Abelaira, H.M.; de Moura, A.B.; de Souza, T.G.; Matos, D.; Goldim, M.P.; Mathias, K.; Garbossa, L.; Petronilho, F.; et al. Acute and Chronic Treatment with Quetiapine Induces Antidepressant-like Behavior and Exerts Antioxidant Effects in the Rat Brain. *Metab. Brain Dis.* **2017**, *32*, 1195–1208. [CrossRef] [PubMed]
88. Sommerfeld-Klatta, K.; Łukasik-Głębocka, M.; Krawczak, E.; Stodolska, A.; Zielińska-Psuja, B. Participation of quetiapine in oxidative stress and inflammation status in the treatment of drug overdose. *Acta Pol. Pharm.* **2023**, *80*, 327–333. [CrossRef] [PubMed]
89. Dietrich-Muszalska, A.; Kolodziejczyk-Czepas, J.; Nowak, P. Comparative Study of the Effects of Atypical Antipsychotic Drugs on Plasma and Urine Biomarkers of Oxidative Stress in Schizophrenic Patients. *Neuropsychiatr. Dis. Treat.* **2021**, *17*, 555–565. [CrossRef] [PubMed]
90. Dietrich-Muszalska, A.; Kontek, B.; Rabe-Jabłońska, J. Quetiapine, Olanzapine and Haloperidol Affect Human Plasma Lipid Peroxidation in Vitro. *Neuropsychobiology* **2011**, *63*, 197–201. [CrossRef] [PubMed]
91. Mani, V.; Alshammeri, B.S. Quetiapine Moderates Doxorubicin-Induced Cognitive Deficits: Influence of Oxidative Stress, Neuroinflammation, and Cellular Apoptosis. *Int. J. Mol. Sci.* **2023**, *24*, 11525. [CrossRef] [PubMed]
92. Stark, A.D.; Jordan, S.; Allers, K.A.; Bertekap, R.L.; Chen, R.; Mistry Kannan, T.; Molski, T.F.; Yocca, F.D.; Sharp, T.; Kikuchi, T.; et al. Interaction of the Novel Antipsychotic Aripiprazole with 5-HT1A and 5-HT 2A Receptors: Functional Receptor-Binding and in Vivo Electrophysiological Studies. *Psychopharmacology* **2007**, *190*, 373–382. [CrossRef] [PubMed]
93. Preda, A.; Shapiro, B.B. A Safety Evaluation of Aripiprazole in the Treatment of Schizophrenia. *Expert Opin. Drug Saf.* **2020**, *19*, 1529–1538. [CrossRef] [PubMed]
94. Prommer, E. Aripiprazole. *Am. J. Hosp. Palliat. Care* **2017**, *34*, 180–185. [CrossRef] [PubMed]
95. Cuomo, A.; Beccarini Crescenzi, B.; Goracci, A.; Bolognesi, S.; Giordano, N.; Rossi, R.; Facchi, E.; Neal, S.M.; Fagiolini, A. Drug Safety Evaluation of Aripiprazole in Bipolar Disorder. *Expert Opin. Drug Saf.* **2019**, *18*, 455–463. [CrossRef]
96. Khanna, P.; Suo, T.; Komossa, K.; Ma, H.; Rummel-Kluge, C.; El-Sayeh, H.G.; Leucht, S.; Xia, J. Aripiprazole versus Other Atypical Antipsychotics for Schizophrenia. *Cochrane Database Syst. Rev.* **2014**, *2014*, CD006569. [CrossRef]
97. Doblado, L.; Patel, G.; Yildiz, R.; Sellinger, L.; Koller, D.; Abad-Santos, F.; Peral, B.; Ben, A.; Monsalve, M. The SGAs Olanzapine and Aripiprazole Inhibit Mitochondrial Respiration and Induce Oxidative Stress. *Free. Radic. Biol. Med.* **2021**, *165*, 58–59. [CrossRef]
98. Dietrich-Muszalska, A.; Kolińska-Łukaszuk, J. Comparative Effects of Aripiprazole and Selected Antipsychotic Drugs on Lipid Peroxidation in Plasma. *Psychiatry Clin. Neurosci.* **2018**, *72*, 329–336. [CrossRef] [PubMed]
99. Eren, I.; Naziroğlu, M.; Demirdaş, A. Protective Effects of Lamotrigine, Aripiprazole and Escitalopram on Depression-Induced Oxidative Stress in Rat Brain. *Neurochem. Res.* **2007**, *32*, 1188–1195. [CrossRef] [PubMed]
100. Mani, V.; Alshammeri, B.S. Aripiprazole Attenuates Cognitive Impairments Induced by Lipopolysaccharide in Rats through the Regulation of Neuronal Inflammation, Oxidative Stress, and Apoptosis. *Medicina* **2023**, *60*, 46. [CrossRef] [PubMed]
101. Kramar, B.; Pirc Marolt, T.; Monsalve, M.; Šuput, D.; Milisav, I. Antipsychotic Drug Aripiprazole Protects Liver Cells from Oxidative Stress. *Int. J. Mol. Sci.* **2022**, *23*, 8292. [CrossRef] [PubMed]
102. Cade, J.F.J. Lithium Salts in the Treatment of Psychotic Excitement. *Med. J. Aust.* **1949**, *2*, 349–352. [CrossRef] [PubMed]
103. Shorter, E. The History of Lithium Therapy. *Bipolar. Disord.* **2009**, *11* (Suppl. 2), 4–9. [CrossRef] [PubMed]
104. Licht, R.W. Lithium: Still a Major Option in the Management of Bipolar Disorder. *CNS Neurosci. Ther.* **2012**, *18*, 219–226. [CrossRef]
105. Leucht, S.; Helfer, B.; Dold, M.; Kissling, W.; McGrath, J.J. Lithium for Schizophrenia. *Cochrane Database Syst. Rev.* **2015**, *2015*, CD003834. [CrossRef]
106. Bschor, T. Lithium in the Treatment of Major Depressive Disorder. *Drugs* **2014**, *74*, 855–862. [CrossRef]
107. Lazzara, C.A.; Kim, Y.-H. Potential Application of Lithium in Parkinson's and Other Neurodegenerative Diseases. *Front. Neurosci.* **2015**, *9*, 403. [CrossRef]
108. Matsunaga, S.; Kishi, T.; Annas, P.; Basun, H.; Hampel, H.; Iwata, N. Lithium as a Treatment for Alzheimer's Disease: A Systematic Review and Meta-Analysis. *J. Alzheimers Dis.* **2015**, *48*, 403–410. [CrossRef] [PubMed]
109. Forlenza, O.V.; de Paula, V.J.; Machado-Vieira, R.; Diniz, B.S.; Gattaz, W.F. Does Lithium Prevent Alzheimer's Disease? *Drugs Aging* **2012**, *29*, 335–342. [CrossRef]
110. Codogno, P.; Meijer, A.J. Chapter 306—Signaling in Autophagy Related Pathways. In *Handbook of Cell Signaling*, 2nd ed.; Bradshaw, R.A., Dennis, E.A., Eds.; Academic Press: San Diego, CA, USA, 2010; pp. 2583–2588.
111. Brown, K.M.; Tracy, D.K. Lithium: The Pharmacodynamic Actions of the Amazing Ion. *Ther. Adv. Psychopharmacol.* **2013**, *3*, 163–176. [CrossRef]
112. Malhi, G.S.; Tanious, M.; Das, P.; Coulston, C.M.; Berk, M. Potential Mechanisms of Action of Lithium in Bipolar Disorder. Current Understanding. *CNS Drugs* **2013**, *27*, 135–153. [CrossRef]

113. Wen, J.; Sawmiller, D.; Wheeldon, B.; Tan, J. A Review for Lithium: Pharmacokinetics, Drug Design, and Toxicity. *CNS Neurol. Disord. Drug Targets* **2019**, *18*, 769–778. [CrossRef] [PubMed]
114. McKnight, R.F.; Adida, M.; Budge, K.; Stockton, S.; Goodwin, G.M.; Geddes, J.R. Lithium Toxicity Profile: A Systematic Review and Meta-Analysis. *Lancet* **2012**, *379*, 721–728. [CrossRef]
115. Rabe-Jabłońska, J.; Dietrich-Muszalska, A. Effects of Lithium on Oxidative Stress. In *Studies on Psychiatric Disorders*; Dietrich-Muszalska, A., Chauhan, V., Grignon, S., Eds.; Springer: New York, NY, USA, 2015; pp. 567–573.
116. De Sousa, R.T.; Zarate, C.A.; Zanetti, M.V.; Costa, A.C.; Talib, L.L.; Gattaz, W.F.; Machado-Vieira, R. Oxidative Stress in Early Stage Bipolar Disorder and the Association with Response to Lithium. *J. Psychiatr. Res.* **2014**, *50*, 36–41. [CrossRef] [PubMed]
117. Banerjee, U.; Dasgupta, A.; Rout, J.K.; Singh, O.P. Effects of Lithium Therapy on Na+-K+-ATPase Activity and Lipid Peroxidation in Bipolar Disorder. *Prog. Neuropsychopharmacol. Biol.* **2012**, *37*, 56–61. [CrossRef]
118. da-Rosa, D.D.; Valvassori, S.S.; Steckert, A.V.; Ornell, F.; Ferreira, C.L.; Lopes-Borges, J.; Varela, R.B.; Dal-Pizzol, F.; Andersen, M.L.; Quevedo, J. Effects of Lithium and Valproate on Oxidative Stress and Behavioral Changes Induced by Administration of M-AMPH. *Psychiatry Res.* **2012**, *198*, 521–526. [CrossRef]
119. Jornada, L.K.; Valvassori, S.S.; Steckert, A.V.; Moretti, M.; Mina, F.; Ferreira, C.L.; Arent, C.O.; Dal-Pizzol, F.; Quevedo, J. Lithium and Valproate Modulate Antioxidant Enzymes and Prevent Ouabain-Induced Oxidative Damage in an Animal Model of Mania. *J. Psychiatr. Res.* **2011**, *45*, 162–168. [CrossRef] [PubMed]
120. Tufekci, K.U.; Alural, B.; Tarakcioglu, E.; San, T.; Genc, S. Lithium Inhibits Oxidative Stress-Induced Neuronal Senescence through miR-34a. *Mol. Biol. Rep.* **2021**, *48*, 4171–4180. [CrossRef] [PubMed]
121. Toplan, S.; Dariyerli, N.; Ozdemir, S.; Ozcelik, D.; Zengin, E.U.; Akyolcu, M.C. Lithium-Induced Hypothyroidism: Oxidative Stress and Osmotic Fragility Status in Rats. *Biol. Trace Elem. Res.* **2013**, *152*, 373–378. [CrossRef] [PubMed]
122. Khairova, R.; Pawar, R.; Salvadore, G.; Juruena, M.F.; de Sousa, R.T.; Soeiro-de-Souza, M.G.; Salvador, M.; Zarate, C.A.; Gattaz, W.F.; Machado-Vieira, R. Effects of Lithium on Oxidative Stress Parameters in Healthy Subjects. *Mol. Med. Rep.* **2012**, *5*, 680–682. [PubMed]
123. Eskandari, M.R.; Fard, J.K.; Hosseini, M.-J.; Pourahmad, J. Glutathione Mediated Reductive Activation and Mitochondrial Dysfunction Play Key Roles in Lithium Induced Oxidative Stress and Cytotoxicity in Liver. *Biometals* **2012**, *25*, 863–873. [CrossRef]
124. Franceschetti, S.; Hamon, B.; Heinemann, U. The Action of Valproate on Spontaneous Epileptiform Activity in the Absence of Synaptic Transmission and on Evoked Changes in [Ca2+]o and [K+]o in the Hippocampal Slice. *Brain Res.* **1986**, *386*, 1–11. [CrossRef]
125. Johannessen, C.U.; Johannessen, S.I. Valproate: Past, Present, and Future. *CNS Drug Rev.* **2003**, *9*, 199–216. [CrossRef] [PubMed]
126. Lloyd, K.A. A Scientific Review: Mechanisms of Valproate-Mediated Teratogenesis. *Biosci. Horiz. Int. J. Stud. Res.* **2013**, *6*, hzt003. [CrossRef]
127. Tomson, T.; Battino, D.; Bonizzoni, E.; Craig, J.; Lindhout, D.; Perucca, E.; Sabers, A.; Thomas, S.V.; Vajda, F.; EURAP Study Group. Dose-Dependent Teratogenicity of Valproate in Mono- and Polytherapy: An Observational Study. *Neurology* **2015**, *85*, 866–872. [CrossRef]
128. Bromfield, E.B.; Dworetzky, B.A.; Wyszynski, D.F.; Smith, C.R.; Baldwin, E.J.; Holmes, L.B. Valproate Teratogenicity and Epilepsy Syndrome. *Epilepsia* **2008**, *49*, 2122–2124. [CrossRef]
129. Gerstner, T.; Bell, N.; König, S. Oral Valproic Acid for Epilepsy--Long-Term Experience in Therapy and Side Effects. *Expert Opin. Pharmacother.* **2008**, *9*, 285–292. [CrossRef] [PubMed]
130. Nanau, R.M.; Neuman, M.G. Adverse Drug Reactions Induced by Valproic Acid. *Clin. Biochem.* **2013**, *46*, 1323–1338. [CrossRef] [PubMed]
131. Marson, A.G.; Sills, G.J. Valproate. In *The Treatment of Epilepsy*; John Wiley & Sons, Ltd.: Hoboken, NJ, USA, 2015; pp. 652–666.
132. Andrade, C. Valproate in Pregnancy: Recent Research and Regulatory Responses. *J. Clin. Psychiatry* **2018**, *79*, 18f12351. [CrossRef] [PubMed]
133. Chateauvieux, S.; Morceau, F.; Dicato, M.; Diederich, M. Molecular and Therapeutic Potential and Toxicity of Valproic Acid. *J. Biomed. Biotechnol.* **2010**, *2010*, 479364. [CrossRef] [PubMed]
134. Gobbi, G.; Janiri, L. Sodium- and Magnesium-Valproate in Vivo Modulate Glutamatergic and GABAergic Synapses in the Medial Prefrontal Cortex. *Psychopharmacology* **2006**, *185*, 255–262. [CrossRef]
135. Sher, Y.; Miller Cramer, A.C.; Ament, A.; Lolak, S.; Maldonado, J.R. Valproic Acid for Treatment of Hyperactive or Mixed Delirium: Rationale and Literature Review. *Psychosomatics* **2015**, *56*, 615–625. [CrossRef] [PubMed]
136. VanDongen, A.M.; VanErp, M.G.; Voskuyl, R.A. Valproate Reduces Excitability by Blockage of Sodium and Potassium Conductance. *Epilepsia* **1986**, *27*, 177–182. [CrossRef] [PubMed]
137. Chaudhary, S.; Parvez, S. An in Vitro Approach to Assess the Neurotoxicity of Valproic Acid-Induced Oxidative Stress in Cerebellum and Cerebral Cortex of Young Rats. *Neuroscience* **2012**, *225*, 258–268. [CrossRef]
138. Salimi, A.; Alyan, N.; Akbari, N.; Jamali, Z.; Pourahmad, J. Selenium and L-Carnitine Protects from Valproic Acid-Induced Oxidative Stress and Mitochondrial Damages in Rat Cortical Neurons. *Drug Chem. Toxicol.* **2022**, *45*, 1150–1157. [CrossRef]
139. Kiang, T.K.L.; Teng, X.W.; Karagiozov, S.; Surendradoss, J.; Chang, T.K.H.; Abbott, F.S. Role of Oxidative Metabolism in the Effect of Valproic Acid on Markers of Cell Viability, Necrosis, and Oxidative Stress in Sandwich-Cultured Rat Hepatocytes. *Toxicol. Sci.* **2010**, *118*, 501–509. [CrossRef]

140. Lee, J.Y.; Maeng, S.; Kang, S.R.; Choi, H.Y.; Oh, T.H.; Ju, B.G.; Yune, T.Y. Valproic Acid Protects Motor Neuron Death by Inhibiting Oxidative Stress and Endoplasmic Reticulum Stress-Mediated Cytochrome C Release after Spinal Cord Injury. *J. Neurotrauma* **2014**, *31*, 582–594. [CrossRef]
141. Suda, S.; Katsura, K.; Kanamaru, T.; Saito, M.; Katayama, Y. Valproic Acid Attenuates Ischemia-Reperfusion Injury in the Rat Brain through Inhibition of Oxidative Stress and Inflammation. *Eur. J. Pharmacol.* **2013**, *707*, 26–31. [CrossRef] [PubMed]
142. Terzioğlu Bebitoğlu, B.; Oğuz, E.; Gökçe, A. Effect of Valproic Acid on Oxidative Stress Parameters of Glutamate-Induced Excitotoxicity in SH-SY5Y Cells. *Exp. Ther. Med.* **2020**, *20*, 1321–1328. [CrossRef] [PubMed]
143. Sommerfeld-Klatta, K.; Łukasik-Głębocka, M.; Kobyłka, S.; Zielińska-Psuja, B. The impact of valproic acid and 2-propyl-4-pentenoic acid on antioxidant status measured by GSH/GSSG ratio and FRAP levels in acute and chronic exposure. *Acta Pol. Pharm. Drug Res.* **2023**, *80*, 335–340. [CrossRef] [PubMed]
144. Tung, E.W.Y.; Winn, L.M. Valproic Acid Increases Formation of Reactive Oxygen Species and Induces Apoptosis in Postimplantation Embryos: A Role for Oxidative Stress in Valproic Acid-Induced Neural Tube Defects. *Mol. Pharmacol.* **2011**, *80*, 979–987. [CrossRef]
145. Fu, J.; Shao, C.-J.; Chen, F.-R.; Ng, H.-K.; Chen, Z.-P. Autophagy Induced by Valproic Acid Is Associated with Oxidative Stress in Glioma Cell Lines. *Neuro. Oncol.* **2010**, *12*, 328–340. [CrossRef] [PubMed]
146. Alrashood, S.T. Carbamazepine. *Profiles Drug Subst. Excip. Relat. Methodol.* **2016**, *41*, 133–321. [PubMed]
147. Pellock, J.M. Carbamazepine Side Effects in Children and Adults. *Epilepsia* **1987**, *28* (Suppl. 3), S64–S70. [CrossRef] [PubMed]
148. Thorn, C.F.; Leckband, S.G.; Kelsoe, J.; Leeder, J.S.; Müller, D.J.; Klein, T.E.; Altman, R.B. PharmGKB Summary: Carbamazepine Pathway. *Pharm. Genom.* **2011**, *21*, 906–910. [CrossRef]
149. Fricke-Galindo, I.; LLerena, A.; Jung-Cook, H.; López-López, M. Carbamazepine Adverse Drug Reactions. *Expert Rev. Clin. Pharmacol.* **2018**, *11*, 705–718. [CrossRef]
150. Wiffen, P.J.; Derry, S.; Moore, R.A.; Kalso, E.A. Carbamazepine for Chronic Neuropathic Pain and Fibromyalgia in Adults. *Cochrane Database Syst. Rev.* **2014**, *2014*, CD005451. [CrossRef] [PubMed]
151. Dailey, J.W.; Reith, M.E.; Yan, Q.S.; Li, M.Y.; Jobe, P.C. Carbamazepine Increases Extracellular Serotonin Concentration: Lack of Antagonism by Tetrodotoxin or Zero Ca^{2+}. *Eur. J. Pharmacol.* **1997**, *328*, 153–162. [CrossRef] [PubMed]
152. Lemos, L.; Fontes, R.; Flores, S.; Oliveira, P.; Almeida, A. Effectiveness of the Association between Carbamazepine and Peripheral Analgesic Block with Ropivacaine for the Treatment of Trigeminal Neuralgia. *J. Pain. Res.* **2010**, *3*, 201–212. [PubMed]
153. Tutanc, M.; Aras, M.; Dokuyucu, R.; Altas, M.; Zeren, C.; Arica, V.; Ozturk, O.H.; Motor, S.; Yilmaz, C. Oxidative Status in Epileptic Children Using Carbamazepine. *Iran J. Pediatr.* **2015**, *25*, e3885. [CrossRef] [PubMed]
154. Varoglu, A.O.; Yildirim, A.; Aygul, R.; Gundogdu, O.L.; Sahin, Y.N. Effects of Valproate, Carbamazepine, and Levetiracetam on the Antioxidant and Oxidant Systems in Epileptic Patients and Their Clinical Importance. *Clin. Neuropharmacol.* **2010**, *33*, 155–157. [CrossRef] [PubMed]
155. Ficarra, S.; Misiti, F.; Russo, A.; Carelli-Alinovi, C.; Bellocco, E.; Barreca, D.; Laganà, G.; Leuzzi, U.; Toscano, G.; Giardina, B.; et al. Antiepileptic Carbamazepine Drug Treatment Induces Alteration of Membrane in Red Blood Cells: Possible Positive Effects on Metabolism and Oxidative Stress. *Biochimie* **2013**, *95*, 833–841. [CrossRef] [PubMed]
156. Erdem Guzel, E.; Kaya Tektemur, N.; Tektemur, A.; Etem Önalan, E. Carbamazepine-Induced Renal Toxicity May Be Associated with Oxidative Stress and Apoptosis in Male Rat. *Drug Chem. Toxicol.* **2023**, *46*, 136–143. [CrossRef] [PubMed]
157. Arora, T.; Mehta, A.K.; Sharma, K.K.; Mediratta, P.K.; Banerjee, B.D.; Garg, G.R.; Sharma, A.K. Effect of Carbamazepine and Lamotrigine on Cognitive Function and Oxidative Stress in Brain during Chemical Epileptogenesis in Rats. *Basic Clin. Pharmacol. Toxicol.* **2010**, *106*, 372–377. [CrossRef]
158. Gasca-Pérez, E.; Galar-Martínez, M.; García-Medina, S.; Pérez-Coyotl, I.A.; Ruiz-Lara, K.; Cano-Viveros, S.; Pérez-Pastén Borja, R.; Gómez-Oliván, L.M. Short-Term Exposure to Carbamazepine Causes Oxidative Stress on Common Carp (Cyprinus Carpio). *Environ. Toxicol. Pharmacol.* **2019**, *66*, 96–103. [CrossRef]
159. Li, Z.-H.; Li, P.; Rodina, M.; Randak, T. Effect of Human Pharmaceutical Carbamazepine on the Quality Parameters and Oxidative Stress in Common Carp (*Cyprinus carpio* L.) Spermatozoa. *Chemosphere* **2010**, *80*, 530–534. [CrossRef]
160. García-Medina, S.; Galar-Martínez, M.; Gómez-Oliván, L.M.; Torres-Bezaury, R.M.D.C.; Islas-Flores, H.; Gasca-Pérez, E. The Relationship between Cyto-Genotoxic Damage and Oxidative Stress Produced by Emerging Pollutants on a Bioindicator Organism (Allium Cepa): The Carbamazepine Case. *Chemosphere* **2020**, *253*, 126675. [CrossRef] [PubMed]
161. Shorvon, S. Oxcarbazepine: A Review. *Seizure* **2000**, *9*, 75–79. [CrossRef]
162. Shorvon, S.D. Drug Treatment of Epilepsy in the Century of the ILAE: The Second 50 Years, 1959–2009. *Epilepsia* **2009**, *50* (Suppl. S3), 93–130. [CrossRef] [PubMed]
163. Tecoma, E.S. Oxcarbazepine. *Epilepsia* **1999**, *40* (Suppl. 5), S37–S46. [CrossRef] [PubMed]
164. Beydoun, A.; Kutluay, E. Oxcarbazepine. *Expert Opin. Pharmacother.* **2002**, *3*, 59–71. [CrossRef] [PubMed]
165. Faught, E.; Kim, H. Oxcarbazepine. In *The Treatment of Epilepsy*; John Wiley & Sons, Ltd.: Hoboken, NJ, USA, 2015; pp. 533–545.
166. Cárdenas-Rodríguez, N.; Coballase-Urrutia, E.; Rivera-Espinosa, L.; Romero-Toledo, A.; Sampieri, A.; Ortega-Cuellar, D.; Montesinos-Correa, H.; Floriano-Sánchez, E.; Carmona-Aparicio, L. Modulation of Antioxidant Enzymatic Activities by Certain Antiepileptic Drugs (Valproic Acid, Oxcarbazepine, and Topiramate): Evidence in Humans and Experimental Models. *Oxid Med. Cell Longev.* **2013**, *2013*, 598493. [CrossRef] [PubMed]

167. Rezaei, S.; Shab-Bidar, S.; Abdulahi Abdurahman, A.; Djafarian, K. Oxcarbazepine Administration and the Serum Levels of Homocysteine, Vitamin B12 and Folate in Epileptic Patients: A Systematic Review and Meta-Analysis. *Seizure* **2017**, *45*, 87–94. [CrossRef] [PubMed]
168. Agarwal, N.B.; Agarwal, N.K.; Mediratta, P.K.; Sharma, K.K. Effect of Lamotrigine, Oxcarbazepine and Topiramate on Cognitive Functions and Oxidative Stress in PTZ-Kindled Mice. *Seizure* **2011**, *20*, 257–262. [CrossRef]
169. Kim, Y.H.; Lee, T.-K.; Lee, J.-C.; Kim, D.W.; Hong, S.; Cho, J.H.; Shin, M.C.; Choi, S.Y.; Won, M.-H.; Kang, I.J. Therapeutic Administration of Oxcarbazepine Saves Cerebellar Purkinje Cells from Ischemia and Reperfusion Injury Induced by Cardiac Arrest through Attenuation of Oxidative Stress. *Antioxidants* **2022**, *11*, 2450. [CrossRef]
170. Park, C.W.; Ahn, J.H.; Lee, T.-K.; Park, Y.E.; Kim, B.; Lee, J.-C.; Kim, D.W.; Shin, M.C.; Park, Y.; Cho, J.H.; et al. Post-Treatment with Oxcarbazepine Confers Potent Neuroprotection against Transient Global Cerebral Ischemic Injury by Activating Nrf2 Defense Pathway. *Biomed. Pharmacother.* **2020**, *124*, 109850. [CrossRef]
171. Kośmider, K.; Kamieniak, M.; Czuczwar, S.J.; Miziak, B. Second Generation of Antiepileptic Drugs and Oxidative Stress. *Int. J. Mol. Sci.* **2023**, *24*, 3873. [CrossRef]
172. Baumann, P. Pharmacology and Pharmacokinetics of Citalopram and Other SSRIs. *Int. Clin. Psychopharmacol.* **1996**, *11* (Suppl. S1), 5–11. [CrossRef]
173. Citalopram Monograph for Professionals. Drugs.com. Available online: https://www.drugs.com/monograph/citalopram.html (accessed on 7 February 2024).
174. Ahmadian, E.; Eftekhari, A.; Fard, J.K.; Babaei, H.; Nayebi, A.M.; Mohammadnejad, D.; Eghbal, M.A. In Vitro and in Vivo Evaluation of the Mechanisms of Citalopram-Induced Hepatotoxicity. *Arch. Pharm. Res.* **2017**, *40*, 1296–1313. [CrossRef] [PubMed]
175. Ilgin, S.; Kilic, G.; Baysal, M.; Kilic, V.; Korkut, B.; Ucarcan, S.; Atli, O. Citalopram Induces Reproductive Toxicity in Male Rats. *Birth Defects Res.* **2017**, *109*, 475–485. [CrossRef] [PubMed]
176. Duan, S.; Fu, Y.; Dong, S.; Ma, Y.; Meng, H.; Guo, R.; Chen, J.; Liu, Y.; Li, Y. Psychoactive Drugs Citalopram and Mirtazapine Caused Oxidative Stress and Damage of Feeding Behavior in Daphnia Magna. *Ecotoxicol. Environ. Saf.* **2022**, *230*, 113147. [CrossRef] [PubMed]
177. Ahmadian, E.; Eftekhari, A.; Babaei, H.; Nayebi, A.M.; Eghbal, M.A. Anti-Cancer Effects of Citalopram on Hepatocellular Carcinoma Cells Occur via Cytochrome C Release and the Activation of NF-kB. *Anticancer. Agents Med. Chem.* **2017**, *17*, 1570–1577. [CrossRef] [PubMed]
178. Herbet, M.; Izdebska, M.; Piątkowska-Chmiel, I.; Poleszak, E.; Jagiełło-Wójtowicz, E. Estimation of Oxidative Stress Parameters in Rats after Simultaneous Administration of Rosuvastatin with Antidepressants. *Pharmacol. Rep.* **2016**, *68*, 172–176. [CrossRef] [PubMed]
179. Gupta, S.; Upadhayay, D.; Sharma, U.; Jagannathan, N.R.; Gupta, Y.K. Citalopram Attenuated Neurobehavioral, Biochemical, and Metabolic Alterations in Transient Middle Cerebral Artery Occlusion Model of Stroke in Male Wistar Rats. *J. Neurosci. Res.* **2018**, *96*, 1277–1293. [CrossRef] [PubMed]
180. Elsworthy, R.J.; Crowe, J.A.; King, M.C.; Dunleavy, C.; Fisher, E.; Ludlam, A.; Parri, H.R.; Hill, E.J.; Aldred, S. The Effect of Citalopram Treatment on Amyloid-β Precursor Protein Processing and Oxidative Stress in Human hNSC-Derived Neurons. *Transl. Psychiatry* **2022**, *12*, 285. [CrossRef]
181. Khanzode, S.D.; Dakhale, G.N.; Khanzode, S.S.; Saoji, A.; Palasodkar, R. Oxidative damage and major depression: The potential antioxidant action of selective serotonin re-uptake inhibitors. *Redox Rep.* **2003**, *8*, 365–370. [CrossRef]
182. DeVane, C.L.; Liston, H.L.; Markowitz, J.S. Clinical Pharmacokinetics of Sertraline. *Clin. Pharm.* **2002**, *41*, 1247–1266. [CrossRef] [PubMed]
183. Cipriani, A.; La Ferla, T.; Furukawa, T.A.; Signoretti, A.; Nakagawa, A.; Churchill, R.; McGuire, H.; Barbui, C. Sertraline versus Other Antidepressive Agents for Depression. *Cochrane Database Syst. Rev.* **2010**, *4*, CD006117. [CrossRef] [PubMed]
184. Li, Y.; Couch, L.; Higuchi, M.; Fang, J.-L.; Guo, L. Mitochondrial Dysfunction Induced by Sertraline, an Antidepressant Agent. *Toxicol. Sci.* **2012**, *127*, 582–591. [CrossRef] [PubMed]
185. Battal, D.; Yalin, S.; Eker, E.D.; Aktas, A.; Sahin, N.O.; Cebo, M.; Berköz, M. Possible Role of Selective Serotonin Reuptake Inhibitor Sertraline on Oxidative Stress Responses. *Eur. Rev. Med. Pharmacol. Sci.* **2014**, *18*, 477–484. [PubMed]
186. Jajoo, A.; Donlon, C.; Shnayder, S.; Levin, M.; McVey, M. Sertraline Induces DNA Damage and Cellular Toxicity in Drosophila That Can Be Ameliorated by Antioxidants. *Sci. Rep.* **2020**, *10*, 4512. [CrossRef]
187. Abdel-Salam, O.M.E.; Youness, E.R.; Khadrawy, Y.A.; Sleem, A.A. Brain and Liver Oxidative Stress after Sertraline and Haloperidol Treatment in Mice. *J. Basic Clin. Physiol. Pharmacol.* **2013**, *24*, 115–123. [CrossRef] [PubMed]
188. Chinnapaka, S.; Bakthavachalam, V.; Munirathinam, G. Repurposing Antidepressant Sertraline as a Pharmacological Drug to Target Prostate Cancer Stem Cells: Dual Activation of Apoptosis and Autophagy Signaling by Deregulating Redox Balance. *Am. J. Cancer Res.* **2020**, *10*, 2043–2065. [PubMed]
189. Lima, M.L.; Abengózar, M.A.; Nácher-Vázquez, M.; Martínez-Alcázar, M.P.; Barbas, C.; Tempone, A.G.; López-Gonzálvez, Á.; Rivas, L. Molecular Basis of the Leishmanicidal Activity of the Antidepressant Sertraline as a Drug Repurposing Candidate. *Antimicrob. Agents Chemother.* **2018**, *62*, e01928-18. [CrossRef]
190. Michalakeas, C.A.; Parissis, J.T.; Douzenis, A.; Nikolaou, M.; Varounis, C.; Andreadou, I.; Antonellos, N.; Markantonis-Kiroudis, S.; Paraskevaidis, I.; Ikonomidis, I.; et al. Effects of Sertraline on Circulating Markers of Oxidative Stress in Depressed Patients with Chronic Heart Failure: A Pilot Study. *J. Card Fail.* **2011**, *17*, 748–754. [CrossRef]

191. Cipriani, A.; Furukawa, T.A.; Salanti, G.; Geddes, J.R.; Higgins, J.P.; Churchill, R.; Watanabe, N.; Nakagawa, A.; Omori, I.M.; McGuire, H.; et al. Comparative Efficacy and Acceptability of 12 New-Generation Antidepressants: A Multiple-Treatments Meta-Analysis. *Lancet* **2009**, *373*, 746–758. [CrossRef]
192. Mierzejewski, P. Wenlafaksyna XR, zastosowanie kliniczne większych dawek (>150 mg). *Psychiatria* **2020**, *17*, 76–79. [CrossRef]
193. Kıvrak, Y.; Güvenç, T.S.; Akbulut, N.; Yağcı, I.; Cığşar, G.; Gündüz, S.; Balcı, B. Accelerated Hypertension after Venlafaxine Usage. *Case Rep. Psychiatry* **2014**, *2014*, 659715. [CrossRef] [PubMed]
194. Ballenger, J.C. Clinical Evaluation of Venlafaxine. *J. Clin. Psychopharmacol.* **1996**, *16* (3 Suppl. 2), 29S–35S; discussion 35S–36S. [CrossRef] [PubMed]
195. Madrigal-Bujaidar, E.; Paniagua-Pérez, R.; Rendón-Barrón, M.J.; Morales-González, J.A.; Madrigal-Santillán, E.O.; Álvarez-González, I. Investigation of the DNA Damage and Oxidative Effect Induced by Venlafaxine in Mouse Brain and Liver Cells. *Toxics* **2022**, *10*, 737. [CrossRef] [PubMed]
196. Ahmadian, E.; Babaei, H.; Mohajjel Nayebi, A.; Eftekhari, A.; Eghbal, M.A. Venlafaxine-Induced Cytotoxicity Towards Isolated Rat Hepatocytes Involves Oxidative Stress and Mitochondrial/Lysosomal Dysfunction. *Adv. Pharm. Bull* **2016**, *6*, 521–530. [CrossRef] [PubMed]
197. Wigner, P.; Synowiec, E.; Czarny, P.; Bijak, M.; Jóźwiak, P.; Szemraj, J.; Gruca, P.; Papp, M.; Śliwiński, T. Effects of Venlafaxine on the Expression Level and Methylation Status of Genes Involved in Oxidative Stress in Rats Exposed to a Chronic Mild Stress. *J. Cell Mol. Med.* **2020**, *24*, 5675–5694. [CrossRef] [PubMed]
198. Mansouri, M.T.; Naghizadeh, B.; Ghorbanzadeh, B.; Amirgholami, N.; Houshmand, G.; Alboghobeish, S. Venlafaxine Inhibits Naloxone-Precipitated Morphine Withdrawal Symptoms: Role of Inflammatory Cytokines and Nitric Oxide. *Metab. Brain Dis.* **2020**, *35*, 305–313. [CrossRef] [PubMed]
199. Khanam, R.; Najfi, H.; Akhtar, M.; Vohora, D. Evaluation of Venlafaxine on Glucose Homeostasis and Oxidative Stress in Diabetic Mice. *Hum. Exp. Toxicol.* **2012**, *31*, 1244–1250. [CrossRef]
200. Lee, H. The Importance of Nutrition in Neurological Disorders and Nutrition Assessment Methods. *Brain Neurorehabil.* **2022**, *15*, e1. [CrossRef]

International Journal of
Molecular Sciences

MDPI

Review

Royal Jelly: Biological Action and Health Benefits

Nada Oršolić [1,*] and Maja Jazvinšćak Jembrek [2,3]

1 Division of Animal Physiology, Faculty of Science, University of Zagreb, Rooseveltov trg 6, HR-10000 Zagreb, Croatia
2 Division of Molecular Medicine, Laboratory for Protein Dynamics, Ruđer Bošković Institute, Bijenička cesta 54, HR-10000 Zagreb, Croatia; maja.jazvinscak.jembrek@irb.hr
3 School of Medicine, Catholic University of Croatia, Ilica 242, HR-10000 Zagreb, Croatia
* Correspondence: nada.orsolic@biol.pmf.hr or norsolic@yahoo.com; Tel.: +385-1-4877-735; Fax: +385-1-4826-260

Abstract: Royal jelly (RJ) is a highly nutritious natural product with great potential for use in medicine, cosmetics, and as a health-promoting food. This bee product is a mixture of important compounds, such as proteins, vitamins, lipids, minerals, hormones, neurotransmitters, flavonoids, and polyphenols, that underlie the remarkable biological and therapeutic activities of RJ. Various bioactive molecules like 10-hydroxy-2-decenoic acid (10-HDA), antibacterial protein, apisin, the major royal jelly proteins, and specific peptides such as apisimin, royalisin, royalactin, apidaecin, defensin-1, and jelleins are characteristic ingredients of RJ. RJ shows numerous physiological and pharmacological properties, including vasodilatory, hypotensive, antihypercholesterolaemic, antidiabetic, immunomodulatory, anti-inflammatory, antioxidant, anti-aging, neuroprotective, antimicrobial, estrogenic, anti-allergic, anti-osteoporotic, and anti-tumor effects. Moreover, RJ may reduce menopause symptoms and improve the health of the reproductive system, liver, and kidneys, and promote wound healing. This article provides an overview of the molecular mechanisms underlying the beneficial effects of RJ in various diseases, aging, and aging-related complications, with special emphasis on the bioactive components of RJ and their health-promoting properties. The data presented should be an incentive for future clinical studies that hopefully will advance our knowledge about the therapeutic potential of RJ and facilitate the development of novel RJ-based therapeutic opportunities for improving human health and well-being.

Keywords: royal jelly; bioactive components; aphytherapy; molecular and cellular activity

1. Introduction

Royal Jelly as Functional Food

Royal jelly (RJ), a viscous product of the beehive, is appreciated as an attractive ingredient for healthy foods. It is secreted by the hypopharyngeal and mandibular glands of worker honeybees (*Apis mellifera*) and used as a food for the bee larvae and the queen. RJ is recognized for its exceptional nutritional value, earning the reputation of a "superfood" whose consumption has numerous health benefits for humans [1–3].

The method for producing RJ is based on artificial larvae grafting. RJ production occurs outside the honeycomb in artificial queen cells made of wax. Worker bee larvae, 12 to 18 h after hatching, are transferred into these cells using an inoculation pen to encourage the bee colony to produce RJ for larval feeding. After 68–72 h (3 days), the larvae are removed from the substrate with tweezers, and the RJ is collected and transferred to a storage bottle. This conventional method, which involves grafting young larvae, is time-consuming, labor-intensive, and limited by the availability of larvae and the technician's vision. A new method for producing RJ eliminates the need for larvae grafting and utilizes a practical and efficient device. The device consists of a plastic worker foundation with regular holes, plastic cell bottoms mounted on a bar that can be inserted into the comb to fill the holes, and into the bottomless plastic queen cups on RJ production bars [3].

In recent years, consumers and the food industry have become increasingly aware of functional foods and how they can contribute to maintaining human health. The important role of a diet in the prevention and treatment of various illnesses is, nowadays, widely accepted. Functional foods can be natural or produced by extracting or replacing one or more ingredients. Furthermore, some ingredients, such as omega-3 fatty acids, vitamins, probiotics, fibers, bioactive peptides, and fitosterols, can be added to the foods to increase their "functionality" or "benefit" [1,2]. Besides RJ, foods with potential health benefits from the beehive include honey, propolis, beebread, and pollen [3,4]. It is recognized that various bee products, including RJ, can have a positive effect on human health. RJ contains a considerable number of essential components, such as proteins, free amino acids, lipids, vitamins, sugars, hormones, and bioactive substances like 10-HDA. Some of the most abundant proteins from RJ are proteins from the family of major royal jelly proteins (MRJPs), antibacterial protein, and 350-kDa protein called apisin, an unique component of RJ that consists of major royal jelly protein 1 (MRJP1) and apisimin [3].

RJ, as the most valued bee product, is not only one of the most attractive functional foods; it can also be used in medicine as a medicinal product. In many countries, it is recommended in pediatrics to geriatric medicine, especially in relation to nutrition and cosmetics. Due to the highly valuable nutritive composition, the consummation of RJ is constantly growing. It can be consumed in different forms, either native or as a functional component of different food products. According to some sources, the annual production of RJ in China, the world's largest producer and exporter, is over 4000 tons, which represents more than 90% of the total production on a global level [5].

Regarding medicinal use, RJ and its biologically active components have gained significant interest due to their potential chemopreventive/protective functions in the maintenance of human health based on their anti-inflammatory and antioxidative properties, as well as food–gene interactions. Bioactive components of RJ, such as polyphenols, vitamins, hormones, and enzymes, are essential for redox reactions and controlling the level of oxidative stress (OS) and OS-induced cell damage and inflammation, factors that lead to the progression of symptoms associated with metabolic syndrome, cancer, aging, and neurodegenerative diseases. Various biological activities and health-promoting properties of RJ are largely assigned to diverse phenolic compounds and glycosides from the RJ, such as pinobanksin, hesperetin, kaempferol, isorhamnetin, isosakuranetin, naringenin, chrysin, acacetin, luteolin, apigenin, and formononetin. These findings directed pharmacological studies towards the beneficial health effects of various RJ components that are capable of interfering with the production of reactive radicals, reduce OS and inflammation, and potentially slow down the onset and progression of numerous chronic diseases.

Nowadays, RJ is being intensively tested, especially in Japan, and many of its effects have been scientifically confirmed. In addition to its use as a cosmetic and dietary supplement, it is considered that RJ has biostimulating and regenerative effects on human health based on its unique chemical composition. However, there is not yet enough data on the effectiveness of RJ and the health benefits for humans. The biological effects of RJ have mainly been studied in experimental animal models and cell cultures rather than in humans. Considering the complexity of RJ, the main approach is to purify and test the biological effectiveness of individual bioactive molecules.

The aim of this review is to collect the latest relevant studies on the use of RJ in the prevention and therapy of numerous diseases associated with oxidative stress and inflammation. These conditions result from the reduced antioxidant capacity of the organism, which contributes to the increase in chronic diseases, including neurological disorders, type 2 diabetes, cancer, aging, cardiovascular damage, acute kidney failure, hypertension, pre-eclampsia, osteoporosis, inflammatory diseases of the liver and intestines, and atherosclerosis, among others. Furthermore, our goal is to highlight the benefits of RJ and its effects on health-issue prevention in both the young and elderly population, especially related to its antimicrobial, antibacterial, immunoregulatory, antidiabetic, and reproductive health improvement properties, wound healing, life extension, slower aging, antilipidemic, antihypertensive, antiviral, and antiparasitic effects, the protection of vital organs such as the brain, heart, liver, and kidneys from toxins and drugs (organo-protective effects—neuroprotective, hepato-renal protective, etc.), neuromodulatory capabilities, stimulation of growth, regulation of healthy cells, antiobesity properties, and memory improvement. We believe that gathering knowledge about the latest molecular mechanisms and pharmacological targets of the active biological components of RJ will enable its wider application and production for the treatment of various diseases, ultimately improving the quality of life, especially for individuals suffering from specific illnesses. These novel findings will enhance the comprehensive understanding and use of RJ, making it more effective in maintaining health. Given the exceptional biological properties of RJ and its use in many areas, from the pharmaceutical and food industries to the manufacturing of cosmetic products, there is a need for its standardization, investigation of qualitative and quantitative properties, and analytic studies of bioactive substances and their transformations during storage and keeping.

2. Chemical Composition of Royal Jelly

RJ is made of 60–70% water; 9–18% proteins (*w*/*w*) (albumin, α, β, γ globulin, glycoproteins, lipoproteins, and 23 amino acids); 7–18% sugars (glucose, fructose, negligible amounts of ribose, maltose, isomaltose, trehalose, neotrehalos, gentiobiose, turanose, and inositol); 3–8% lipids (*w*/*w*) (sterols and glycerols, wax, neutral fats, fatty acids, phospholipids, phenolic lipids, and free organic acids), 0.7–1.5% minerals (K, Na, Ca, Mg, Cu, Fe, Mn, Zn, Si, Cr, Ni, Ag, Co, Al, As, Hg, Bi, Au, S, and P), and vitamins (B_1, B_2, B_3, B_5, B_6, B_7, B_9, B_{12}, E, D, A, K, and C, 336–351 mg/100 g) [2,3,5–7]. The chemical composition, especially the sugar content in RJ, is highly variable and depends on the geographical origin, plant species, bee species, season, and method of collection. RJ also contains various previously mentioned phenolic compounds, flavonoids, organic acids, enzymes (amylase, invertase, catalase, acid phosphatase, and others), neurotransmitter acetylcholine and its precursor choline, as well as sex hormones (estradiol, testosterone, and progesterone). In addition to proteins and peptides, RJ contains a large amount of free amino acids, such as lysine, proline, cystine, aspartic acid, valine, glutamic acid, serine, glycine, cysteine, threonine, alanine, tyrosine, phenylalanine, leucine, isoleucine, and glutamine. As mentioned, RJ is also rich in lipids that account for 15–30% of the lyophilized product. The lipid content predominantly encompasses fatty acids (more than 80%) that are followed by phenols (4–10%), waxes (5–6%), steroids (3–4%), and phospholipids (0.4–0.8%). The most abundant are medium-chain fatty acids (MCFAs), such as (10-HDA) sebacic acid and 9-hydroxy-2-decenoic acid. 10-HDA is the main constituent (app. 21 mg/g RJ) that is also regarded as a marker of quality and freshness [8–11].

In addition to phenolic compounds, pharmacological effects of RJ are also attributed to 10-HDA, royalisin, apisin, and some antimicrobial proteins [12,13]. According to Furusawa et al. [10], apisin is a hetero-oligomer containing MRJP1 (55 kDa protein) and apisimin (5 kDa protein). The apisin content in RJ is fairly constant (i.e., 3.93 to 4.67 *w*/*w*%) and can be used as a quality standard of RJ. The main compounds from RJ are shown in Table 1.

Proteins and peptides are the second most abundant components of RJ. The main proteins are MRJP1 (royalactin) to MRJP9 (more than 80% of the protein content, molecular weights between 49 to 87 kDa), whereas the most often-found peptides in RJ are apisimin, royalisin, apidaecin, defensin-1, and jelleins [13–16]. Proteins represent more than 50% of dry matter [13–16] and have a specific physiological role in queen bee development. MRJPs include numerous essential amino acids, like ovalbumin and casein [17–22]. Proteins from the MRJP family, from MRP1 to MRP9, are the main soluble proteins (31%) of RJ [17–19]. MRJP 1 is a weakly acidic glycoprotein (55 kDa) that forms oligomers of 350 or 420 kDa [19,20]. MRJP 2, MRJP3, MRJP4, and MRJP 5 are glycoproteins of 49 kDa, 60–70 kDa, 60 kDa, and 80 kDa, respectively) [22].

Table 1. Key components and their content in fresh and lyophilized royal jelly.

Contents	Fresh Royal Jelly (%)	Lyophilized Royal Jelly (%)	References
Water	60–70	<5	[2,3,5–23]
Lipids	3–8	8–19	
10-hydroxy-2-decenoic acid (10-HDA)	>1.4	>3.5	
Proteins	9–18	27–41	
Fructose + glucose + sucrose	7–18	-	
Fructose	3–13	-	
Glucose	4–8	-	
Sucrose	0.5–2.0	-	
Minerals	0.7–1.5		
Ash (dry weight)	0.8–3.0	2–5	
pH	3.4–4.5	3.4–4.5	
Acidity (mL 0.1N NaOH/g)	3.0–6.0	-	
Furasine (mg/100 g protein)	<50	-	

In one study that investigated the protein composition of RJ, 134 proteins were identified by gel-based and gel-free proteomics [20,22–24]. MRJPs were the main protein components of RJ, together with some proteins participating in the carbohydrate metabolism, such as glucose oxidase, predecessor-glucosidase, and glucose dehydrogenase. The study revealed 19 new proteins that were predominantly grouped in three functional categories: redox proteins, protein-binding proteins, and lipid-transporting proteins. The important physiological functions of RJ proteins have been demonstrated in numerous studies [16–25]. For example, some MRJPs stimulate cell proliferation [26–34], while others inhibited bisphenol A-induced proliferation of human breast cancer cell lines [34]. MRJP1 and MRJP2 stimulate mouse macrophages and the release of tumor necrosis factor α (TNF-α) [35], while MRJP 3 modulates the immune response by suppressing the production of interleukin (IL)-4, IL-2, and interferon γ (IFN-γ) in T-lymphocytes [36,37]. Yet another protein primarily identified in RJ is apolypophorin III-like protein, a lipid-associated protein that transfers lipids in aqueous environments in the form of a protein–lipid complex [38].

3. Royal Jelly as Nutrient for Queen and Larvae

RJ, a yellowish-white, creamy liquid, is a special food for queen bees and larvae in the hives. All larvae are fed with RJ, but only for the first three days. Afterwards, only those larvae that will become queens are fed with RJ, as well as adult queens [3,39–42]. The bee queens are approximately two times larger and live 10 times longer than worker bees. The difference in feeding, particularly during the larval stage, is considered as the main contributing factor to their exceptional fertility, morphology, lifespan, and behavior, including their memory abilities, compared to worker bees [39]. There are three types of royal jelly: worker jelly, royal (queen) jelly, and drone jelly. Royal jelly is white, acidic (pH 3.6–4.2), and of a specific flavor. Compared to worker and drone jelly, the Queens' royal jelly contains 10 times more pantothenic acid, biopterine, and neobiopterine. During the development of the worker and drone larvae, the glucose-to-fructose ratio changes from 0.1 to 0.7, while in the queen's royal jelly it remains constant, 1.2–2.5. Kamakura [43] has demonstrated that egg differentiation into queen or worker bees is determined by the intake of royal jelly; more precisely, royalactin (MRPJ1), a 57 kDa protein of RJ, promotes larvae differentiation into queens. Royalactin increases the size of the body and ovary size, and reduces the developmental time of queens. The effects of royalactin on body size are mediated by p70 S6 kinase, the increased activity of mitogen-activated protein kinase (MAPK), and a shortened developmental time, whereas an increased concentration of the juvenile hormone affects the development of ovaries. All these effects during the bee larvae differentiation into queens are triggered through the activation of the epidermal growth factor receptor (EGFR) signaling pathway [30,43,44].

During the spring, a queen that is well-mated and well-fed can lay app. 1500 eggs per day. At every moment, she is surrounded by worker bees who take care of her needs. They provide queen with the food and dispose of her waste. The queen bee has no direct control over the hive. She serves as the reproducer and is able to determine the sex of the eggs she lays, i.e., a fertilized (female) or unfertilized (male) egg, depending on the width of the cell. To fertilize the egg, the queen selectively releases the sperm stored in her spermatheca when the egg passes the oviduct [45]. In queenless honey bee colonies, bee workers that are fed with the RJ-rich diet may acquire queen-like properties and increased fertility (through ovarian development). In particular, the consumption of tyrosine in RJ increases brain levels of dopamine and tyramine and promotes the transition from normal to reproductive workers. The activation of EGFR also regulates this process by increasing the production of the juvenile growth-enhancing hormone (4–8 mM in RJ). Furthermore, RJ improves the memory and survival of bee workers due to its high concentration of acetylcholine. The permanent expression of the DNA methyltransferases 3 (*DNMT3*) gene which encodes DNA methyltransferase and has an important role in the formation of long-term memory further contributes to the extraordinary cognitive performances of queen bees [46,47].

During the queen honeybee and larvae development, MRJPs from the RJ are an important source of certain essential amino acids, whereas lipids are responsible for biological activities related to the development strategies of the colony [48]. Besides providing various nutrients, the ideal viscosity of RJ ensures that developing queen larvae are kept in place. This consistency of RJ is dependent on a protein–sterol complex made of two proteins and a sterol, MRJP1, apisimin, and 24-methylenecholesterol (24MC), respectively. The complex contains four MRJP1 molecules that surround four molecules of apisimin and eight molecules of 24MC. The viscosity of the complex is pH-dependent. A low pH increases the viscosity of RJ due to the formation of the fibrillar structures of the complex. Interestingly, proteins of the complex are produced by hypopharyngeal glands, whereas acidic conditions are achieved by mandibular glands that secrete fatty acids. The formation of fibrils also depends on the 10-HDA secreted from the mandibular glands. In queen-right colonies, workers predominantly produce 10-HDA and 10-HDAA by their mandibular glands, while the main components of the mandibular glands of the queen are (E)-9-oxodec2-enoic acid (9-ODA) and (E)-9-hydroxydec-2-enoic acid (9-HDA) that constitute a queen mandibular pheromone [49]. 10-HDA, a fatty acid, can account for up to 5% of RJ composition and may act as a histone deacetylase (HDAC) inhibitor. During the development and adult life of bees, there is a strong link between the queen–worker differentiation, OS, longevity, and dietary levels of metal cations, including zinc, iron, and potassium, based on the modulation of HDAC activity by these chemical species [50]. Among other possible mechanisms, a regulation of HDAC3 activity by metal cations and 10-HDA may represent possible epigenetic mechanisms of queen–worker bee differentiation. Therefore, various metals at different levels in RJ and worker bee jelly potentially may affect plasticity in caste differentiation and behavior through epigenetic regulation. Reducing sugars in RJ are also thought to contribute to the epigenetic effects by activating the insulin-like growth factor 1 (IGF-1) and mammalian target of rapamycin (mTOR) signaling cascades. Thus, they stimulate differentiation into queens through the increased intake of food and essential nutrients [51]. Moreover, as concentrations of various trace elements and minerals are found to be fairly constant in RJ samples of different botanical and geographical origin, it has been suggested that RJ, viewed as a form of insect lactation, shows homeostatic adjustments similar to mammalian milk.

4. RJ Values in Human Nutrition and as a Nutraceutical

The importance of RJ from the perspective of human nutrition is relatively small. Considering a daily intake of 2 g of RJ, the proteins, lipids, carbohydrates, and minerals present in RJ do not contribute significantly to the recommended daily intake (RDI). On the other hand, there is a small contribution of the vitamins B1, B2, B6, and biotin (B7). In addition, RJ is one of the best sources of pantothenic acid (vitamin B5) which is needed to release energy from food. B5 is the most abundant vitamin in RJ (52.8 mg/100 g), followed by niacin (B3) (42.42 mg/100 g). A B5 deficiency increases susceptibility to infections, bad mood, and gastrointestinal problems. All B-group vitamins help in the conversion of proteins, carbohydrates, and fats into energy. B vitamins are also important for healthy skin, hair, and eyes, the proper functioning of the nervous system and liver, a healthy digestive tract, the production and differentiation of all blood cells, especially erythrocytes, and the production of steroid hormones in the adrenal glands. Hence, the mentioned vitamins are important components that increase the nutritional value and the health-promoting potential of RJ.

As already mentioned, the concentrations of trace and mineral elements are quite constant in different RJ samples. In fresh RJ, the ash content is 0.8–3%, while in dry RJ it is 2–5%. The ash contains different minerals—K^+, P^{3-}, S^{2-}, Na^+, Ca^{2+}, Al^{3+}, Mg^{2+}, Zn^{2+}, Fe^{2+}, Cu^+, and Mn^{2+}—as well as trace elements including Ni, Cr, Sn, W, Sb, Bi, and Ti. Trace elements and minerals play a key role in the biomedical activities associated with RJ, participating in various biological effects. The most abundant microelements in RJ are Zn, Fe, Cu, and Mn [3,11,52].

The presence of potassium as the main macroelement should be highlighted (321.1–357.4 mg/100 g,), followed by phosphorus (338.4–412.1 mg/100 g), sulfur (153.2–169.3 mg/100 g), calcium (22.8–24.0 mg/100 g), magnesium (44.0–50.4 mg/100 g), and sodium (0.3–13.8 mg/100 g) [52–56]. Potassium regulates the fluid balance, decreases the blood pressure, regulates the electrical activity of the muscle cells and heart, and improves the bone mineral density [53,54].

Ca is important for the bone mineral density and bone mineral content. The intake of calcium is usually insufficient at all ages which has adverse effects on bone health, weight gain, and fat accumulation. In contrast, diets rich in calcium can prevent fat accumulation, regulate blood pressure and premenstrual syndrome, and reduce the risk of colon cancer [54–56]. Mg also helps with high blood pressure, cardiovascular diseases, osteoporosis, and diabetes, whereas Zn supports growth, development, and immune functions. Iron participates in various metabolic processes, such as oxygen transport, DNA synthesis, and electron transport [54].

As previously emphasized, MRJP1 is the main protein from RJ which may exist in monomeric (55 kDa) and oligomeric forms. Many lines of evidence indicate that MRJP1 has a wide range of pharmaceutical effects on human health. It shows wound healing and antibacterial, antifungal, hypocholesterolemic, antitumor, and immune-enhancement activities [3,7,13,48,57]. In addition, MRJP 1–5 are important sources of 10 essential amino acids (Arg, His, Ile, Leu, Lys, Met, Phe, Thr, Trp, and Val), MRJP2, MRJP3, and MRJP5 provide the nitrogen supply, while MRJP 6–9 do not have a nutritional value. MRKP5 has the highest content of essential amino acids (51.4%), followed by MRJP1 (48%) and MRJP2 (47%) [3,57].

It has been mentioned that RJ contributes to the unique qualities of bee queens, including their excellent learning and memory abilities. In animal models of aging and Alzheimer's disease (AD), RJ was able to enhance learning and memory retention, as well as prevent and treat cognitive deficits. In preclinical studies, in animal models and in cell lines, RJ, enzyme-treated RJ (eRJ), 10-HDA, RJ peptides, and MRJPs were effective against AD pathology by interfering with protein misfolding, amyloid synthesis, and amyloid clearance. Furthermore, RJ promoted neuronal survival and functioning by targeting inflammation, OS, mitochondrial dysfunction, disturbed proteostasis, amyloid β (Aβ) toxicity, Ca-mediated excitotoxicity, and bioenergetic failure. In clinical trials, RJ was effective against high blood pressure, diabetes, multiple sclerosis, infertility, menopausal symptoms, and even cancer [58,59].

Based on all these findings, [60] RJ has a great potential for the development of novel dietary supplements with valuable nutritional and bioactive properties. For example, the addition of RJ improved the probiotic viability and antioxidant, antimicrobial, and anticancer activities of fermented milk. When compared to the control fermented milk, milk supplemented with 1% of RJ preserved more *Lactobacillus helveticus* Lh-B02 during the 21 days of cold storage. *Lactobacillus helveticus* may improve the antioxidant status and immunological response of the host, produce bioactive peptides, and enhance the bioavailability of the nutrients' production of biopeptides. Fermented milks with 0.5%, 1%, and 1.5% RJ have shown better radical scavenging activity (30.15%, 45.13%, and

58.36%, respectively) compared to fermented milk (27.62%). Fermented milk with 1.5% RJ demonstrated the best anticancer and antibacterial properties, but milk with 1% RJ had the best sensory acceptability (in terms of flavor, appearance, and color). Increasing the RJ content from 1.0% to 1.5% significantly improved the antimicrobial activities against *Staphylococcus aureus* ATCC 25923, *Candida albicans* ATCC 10231, *Aspergillus niger* NRRL 326, and *Aspergillus flavus* NRRL 1957. All fermented milks containing RJ (0.5–1.5%) have shown anticancer activity and the inhibited growth of various cancer cell lines, such as MCF-7, HepG2, HCT-116, and MCF7-12F, perhaps due to the presence of 10-HDA. The authors suggested that probiotic fermented milk with 1.5% RJ could be a promising option for developing novel functional symbiotic milk with health-promoting effects [60,61].

It is worth mentioning the numerous polyphenolic components of RJ, along with various glycosides, which have huge potential to contribute to human health [62–67]. However, many of these claims still need scientific evidence from clinical trials. The most important bioactive components of RJ and their functional roles are shown in Table 2.

Table 2. Bioactive components of royal jelly and their functional activity. n.d.: Not determined.

Bioactive Component	Fresh Royal Jelly (%)	Lyophilized Royal Jelly (%)	Functional Activities	References
Proteins				
MRPJ1 (Alternative name: Royalactin, apalbumin 1, D III)	5.89%		Antimicrobial, antibacterial, antifungal, wound healing, antiproliferative, antioxidant, anti-inflammatory, antitumoral, immunomodulatory, hypocholesterolemic, anti-hypertensive, proliferation of intestinal epithelial cells (IEC-6), increase in lifespan in invertebrates, proliferation rat hepatocytes, larvae differentiation into queen via epidermal growth factor signaling, self-renewal of stem cells, proliferation of human monocytes and Jurkat lymphoid cell	[2,3,12,14,18,48,63] [3,7,13,26,31,48,57] [7,13,29,58,68–76] [13–15,17,19,69] [27,28] [31] [11,26,53] [26] [11,30,43,44,47,48] [11,26,30] [33,35,44]
MRPJ2 and isoform (Alternative name: Apalbumin 2)	1.41%		Antimicrobial, antibacterial, antifungal, antiviral, wound healing, antioxidant, antitumoral, anti-allergic, hepato-renal protective, promotione of caspase-dependent apoptosis, inhibition of bcl-2 and p53 expression in HepG2 cells	[2,3,12,14,18,48,63] [26,31] [29,62–68] [31,37] [60,61]
MRPJ3	1.66%		Wound healing, anti-allergic, anti-aging, anti-inflammatory, antitumoral, immunoregulatory effect, modulation of immune responses of T cells, suppression of proinflammatory cytokine secretion, decrease of IL-4, IL-2, and IFN-γ in vitro and anti-OVA IgE and IgG1 in vivo	[26,31] [31,37] [53] [34,36,69–71] [13,37]

Table 2. *Cont.*

Bioactive Component	Fresh Royal Jelly (%)	Lyophilized Royal Jelly (%)	Functional Activities	References
MRPJ4	0.89%		Antimicrobial	[2,3,12,14,18]
MRPJ7	0.51%		Wound healing	[14,17,19,26]
Enzymes				
Glucose oxidase		0.08%	Carbohydrate metabolism, antibacterial	[3,5,15]
Gluco-cerebrosidase			Hydrolysis glucosylceramide	[22,53]
Alpha-glucosidase			Hydrolysis of polysaccharides and oligosaccharides into monomers	[22,53]
Antimicrobial peptides and proteins				
Royalisin	0.83%		Antimicrobial, antibacterial, antifungal, inhibition of Gram-positive bacteria through damage to cell walls and cell membranes	[12–16,48,63,68]
Apisimin	0.13%		Antibacterial, increases the proliferation and stimulation of human monocytes	[9,10,12,17,48] [21,33]
Yelleines I-III	0.37%		Antimicrobial, antibacterial, inhibition of yeast, Gram-positive and Gram-negative bacteria, cell degranulation, hemolysis, increase immune response	[13–16,48,63,68]
Yelleine IV	-		Antimicrobial	[48]
Venom protein 2	-		Protection of larvae from diseases infection	[48,63]
Apolipophorin-III-like protein	0.08%		Antimicrobial, immunoregulatory effect, stimulation of immune response	[48,63]
Lipids and fatty acids				
10-hydroxy-2-decenoic (10-HDA),	0.75–3.39%		Immunomodulatory, antioxidant, antiaging, neurotrophic and neurogenesis inductor, anti-inflammatory functions, antimicrobial, antibacterial, estrogenic, antialergic, antiosteoporetic, antitumor activity, activation of TRPA1 and TRPV1 receptors and increased longevity in *C. Elegans*, anti-ultraviolet B properties and skin protection, decrease of IL-6 production by reducing expression of IκBζ in RAW264 cells, inhibition of NO production through the inhibition of NF-κB activation	[13,67,69,76,77] [7,52,53,62,68] [53,67] [4,58,68] [7,13,58,62,63,68,69] [48,67,68] [28,58] [7] [35,58] [7,34,60,61] [52,53,59] [59] [48,63,68] [13,58,69]

Table 2. *Cont.*

Bioactive Component	Fresh Royal Jelly (%)	Lyophilized Royal Jelly (%)	Functional Activities	References
10-hydroxydecanoic acid (10-HDAA)	0.78–1.05%		Anti-inflammatory, estrogenic, activation of TRPA1 and TRPV1 receptors	[67,68] [28,60] [52,53,59]
8-hydroxy octanoic acid	0.18–0.39%		Varroa-repellent	[3,35,67,68]
3-hydroxydecanoic acid	0.05–0.09%		Antifungal	[3,5,35,67,68]
3,10-dihydroxydecanoic acid	0.26–0.46%		Immunomodulatory, stimulation of dendritic cell, differentiation, inhibition of the proliferation of allogeneic T cells and dendritic cell-dependent production of IL-2	[22,23,35]
9-hydroxy-2-decenoic acid	0.07–0.15%		Signal components (pheromone) of honeybee queen	[35,49,50]
1,10-decanedioic acid (sebacic)	0.15–0.24%		Estrogenic, anti-inflammatory, hypotensive	[28,53] [36,68,69] [8,23]
2-Decenedioic	0.18–0.33%	<0.1–3.6%	Anti-inflammatory	[36,68,69]
Phenols	0.24–0.6%	4–10%	Antioxidant	[8–11,62–67]
Phenolic Acids				
Ferulic acid Chlorogenic Acid Caffeic Acid	68.42 mg/100 g 37.61 mg/100 g 5.14 mg/100 g		Antioxidant, anti-inflammatory, and antiviral properties	[62,63]
Flavonoids				
Quercetin Naringin Hesperetin Galangin	16.13 mg/100 g 0.47 mg/100 g 0.85 mg/100 g 0.51 mg/100 g		Anticancer, antioxidant, anti-inflammatory, and antiviral properties, neuroprotective and cardio-protective	[62–67]
Waxes	0.3–0.36%	5–6%	-	
Steroids 24-methylene cholesterol Phospholipids	0.18–0.24% 6.06 mg/lipid 0.02–0.04%	3–4% (0.4–0.8%)	Effects on collagen synthesis Estrogenic -	[2,3,28]
Carbohydrates				
Fructose + glucose + sucrose Fructose glucose	7–18% 3–13% 4–8%	90% of the total sugar 2.3–7.6% 2.9–8.1%	Act as an energy source, help in control of blood glucose and insulin metabolism, participate in cholesterol and triglyceride metabolism, and help with fermentation	[2,3,5–7,52]
Sucrose	0.5–2.0%	<0.1–3.6%	Increases mental alertness, memory, reaction readiness, attention and the ability to solve mathematical problems, as well as reducing the feeling of fatigue	[2,3,5–7,52]

Table 2. *Cont.*

Bioactive Component	Fresh Royal Jelly (%)	Lyophilized Royal Jelly (%)	Functional Activities	References
Trehalose, maltose, erlose, melibiose, ribose gentiobiose, isomaltose, raffinose, and melezitose			Modulate glucose homeostasis, reduce bone resorption and inflammation, induce autophagy and alleviate Huntington's disease, neurodegenerative and cardiometabolic diseases, enhance resistance to oxidative stress	[2,3,5–7,52]
Vitamins				
Vitamin A	1.10 mg/100 g		Helps form and maintain healthy teeth, skeletal and soft tissue, mucus membranes, and skin, reproduction, immunity, maintenance of the visual system, and epithelial cellular integrity	[2,3,5–7]
Vitamin B1	2.06 mg/100 g		Transketolation, metabolism of fats, proteins, and nucleic acids	[2,3,5–7]
Vitamin B2	2.77 mg/100 g		Precursor of FMN and FAD	[2,3,5–7]
Niacin (B3)	42.42 mg/100 g		Increase HDL	[2,3,5–7]
Vitamin B5 (Pantothenic acid)	52.80 mg/100 g		Constituent of coenzyme A, plays a role in breaking down fats and carbohydrates for energy, crucial for red blood cell production, production of sex and stress-related hormones from the adrenal glands, reduces cholesterol levels	[2,3,5–7]
Vitamin B6	11.90 mg/100 g		Plays a role in cognitive development through the biosynthesis of neurotransmitters and in maintaining normal levels of homocysteine, an amino acid in the blood, gluconeogenesis and glycogenolysis, immune function, and hemoglobin formation, transamination, and decarboxylation of amino acids	[2,3,5–7]
Vitamin B9 (Folic acid)	0.40 mg/100 g		Helps to form DNA, RNA, and protein metabolism, rapid growth during pregnancy and fetal development, supports healthy blood cells, plays a key role in breaking down homocysteine, DNA biosynthesis, and methylation	[2,3,5–7]
Vitamin B12	0.15 mg/100 g		Plays an essential role in red blood cell formation, cell metabolism, nerve function, and the production of DNA, the molecules inside cells that carry genetic information	[2,3,5–7]
Vitamin C (Ascorbic acid)	2.00 mg/100 g		Antioxidant activity, form blood vessels, cartilage, muscle, and collagen in bones	[2,3,5–7]

Table 2. *Cont.*

Bioactive Component	Fresh Royal Jelly (%)	Lyophilized Royal Jelly (%)	Functional Activities	References
Vitamin D	0.2 mg/100 g		Calcium and phosphorus absorption, essential for the bones and teeth, the immune system, brain health, and for regulating inflammation	[2,3,5–7]
Vitamin E	5.00 mg/100 g		Antioxidant activity	[2,3,5–7]
Free amino acid				
Lysine Proline Cysteine aspartic acid valine, glutamic acid, serine, glycine, cysteine, threonine, alanine, tyrosine, phenylalanine, hydroxyproline, leucine-isoleucine, and glutamine	62.43 mg/100 g 58.76 mg/100 g 21.76 mg/100 g 17.33 mg/100 g less than 5 mg/100 g		Prevent chronic fatigue, help maintain skin, hair, nails, bones, joints, hormonal regulation, sexual vitality, weight regulation, body vitality, recovery from illness, stimulation of the immune system, health of the cardiovascular system	[3,57,64,65]
Minerals				
Macroelements	321.1–357.4 mg/100 g			
Na	0.30–13.8 mg/100 g		Helps maintain normal blood pressure, supports the work of your nerves and muscles, and regulates your body's fluid balance	[54,55]
K	321.1–357.4 mg/100 g		Regulates fluid balance, decreases blood pressure, regulates electrical activity of muscle cells and heart, and improves bone mineral density	[53,54]
Ca	22.8–24.0 mg/100	14.5–113	Effect on bone mineral density and bone mineral content, prevent fat accumulation, regulate blood pressure and premenstrual syndrome, and reduce the risk of colon cancer	[57,58]
Mg	44.0–50.4 mg/100		Helps with high blood pressure, cardiovascular diseases, osteoporosis and diabetes, reduces the inflammatory processes, improves glucose and insulin metabolism, and normalizes the lipid profile	[52–56]
P	338.4–412.1 mg/100		Plays key roles in regulation of gene transcription, activation of enzymes, maintenance of normal pH in extracellular fluid, and intracellular energy storage, helps in the formation of bones and teeth	[52–56]

Table 2. *Cont.*

Bioactive Component	Fresh Royal Jelly (%)	Lyophilized Royal Jelly (%)	Functional Activities	References
S	153.2–169.3 mg/100		Plays role in formation of collagen and keratin proteins, responsible for wound healing and for the health of the skin, hair, nails, and connective tissue, is important for proper development of cartilage and tendons, participates in detoxification processes, blood coagulation, and the production of some bile of acids	[52–56]
Microelements				
Fe	n.d.		Oxygen transport, DNA synthesis, and electron transport, metabolic processes and energy, regulates macrophage polarization, activity and function of neutrophils, NK, T, and B cells	[3,11,50,52]
Mn	0.01–0.08 mg/100		Oxidative phosphorylation, fatty acids, and cholesterol metabolism, mucopolysaccharide metabolism, and urea cycle	[3,11,52]
Zn	2.07–2.58 mg/100		Supports growth, development, and immune functions	[3,11,52]
Cr	0.03–0.15 mg/100		Helps control whole body metabolism, utilizes energy, controls body sugar, and body function.	[3,11,52]
Cu	0.31–0.39 mg/100		Supports energy production, iron metabolism, neuropeptide activation, connective tissue synthesis, and neurotransmitter synthesis, angiogenesis, neurohormone homeostasis, and regulation of gene expression, brain development, pigmentation, and immune system functioning, defense against oxidative damage	[3,11,50,52]

5. Biological Function of Royal Jelly

The biological role of RJ as a functional food refers to its bioactive components and their antioxidant and anti-inflammatory properties, its effects on beauty and aging delay, immunity, memory, chronic inflammatory diseases, wound healing, diabetes, obesity, hypertension, osteoporosis, reproduction, antimicrobial properties, anti-allergic/allergic properties, as well as antitumor properties and protection against the accompanying toxic effects of chemotherapy and radiation. The biological and pharmacological effects of RJ have been shown in cell cultures, animal models, and human experiments.

5.1. Antioxidant and Anti-Inflammatory Activity of RJ

The most important antioxidants in RJ are flavonoids and phenolic compounds. As determined by the study of Nabas et al. [62], RJ contains 23.3 ± 0.92 gallic acid, equivalent (GAE) µg/mg of the total phenolic components, and 1.28 ± 0.09 rutin equivalent (RE), µg/mg of the total flavonoids. The flavonoids of RJ are an important group of phenolic compounds with a pronounced ability to scavenge free radicals. They can be differentiated into four groups: (i) flavanones, e.g., pinocembrin, hesperetin, isosakuranetin, and naringenin; (ii) flavones, e.g., acacetin, apigenin and its glucoside, chrysin, and luteolin glucoside; (iii) flavonols, e.g., quercetin, galangin, fisetin, isorhamnetin, and kaempferol glucosides; and (iv) isoflavonoids, e.g., coumestrol, formononetin, and genistein [62,63]. Fatty acids and their esters, including octanoic acid, benzoic acid, 2-hexenedioic acid and its esters, and dodecanoic acid and its ester, known as 1,2-benzenedicarboxylic acid, contribute to the antioxidant capacity of RJ as well [7,13,64,65]. In addition, the antioxidant activity of RJ may be related to the presence of free amino acids [63,65]. Furthermore, the antioxidant capacity and the total amount of polyphenols are dependent on the time of the collection of RJ; the best antioxidant properties were detected after 24 h [62,63].

The antioxidant abilities of RJ were investigated by various methodological approaches, including the scavenging of 1,1-diphenyl-2-picrylhydrazyl (DPPH), hydroxyl and superoxide radicals, reducing power, and the inhibitory effect on superoxide dismutase activity and linoleic acid oxidation. The antioxidant abilities of RJ were also dependent on the larval age and time of collection. Depending on the time of harvest (24–72 h after the larval transfer), the DPPH radical scavenging ability was between 43.0 and 62.8%, the inhibition of the superoxide radicals was in the range 23.9 to 37.4%, those of hydroxyl radicals varied from 48 to 68%, and linoleic acid oxidation was reduced by 8.6–27.9%. Furthermore, RJ harvested 24 h after the larval transfer has shown the highest reducing power, while the most significant effect on SOD activity was observed for RJ collected 72 h after transfer. These findings indicate that superoxide radicals' scavenging and SOD inhibition are likely mediated by different compounds from RJ. The antioxidant properties of RJ have also been demonstrated in vivo. Mice that were fed RJ had reduced levels of 8-hydroxy-2-deoxyguanosine (8-OHdG), a marker of oxidative DNA damage, in the kidneys and serum [62,64,65].

Interestingly, di- and tri-peptides obtained by the hydrolysis of RJ proteins have also demonstrated the antioxidant properties, especially regarding hydrogen peroxide-scavenging. However, the metal-chelating activity and scavenging of superoxide radicals were not observed. From 29 hydrolyzed peptides, 12 peptides with 2–4 residues have demonstrated prominent antioxidative properties, of which the dipeptides Lys-Tyr, Arg-Tyr, and Tyr-Tyr have shown strong scavenging activity through the donation of a hydrogen atom of the phenolic hydroxyl group of Tyr residues [64,65]. Similarly, MRJPs have shown a DPPH radical-scavenging ability and have protected DNA against oxidative injury [29,66]. In another study, recombinant MRJPs from *Apis cerana* (AcMRJPs) protected NIH 3T3 cells from OS-induced apoptosis by reducing caspase-3 activity. AcMRJPs also demonstrated an antioxidative effect and protected DNA from oxidative damage in an in vitro assay [66].

Furthermore, the antioxidative effects of RJ have been demonstrated in liver and kidney tissues exposed to various harmful stimuli with pro-oxidant activity. RJ reduced the extent of lipid peroxidation and improved the activities of the key antioxidative enzymes glutathione reductase (GR), glutathione peroxidase (GPx), superoxide dismutase (SOD), and catalase (CAT). The activation of the transcription factor nuclear factor erythroid 2-related factor 2 (Nrf2) has been recognized as one of the most important mechanisms underlying the antioxidative activity of RJ. Nrf2 regulates cellular redox balance and offers protection against toxic and oxidative insults by controlling the expression of genes involved in the oxidative stress response and drug detoxification [67]. In particular, its transcriptional activation improves its resistance to oxidative stress, chemical carcinogens, and inflammatory challenges. Chi et al. [67] demonstrated that RJ induces the transcriptional expression of Nrf2 and its target genes heme oxygenase (HO-1) and GPx1, suggesting that RJ activates the Nrf2–HO-1 pathway to improve antioxidant defense. Moreover, changes in the gene expression profiles were paralleled with the improved activity of enzymatic antioxidants in the liver. It has been suggested that the phenolic components of RJ are likely responsible for the observed induction of Nrf2 expression at the gene level (Figure 1).

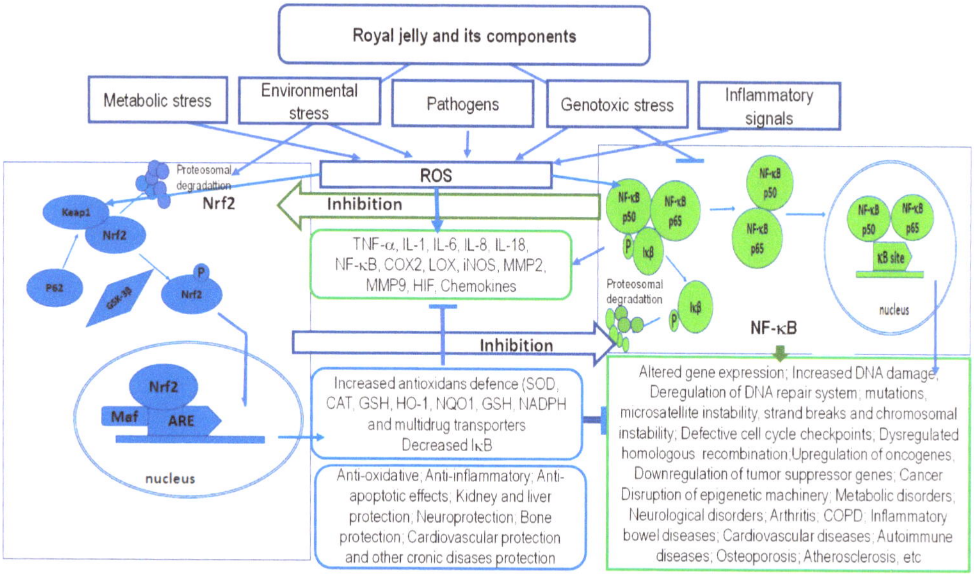

Figure 1. Modulation of Nrf2 and NF-κB signaling pathways by royal jelly (RJ). RJ reduces reactive oxygen species (ROS)-induced tissue damage and toxicity by modulating Nrf2 and NF-κB signaling pathways. Nrf2 and NF-κB are important regulators of the body's response to oxidative stress and inflammation. The figure shows potential molecular mechanisms of RJ action via Nrf2 and NF-κB pathways and important effects on harmful exogenous and endogenous factors, as well as interplay between Nrf2 and NF-κB signaling. NF-κB functions as a homo- or heterodimer derived from one or more of the five members of the NF-κB family (RelA/p65, RelB, cRel, NF-κB1 or p50, and NF-κB2 or p52), and is activated by stimulus-dependent inhibitor degradation, post-translational modifications, nuclear translocation, and chromatin-binding. The activated NF-κB drives the pro-inflammatory response that plays an important role in the pathogenesis of chronic inflammatory diseases. In the nucleus, p65 coordinates gene transcription by recruiting coactivators (e.g., CREB-binding proteins (CBP)) or corepressors (e.g., histone deacetylases (HDACs)). Nrf2 and NF-κB compete for the CBP-binding in the nucleus; which transcription factor will bind to CBP depends on the relative amounts of translocated Nrf2 and NF-κB. In addition, NF-κB recruits HDAC3 which deacetylates Nrf2, reduces Nrf2 levels, and inhibits expression of ARE-dependent genes.

The inflammatory response is also characterized by the orchestrated activation of intracellular signaling pathways that regulate the expression of various pro- and anti-inflammatory mediators. The activation of the transcription factor NF-κB is widely implicated in various inflammatory diseases. NF-κB regulates the expression of proinflammatory molecules, including cytokines, chemokines, and adhesion molecules. Consequently, the activation of the canonical NF-κB pathway largely contributes to the pathogenesis of chronic inflammatory diseases such as atherosclerosis, asthma, chronic obstructive pulmonary disease (COPD), inflammatory bowel disease (IBD), multiple sclerosis (MS), rheumatoid arthritis (RA), ulcerative colitis, and others. On the other hand, RJ is able to modulate levels of the main inflammatory mediators, including the aforementioned cytokines, chemokines, and adhesion molecules, thereby attenuating the inflammatory response. The anti-inflammatory abilities of RJ are mediated by various mechanisms. Besides inhibiting the production of pro-inflammatory cytokines, RJ also suppresses the NF-κB signaling pathway and modulates immune cells' functions (see Figure 1).

Regarding individual compounds, the anti-inflammatory effects of RJ are attributed to 10-HDA, 10-HDAA, and sebacic acid (SA). The anti-inflammatory effect of 10-HDA, the main lipid component of RA, has been demonstrated by many studies. Thus, Jang and colleagues [68] have investigated the effects of 10-HDA on the production of TNF-α, IL-1β, IL-8, and IL-1ra in WiDr cells. 10-HDA inhibited the production of TNF-α, IL-1β, IL-8, and NF-κB but increased the amount of IL-1ra. The inhibitory effects (81.79%) on the production of TNF-α were observed at a 3 mM concentration of 10-HDA. Thus, the results indicate that 10-HDA has the ability to suppress the secretion of pro-inflammatory cytokines and increase the production of anti-inflammatory cytokines. Enzyme-treated RJ (ERJ) has also shown the anti-inflammatory and immune-promoting properties. ERJ decreased the levels of TNF-α, IL-1, IL-6, IL-10, IFN-γ, and IL-12, and increased the proliferation of B- and T-lymphocytes and natural killer cells (NK-cells). In another study, 10-HDA greatly reduced the expression of pro-inflammatory cytokines (IL-1, IL-6, cyclooxygenase 2 (COX-2), and monocyte chemoattractant protein-1 (MCP-1)) and the activation of the NF-κB and c-Jun N-terminal kinase (JNK) pathways. Furthermore, 10-HDA can act as an HDAC inhibitor and has the ability to inhibit the proliferation of fibroblast-like synoviocyte (FLS) cells induced by RA, a systemic chronic inflammatory disease [13,69]. The anti-inflammatory effects of MRJP3 or its C-terminal tandem pentapeptide repeats (TPRs) were also reported. They inhibited the expression of TNF-α and IL-6 mRNAs in lipopolysaccharide (LPS)-stimulated THP-1 cells. The anti-inflammatory activity of MRJP3 and its ability to suppress the production of the pro-inflammatory cytokines has also been observed in mice [36,69–71].

By activating the Nrf2 pathway, RJ increases the antioxidant capacity and inhibits the inflammatory response mediated by NF-κB, reducing the organ toxicity induced by endogenous and exogenous factors. RJ directly or indirectly activates Nrf2 signaling, prevents IκBα degradation, increases expressions of HO-1, and inhibits the activation of NF-κB. In the nucleus, Nrf2 heterodimerizes with small Maf proteins (MafF, MafG, and MafK) and binds to the antioxidant responsive element (ARE). Through the activation of the Nrf2 pathway, RJ increases the cellular antioxidant defense, promoting the resistance to the toxic effects of various stressors and drugs. In addition, RJ may increase the activation of the Nrf2 pathway and ARE gene transcription by increasing the free CBP levels, and by reducing the recruitment of HDAC3 to the ARE region. Furthermore, RJ may inhibit the nuclear translocation of NF-κB.

Note: ARE, antioxidant responsive element; CAT, catalase; CBP, CREB-binding proteins; HDACs, histone deacetylases; COPD, chronic obstructive pulmonary disease; COX-2, Cyclooxygenase-2; GSH, glutathione; GSK-3β; glycogen synthase kinase-3β; HIF, hypoxia-inducible factor; HO-1, heme oxygenase 1; IκB, Nuclear factor of kappa light polypeptide gene enhancer in B-cells inhibitor; iNOS, inducible nitric oxide synthase; Keap1, kelch-like ECH-associated protein 1; LOX, Lipooxygenase; Maf, Maf proteins (MafF, MafG, and MafK); MMP-9, matrix metalloproteinase 9; NADPH, nicotinamide adenine dinucleotide phosphate; NF-κB, nuclear factor kappa-light-chain-enhancer of activated B cells; NF-κB1 (also named p50), NF-κB2 (also named p52), *NQO1*, NAD(P)H quinone oxidoreductase 1; Nrf2, nuclear factor-erythroid 2-related factor 2; RelA (p65), ROS, reactive oxygen species; SOD, superoxide dismutase; and TNF-α, tumor necrosis factor alpha.

Ulcerative colitis (UC) and Crohn's disease (CD) are inflammatory bowel diseases (IBD) with a complex etiology resulting from interactions of genetic, environmental, and microbial factors.

The effects of RJ have been investigated in several animal models of colitis. Colitis is induced by either 2, 4, 6-trinitrobenzene sulfonic acid (TNBS), dextran sulfate sodium (DSS), or acetic acid (AA). RJ exhibited anti-inflammatory, antioxidant, and regenerative effects and improved the colonic mucosal barrier and intestinal gut microbiota. In rats with AA-induced colitis, treatment with RJ alleviated the damage of the colon tissue and the number of colonic CD3+CD45+ T cells and mast cells, without affecting the number of CD68+ macrophages and CD5+T cells. RJ also stimulated the production of the anti-inflammatory cytokine IL-10 and GPx activity. In rats with TNBS-induced colitis, supplementation with RJ also reduced CD3+, CD5+, CD8+, and CD45+ T cells, the production of pro-inflammatory cytokines IL-1β and TNF-α, and the levels of COX-2 and NF-κB. In the DSS-induced mouse model of colitis, treatment with RJ (2.0 g/kg) improved symptoms, reduced the apoptosis of colonic cells, and decreased intestinal permeability by upregulating the expression of the tight-junction protein, goblet cells, and their product, glycoprotein mucin 2 (MUC2). RJ also reduced the expression of proinflammatory cytokine IL-6 and increased the levels of anti-inflammatory cytokine IL-10 and antibody sIgA, which has an important role in mucosal immunity. RJ also improved DSS-induced changes in the relative abundance of various bacterial strains in the colon, including *Parabacteroides, Proteobacteria* (*Gammaproteobacteria, Enterobacteriales,* and *Enterobacteriaceae*), *Escherichia Shigella,* and *Muribaculum.* These results indicate that RJ might reduce colon damage by reducing intestinal inflammation [72]. In another study, in mice fed with RJ, RJ increased the relative abundance of *Lachnospiraceae_NK4A136_group, Prevotellaceae,* and *Bacteroides* and decreased the relative abundance of Alistipes [73].

All-together, increasing evidence suggests that RJ not only stimulates immunity and antioxidative activities, but also regulates the composition and structure of the gut microbiota. The gut barrier has an important role in transporting nutrients and metabolites across the epithelial cells and prevents damage by intraluminal substances [68,72,74].

It has been shown that RJ proteins may regulate immune function by stimulating macrophage activity and by reducing the levels of inflammatory mediators [75]. Thus, in immunodeficient cyclophosphamide-treated mice, the monomeric MRJP1, MRJP2, and MRJP3 proteins increased the number of murine macrophages, stimulated the immune response, and improved the composition of intestinal flora [76]. In particular, MRJPs affected the development of the spleen and liver, the number of leukocytes in the peripheral blood, the immunoglobulin content, cytokine levels, and the proliferation ability of spleen T- and B-lymphocytes.

In another study performed in *db/db* mice, RJ improved gut microbiota dysbiosis and intestinal and liver inflammation. It also regulated the expression of genes involved in nutrient absorption in the small intestine, increasing the excretion of saturated fatty acids in feces and the number of short-chain fatty acid (SCFA)-producing intestinal bacteria, altogether improving the atrophy of the intestinal mucosa. In general, SCFAs are end-products of the fermentation of non-digestible carbohydrates by gut microbiota. They are the main nutritional source for epithelial cells and are accordingly important for colon health. In addition to increasing mucus production and strengthening the tight junctions between the intestinal epithelial cells, SCFAs also cause an increase in mucin expression in goblet cells. Furthermore, SCFAs bind to the free fatty acid receptor and inhibit the activation of NF-κB [77], suppressing the secretion of pro-inflammatory cytokines like IL-1, IL-12, and TNF-α [78–80]. These cytokines further impact innate lymphoid cells (ILC1 and ILC3) and the production of their cytokines, including NF-α, IFN-γ, IL-17, and IL-22, leading to inflammation and cytotoxicity.

According to Kobayashy et al. [80], RJ can help in non-alcoholic fatty liver disease (NAFLD). Besides improving gut dysbiosis and inflammation, RJ increases the excretion of saturated palmitic acid in the feces, thus decreasing its content in the blood and liver, and increases the content MCFAs in the liver. In RJ, four main MCFAs have been identified: 10-HDA, 10 HDAA, 2-decenedioic acid (2-DA), and sebacic acid (SA). This finding is important as it is recognized that a high content of saturated fatty acids in a diet may increase the secretion of IL-12 from macrophages, induce mitochondrial damage, and sustain chronic low-grade inflammation, contributing to the pathogenesis of metabolic disorders, muscular atrophy, progressive liver inflammation, and cardiovascular diseases [77–80]. NAFLD pathogenesis is related to the "two-hits" hypothesis, which suggests that steatosis develops into nonalcoholic steatohepatitis (NASH) through excessive free fatty acids (FFAs), hyperinsulinemia, and lipid peroxidation [81]. The disturbance of the circadian rhythm and its Period genes (*Pers*) is associated with disruption of metabolic activity, increased fat storage, and a decrease in its consumption, ultimately causing hepatic steatosis which exacerbates the development of NAFLD [82]. According to You et al. [82], RJ could decrease the body and liver weights, improve cholesterol levels, downregulate ALT and AST levels, and combat NAFLD in OVX rats. The preventive effect of RJ may align with its strong antioxidative activity and its capacity to ameliorate the disturbances of the circadian genes, *Per1* and *Per2*. In another study, the protective effect of RJ was demonstrated against NAFLD due to its antioxidant and anti-inflammatory effect, as well as regulating the metabolism of FAs such as α-linolenic acid, linoleic acid, and arachidonic acid, and the biosynthesis of unsaturated fatty acids [83]. Felemban and coauthors [84] revealed that the chronic feeding of RJ to HFD-fed rats not only reduced the gain in weight and improved insulin resistance (IR), but also attenuated hyperglycemia and alleviated hepatic damage and steatosis. In addition, this study showed that the antidiabetic and anti-steatosis mechanisms by which RJ acts involve at least antioxidant potential, as well as the activation of the hepatic AMPK signaling-mediated upregulation of PPARα (fatty acid oxidation) and the suppression of SREBP1/2 (de novo lipogenesis) The treatment with RJ also reduced the serum levels of liver function enzymes, interleukin 6 (IL-6), tumor necrosis factor-α (TNF-α), and leptin, but significantly increased the serum levels of adiponectin. In addition, 10-HDA inhibits matrix metalloproteinases (MMPs) which degrade matrix and non-matrix proteins, resulting in tissue aging (e.g., skin) and chronic inflammatory diseases such as rheumatoid arthritis (RA) [85].

RA is an autoimmune inflammatory disease with an unclear etiology. The hallmarks of RA are hyperplasia and persistent inflammation of the synovial membranes, which penetrate deep into the bone and articular cartilage. The damage of bone and cartilage in RA joints is attributed to MMPs produced by the rheumatoid arthritis synovial fibroblasts (RASFs). MMP-1 (collagenase 1) and MMP-3 (stromelysin 1) are particularly important proteases in RA-associated tissue degradation. TNF-α is one of the well-known cytokines that stimulates the production of MMPs by activating the MAPK signaling pathways. The regulation of MMPs' production is achieved through the activation of JNK, p38, and NF-κB in synovial tissue and cultured RASFs. It has been shown that 10-HDA from the RJ may reduce joint destruction in RA. 10-HDA exerted its effects by reducing the TNF-α-induced gene expression of MMP-1 and MMP-3, and by inhibiting the activation of the p38 and JNK/AP-1 signaling pathways. On the contrary, it had no effect on the TNF-α-induced activation of the extracellular signal-regulated kinase (ERK) cascade, NF-κB activity, or IκBα degradation [85]. These findings also indicate that the inhibition of the p38 and JNK pathways could be a possible therapeutic target against inflammation-related joints' destruction in RA [85].

Overall, the anti-inflammatory effects of SA, 10-had, and 10-HDAA are not related only to the regulation of proteins involved in MAPK and NF-κB signaling [86,87]. They also may affect estrogen signaling by stimulating the activity of estrogen receptors (ER), ERα and ERβ [35], potentially exerting beneficial effects on the bones, muscles, and adipose tissue in a sex-dependent manner. Another study demonstrated that the inhibitory effect of 10-HDA on the proliferation of fibroblast-like synoviocytes was mediated by its ability to act as an HDAC inhibitor and downregulate the PI3K–AKT pathway. It also increased the expression of genes involved in cytokine–cytokine receptor interactions [88].

Multiple sclerosis (MS), also a chronic inflammatory disease, affects about 250,000 to 350,000 individuals in the USA and markedly reduces their quality of life. Demyelinating lesions in the brain, spinal cord, and optic nerve are typical hallmarks of MS. Oshvandi et al. [89] showed that supplementation with RJ can be beneficial in improving quality of life; following a 90-day period of supplementation, the patients' activity was increased. In another study, Seyyedi et al. [90] have reported that the consumption of RJ, through its estrogenic effect and reduced vaginal atrophy, improves the quality of life of postmenopausal women [90,91]. The anti-inflammatory effect of RJ was also confirmed in experimental autoimmune encephalomyelitis (EAE), an animal model of MS. RJ and 10-HDA reduced demyelination, regulated the polarization of Th17 and Th1 cells, and attenuated the infiltration of the peripheral immune cells into the CNS. In addition to RA and MS, RJ can be useful in other human autoimmune diseases such as Graves' disease and lupus erythematosus by strengthening the immune system.

RJ, MRJP3, or its C-terminal TPRs sequence may exert anti-inflammatory effects by inhibiting the production of pro-inflammatory cytokines TNF-α, IL-1β, IL-2, IL-6, and IL-33. This has been shown in various conditions, including herpes stromal keratitis (HSK) caused by *Herpes simplex virus* type 1 (HSV-1), LPS-stimulated THP-1 cells, formalin-induced rat paw edema, and nanoparticle-induced inflammation of the skin, gastrointestinal and respiratory tract, and cardiovascular system [92,93].

Environmental and occupational exposure to heavy metals, such as Cd, has been tightly linked to the ROS-induced oxidative damage of proteins, lipids, carbohydrates, and DNA, which underlies the development and progression of pathological changes in many diseases. Exposure to Cd also induces apoptotic events and modulates the ratio of pro- and anti-apoptotic proteins. In addition, Cd results in massive inflammation through the excessive release of pro-inflammatory mediators, like IL-1β, TNF-α, and nitric oxide (NO) [94]. It has been shown that RJ markedly reduces Cd-induced oxidative damage in mouse testes via the Nrf2 pathway [95]. By increasing Nrf2 and homoxygenase-1, RJ also protected the lymphocytes, liver, kidney, and heart tissue against drug- or toxin-induced oxidative injury [96]. In 6-hydroxydopamine-induced cell death, Nrf2 translocation to the nucleus and the enhanced expression of antioxidant and detoxifying enzymes were induced by 4-hydroperoxy-2-decenoic acid ethyl ester (HPO-DAEE), a lipid component of RJ [97].

5.2. *Royal Jelly, Beauty, and Postponement of Ageing*

The majority of the aging process is conditioned by the genetically programmed weakening and failure of the homeostatic mechanisms. Various stressors may induce the senescence process (see Figure 2), especially OS, mitochondrial dysfunction, ER stress, and epigenetic stress, leading to irreversible DNA damage and the activation of molecular mechanisms of aging associated with p53 regulation. The cell's DNA damage response (DDR), particularly to double-strand breaks (DSB), results in p53 phosphorylation, p21 activation, and cell cycle arrest [98–102].

Continuous OS and chronic inflammation are associated with many cellular and molecular changes: damage of the main biological molecules, loss of enzymatic activity, mitochondrial dysfunction, reduced proteostasis, genome instability, weakened repair mechanisms, telomere shortening, epigenetic modifications, and the disturbance of gene expression and signaling pathways. In addition, these changes include the loss of intercellular communication, immunosenescence and dysfunction of effector functions of T and B cells, decrease in the antigen-presenting functions, exhaustion of stem cells, low-grade inflammation and increased cytokine release, dysbiosis of intestinal microbiota and alternations in intestinal permeability, and ultimately, cellular aging (see Figure 2).

Cellular senescence is induced by critically short telomeres, triggering the permanent activation of DDR and cell cycle arrest. The DDR is a well-known activator of the senescence-associated secretory phenotype (SASP) which is characterized by the increased expression of an array of pro-inflammatory factors, mostly in an NF-Kb-dependent manner, such as IL-6, IL-8, IL-1β, monocyte chemoattractant protein (MCP)-1, MCP-2 and MCP-4, growth factors like the human growth factor (HGF) and fibroblast growth factor (FGF), various proteases like MMPs, and secreted insoluble proteins/extracellular matrix proteins (ECM). Senescent cells disrupt the homeostasis and function of tissues and organs, resulting in the loss of tissue regeneration and the reduced function of stem cells. SASP components can induce tissue fibrosis in certain epithelial tissues, whereas the infiltration of macrophages and lymphocytes, fibrosis, and cell death are recognized as the cause of numerous diseases associated with aging [98–102].

Therefore, the antioxidant, anti-inflammatory, and antisenescence properties of RJ as well as the modulation of cellular senescence by targeting Nrf2 activation can be a promising preventive strategy against cancer and other degenerative diseases (NAFLD, neurodegenerative diseases, aging, heart diseases, and cardiovascular diseases) [58,100–103].

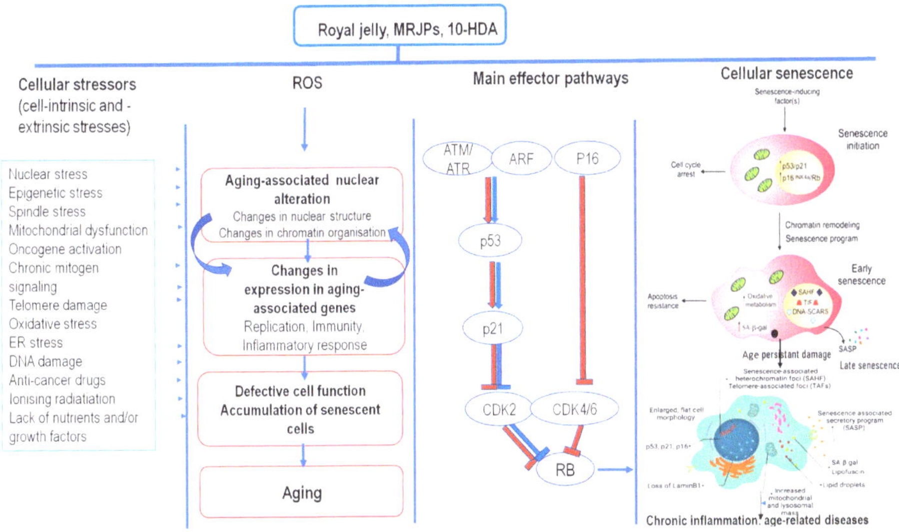

Figure 2. Anti-senescence effect and molecular mechanisms of royal jelly (RJ) and its components on cellular senescence, healthy aging, and longevity induced by endogenous and exogenous factors. Cellular senescence is triggered by various intrinsic and extrinsic stimuli such as ROS, inflammation, mitochondrial dysfunction, genotoxic stress, irradiation and chemotherapeutic agents, telomere shortening, irreversible DNA damage, or signals such as oncogene activation or the overexpression of pluripotency factors. These stressors initiate various cellular signaling cascades, ultimately resulting in the activation of p53, p16Ink4a, or both. Their activation induces cell cycle arrest by inhibiting cyclin D–Cdk4/6 and cyclin E–Cdk2 and prevents Rb inactivation, resulting in continuous repression of E2F target genes required for S-phase. ARF can inhibit MDM2 and stabilize p53, which leads to the arrest of the cell cycle and cellular aging and the possibility of repairing minor damages. Accordingly, senescence is associated with several molecular and phenotypic alterations, such as senescence-associated secretory phenotype (SASP), cell cycle arrest, DNA damage response (DDR), senescence-associated β-galactosidase, morphogenesis, and chromatin remodeling. The anti-senesce effects of RJ and its component (MRJPs, 10-had, and RJPs) is the result of the interplay between several genes involved in downregulation of insulin/insulin-like growth factor-1 signaling (IIS) and targeting of rapamycin (mTOR), upregulation of the epidermal growth factor (EGF) signaling, dietary restriction, and enhancement of antioxidative capacity via Nrf2 activation. These signaling pathways affect cellular processes associated with longevity: DNA repair, autophagy, antioxidant activity, anti-inflammatory activity, stress resistance, and cell proliferation. In addition, RJ suppresses cellular senescence by upregulation of SOD1 and downregulation of Mtor and catenin beta like-1, and by regulating the expression levels of p53, p16, and p21. The life-expanding effect of RJ possibly originates from its antioxidant and anti-inflammatory properties, which can promote healthy aging by improving glycemic status, lipid profiles, and oxidative stress and hence can prevent the occurrence of various debilitating metabolic diseases. Furthermore, it should be noted that RJ contains epigenetically active compounds that inhibit DNMT3 or HDAC3, thus changing the epigenetic information generated in response to exogenous and endogenous factors during the aging process. Note: ATM, Ataxia telangiectasia mutated; ATR, Ataxia telangiectasia mutated and Rad3 related; BDNF, brain-derived neurotrophic factor; CDK2, Cyclin-dependent kinase 2; CDK4/6, Cyclin-dependent kinase 4 and 6; ER stress, Endoplasmic reticulum stress; NGF, nerve growth factor; Nrf2, nuclear factor-erythroid 2-related factor 2; p21 and p16, cyclin dependent kinase (CDK) inhibitors; Rb, retinoblastoma protein; ROS, Reactive oxygen species; SA-β-gal, senescence-associated β-galactosidase; SAHF, Senescence-associated heterochromatin foci; SASP, Senescence-associated secretory phenotype; TAFs, telomere-associated foci.

A daily intake of RJ can extend the lifespan of bees and other species, including nematodes, crickets, or mice. This effect is attributed to proteins and lipids from royal jelly and MRJPs. In *Drosophila melanogaster*, RJ extended longevity by promoting the epidermal growth factor (EGF) receptor-mediated pathway [104]. Royalactin (MRJP1) also stimulated EGF and epidermal growth factor receptor (EGFR) pathways in *Caenorhabditis elegans* [105]. Wang et al. [106] found that royal jelly and an enzyme-treated RJ (RJ/eRJ)-mediated lifespan extension requires insulin/IGF-1 signaling and the activities of the DAF-16, SIR-2.1, HCF-1, and FTT-2, a 14-3-3 proteins. These findings reveal that RJ/eRJ supplementation triggers a sophisticated regulatory mechanism, mediated by the interplays of DAF-16, SIR-2.1, HCF-1, and 14-3-3, to fine-tune DAF-16 activities and thereby promote prolongevity and stress responses in *C. elegans*. DAF-16 is a key regulator of stress responses; the DAF-16 target genes (sod-3, mtl-1, and F21F3.3) which promote *C. elegans'* response to oxidative stress, heavy metals, and heat shock. Thus, RJ and eRJ consumption increased the lifespan, health span, and the tolerance of *C. elegans* to oxidative stress, ultraviolet irradiation, and heat shock stress. Earlier studies reported that DAF-16/FOXO, SIR-2.1/SIRT1, FTT-2, HCF-1, and 14-3-3 proteins are evolutionarily conserved from *C. elegans* to mammals, and that these findings may have immediate implications in utilizing RJ/eRJ as aging-intervention means to prolong one's health span and combat age-related diseases in higher-order organisms, including humans. In addition, 10-HDA can increase the lifespan of *Caenorhabditis elegans* through dietary restriction and the targeting of rapamycin (TOR) signaling [107]. Moreover, the long-term use of RJ in D-galactose-induced mice prevented age-related weight loss, improved memory abilities, and delayed thymus atrophy. It also reduced muscle cell atrophy and, consequently, increased the mobility and physical condition of mice [52,108–110]. In humans, the intake of RJ can also delay aging and the development of some age-related disorders, improve the quality of life during aging, and significantly delay age-related motor dysfunctions [52,110]. In human cell cultures, lipid components of RJ inhibited the aging process through the upregulation of EGF signaling and downregulation of insulin-like growth factors (IGF) [5,109–111]. In mouse embryonic stem cells, it was shown that royalactin can maintain pluripotency by activating a ground-state pluripotency-like gene network [44]. Furthermore, the same authors discovered Regina, a mammalian structural analog of royalactin that can promote ground-state pluripotency in mouse embryonic stem cells, indicating the possibility of using royalactin as a regenerative therapy.

Salazar-Olivio and Paz-Gonzales [112] also have shown that RJ proteins can have an effect in the postponement and prevention of ageing. In their study, RJ have promoted proliferation in insect cell cultures. Likewise, Watanabe et al. [33] have demonstrated the mitogenic effect of RJ on a human monocyte cell line (U-937 cells) and its ability to increase the synthesis of DNA and albumins in liver cells [113]. It is believed that RJ contains growth factors or hormones that stimulate cell growth. Taken together with the finding that certain protein fractions of RJ increase the synthesis of new adhesion molecules, this confirms the cosmetic efficacy of royal jelly [26,114]. Kawano et al. [114] demonstrated that RJ can reduce the expression of miR-129-5p and can prevent the photoaging of skin. It is possible that the effect of miR-129-5p a is not only involved in increasing the number of cells, but can prevent skin aging through the regulation of its target genes. Many genes are predicted as putative targets of miR-129-5p including calcium signaling-related molecules, such as the calcium channel, voltage-dependent, γ subunit 2 (CACNG), calcium/calmodulin-dependent protein kinase II inhibitor 1 (CAMK2N1), FK506-binding protein 2, 13 kDa (FKBP2), and calmodulin 1 (phosphorylase kinase, delta) (CALM1).

The skin is the largest organ that covers the entire surface of the body. The main function of the skin is to protect organism from environmental insults [115]. In order to fulfil its function, the skin can initiate a defense process targeted at tissue repair and pathogen removal [115]. However, an estrogen deficiency and decrease in collagen during menopause and natural aging reduce skin elasticity and strength. RJ constituents, especially 10-HDA, can reduce cell aging and stimulate the production of procollagen type I and transforming growth factor-1 (TGF-β1) [109,110,116–121]. Similarly, MRJP promotes cell proliferation, affects the telomere length, and reduces aging [109,111]. Furthermore, Koya-Miyata et al. [119] have shown a beneficial effect of RJ on collagen production in skin fibroblasts and an isolated active substance named the collagen production-promoting factor. The pharmaceutically active ingredients of RJ in collagen production were 10H-2DA and 10-HDA. These acids in the presence of ascorbic acid promote the production of TGF that further increases collagen production. It still remains unknown if these acids influence enzymes involved in collagen synthesis as well (prolyl hydroxylase and lysyl hydroxylase).

RJ is appreciated today as a protective agent against skin aging. Experiments performed in ovariectomized rats have indicated its ability to increase collagen production [117,120]. Following the administration of 1% RJ to female Sprague–Dawley rats without estrogen, the skin level of the type I procollagen protein was returned almost to normal values. Hence, according to the data provided, it seems that RJ could be an effective dietary supplement against the natural aging process of postmenopausal skin, but further clinical research is needed to confirm this [120].

Of note, collagen is a predominant fibrous protein of extracellular matrix and the main protein in connective human tissue, making about 3–6% of total body proteins. The functional properties of skin are largely dependent on the integrity of dermal collagen. Alterations in the level of collagen settling are observed during wound healing, bone development, and ageing. Hence, collagen metabolism control is important not only from a cosmetic perspective, but also for therapeutic applications.

In a recent study, Khani-Eshratabadi et al. [121] have shown the potential anti-apoptotic effects on RJ in different rat tissues (brain, liver, kidney, and lymphocytes) by regulating the levels of Bax, Bcl-2, and telomerase enzymes. In rats treated with RJ, there was a trend towards a telomerase increase, the significant effect on the reduction of the Bax/Bcl-2 ratio, and the improved survival rate of the liver, kidney, and especially brain cells at a dose of 300 mg/kg. A similar effect was obtained in a study conducted by Jiang et al. [111]. The treatment of a human embryonic lung fibroblast cell line (HFL-I) with different concentrations of MRJPS (0.1–0.3 mg/mL) had beneficial impacts on proliferation, senescence, and the telomere length. The antisenescence effects of MRJPs were associated with the upregulation of SOD1 and downregulation of the mTOR, catenin beta like-1 (CTNNB1), and transcription factor 53 pathways, which altogether had a stimulatory effect on DNA and protein synthesis. Likewise, in human lymphocytes exposed to the genotoxic chemotherapeutic compound doxorubicin, the beneficial effects of RJ were associated with the increased hTERT/BAX ratio, indicative of greater longevity [122].

Immunity is also affected by aging; aging reduces cell proliferation, the production of new naive lymphocytes, and the production of cytokines in the defense process, especially interleukin 2 (IL-2) [101,102]. Immunosenescence is a process associated with aging that leads to the dysregulation of cells of innate and adaptive immunity and the reduced ability of the immune system to respond to foreign antigens and maintain tolerance to self-antigens. Immunosenescence is characterized by a reduced proliferation capacity, telomere shortening, and increased resistance to the apoptosis of CD28+ T-lymphocytes in general [101,102,123]. In the elderly, the repertoire of naive CD4+ and CD8+T cells along with cytokine production is severely affected with alterations in memory B cells and antibody production [101,102,123], which results in high susceptibility to infection, cancer, and autoimmune diseases, and a reduced response to vaccinations. Bouamama et al. (124) demonstrated some mechanisms that delay PBMCs' cell senescence in vitro by RJ through enhancing their cell proliferating ability, MDA, GSH, IL-2, IL-6, IL-4 cytokines, and NO release. The immuno-enhancing potential and anti-immunosenescence effects of royal jelly may play a primordial role in the health of the elderly to corroborate and combat pathological aging by improving the immune functions, enhancing PBMCs' proliferation along with the cytokine release [123–125].

Inoue and co-authors [126] have shown that RJ can increase the lifespan of C3H/HeJ mice by reducing oxidative damage. The theory of «free radicals and ageing» is widely known; ROS production results in the overall damage of the cell [4,127,128] and its consequences include the modifications of cell proteins, lipids, and DNA. The results of many studies indicate the important contribution of the increased oxidative DNA damage to the ageing of the cell and organism. In fact, it is considered that DNA damage is the cause of ageing and degenerative diseases related to ageing, including tumors, heart diseases, and cardiovascular diseases (Figure 2). Mutations, a consequences of oxidative damage, shorten one's lifespan. In the aforementioned study on C3H/HeJ mice, dietary supplementation with RJ increased mice survival by 50%. The authors found that the mechanism of protection was not based on the free radical scavenging ability of RJ, but on the suppression of oxidative DNA damage, perhaps through reduced chronic inflammation [103–105,126,129–131].

In addition, the accumulation of senescent cells in the tumor microenvironment can drive tumorigenesis in a paracrine manner through the SASP. Hatson et al. [132] suggested that senescent macrophages play an important role in the initiation and progression of lung cancer, and may be a potential target in cancer prevention strategies. It seems that the clearance of senescent macrophages can ameliorate tumorigenesis in KRAS-driven lung cancer. It has been suggested that SASP can reinforce senescence-induced cell cycle arrest by autocrine or paracrine mechanisms and can modulate the tissue microenvironment by paracrine pathways. For example, 16INK4a-expressing macrophages express many pro-tumorigenic SASP factors unique to a tumorigenic lung (i.e., Bmp2, CCL2, CCL7, CCL8, CCL24, CXCL13, and IL-10) and may represent important mediators of paracrine pro-tumorigenic effects. Chemokines CCL7, CCL24, and CXCL13, as well as IL-10 and Bmp2, exert pro-tumorigenic effects in a variety of cancers, promoting the invasiveness, metastasis, and stemness of cancer cells. Furthermore, the senescent cells may contribute to the formation of an immunosuppressive tumor microenvironment (TME) (rich in Tregs and low in CD4+ and CD8 + T cells), which can be switched toward an immunostimulatory TME (low in Tregs and high CD4+ and CD8 + T cells) through the clearance of senescent cells. On the other hand, macrophage depletion or a colony stimulating factor 1 receptor (CSF1R) signaling blockade disturb the intratumoral vascular network and reduce food and oxygen delivery to the tumor cells [98,132–134]. RJ compounds display their anticancer effects through a number of mechanisms such as controlling reactive oxygen species (ROS)-scavenging enzyme activities, suppressing the cell cycle, and promoting the apoptosis and inhibition of the proliferation of cancer cells, as well as their antimetastasis, antiangiogenic, etc., effects. The antioxidant, anti-inflammatory, anti-stress, immuno-enhancing potential, and anti-immunosenesence effects of RJ as well as the modulation of cellular senescence by Nrf2 activation can be a good preventive strategy in preventing the occurrence of cancer and other degenerative diseases.

5.3. *Royal Jelly and Its Effect on Brain Cells*

The ongoing rise in the elderly, particularly in Western countries, is one of the major worldwide problems today. The decline of cognitive abilities and increase in neuropsychiatric disorders, such as Alzheimer disease (AD) and depression, are closely related to aging. AD is a neurodegenerative disease characterized by intracellular aggregates of neurofibrillary tangles (NFTs) made of hyperphosphorylated and truncated tau proteins, and the extracellular deposition of amyloid beta (Aβ) peptides generated through the proteolytic cleavage of the amyloid precursor protein (APP) [135,136]. The accumulation of Aβ plaques activates microglial cells and the immune response, leading to increased OS, elevated intracellular Ca^{2+} levels, and a local inflammatory reaction, contributing to neurotoxicity. On the other hand, due to the selective loss of cholinergic neurons, acetylcholine (Ach), a neurotransmitter with a critical role in learning and memory, is depleted in AD patients. Levels of brain-derived neurotrophic factor (BDNF) are also reduced in patients with severe AD. BDNF is involved in learning and memory due to its important role in neuronal plasticity. In addition, BDNF inhibits cytokine production through its direct anti-inflammatory effect on microglial cells [137].

According to papers [58,138–152], RJ has many beneficial effects on cognition and AD pathology, including the improvement of memory, neuroprotection and regulation of neurotrophins, regulation of neurotransmission, regulation of brain energy metabolism, protection against oxidative stress and neuroinflammation, reduction of apoptosis, attenuation of Aβ-induced neurotoxicity, and improvement of hormonal and metabolic abnormalities associated with cognitive impairment (see Figure 3).

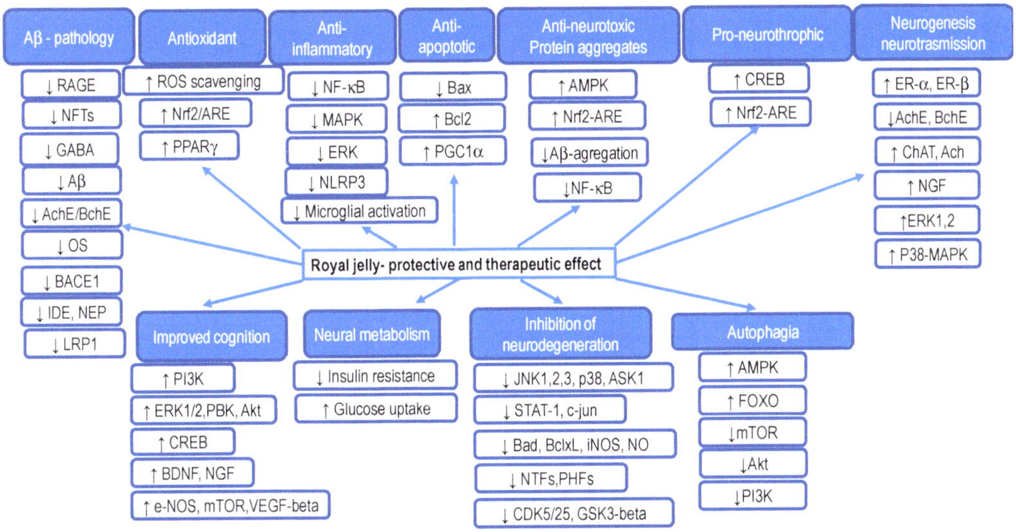

Figure 3. The possible protective and therapeutic mechanisms of royal jelly and its components in neuroprotection, cognitive performance, and suppression of neurodegeneration. Note: Aβ, amyloid beta; ACh, acetylcholine; AChE, acetylcholinesterase; AMPK, AMP-activated protein kinase; ARE, antioxidant responsive element; BACE1, beta-site APP cleaving enzyme 1; Bax, Bcl-2-associated X protein; BChE, butyrylcholinesterase; Bcl-2, B-cell lymphoma-2; BDNF, brain-derived neurotrophic factor; ChAT, choline acetyltransferase; CREB, cAMP-response element (CRE)-binding protein; ER β and α, estrogen receptors β and α; ERK, extracellular signal-regulated kinase; ERK1/2, extracellular signal-regulated kinase 1 or 2; eNOS, endothelial nitric oxide synthase; FOXO, forkhead box O transcription factor; GABA, gamma-aminobutyric acid; IDE, insulin-degrading enzyme; JNK, c-jun N-terminal kinase; LRP-1, low-density lipoprotein receptor-related protein; MAPK, mitogen-activated protein kinase; mTOR, mammalian target of rapamycin; NEP, neprilysin; NF-κB, nuclear factor-kappa B; NFT, neurofibrillary tangles; NGF, nerve growth factor; NLRP3, nucleotide-binding domain and leucine-rich repeat-containing protein 3; Nrf2, nuclear factor-erythroid 2-related factor 2; OS, oxidative stress; p38, p38 protein kinases; PI3K, phosphatidylinositol 3-kinase; PGC-1α, peroxisome proliferator-activated receptor-γ coactivator 1-a; PPAR-γ, peroxisome proliferator-activated receptor; RAGE, receptor for advanced glycation end-products; VEGF, vascular endothelial growth factor; ↑ upregulated; ↓ downregulated.

Many studies have highlighted the important role of neurotropic factors in the etiology and/or development of AD and other age-related diseases, suggesting that the increased synthesis of neuropeptide factors can be a promising avenue in the prevention of these diseases. Hashimoto et al. [153] have found that RJ selectively stimulates the mRNA expression of the glial cell line-derived neurotropic factor (GDNF) and neurofilament H, an axonal marker, in the hippocampus of adult mice. The neuroprotective effects of GDNF have been demonstrated in various conditions. Thus, the exogenous addition of GDNF protects the nigrostriatal dopaminergic terminals from neurodegeneration and ameliorated damage induced by cerebral ischemia and traumatic brain injury. These observations suggest that GDNF could be a promising approach in the protection and treatment of neurological diseases. However, further studies are needed of other RJ-induced active components with the effects on brain functions such as learning and memory. A better understanding of the biological effects of RJ at the molecular level likely will contribute towards more effective protection, as well as therapy for some neurological diseases, and to the more efficient use of RJ in healthcare.

The beneficial effects of RJ on cognition and AD-related pathologies have been demonstrated in various models, including copper- and cholesterol-fed rabbits [150], hippocampal neurons exposed to streptozotocin [151] and trimethyltin [154], and double transgenic APP/PS1 mice harboring mutations associated with early-onset AD (chimeric mouse/human APP (Mo/HuAPP695swe) and human presenilin 1 lacking exon 9 (PS1-dE9)) [145]. You et al. [145] argued that RJ may serve as a functional food for AD pathology. They found that the administration of RJ at a dose of 300 mg/kg/d for 3 months improved behavioral impairments and reduced the accumulation of Aβ in APP/PS1 mice. RJ also alleviated JNK-mediated apoptosis by suppressing oxidative stress. The authors suggested that RJ exerts protective effects on learning and memory by inhibiting or repairing AD-related hippocampal and cortical lesions. Importantly, the hippocampal levels of cAMP, p-PKA, p-CREB, and BDNF levels were significantly increased in RJ-treated mice, indicating the important effects of RJ on the cAMP/PKA/CREB/BDNF pathway in ameliorating cognitive decline. RJ also improved spatial learning and memory abilities in normally aged rats, as evidenced by the better performance in the Y-maze [139], Morris Water Maze test, passive avoidance test [103,151,154], and open field test [108].

Oxidative stress increases the amount of amyloid precursor protein (APP) and then further aggravates the AD pathology [145,155]. It is confirmed that oxidative stress is a therapeutic target of RJ in AD [138]. Some component derived from RJ as 10-HDA may be used to treat age-related neurodegenerative disorders; it stimulates neuronal differentiation from progenitor cells (PC12) through mimicking the effect of brain-derived neurotrophic factor (BDNF)] [156]. 10-had, in addition to stimulating neurogenesis via neural stem/progenitor cells, easily crossed the blood–brain barrier (BBB) and exerted unique neuromodulatory activity due to its smaller size [156]. In addition, it possesses neuroprotective effects against glutamate- and hypoxia-induced neurotoxicity [157]. Furthermore, AMP N1-oxide, the unique active nucleotide component present in RJ, has been shown to exhibit neurogenic and neurotrophic activities. AMP N1-oxide stimulates neurite outgrowth and induces the differentiation of PC12 cells into neurons through the activation of two signaling pathways: MAPK/extracellular signal-regulated kinase 1 or 2 (ERK1/2) and the phosphatidylinositol 3-kinase/Akt pathway. AMP N1-oxide promotes neurite outgrowth activity via adenylate cyclases coupled to adenosine A2A receptors crucial for neural development and the regulation of synaptic plasticity. It seems that AMP N1-oxide and 10-HDA are active components in RJ that reduce the deposition of Aβ by regulating the production, degradation, and clearance process, and in this way, they mitigate cognitive deficits and Aβ accumulation in the APP/PS1 mouse model [157].

A recent study by Aslan et al. [158] has shown that RJ (applied at a dose of 100 mg/kg bw during 56 days) prevented fluoride-induced brain damage via anti-oxidative effects. In addition, RJ reduced fluoride-induced increases in the expression of Bcl-2, NF-κB, and COX-2, and normalized the levels of caspase-3, caspase-6, Bax, and Erk.

Chen et al. [159] showed that supplementation with MRJPs improves the cognitive abilities of aged rats. MRJPs enhanced the metabolic activity of the brain by increasing the levels of glucose and phosphoenolpyruvic acid. The metabolomic analysis of the urine of MRJPs-fed rats did not show a significant difference compared to young rats. The main changes induced by MRJP supplementation were related to an increased level of nicotinic acid mononucleotide (NaMN), the precursor of NAD+, and xanthosine, which is important for the nucleic acid metabolism and DNA repair in old rats. MRJP proteins also increased the production of cysteic acid and other neuroprotective molecules in aged rats.

As previously mentioned, Aβ is produced from the APP through the amyloidogenic pathway. The first cleavage of APP is made by β-secretase (BACE1) which generates soluble APP peptide-β (sAPPβ) and C-terminal fragment-β (CTFβ). CTFβ is further cleaved by γ-secretase to yield hydrophobic Aβ polypeptides (predominantly Aβ40 and Aβ42). In N2a/APP695 neuroblastoma cells, crude royal jelly peptides (RJPs), obtained by the digestion of RJ proteins, reduced the production of Aβ40 and Aβ42 peptides by downregulating BACE1. Thus, RJPs could have the potential for ameliorating AD-related Aβ pathology [139].

Taken together, numerous studies have shown that RJ has an effect on various pathophysiological mechanisms related to cognitive decline and AD. RJ acts through neurotrophic, antioxidant, anti-inflammatory, antiapoptotic, and antiamyloidogenic mechanisms, delaying the onset of AD, slowing down its progression, and stimulating the recovery process.

Ali and Kunugi [59] summarized the main mechanisms of the RJ action contributing to the improvement of cognitive abilities and alleviation of Aβ pathology: (i) RJ reduces the influx of Aβ through the BBB by inhibiting the receptor for advanced glycation end-products (RAGE) which also acts as the receptor for Aβ, (ii) RJ prevents APP cleavage by inhibiting BACE1, and (iii) RJ facilitates the clearance of Aβ. In addition, predominantly by activating the AMPK signaling cascade, RJ stimulates autophagy and antioxidative defense, and suppresses inflammation. RJ and its lipid components also bind to estrogen receptors and increase the production of neurotrophic factors like NGF and BDNF and stimulate ACh production, neurogenesis, and synaptic plasticity.

Hattori et al. [154,156] have shown the effect of RJ and 10H2DA on the neurogenesis of neural progenitor/stem cells (NSCs) in vitro. NSCs have a self-regenerative ability and potential to differentiate into neurons, astrocytes, and oligodendrocytes. RJ stimulated the differentiation of all types of brain cells (neurons, astrocytes, and oligodendrocytes), whereas 10H2DA stimulated the production of neurons but reduced the differentiation of astrocytes. Hence, the RJ-induced activation of NSCs could be a relevant target for the treatment of AD and other neurodegenerative conditions.

5.4. Royal Jelly and Diabetes

RJ contains compounds functionally and structurally similar to insulin [160]. Moreover, as one of the most powerful therapeutic formulations with regenerative features, RJ may regenerate damaged pancreatic cells and prevent the development of diabetes [60,161–165]. The regeneration of pancreatic cells and preservation of insulin levels are key factors in lowering blood glucose [160–164]. In the Otsuka Long–Evans Tokushima Fatty (OLETF) rat model of type 2 diabetes, the long-term usage of RJ was effective in the prevention of insulin resistance [166]. Research by Zamami and colleagues also confirmed that RJ can reduce the index of insulin resistance (HOMA-IR), although not the blood glucose in rats [167]. The authors suggested that antioxidant peptides present in RJ are responsible for insulin resistance [162,167–169]. Overall, the beneficial effects of RJ observed in an animal model of diabetes include: (i) the improvement of the antioxidative properties of plasma; (ii) the reduction of biochemical parameters (alanine transaminase (ALT), aspartate aminotransferase (AST), and alkaline phosphatase (ALP)) and fasting blood glucose (FBG), and (iii) the reversal of histopathological changes in rat reproductive tissue (the tubular differentiation index, number of mononuclear immune cells, thickness of tunica albuginea, diameter of seminiferous tubules, Johnsen score, spermiogenesis index, Sertoli cell index, and meiotic index).

In healthy volunteers, RJ significantly reduced serum glucose levels 2 h after ingestion [170]. The same results are observed in diabetic patients [170,171]. In particular, RJ intake (3 g per day) reduced serum glucose, increased serum apolipoprotein (Apo)A-I, and modified the ApoB/ApoA-I ratio following 8 weeks of supplementation. Of note, ApoB is significantly increased in patients with type 2 diabetes. However, increases in ApoA-I are more important compared to decrease in ApoB regarding the risks for coronary heart disease in diabetic patients. Moreover, the ApoB/ApoA-I ratio is a better predictor of cardiovascular disease compared to low- and high-density lipoprotein cholesterol (LDL-C and HDL-C, respectively) [172]. Hence, it is likely that RJ contains biologically active substances with insulin-like activity. Similarly, Pourmoradian et al. [173] demonstrated that supplementation with RJ (1000 mg once a day during 8 weeks) decreases FBG and serum glycosylated hemoglobin (HbA1c) levels and increases the insulin concentration in patients with type 2 diabetes. They also observed the antioxidant effect of RJ evidenced through the significant increase in SOD and GPx activities in erythrocytes and a decrease in the MDA concentration. An increase in the total antioxidant capacity and a decrease in insulin resistance after RJ supplementation in patients with type 2 diabetes was also shown by Shidfar et al. [174]. They suggested that RJ can ameliorate insulin resistance via an antioxidant effect and may be beneficial for diabetic patients. Diabetes, as well as other pathophysiological conditions such as hypertension and atherosclerosis, is accompanied with the impairment of peripheral circulation [168,175] and organ injury (e.g., heart, kidney, and brain) due to decreased blood flow. On the other hand, it has been shown that 10H2DA from RJ exerts vasodilatory activity, and consequently, antihypertensive effects in an in vitro assay. Moreover, RJ exerted transient vasodilating effects on canine femoral arteries, which may be relevant for the treatment of diabetic foot ulcers. However, clinical trials did not show thensuperiority of 5% topical RJ compared to the placebo for the treatment of diabetic foot ulcers [175]. Contrary to Siavash et al. [175], Yakoot et al. [176] showed that the new patented topical ointment PEDYPHAR®, composed of natural RJ and panthenol, in an innovative, enriched alkaline base, is an effective and safe cream for the treatment of diabetic foot infections. Some of the possible mechanisms of positive actions of RJ and its components are: (i) the powerful antibacterial activity of royalisin against Gram + bacteria including methicillin-resistant *Staphylococcus aureus* at very low concentrations; (ii) the strong antimicrobial, neurogenic, and angiogenic activities of 10-HDA; (iii) the effect of RJ on the differentiation of all types of nerve cells (neurons, astrocytes, and dendrocytes) and an increase in mRNA expression of the potent glial cell line-derived neurotrophic factor; (iv) the stimulation of neurogenesis with the active compound of RJ, AMP N1-oxide, by stem cells through the activation of the signal transducer and activator of transcription 3; (v) the production of type I collagen and bone formation through action on osteoblasts; and (vi) the expression of the vascular endothelial growth factor gene. Panthenol, on other hand, enhanced the oxidative phosphorylation of pyruvate and fatty acid carnitine esters and increased the activity of carnitine palmitoyltransferase. Nevertheless, RJ promoted wound healing in an animal model of diabetes. In addition, it has been shown that RJ induces vasorelaxation by increasing NO production [177]. In particular, it was found that some RJ components act as muscarinic receptor agonist(s), most likely ACh, and induce vasorelaxation by releasing NO from the vascular endothelium of healthy rats. The authors concluded that the vasodilatory ability of RJ may increase the blood mass and blood flow, without affecting systemic circulation. This further implies that RJ may be used to improve the peripheral circulation in healthy individuals, but further studies are needed to clarify the effects (if any) of RJ on the peripheral circulation in patients with severe endothelial dysfunction, such as hypertension and atherosclerosis.

5.5. Positive Effect of RJ on Overweight and Obesity

Obesity is one of the major health problem worldwide. Moreover, it is associated with increased cardiovascular risk factors such as dyslipidemia, glucose intolerance, and hypertension [178]. A social context that encourages a sedentary lifestyle, easy, 24 h availability to high-energy food, and large portion sizes, are all components of the obesogenic environment, which is a contributing factor to obesity [179].

According to Vajdi et al. [180] supplementation with RJ reduces body weight (BW) and the body mass index (BMI) at the dosages <3000 mg/day. On the other hand, as mentioned previously, numerous data show that dietary supplementation with RJ improves oxidative stress, inflammation, lipid metabolism, and insulin sensitivity [167–169], suggesting its potential use in the prevention of obesity-related metabolic disorders.

In the study of Yoneshiro et al. [181], C57BL/6J mice were fed with four different regimes for 17 weeks: a normal diet (ND), high-fat diet (HFD), HFD with 5% RJ, and HFD with 5% honey bee larva powder (BL). In contrast to BL, RJ ameliorated HFD-induced obesity, hyperglycemia, and hyperinsulinemia, as well as hepatic steatosis by stimulating thermogenesis in brown adipose tissue (BAT). In particular, RJ reduced fat accumulation in white adipose tissue (WAT), increased the thermogenic capacity of BAT, and normalized glucose levels regardless of energy intake and physical activity. The increase in the BAT thermogenic capacity was accompanied with the increased gene and protein expression of mitochondrial uncoupling protein 1 (UCP1) and COX-IV, and increased mitochondrial biogenesis. Hence, RJ may be a novel promising food ingredient to combat obesity and metabolic disorders because it exerts its effects on fat accumulation and hepatic triglycerides without modifying food intake. The authors hypothesized that the activation of the transient receptor potential (TRP) channels' sympathetic nervous system (SNS)-BAT axis by hydroxydecenoic acid (HDEA) and hydroxydecanoic acid (HDAA) could be the mechanism by which RJ reduces the accumulation of body fat and restores glucose homeostasis. In vitro, HDEA and HDAA stimulate cold-sensitive TRP channels [182]. Based on the mechanism of action of capsinoids that activate TRP channels on sensory neurons in the gastrointestinal tract, enhancing the firing of sympathetic nerves connecting to BAT and thereby increasing thermogenesis [182], the authors speculated that the effects of 10-hydroxy-Trans- 2-decenoic acid (10-HDAE) and 10-HDAA are mediated via TRP channels. BL, which does not contain HDEA or HDAA, had no apparent effect on HFD-induced changes in body weight, blood glucose, and insulin, suggesting that the effects of RJ on BAT thermogenesis were indeed mediated by 10-HDAE and 10-HDAA. Similar results were obtained in obese rats. RJ reduced adiposity, promoted the browning of WAT, and activated BAT thermogenesis by upregulating UCP-1. The expression of the PR domain containing 16 (PRDM16), a modulator of BAT development, was also increased, as well as the expression of p38, bone morphogenetic protein 8B (BMP8B), and CREB1, which are also important for WAT remodeling and BAT activation. The benefits of RJ might be attributed to an increased oxygen metabolism, cellular respiration, and oxidative phosphorylation. In addition, 10-HDA from RJ stimulated thermogenesis and energy expenditure by activating TRPA1 (transient receptor potential Ankyrin 1) and TRPV1 (vanilloid1) channels [180].

In obese/diabetic KK-Ay mice, the effect of RJ supplementation on the enhanced lipolysis and reduced body weight was associated with the increased expression of peroxisome proliferator-activated-alpha (PPAR-α). RJ supplementation in mice on a high-fat diet also reduced inflammation, increased levels of irisin, a myokine whose levels are increased in obese individuals, and promoted the metabolic thermogenesis of BAT [180,181,183–186].

The hypocholesterolemic efficacy of RJ is yet another important factor when considering its potential use for overweight and obesity. The cholesterol-lowering effects of RJ are mainly attributed to its proteins, particularly MRJP1 and MRJP2. MRJP1 binds bile acids and increases cholesterol excretion by lowering the solubility of cholesterol in the jejunum [187]. Furthermore, MRJP may interfere with the reabsorption of bile acid in the ileum, which could ultimately increase the excretion of fecal steroids. Moreover, RJ increased leptin levels in obese adults. Leptin is a hormone that inhibits hunger and regulates energy balance.

Petelin and co-authors [188] have summarized the most significant positive effects of RJ in overweight adults: RJ decreases the levels of cholesterol and C-reactive protein, the inflammatory marker, and increases the levels of adiponectin, an anti-inflammatory marker. Furthermore, RH strengthens the total antioxidant capacity of the serum and increases the levels of bilirubin, an endogenous antioxidant bilirubin, and the levels of leptin, which acts as a satiety signal [188]. In addition, 10-HDA inhibits adipogenesis through the downregulation of key adipogenic transcription factors such as PPARγ, FABP4, CEBPα, SREBP-1c, and Leptin. According to Pandeya and co-authors [189], RJ may be a potential drug in the treatment of obesity, given that the anti-adipogenic effect of 10-HDA on 3 T3-L1 adipocytes occurs via two mechanisms: the inhibition of the cAMP/PKA pathway and the inhibition of p-Akt- and MAPK-dependent insulin signaling pathways.

5.6. Effectiveness of RJ in Reducing Blood Pressure and Protection of Vascular System and Heart

Hypertension is one of the strongest risk factors for cardiovascular diseases in the elderly population and a major risk factor for global disease burden. It may cause the infarction of the myocardium, heart failure, and stroke. There is also a link between hypertension and obesity, dyslipidemia, and insulin resistance, i.e., the metabolic syndrome.

The antihypertensive properties of RJ have been investigated by Tahir et al. [190]. They reported the effects of *trans*-2-octenoic acid and 10-HDA in the control of blood pressure. However, the hypotensive effect of unsaturated fatty acids could be questionable in vivo due to the instability of these acids in the digestive system. Matsui et al. [191] have studied the physiological functions of RJ in spontaneously hypertensive rats. Some peptides from RJ, obtained by enzymatic hydrolysis in the digestive system, act as angiotensin I-converting enzyme (ACE) inhibitors. In general, blood pressure is regulated by the renin-angiotensin system which has an important physiological role in the circulatory system and/or local organs. ACE inhibitor peptides, e.g., IY, VY, and IVY, obtained from protease-treated RJ, are resistant to stomach and bowel proteases. These peptides can control the excretion of other active compounds regulating blood pressure, such as NO, endothelin, or prostaglandins. The antihypertensive effect of RJ peptides has been demonstrated by Tokunaga et al. [192] in spontaneously hypertensive rats, indicating that RJ can be appreciated as a functional food for regulating blood pressure in people with hypertension. Moreover, the intake of RJ hydrolysates reduces a high cholesterol level and increases hemoglobin values in humans, thus having a positive effect on organism homeostasis [187,193–197]. Kashima et al. have identified MRJP1, MRJP2, and MRJP3 as bile acid-binding proteins from RJ [187]. Moreover, the positive effect of MRP1 on hypercholesterolemia was accompanied with the inhibition of corticosterone synthesis. The cholesterol-lowering effect of MRJP1 was due to its ability to interact with bile acids and increase their excretion. MRJP1 also showed a tendency of increasing fecal cholesterol excretion. In addition, it stimulated the hepatic cholesterol catabolism. Interestingly, MRJP1 exhibited better hypocholesterolemic activity than β-sitosterol in rats. Moreover, MRP1 reduced the absorption of cholesterol in Caco-2 cells which are used as a model of intestinal absorption in humans. Hence, it has been suggested that MRJP1 decreases the cholesterol micellar solubility. By suppressing the cholesterol micellar solubility, and due its high bile acid-binding capacity, it is likely that MRJP1 inhibits cholesterol absorption in the jejunum and the reabsorption of bile acids in the ileum, altogether lowering the serum cholesterol level. Pan et al. [197] have shown that RJ may cause hypotension and vasodilation by increasing NO production. They investigated the mechanisms underlying the hypotension and vasorelaxation effects of RJ in spontaneously hypertensive rats (SHR) and the isolated rabbit thoracic aorta rings model. In their study, RJ reduced systolic and diastolic blood pressure with little effect on the heart rate, and increased NO levels. Furthermore, RJ contains muscarinic receptor agonists, likely Ach or Ach-like substances, and induces vasorelaxation by activating the NO/cGMP pathway and calcium channels. Hence, the authors concluded that the oral administration of RJ reduces blood pressure due to the RJ-induced effect of NO on arterial vasodilation. Accordingly, L-NAME (nonselective eNOS inhibitor) and indomethacin (nonspecific COX inhibitor) attenuated this vasodilatory effect, further indicating that some components of RJ act on the muscarinic receptor of vascular endothelial cells and stimulate the release of NO and prostacyclin (PGI2) which act as vasodilators by increasing the cGMP levels. Of note, it has been estimated that RJ contains around 1000 μg/g of ACh [177]. The lack of effect of RJ on the heart rate was explained by two opposite mechanisms that act. While ACh slows down the heart rate, acting on the cardiac muscarinic receptor too, adrenaline speeds up the heart rate via the cardiac beta1 receptor. In addition to ACh-like components, other components from RJ may have effects on blood pressure, including 10-HDA, 10-HDAA, sebacic acid, MRPJPs such as MJP1, and ACE-inhibiting peptides [197].

The cholesterol-lowering effect of RJ has already been mentioned. High blood cholesterol is a risk factor for heart and vascular diseases. These include atherosclerosis, high blood pressure, and other vascular diseases, as well as heart attacks, angina pectoris, and other heart diseases. It also increases the risk of stroke and diabetes. Therefore, it is of great importance that RJ reduces the cholesterol levels in animals and atherosclerosis in humans [193–195]. Furthermore, it regulated the lipid metabolism in rats and prevented atherosclerosis in rabbits fed with cholesterol-rich food [197]. More importantly, the oral use or injection of RJ reduced serum lipids and cholesterol in arteriosclerotic patients with moderately high cholesterol levels. Vittek [195] reported the effect of RJ on the reduction of total lipids (around 10%) in serum and the liver, but also on the lowering of the cholesterol level (for 14%). RJ was used at a dose of 5–100 mg daily during at least 2 to 3 months.

The main lipids in plasma are cholesterol, triglycerides, and phospholipids. Lipoproteins, the macromolecular particles made of lipids and proteins, transport cholesterol and tryglicerides through the body. Low-Density Lipoproteins (LDLs) are the main carriers of cholesterol. Therefore, a high level of cholesterol in serum is usually related to abnormally high levels of LDL cholesterol. High LDLs can result from their overproduction or due to the inadequate removal of Very-Low-Density Lipoproteins (VLDLs), an LDL precursor in the hepatic route. Whereas LDLs contain more cholesterol, VLDLs have a higher percentage of triglycerides. There are several categories of VLDLs depending on their size [198]. In plasma, large VLDL particles are eliminated or catabolized to small VLDLs through the lipolysis of triglycerides by lipoprotein lipases attached to the endothelia. Therefore, the VLDL metabolism is one of the regulatory factors of the LDL cholesterol concentration in the blood. Furthermore, VLDLs increase LDLs which have atherogenic properties. Guo et al. [194] have shown that the intake of RJ decreases the total levels of cholesterol and LDLs by decreasing the levels of small VLDLs. Recently, it was suggested that small VLDLs are a powerful independent predictor of atherosclerosis progression and more directly involved in progression than LDLs, which are usually considered the main atherogenic lipoproteins. In addition to the previously explained mechanism of the hypocholesterolemic effect of MRJP1 through the interactions with bile acids and increased excretion of fecal bile acids and fecal cholesterol [197], RJ and MRJPs exert a cholesterol-lowering effect by affecting the cholesterol catabolism in the liver. Moreover, MRJPs may induce the gene expression of the low-density lipoprotein receptor (LDLR) and decrease the expression of the genes involved in cholesterol biosynthesis, such as squalene epoxidase and the sterol regulatory element-binding protein [199–201]. RJ proteins including royalisin and degradation products of MRJP1/MRJP3 may have therapeutic beneficial effects on atherosclerosis owing to the reduction of plaque inflammation. These proteins can bind to LDLs and Ox-LDLs and inhibit macrophage proliferation regardless of the presence or absence of LDLs and Ox-LDLs in vitro. According to Sato et al. [199], royalisin and the degradation products of MRJP1 and MRJP3 were bound with an approximately six-times higher affinity to LDLs than to Ox-LDLs, and the authors suggest that further research on RJ proteins may lead to the discovery of new anti-atherosclerotic drugs. It has been shown that RJ can induce the upregulation of cholesterol 7-α-hydroxylase (CYP7A1), a key enzyme for hepatic cholesterol degradation. Therefore, the regulation of CYP7A1 gene expression could be an important strategy against hypercholesterolemia and atherosclerosis.

The daily intake of RJ may help to normalize HDL-C, LDL-C, and total cholesterol (TC). In healthy volunteers, an intake of RJ (6 g/day during 4 weeks) decreased LDL-C and TC without affecting HDL-C and TG levels. In another study, Lambrinoudaki et al. [202] analyzed cardiovascular risk markers in postmenopausal women after three months of RJ administration (150 mg daily). They observed prominent changes in lipid parameters. HDL-C values were increased, whereas levels of LDL-C and total cholesterol (TC) were reduced. According to recently performed meta-analyses related to studies with a long-term follow-up, RJ reduces TC and LDL-C levels, but does not improve TG and

LDL-C values. The cholesterol-lowering effect of RJ could be mediated by its estrogenic activity. The estrogenic action of RJ and 10-HDA have been shown in cultured cells and in rats [28,203]. On the other hand, it is well known that estrogen and estrogen modulators may reduce serum cholesterol levels in rats [28,127,203,204] However, purified MRJP1 also showed a hypocholerostemic effect which was, therefore, independent of the estrogenic effect of 10-HDA [187]. Altogether, these findings indicate the possibility of using RJ as an anti-atherogenic functional food.

5.7. Estrogen Effect of Royal Jelly

Mishima et al. [28] have shown the weak estrogenic effect of RJ. In MCF-7 breast cancer cells with estrogen receptors, RJ increased the proliferation rate. The effect was counteracted with tamoxifen, a chemotherapy drug that acts as an antagonist of the estrogen receptor. Furthermore, the subcutaneous injection of RJ restored the expression of the gene for the vascular endothelial growth factor (VEGF) in ovariectomized mice. Estrogen has an essential role in the bone metabolism, particularly in women. Accordingly, a lack of estrogen is the main factor of bone loss and the development of osteoporosis in postmenopausal women, whereas the dietary intake of phytoestrogens has been suggested as an option in the prevention of osteoporosis [127,204,205]. For example, in osteoblastic MC3T3-E1 cells, the soy isoflavones, genistein and daidzein, increased mineralization, likely through their estrogenic properties [205]. RJ stimulated the proliferation of the same cells, as well as the production of type I collagen. The long-term oral intake of RJ also increased the ash content of the tibiae in female mice, indicating that it may stimulate bone formation by acting on osteoblasts. Besides increasing the tibial weight, RJ also induced the expression of genes participating in the formation of the extracellular matrix. The same effects have been observed in a rat model, suggesting that RJ may be used as a dietary supplement in osteoporosis prevention [87,206].

The daily use of RJ improved ovarian hormone secretion, follicle development, and oocyte maturation, ameliorated the redox status in the oocytes, and activated the glucose pathway in cumulus cells, leading to the improvement of the fertility parameters, at least in rats. In ovariectomized rats, it has been shown that RJ competes with E2 for binding to ERα and ERβ, but with a weaker affinity compared to phytoestrogens. However, despite their weak affinity, RJ may restore VEGF expression.

According to Suzuki et al. [207], some lipid components from RJ (10-HDA, 10-HDAA, 10-HDAE, and 24-methylenecholesterol) inhibited the binding of 17β estradiol to ERβ, but were without the effect of binding to ERα. Husein and Kridli [208] as well as Huseini and Haddad [209] have confirmed the effect of RJ on the reproductive potential in sheep. RJ combined with progesterone can increase the reproductive potential in sheep. Ovulation was advanced, and follicular growth and estradiol secretion were increased. Similar data were obtained in laying hens where RJ at doses of 100 or 200 mg/kg body weight attenuated the negative effects of senescence, improved the morphology of the reproductive tract, stimulated follicular growth and the rate of egg production, and improved the internal egg quality parameters in elderly laying hens [210].

In addition, RJ has an important role in the regulation of the hormonal balance. It increases the production of testosterone and estrogen. 10-HDA in particular may improve the hormonal balance by enhancing the production of the ovulation hormones and by preserving the follicular pool [211].

Luteinizing hormone (LH) and follicle-stimulating hormone (FSH) are gonadal hormones important for reproduction and aging. They are regulated by estrogen and inhibin. In young women, high estrogen levels maintain an increased level of FSH and a decreased level of LH [121,211]. In menopause, the reduction in the follicle size results in abnormal FSH secretion. RJ in the diet may improve these changes as the presence of 10-HDA increases estrogen production and maintains low levels of FSH and LH in the serum. As mentioned previously, 10-HDA also prevents follicular depletion and improves hormonal regulation [211]. RJ (1 g/kg) can reduce premenstrual symptoms and improve quality of life in the menopause and postmenopause phase by relieving genito-urinary syndromes. Furthermore, RJ can alleviate postmenopausal symptoms such as hot flushes, night sweats, and other symptoms. In addition, menopause is characterized by estrogen depletion which affects the autonomic nervous system, leading to the development of neurodegenerative diseases like Alzheimer's disease, mood disorders (e.g., anxiety, depression), headaches, and low-back pain. Through its estrogenic activity, RJ significantly reduces these symptoms without side effects.

It should be emphasized that the content of antioxidants in RJ may overcome free-radicals-induced oxidative stress in women before getting pregnant. Good nutrition before conception can reduce the risk of complications at the time of conception that could threaten the health of the offspring. Stress that occurs in women during preconception may greatly affect the health of the mother and cause menstrual disorders, polycystic ovary syndrome (PCOS), and infertility. Oxidative stress in preconceived women can be treated with non-pharmacological therapy, one of which is RJ. Up to 20% of women of reproductive age are diagnosed with PCOS. PCOS is an endocrine disorder characterized by high androgens and ovulatory dysfunction, which consequently leads to infertility and mental illness such as anxiety and depression. Hamid et al. [212] investigated the effect of RJ, applied at doses of 100 mg/kg, 200 mg/kg, and 400 mg/kg over a period of 4 weeks, on the hormonal profile of PCOS animal models. The most effective dose of RJ was 200 mg/kg which improved the regularity of the estrus cycle, histology and ovarian function, the level of reproductive hormones (LH, testosteron, FSH, and estradiol), as well as the antioxidant status of the ovaries (MDA, total antioxidant capacity (TAC), GPx). The authors suggested that royalactin is responsible for the histological changes of the ovaries. Furthermore, data showing the protective effect of RJ on the liver and kidneys through the reduction of lipid peroxidation and increased the GSH content, as well as the presence of 10-HDA which has an anti-inflammatory effect, indicating the potential of RJ in reducing oxidative stress. In addition, the positive effect of RJ could be due to its effect on the accelerated growth and development of follicles that secrete estradiol to stimulate the uterus, increasing the level of LH and triggering ovulation [213]. MRJP1 from RJ, through its hypocholesterolemic activity, may reduce the synthesis of corticosterone, which further may affect the energy regulation, immune reactions, and stress response. Moreover, MRJPs increase the estrogenic activity and antioxidant potential of the reproductive system, upregulate the gene expression of the estrogen receptor beta (ER beta), and stimulate hormone secretion and ovary development in female mice [214].

5.8. *Effect of Royal Jelly on Spematogenesis*

RJ improves fertility in both men and women. In men, it increases the quality of the sperm, whereas in women, it increases the quality of the ovules. Previous studies have shown that RJ increases the levels of male hormones, improves the sperm count, motility and morphology, and reduces the damage of the reproductive tract induced by various toxic stimuli. Shahzad et al. [215] showed that RJ (0.1–0.3%) protects spermatozoa during freezing and increases their mobility. The increased motility of sperm after freezing may be due to the high antioxidant capacity of RJ, as well as the presence of active biological amino acids such as aspartic acid, cysteine, glycine, cysteine, tyrosine, leucine, lysine, isoleucine, and valine. Thus, it is hypothesized that proline may protect cell membranes from stressful conditions, while cysteine, a powerful antioxidant, may neutralize free radicals and participate in glutathione synthesis during the freezing period [215]. RJ showed potent antioxidant activity against Cd-induced oxidative damage in the testicular tissue. Cd-induced testicular dysfunction was accompanied with increased LPO and nitrate/nitrite levels and the reduced activity of cellular antioxidant and detoxifying molecules, including GSH, GPx, glutathione reductase, SOD, CAT, and Nrf2. Moreover, RJ supplementation downregulated the gene expression of the cytochrome P450 4A14 (CYP4A14) which stimulates the production of intracellular free radicals and catalyzes lipid peroxidation. The antioxidative effect of RJ observed in Cd-induced oxidative stress was likely mediated through the upregulation of Nrf2. Nrf2 provides protection against ROS via different mechanisms, including the increase in GSH synthesis, the upregulation of antioxidant and detoxifying enzymes, and the degradation of superoxide and peroxide radicals by GPx and SOD. In another study performed in male rabbits, RJ applied at a dose of 150 mg/kg body weight showed positive effects on libido, glucose, blood testosterone, plasma total proteins, fertility, and sperm production and quality [216]. The protective effect of RJ on hormonal parameters has also been observed in aluminum chloride (AlCl3)-induced toxicity. RJ attenuated the AlCl3-induced changes of gonadotropin levels (FSH, LH) and testosterone, as well as levels of the thyroid-stimulating hormone (TSH), thyroxine (T4), triiodothyronine (T3), and the T3/T4 ratio [217]. AlCl3 also resulted in oligospermia, hypoplasia, constriction of the blood vessels, and exfoliation of tubules. These changes were similarly attenuated by RJ. Finally, RJ was beneficial in adult rats that received hydrogen peroxide (oxidative stress inducer). RJ improved the number of spermatozoa, percentage of live spermatozoa, testosterone level, and levels of glutathione and malondialdehyde [218, 219]. RJ treatment at a dose of 100 mg/kg/day for 4 weeks protected the testicular structure from the damaging effect of diabetic oxidative stress through its antioxidant effect, thus preserving male fertility [218].

5.9. *Royal Jelly and Osteoporosis*

A few studies have investigated the effects of RJ on the bone metabolism and related cellular functions. Bone loss has become a major problem in postmenopausal women with significant morbidity and mortality. In both postmenopausal women and ovariectomized rats, bone loss is a result of an ovarian hormone deficiency. The study of Kafadar et al. [220] has shown that RJ and bee pollen reduce osteoporotic bone loss in an oophorectomized rat model. The total body bone mineral density (BMD) was similar in all groups, whereas BMD of the lumbar spine and proximal femur were higher in animals that received RJ or bee pollen. The calcium and phosphate levels in bone tissue were also higher in RJ and bee pollen groups, suggesting that both RJ and bee pollen could be beneficial in clinical practice. Hatori et al. obtained similar results [221]. They studied the effects of royal jelly protein (RJP) on the bone mineral density and strength in ovariectomized Sprague–Dawley rats that received RJ for 8 weeks. RJP reduced the BMD decrease in the lumber spine and proximal tibia and improved bone strength. These findings indicate that RJP is an option for suppressing trabecular bone loss in ovariectomized rats and that RJP may prevent bone abnormalities induced by a sex hormone deficiency. Tsuchiya et al. [206] demonstrated that 10-HDA, a key RJ constituent, protects against bone loss by suppressing osteoclastogenesis. In particular, the binding of 10-HDA to free fatty acid receptor 4 (FFAR4) inhibited the activation of the NF-κB pathway in osteoclasts (see Figure 4). This further inhibited the induction of the nuclear factor of activated T cells c1 (NFATc1), a key transcription factor for osteoclast differentiation [206]. The authors suggested that 10-HDA inhibits osteoclast differentiation and function by suppressing the NF-κB signaling pathway and its downstream molecules including NFATc1, CtsK, TRAP, V-ATPase D2, and MMP-9 through the FFAR4. Considering that FFAR4 is implicated in various pathological and physiological processes, including inflammation, the secretion of glucagon-like peptide-1, adipocyte differentiation, insulin sensitization, the regulation of appetite, and tumor progression, FFAR4 represents a promising target not only for osteoporosis, but also for the treatment of obesity-related metabolic disorders, such as cancer. It was also shown that RJ reduces ovariectomy-induced bone loss by suppressing osteoclastogenesis through the inhibition of RANKL (receptor activator of nuclear factor-kB (NF-κB) ligand)-induced osteoclastogenesis [206]. On the contrary, Shimizu, et al. [222] suggested that the main effect of RJ is not the prevention of bone loss, but the improvement of bone strength.

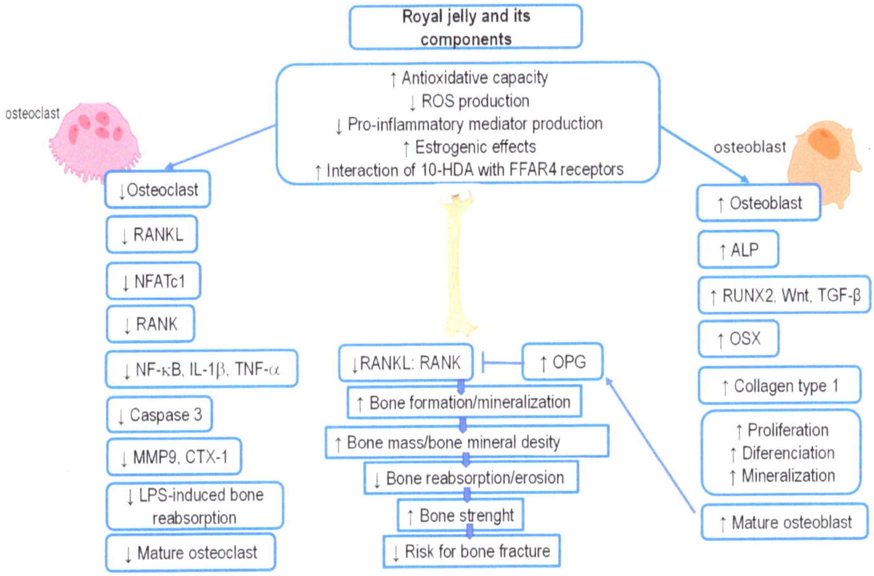

Figure 4. The effects of royal jelly (RJ) and its components on bone mineral density and strength. The key mechanisms of RJ action are based on increasing the antioxidant capacity, reducing oxidative stress, and regulating the production of inflammatory mediators, estrogenic activity, and interaction of 10-HDA with FFAR4 receptor. RJ and its components, such as 10-HDA, have an inhibitory effect on osteoclast differentiation and function by suppressing the NF-κB signaling pathway and its downstream molecules including NFATc1, CtsK, TRAP, V-ATPase D2, and MMP9, via FFAR4. Moreover, the inhibitory effect of RJ on ROS reduces RANKL, TRAP, NF-B, and caspase-3 activities in osteoclasts. RJ upregulates Runx2, Wnt, TGF-β, Osterix, Osteocalcin, and ALP by inhibiting accumulation of ROS. This contributes to the increased bone formation/mineralization and decreased bone resorption, resulting in increased bone mass, bone mineral density, and bone strength, and decreased risk of bone fractures. Note: 10-HDA, 10-hydroxy-2-decenoic acid; BMD, bone mineral density; CTX, C-terminal telopeptide; FFAR4, free fatty acid receptor 4; IL-1β, interleukin 1 beta; LPS, lpopolysaccharide; RANK, receptor activator of nuclear factor-κB; RANKL, receptor activator of NF-kB ligand; RUNX2, runt-related transcription factor 2; NFAT c1, nuclear factor of activated T cell; MMP-9, matrix metalloproteinase 9; NF-κB, nuclear factor-kappa B; OPG, osteoprotegerin; Osx, Osterix, transcription factor; TGF-β, transforming growth factor;TNF-α, tumor necrosis factor alpha. ↑ upregulated; ↓ downregulated.

Moreover, the weak estrogen-like activity of RJ has been shown in cultured osteoblasts [38,86]. As post-menopausal osteoporosis is mainly caused by the reduced production of estrogen, it is likely that the estrogen-like activity of RJ may help in alleviating post-menopausal osteoporosis [121,223–225]. Since RJ also contains the testosterone, it may also be effective in men's osteoporosis induced by a lack of androgen. Besides estrogen-like activity, RJ stimulates the migration of dermal fibroblasts, increases the production of collagen [29,66], and improves muscle mass, strength, and function. The underlying mechanisms behind the effects on skeletal muscles likely include anti-inflammatory and anti-oxidative properties, improved metabolic regulation, the activation of muscle stem cells, increased blood supply, the suppressed expression of catabolic genes, and the stimulation of peripheral neuronal regeneration [52,58,103,108,147]. Therefore, natural products that do not show significant side effects, such as RJ, can be used as an alternative or adjuvant therapy for the treatment of osteoporosis. Due to its estrogen-like effect, RJ may also decrease the risk of osteoporotic fractures.

5.10. Anticancer Effectiveness of Royal Jelly and Hematopoiesis Stimulation

The anticancer effect of RJ has been investigated in various models, such as $6C_3HED$ lymphosarcoma, TA_3 mammary carcinoma, Ehrlich ascites carcinoma, leukemia in AKR mice, sarcoma 180, Solid Ehrlich carcinoma, lymphatic L1210, and P388 leukemia [226–229]. The effect of RJ was observed in slow-growing tumors but not in fast-growing ones. The anticancer activity was attributed to 10-HDA and saturated dicarboxylic acids (succinic, glutaric, adipic, pimelic, suberic, azelaic, and sebacic acid). Oršolić et al. [228,229] have shown that RJ reduces the number of tumor nodules only if administered together with tumor cells. Furthermore, they showed that RJ has significant immunostimulatory properties [230]. Similarly, Kimura [231] demonstrated the inhibitory effect of RJ (at doses of 300 or 600 mg/kg) on tumor growth and/or metastasis in the liver or lungs. Although the antitumor activity of RJ has been confirmed in many studies, its antimetastatic effect may depend on the method of administration, and consequently, on the close contact of RJ, especially 10-HDA, with tumor cells. Thus, in contrast to intravenous administration, the intraperitoneal or subcutaneous application of RJ had no effect on the formation of lung metastases [228]. In particular, RJ inhibited tumor-induced angiogenesis and/or stimulated the immune response by enhancing the production of T lymphocytes involved in the elimination of viruses and tumor cells [232]. In B16F1 melanoma cells, the antiproliferative effect of RJ was achieved through the inhibition of microphthalmia-associated transcription factor and tyrosinase-related protein 1 (TRP-1) and TRP-2, which ultimately suppresses melanin production [233]. Accordingly, RJ reduced skin pigmentation in mice which further indicates its potential for the production of skin care products [233]. In another study, a derivative of 10-HDA, 4-hydroperoxy-2-decenoic acid ethyl ester (HPO-DAEE), induced the apoptosis of A549 human lung cancer cells by activating the ROS-ERK-p38 and C/EBP homologous protein (CHOP) pathways [234,235]. Hence, the pro-apoptotic effect of HPO-DAEE was, at least partially, dependent on signaling pathways related to endoplasmic reticulum stress [235]. Moreover, 10-HDA has been recognized as an inhibitor of MMPs. Under inflammatory conditions, these endopeptidases are activated by proteolytic cleavage. They degrade matrix and non-matrix proteins and promote angiogenesis, the infiltration of cancer cells, and metastasis. The anticancer effects of RJ have also been demonstrated on HeLa cells (cervical cancer in women), particularly for the protein fraction RJP30 that induced 50% cytotoxicity [112], as well as in Lewis lung carcinoma and colorectal adenocarcinoma cells [231,236] where the effect was attributed to 10-HDA. The efficacy of 10-HDA was also reported in transplantable leukemia in AKR mice and various ascitic tumor cell lines in mice. As mentioned in previous sections, 10-HDA acts as a potent HDAC inhibitor and suppresses proliferation by inhibiting PI3K/Akt signaling [47,88]. The lipophilic extract of RJ demonstrated the antiproliferative effects in human neuroblastoma cells (SH-SY5Y) and human glioblastoma (U373) [237,238]. Treatment with a high dose of RJ significantly increased the apoptotic cell population of both SH-SY5Y-human neuroblastoma and U373-human glioblastoma and arrested the cell cycle at the G0–G1 phase in SH-SY5Y cells and at G2–M in U373 cells. Furthermore, 10-HDA and 4HPO-DAEE inhibited the proliferation of leukemia cells THP-1 by inhibiting HDAC activity. In general, HDAC inhibitors are strong anti-inflammatory drugs [68,239]. Accordingly, in human colon cancer cells (WiDr cells), the production of pro-inflammatory cytokines IL-8, IL-1β, and TNF-α was modulated by 10-HDA [68]. Levels of IL-8 were largely attenuated following treatment with 3 mM 10-HDA, whereas levels of IL-1β and TNF-α were only slightly, although significantly, decreased. On the other hand, RJ increased the amount of IL-1ra. Hence, it seems that RJ may be effective in controlling chronic inflammation and carcinogenesis due to its ability to inhibit NF-κB and the production of TNF-α, IL-1β, and IL-8. In addition, in J5 cells (human hepatocellular carcinoma), RJ interfered with the activation of arylamine carcinogens. RJ inhibited the N-acetylation of 2-aminofluorene (2-AF), i.e., it inhibited the activity of N-acetyltransferases and the generation of 2-AF metabolites [240]. Of note, it has been shown that N-acetyltransferases are involved in chemical carcinogenesis as higher N-acetyltransferase activity increases sensitivity to the mutagenic effects of arylamines.

Taken together, the pharmacological effects of 10-HDA are mainly mediated through the anti-tumor activity, inhibition of angiogenesis, and immunomodulatory properties.

A study by Abu-Serie and Habashy [241] revealed the potent anticancer effect of MRJP2 and its isoform X1. These proteins induced caspase-dependent apoptosis, the reduced expression of Ki-67, a marker for proliferation, and the regulated expression of Bcl-2 and p53 in HepG2 cells. In fact, MRJP2 increased the number of early and late apoptotic cells more than doxorubicin. Therefore, the authors suggested that MRJP2 and X1 can be a promising strategy against hepatic cancer [241].

The effects of RJ have also been studied in Ehrlich solid and ascites tumors (EST and EAT) [242,243]. Albalawi et al. showed that the treatment of EST-suffering mice with RJ at the doses of 200 and 400 mg/kg causes a significant reduction in the tumor volume and inhibition rate, body weight, tumor markers such as the serum level of alpha-fetoprotein (AFP), and carcinoembryonic antigen tumors (CAE). In addition to tumor markers (AFP and CAE), a decrease in the serum level of the liver and kidneys, LPO and NO, TNF-α level, as well as the expression level of Bcl-2 was observed in the RJ-treated group compared to the control EST group. The level of antioxidant enzymes of GPx, CAT, and SOD and the expression level of caspase-3 and Bax genes was significantly increased in RJ-treated groups.

Cells of EAT grow fast in most mice strains and disturb various hematopoietic and immune parameters, causing the host's death even in the presence of a small number of cancer cells. EAT reduces the number of granulocyte–macrophage colonies in the spleen and the induction of natural suppressor cells. Phagocytes, especially macrophages and neutrophils, play an important role in host defense against tumor growth. One of the main characteristics of these cells is their ability to migrate inside the inflamed area. Animal model studies have shown that tumor cells can produce factors that impair the inflammatory response, promoting tumor growth. More precisely, tumor cells can stimulate the suppressor activity of the host macrophages. Macrophages have a dual role in cancer, which is a result of their plasticity in response to environmental conditions. Macrophages can kill tumor cells, mediate cellular cytotoxicity and antibody-dependent phagocytosis, induce vascular damage and tumor necrosis, and activate innate or adaptive tumor resistance mechanisms mediated by lymphoid cells. In contrast, tumor cells can evade macrophage cytotoxicity and redirect macrophage activities to contribute to cancer progression and metastasis. Besides the inappropriate accumulation of phagocytes in the inflamed areas, other cellular functions are also disturbed in tumor carriers, including the reaction of granulocyte–macrophage colonies on the colony activation factor. In that regard, treatment with RJ (at doses 0.5, 1, and 1.5 g/kg) did not increase the number of bone marrow cells and granulocyte–macrophage colonies in the spleen of the healthy mice, whereas in EAT-bearing mice, the number of bone marrow cells and number of cells in peripheral circulation were increased. The increased number of long-living stem cells, as well as the number of granulocyte macrophage colonies, have been observed in cell cultures treated with RJ. Thus, RJ may enhance the host resistance against tumors through stimulating macrophage function, antibody production, and immunocompetent cell proliferation. RJ pre-treatment to EAT-bearing mice also increased the phagocytic function of macrophages, the activity of T cells, and the activity of B cells. Furthermore, RJ pretreatment effectively decreased the proliferation of EAT cells in the peritoneal fluid and decreased the viability of EAT cells in vitro. The size of the solid Ehrlich tumor in the thigh muscle of the mice was also significantly reduced [226].

It has been shown that RJ promotes macrophage recovery, their number, and activity. Accordingly, the improved recovery of hematological parameters in EAT-bearing mice was reflected in prolonged survival. In general, tumor associated macrophages (TAM) stimulate tumor growth and inhibit the activity of NK cells and T lymphocytes [36,37,243]. This indicates that certain RJ components prevent the tumor-induced suppression of macrophages and stimulate their immunomodulatory activity, consequently increasing the control of tumor growth and spread. RJ has the ability to protect against macrophages immunosuppression caused by tumor secreting substances. RJ inhibited the increase in prostaglandin (PGE_2) by 30%, which inhibited the tumoricidal activity of macrophages. PGE_2 alters the immunological response including the mitogenesis of T lymphocytes, cytokine production, and tumor cytotoxicity mediated by macrophages and NK cells. Furthermore, RJ can inhibit the production of anti-inflammatory cytokines, such as TNF-α, IL-6, and IL-1, without reducing the cytotoxic effect of macrophages stimulated with LPS and/or LPS + IFN-γ [36]. Bincoletto et al. [243] argued that the RJ-induced reduction of PGE_2 in EAT-bearing mice is the main reason for their survival. RJ is capable of modifying the biological response, reducing myelosuppression, and increasing the antitumor effect. The results of our studies on rats confirm those claims [227–230]. In LPS + IFN-γ-stimulated macrophages, RJ (2.5 mg/mL) reduced PGE_2 synthesis by 63% in comparison to control macrophages [36]. These results also indicate the possibility of the effective use of RJ as a food supplement for increasing quality of life in patients with autoimmune diseases such as rheumatoid arthritis and inflammatory bowel diseases. The inhibition of PGE2 is important as PGE2 is involved in the process of carcinogenesis. PGE2 promotes the proliferation and invasion of tumor cells and inhibits the apoptotic process in various types of cancers [244,245]. In addition, it regulates the proliferation of lymphocytes and suppresses the tumoricidal activity of normal macrophages. On the contrary, RJ reverses myelosuppression in mice with EAT, promotes the hematopoietic function of the spleen, reduces PGE2 production, and prolongs the survival of mice. The inhibition of PGE2 synthesis reactivates the immune system response, stimulates the mitosis of T lymphocytes and lymphokine production, and increases the tumor-killing activity of macrophages and natural killer cells [229,243]. The stimulation of monocyte–macrophage cells was confirmed in the research of Wang et al. [246] who used RJ to stimulate human monocytic cells (MNC). After MNC stimulation, their filtered conditioning medium (MNC-CM) was used to treat U937 cells. Four conditioned media inhibited U937 cell growth by 25.9–50.6%. CD11b and CD14 expressions on the treated U937 cells were increased by 38.1–49.8% and 43.4–52.0%, respectively. In this way, Wang et al. [246] confirmed that RJ stimulates human mononuclear cells to secrete cytokines (IL-1β, TNF-α, and IFN-γ) and NO in MNC-CM, which inhibit the growth of U937 cells and induce their differentiation, which can be a natural and alternative pathway in the treatment of leukemia.

A 350 kDa glycoprotein (apisin) has been identified as an RJ component that stimulates the proliferation of human monocytes. The protective effect of RJ on hematopoiesis has also been observed in mice irradiated with X-rays [247–249]; RJ prevented the radiation-induced damage of stem cells. The immunostimulatory properties of RJ combined with propolis (product called "Apinhalin") have been observed in granulocytopoiesis and lymphopoiesis following irradiation with the dose of 3 Gy and/or 5 Gy. The regeneration of cells was observed after only 10 days in comparison to the control group [250]. Moreover, RJ stimulated the production of antibodies and the proliferation of immunocompetent cells [230].

RJ also inhibited the bisphenol A-induced proliferation of human breast cancer cells (MCF-7) [34]. Bisphenol A is an environmental estrogen widely used in the production of polycarbonate plastics and polyepoxide. It is an endocrine disruptor that shows a weak binding affinity for estrogen receptors. Consequently, it negatively affects human health, especially in women [251]. In MCF-7 breast cancer cells, RJ prevented the stimulatory effect of bisphenol A on cell proliferation. The authors suggested that RJ inhibited estradiol-induced intracellular signaling events, not the binding of estradiol to the estrogen receptor.

In the renal cell carcinoma (RCC) model, it was shown that 10-HDA suppresses tumor growth, invasion, and metastasis through its strong anti-inflammatory effect. 10-HDA inhibited the secretion of TNF-α which promotes the proliferation of cancer cells and their malignant transformation. More importantly, the reduced concentration of TNF-α and TGF-β following RJ intake reduced the paraneoplastic syndrome in RCC patients [252]. Thus, the anti-cancer and anti-inflammatory action of 10-HDA was mediated through the reduced production of pro-inflammatory cytokines (TNF-α, IL-1β, and IL-8). Another fatty acid from RJ, 3,10-dihydroxydecanoic acid, stimulated the maturation of monocyte-derived dendritic cells and their Th1 polarizing capability, overall increasing the anti-cancer response [253]. Furthermore, 10-HDA may reduce the tumor vascularization. In addition, it has confirmed that RJ nanoparticles can alleviate the experimental model of breast cancer through suppressing regulatory T cells and upregulating Th1 cells [254]. Furthermore, new research from Xu and co-authors confirms that RJA exerts antitumor effects by affecting the glycolytic pathway in Human hepatocellular carcinoma (HCC) through the lactate modification pathway [255].

In a 4T1 breast cancer mice model, RJ also reduced the tumor weight, particularly when applied as a prophylactic treatment. The anticancer effect was accompanied with the increased SOD activity, total antioxidant capacity (T-AOC), and glutathione reductase activity in the liver, kidneys, and serum [256].

5.11. RJ as Protective Agent against Pro-Oxidants' Toxicity and Chemo- and Radiotherapy Side Effects

Cytostatics have multiple effects on tumor cells: they prevent cell division, stop the division of already-dividing cells, induce spontaneous cell death, and reduce the growth of blood vessels that consequently decreases the delivery of food and oxygen into the tumor tissue. As cytostatics are not selective, they also act on healthy cells, causing various unwanted effects. All cytostatics cause side effects, some of which are common to all cytostatics, and others specific to individual cytostatics.

The most important unwanted consequences or side effects of chemotherapy are: bone marrow suppression (myelosuppression or myelotoxicity); weakness, nausea, and vomiting; oral mucositis (inflammation of the mucous membranes in the mouth and throat), stomatitis (inflammation of the membranes and tissues in the oral cavity and the entire mucosa of the digestive tract), and esophagitis (inflammation of the mucous membrane of the esophagus); diarrhea and dehydration; constipation; allergic reactions and anaphylaxis; hair loss; extravasation (exit of cytostatics from the blood vessel into the surrounding tissue); changes in the sense of taste; anemia due to the reduced number of erythrocytes, shortness of breath, and chronic fatigue; bleeding and bruising as a result of thrombocytopenia; phlebitis (inflammation and the formation of clots in superficial veins); increased infection risk (due to the reduced number of leukocytes); febrile neutropenia (a result of a reduced number of granulocytes); cardiac toxicity, nephrotoxicity, and bladder damage; pulmonary toxicity; neurological toxicity; gonadal dysfunction; hepatotoxicity; induction of secondary tumors; and tumor rapid disintegration (lysis) syndrome, among others [257]. The side effects can be as detrimental as the cancer itself and may greatly reduce one's quality of life. Moreover, the addition of other drugs to ameliorate the side effects of the anticancer therapy may trigger other health hazards. The polypharmacy may result in predictable and unexpected drug–drug interactions, posing the additional risk to the patient's health [258].

One of the main challenges in cancer therapy is to find effective drugs with minimal adverse effects. In that regard, natural products may minimize the unwanted side effects. They also may act synergistically with standard therapy, improve the efficacy of cytostatics, and improve the quality of life of cancer patients [252,253,257–259]. Moreover, natural products, such as RJ, are readily available, economical, and relatively safe.

Many beneficial effects of RJ in chemotherapy-induced toxicity have been reported. RJ protected lymphocytes against doxorubicin-induced genotoxicity. It improved the antioxidative response and increased the Nrf2/Bax and Bcl-2/Bax ratio [97,252,260–262]. Moreover, RJ inhibited the expression of caspase-3 and increased the expression of the anti-apoptotic protein Bcl-2 in the liver and kidneys of the cisplatin-treated rats [263,264]. On the contrary, RJ downregulated the expression of Bax in rats treated with cyclophosphamide [265]. It is likely that the anti-apoptotic effect of RJ might be assigned to its antioxidant capacity [260–266].

Previous studies have indicated that MRJPs contribute to the regulation of immune functions by stimulating macrophages and by attenuating the production of inflammatory mediators, at least in animal models [242]. Wang et al. [76] suggested that MRJPs promote immune functions in cyclophosphamide-induced mice by increasing the number of white blood cells, the production of anti-inflammatory cytokines IL-4 and IL-6, and the proliferation ability of T/B-lymphocytes in the spleen by modulating the composition of the immune-associated intestinal flora. The protective effect of RJ against cyclophosphamide-induced thrombocytopenia, as well as bone marrow, spleen, and testicular damages in rats, was confirmed by Khazaei and coauthors [267]. RJ pretreatment normalized the number of platelets, white and red blood cells, serum levels of platelet factor 4 (PF4), nitric oxide (NO) and ferric-reducing antioxidant power (FRAP), levels of serum biochemical factors, and histological structures of bone marrow, spleen, and testes [267]. Furthermore, RJ and 10-HDA reduced the weight loss in the body, thymus, and spleen of the cyclophosphamide-induced mice, improved the thymus/spleen indexes, stimulated the pathways involved in DNA/RNA/protein activities, restored the proliferative ability of cells in the thymus and spleen, and promoted the activities of the T and B lymphocytes [268]. It seems that RJ provides protection to many tissues and organs injured by chemotherapy, especially the liver and kidneys, through its antioxidant, anti-inflammatory, and anti-apoptotic activities.

Furthermore, RJ can modulate oxidative stress and apoptosis in the liver and kidneys of rats treated with cisplatin. Thus, prophylaxis with RJ significantly reduced the severity of lipid peroxidation in the liver and kidneys. It is considered that the biologically active, free amino acids such as aspartic acid, L-cysteine, cystine, tyrosine, glycine, lysine, leucine, isoleucine, and valine mediate the antioxidative effects of RJ [269]. In addition, the beneficial effect of RJ on the antioxidative status is visible through the increased GSH content and increased activities of antioxidative enzymes GPx, glutathione–S–transferase and SOD. In addition to the positive effects of RJ on chemotherapy-induced cellular damage, RJ ameliorated the damage of liver cells induced by exposure to tetrachloromethane, cadmium, and paracetamol and reduced the genotoxic and nephrotoxic effects of these chemicals [95,270,271]. ROS produced during the toxic attack of these compounds resulted in lipid peroxidation and DNA and protein oxidation. However, RJ inhibited lipid peroxidation and preserved the structure of the biological membranes, membrane potential, and permeability for various ions.

Different mechanisms of the action of RJ have been elucidated following treatment with compounds such as cyclophosphamide, bleomycin, doxorubicin, 5-fluorouracil (5-FU), thymoquinone, cisplatin, hydroxyurea, temozolomide, interferon alpha, and GE132 plus (a nutraceutical supplement) [250,251,263,265,272]. Thus, RJ reduced genotoxicity and DNA damage when used with cyclophosphamide. Following treatment with 5-FU, RJ reduced the cell viability and IC50 of 5-FU in colorectal cancer cells [273,274]. It is also capable of initiating apoptotic events in breast or liver and kidney cancer cells in animals treated with thymoquinone or cisplatin, respectively [269,275]. When combined with GE132, interferon alpha, or temozolomide, RJ increased the efficacy of these drugs, further exacerbating their anti-proliferative action [276,277]. Numerous studies have demonstrated the synergistic effect of RJ and chemotherapeutic drugs. When applied together, they increase the death of tumor cells, strengthen the protection by immune cells, and protect cells exposed to harmful drugs such as kidney and liver cells.

Radiotherapy is an important therapeutic modality in cancer therapy. The main objective of radiation treatment is to apply an effective dose of ionizing radiation to eliminate cancer cells in a well-defined cancer volume, with minimal side effects to the surrounding healthy tissue. However, the generation of free radical metabolites may lead to the injury of normal tissue, limiting the effectiveness of the therapy. RJ has shown the anti-inflammatory, DNA-protective, and anti-tumor effects in animal models. It may largely reduce the adverse effects of reactive species and limit the cellular damage induced by reactive oxygen and nitrogen species derived through radiotherapy or chemotherapy. In the adult male Sprague–Dawley rats, exposure of the whole body to irradiation induced prominent liver failure, characterized by a marked increase in serum AST, ALT, cholesterol, and triglyceride levels, and with the increased production of MDA and reduced levels of GPx, CAT and SOD in the lung and liver tissue. Pre- and post-treatment with RJ markedly decreased the oxidative stress parameters and ameliorated changes of biochemical parameters, increasing the antioxidant activities [249,278]. The authors suggested that the protective effect of RJ in irradiated animals may be due to the improved activity of endogenous antioxidants, the free radical scavenging activity of RJ, and decreased lipid peroxidation. In addition, the antioxidative, as well as the anti-inflammatory effects of RJ, may be achieved through the increased expression of Nrf2 and decreased levels of NF-κB and pro-inflammatory cytokines. The data of Sarhan et al. [279] have shown that the whole-body gamma exposure of rats by fractionated doses (5×2 Gy) resulted in hyperlipidemia and increased serum levels of TC, TG, and LDL-C, together with the significant decrease in HDL-C. The GSH content and SOD activity were decreased, as well as MDA, creatinine kinase-MB (CK-MB), and cardiac troponin I (cTnI). In addition, the histopathologic changes were observed in the heart tissue. In rats supplemented with RJ (250 mg/kg/day), these changes were reduced. Furthermore, RJ may improve the symptoms of oral mucositis and shorten the healing time [280,281]. Rafat et al. [248] also demonstrated the radioprotective effect of RJ. RJ prevented radiation-induced apoptosis in human peripheral blood leukocytes. The blood samples were taken on days 0, 4, 7, and 14 from healthy male volunteers that received a 1000 mg RJ capsule per day for 14 consecutive days. Samples were then exposed to the 4 Gy X-ray. RJ modified the radiation-induced apoptosis of peripheral blood leukocytes, likely through its antioxidant properties and free radical scavenging ability. RJ-mediated protection against the mutagenic effect of Adriamycin and gamma radiation was investigated by El-Fiky et al. [282]. The study showed that pretreatment with RJ reduces DNA fragmentation at two days after gamma radiation at a level $p < 0.01$, reaching $p < 0.001$ at days 4, 7, and 14 after exposure. However, the effects of RJ were not significant in the combined treatment (Adriamycin plus gamma radiation), except for the total number of structural aberrations at day 2 (changes were decreased at $p < 0.05$). Fatmawati et al. [283] reported the protective effect of RJ against UV radiation in Wistar rats exposed to 40 Watt UV-B lamps for 2 h daily during two weeks. RJ was applied as a cream (at concentrations of 2.5%, 5%, and 10%) and protected the skin from UV rays. RJ reduced inflammatory processes and strengthened the antioxidant defense. The highest dose of RJ significantly increased Nrf2 levels and decreased the expression of NF-κB and TNF-α.

The effects of RJ and 10-HDA on UVB-induced photoaging were tested by measuring procollagen type I, TGF-β1, and MMP-1. In UVB-irradiated human skin fibroblasts treated with RJ and 10-HDA, procollagen type I and TGF-β1 were increased, whereas changes in MMP-1 were not observed. It was suggested that potentially RJ could be effective in skin protection from UVB-induced photoaging through enhanced collagen production [117,284].

Apart from chemotherapy and radiation, previous studies reported the in vivo protective and antioxidative roles of RJ against CCl4, oxymetholone, paracetamol, celecoxib, and fumonisin-induced liver and kidney injury, without identifying the responsible components [270,285–291].

5.12. Antimicrobial Activity of Royal Jelly

Due to the huge problem of the rising resistance of microorganisms to known antibiotics, there is an urgent need for novel antibiotics with the advanced mechanisms of action on which microorganisms cannot develop resistance. In this decade, molds and bacteria have been investigated as the source of new antibiotics. Insects only recently became interesting to scientists as fat tissue and other insect cells produce numerous antimicrobial peptides that can be found in their hemolymph. Antimicrobial peptides (AMPs) are also present in RJ [48,63,68,292–300]. In addition to antibacterial activity, these peptides show antiviral, antitumoral, immunoregulatory, and hepatoprotective effects as well. The cationic AMPs interact with the negatively charged membranes of various microorganisms and change their membrane electrochemical potential, which ultimately ends in bacterial death due to the disturbance of membrane integrity. Some examples of AMPs are royalisin, jelleines, and aspimin which are present in RJ in small amounts [293]. Peptides present in insects impact bacteria through several mechanisms: (i) creating peptide monomers that join and form big transmembraneous channels in the bacterial wall, and (ii) creating peptides that act as detergents and destroy the bacterial cell wall. Based on the spectrum of activity, the AMPs can be grouped into three categories: (i) peptides that are effective only against bacteria and not towards normal cells of mammals and fungi (selective peptides), (ii) peptides that are effective against bacteria, but also against normal mammalian cells and potentially fungi, and (iii) peptides that are effective exclusively against fungi [294]. The key AMPs found in RJ are defensins, the cysteine-rich (cationic) peptides, such as royalisin. Royalisin is an amphipathic peptide that makes up to 6.5% of the total protein content in RJ. The primary structure of royalisin is composed of 51 amino acids, of which six cysteines form three disulfide bonds [68,295]. These bonds are important for the high stability of royalisin at a low pH and high temperature. The molecular weight of the protein is 5.5 kDa. In addition to royalisin, 10-HDA contributes to the antibacterial activity of RJ [68]. 10-HDA showed prominent bactericidal activity towards animal- and human-specific pathogens, including several strains of *Staphylococcus* (*S. aureus, S. alactolyticus, S. intermedius B, S. xylosus,* and *S. cholearasuis*), *Vibrio parahaemolyticus*, and hemolytic *Escherichia coli* [68]. The antibacterial activity of royalisin and 10-HDA have been reported in both Gram-positive and Gram-negative species of bacteria [48,63,68,292–295]. These two antibacterial components are important for bees themselves.

Using reverse-phase HPLC 4, Fontana et al. [296] have isolated Jelleine-I-IV, yet another antibacterial peptide from RJ. Jelleine-I-III were effective against yeast, Gram-positive, and Gram-negative bacterial species while Jelleine-IV did not show antibacterial activity. The primary structure of jelleines do not show similarity with other antimicrobial peptides produced by honeybees such as hymenoptaecin, abaecin, apidaecin, and royalisin. Han et al. [297] have studied the antibacterial activities of Jelleine-II and artificially phosphorylated Jelleine-II in one threonine residue against *Paenibacillus larvae, Staphylococcus aureus, Bacilus subtilis, Pseudomonas aeruginosa,* and *Escherichia coli*. The native form of the Jelleine-II showed antibacterial properties, whereas the activity of the phosphorylated form was markedly decreased. It was concluded that phosphorylation adds the negative charge into the peptide, decreasing the antibacterial function. The hydrophobic residues present in jelleines and royalisin are crucial for the observed antimicrobial properties as they modify the functions of bacterial membranes. On the contrary, the halogenation of jellines increased the binding affinity to the bacterial wall and improved the antimicrobial and antibiofilm activity 1- to 8-fold. The proteolytic stability was also improved by 10- to 100-fold. The halogenation of chlorine-, bromine-, and iodine-jelleine-I was more effective than fluorine-jelleine-I [292,298,299]. The antibacterial activity of halogenated derivatives of jelleine-1 (applied at 1 μM to 256 μM) was confirmed against *Staphylococcus aureus, Bacillus subtilis, Staphylococcus epidermidis, Escherichia coli, Pseudomonas aeruginosa, Klebsiella influenza,* and *Cronobacter sakazakii* at 10^5 to 10^6 CFU/mL. The apolipophorin III-like protein from RJ also contributes to its antimicrobial activity. The apolipophorin III-like protein is a lipid-binding protein that binds to the components of the bacterial cell wall. The antibacterial effect of the glucose oxidase present in RJ also needs to be emphasized. This enzyme catalyzes the oxidation of glucose into hydrogen peroxide which shows antimicrobial activity.

In addition to AMPs, the antimicrobial properties of RJ could be assigned to royalactin (MRJP1). MRJPs demonstrate strong antimicrobial and bactericidal activities even against the most drug-resistant bacterial strains such as methicillin-resistant *Staphylococcus aureus, Pseudomonas aeruginosa,* and *Klebsiella pneumoniae*, vancomycin-resistant *Enterococci*, as well as extended-spectrum β-lactamase-producing *Proteus mirabilis* and Escherichia coli [48,63,296,300]. Besides being antibacterial, MRJP1 also has antifungal and immunostimulatory properties. Due to the negatively charged surface, even at a neutral pH, the oligomer form of MRJP1 (280–420 kDa), called apalbumin, has better storage stability and resistance to heat than the monomeric form. The antibacterial activity of MRJP2 was also reported. The effect on *Paenibacillus larvae* was likely due to the presence of the peptides apidaecin and hymenoptaecin [48,295]. MRJP1 and MRJP2 have a different pattern of glycosylation [295,300,301]. At least for *Paenibacillus larvae*, the glycosylation may affect the antimicrobial activity of MRJP2 [295]. In yet another study, glps, the glycoprotein fraction isolated from honey, was capable of permeabilizing and agglutinating the bacterial membrane. Mass spectroscopy revealed that glps resembles the MRJP1 precursor-harboring jelleins 1, 2, and 4. The authors suggested that high-mannose N-glycans mediate the lectin-like effect of MRJP1, while jelleins contribute to membrane permeabilization [301]. Interestingly, exosome-like extracellular vesicles (EVs) have been found in honey. These vesicles contain MRJP1, defensin-1, and jellein-3 and show antibacterial and antibiofilm activity against oral streptococci which indicates their potential in the prevention of dental caries [302,303]. In closure, the MRJPs demonstrate powerful antimicrobial and bactericidal activities, even against the highly resistant strains such as MRSA, *Pseudomonas aeruginosa*, *Klebsiella pneumoniae*, vancomycin-resistant Enterococci, as well as *Proteus mirabilis* and *Escherichia coli* that produce extended-spectrum beta lactamase [63,300].

The phenolic components of RJ are also important for its antimicrobial activity via various mechanisms. The main components of RJ that contribute to antioxidant and antimicrobial activity are flavanones (naringenin, naringin, hesperetin, isosacuranetin, and pinocembrin), flavones (chrysin, luteolin glucoside, acacetin, apigenin, and its glycoside), flavonol (quercetin, kaempherol, galangin, fisetin, and isorhamnetin), and isoflavones [62,63]. Phenolic components may cross the microbial cellular membranes and impair membrane fluidity. Interactions with membrane enzymes and proteins may result in the flow of protons in the opposite direction and disturb cellular activities such as energy production, membrane transport, and other metabolic regulatory functions. Phenolic compounds also inhibit the synthesis of DNA and RNA and protein translation, and may suppress microbial virulence factors [304,305]. They can also degrade the cell wall and cytoplasmic membranes, induce the leakage of the cellular content, and change fatty acid and phospholipid constituents. Furthermore, they act synergistically with antibiotics, thus increasing their effectiveness and reducing the dose. Besides showing their antibacterial effect, phenolic components also inhibit the growth of protozoa, food-related pathogens, and fungi. The antifungal properties of RJ have been shown against *Aspergillus fumigants*, *Aspergillus niger*, *Candida albicans*, and *Syncephalastrum racemosum* [304]. Finally, high concentrations of RJ are effective against *Pseudomonas Aeruginosa* which may be important when using RJ in the wound healing process [304].

Furthermore, RJ can inhibit the growth of *Trypanosoma cruzi*, a parasitic protozoan. Its activity has been confirmed for another parasite, dysenteric amoeba. It effects flu viruses as well. Multiple small doses of royal jelly increase resistance to stress in laboratory animals while high doses are lethal. Antibacterial and bactericidal properties have been proven against the species *Bacillus alvei*, *Streptococcus haem*, *Staphylococcus aureus*, *Proteus vulgaris*, *Micrococus*, and *Listeria monocytogene* [101,292–300,306].

It is interesting that RJ was used as an adjuvant for the HIV-1 multi-epitope vaccine candidate. It was supposed that the components of RJ act as immunopotentiators and promote the Th1 immune response. RJ applied alone stimulates cellular and humoral immune responses, but shows synergistic effects when combined with alum, thus improving the immunologic parameters such as the production of total antibodies and IgM, IgG1, IgG2a, and IgG2b isotypes. As an adjuvant, RJ stimulated lymphocyte proliferation and the release of IFN-γ which further activated TCD8+ and TCD4+ lymphocytes in the fight against viral infections. The induction of the Th1 response is crucial for combating viral infections such as HIV-1. 10-HDA was the main component of RJ for the production of the Th1 cytokine pattern in human monocyte-derived dendritic cells. It seems that T cells stimulated with RJ may stimulate B lymphocytes to produce antibodies. RJ can induce the production of all isotypes of antibodies, i.e., the poly-isotypic humoral immune response, indicating a better biological response [307]. In addition to RJ, purified MRJPs of *Apis mellifera* also showed powerful antiviral activity against HCV, HIV, and SARS-CoV-2 [305–311]. The antiviral effects of MRJP2 and its isoform X1 have been studied by the computational tools and 3D structure of the SARS-CoV-2 proteins (from the Protein Data Bank) which includes papain-like protease (non-structural protein nsp3), 3CL protease (nsp5), the nsp5-inhibitor complex, and RNA replicase (nsp9). The RNA-dependent RNA polymerase (nsp12)-cofactor (nsp7-nsp8) complex and the methyltransferase (nsp16)-cofactor (nsp10) complex were also involved. MRJP2 and MRJP2 X1 exerted inhibitory effects on SARS-CoV-2 non-structural proteins (main and papain proteases, RNA-dependent RNA polymerase, RNA replicase, and methyltransferase). The obtained results suggest that functional food proteins could be effective in the prevention of the SARS-CoV-2 cell-attachment. The antiviral action was assigned to their sialidase activity and ability to interact with the binding sites of the angiotensin converting enzyme-2 (ACE2) on the viral spike. The docking studies indicated that the inhibitory activity of MRJP2 and MRJP2 isoform X1 was based on their ability to bind to the active sites or the cofactor-binding site on the viral non-structural protein nsp3, nsp5, nsp9, nsp12, and nsp16. Therefore, the RJ proteins could be effective in the prevention of the severe complications of the disease in the lungs, such as hypoxia, and in the prevention of inflammation and thrombosis. In conclusion, RJ proteins have an important role both in the prevention of viral replication and in the prevention of life-threatening complications [308].

5.13. Wound-Healing Activity of Royal Jelly

Wound healing is a programmed biological process involving inflammation and cell proliferation, differentiation, and migration, as well as numerous intracellular and extracellular components, like inflammatory mediators (cytokines and chemokines), growth factors, and ATP, among others [312]. In the process of wound healing, the proliferation and differentiation of fibroblasts are critical for the formation of the granulation tissue and connection of wound edges. The proliferation and migration of keratinocytes from the wound enables re-epithelialization, protecting the wound from infection and desiccation. Macrophages are also important for wound healing by dampening inflammation. They produce various regulators that promote an inflammatory response and remove bacteria and necrotic tissue through the phagocytic activity [36,313–317].

In general, it has been shown that RJ and its components promote wound healing at both animal and cellular levels [318–326]. Some components of RJ show anti-inflammatory effects (SA, 10-HDA, and 10-HDAA), some components promote proliferation and migration (MRJPs, especially MRJP2, MRJP3, and MRJP7), whereas some components stimulate regenerative activities (royalactin, royalisin, and 10-HDA) [313–325].

In streptozotocin-induced diabetic rats, the wound-healing activity of RJ was attributed to its royalisin-mediated antimicrobial effects, the anti-inflammatory action, and the ability to reduce exudation and collagen formation in granulation tissue [313,314]. Kohno et al. [36] suggested that the anti-inflammatory actions of RJ on the inhibition of the proinflammatory cytokine are released by activated macrophages as well as the scavenging activity. In streptozotocin-induced diabetic rats, RJ also shortened the time required for the recovery of desquamated skin lesions [313,314]. El-Gayar et al. [314] have shown the wound healing effect of RJ in a rat model of an MRSA skin infection. In another study, Lin et al. [315] have tested the wound healing efficacy of different RJ samples in excisional full-thickness wounds. The most potent was *Castanea mollissima* Bl RJ. This type of RJ accelerated wound repair by promoting the proliferative and migratory abilities of keratinocytes by 50.9% and 14.9%, respectively. Furthermore, *Castanea mollissima* Bl RJ inhibited the production of nitric oxide by 46.2%, and promoted cell growth by increasing the levels of TGF-β by 44.7%. On the contrary, for *Brassica napus* L., RJ ameliorated inflammation by reducing the secretion of TNF-α by 21.3%. Hence, in complicated wound models, such as MRSA skin infections, diabetic foot ulcers, and infected cutaneous wounds, RJ could be considered as an option for wound care. Further research should explore in more details the range of applications of a particular type of RJ in chronic wounds, and identify specific components of RJ that promote wound healing.

Patients undergoing radiotherapy and chemoradiotherapy for the treatment of head and neck cancers are often faced with oral mucositis, usually accompanied with the ulcerations of the oral mucosa. Oral mucositis develops in 15–40% of patients treated with standard chemotherapy, and in all patients receiving radiation therapy as part of the head and neck cancer treatment, oral mucositis occurs at some degree. These patients also may experience pain, dysphonia, and dysphagia. Tissues with the most prominent mitotic activity, such as oral mucosa, are rapidly affected by radiation. A quick response is also characteristic for chemotherapeutics such as cisplatin, S-1, nedaplatin, and docetaxel. The level of normal tissue damage following chemoradiotherapy depends on the dose, fractionation schedule, and volume of the treated tissue. A beneficial effect of RJ in reducing chemoradiotherapy-induced oral mucositis in head and neck cancer patients and animal models was also observed [326–331]. For example, the application of RJ films (10% and 30%) accelerated recovery from a 5-FU-induced injury by showing the free radical-scavenging activity and by reducing the myeloperoxidase activity and production of pro-inflammatory cytokines in hamsters [327,329,330]. Erdem and Güngörmüş [280] performed studies in patients undergoing radiotherapy and chemotherapy. They reported a significantly shorter mean time for the resolution of oral mucositis in the RJ group. These data suggest that RJ possesses a healing effect against the chemotherapy- and radiotherapy-induced oral mucositis that is largely mediated by the anti-inflammatory and anti-oxidative activities of RJ [328,331].

Chen et al. [332] have found that MRJPs from RJ could induce the proliferation of human cells and could replace the fetal bovine serum in culture media. The growth-promoting activity was confirmed in many cell lines, including human embryonic lung fibroblasts (HFL-I) [111], human monocytes (U-937 and HB4C5) [21], human lymphoid cells (U-937, THP-1, U-M, HB4C5, and HF10B4) [33,246,332], human keratinocytes [26], human microvascular endothelial cells (HMEC-1) [115], the primary culture of rat hepatic cells [26,27], rat small intestine epithelial cells [74], murine fibroblasts (NIH-3T3) [29], stem cells [30], monocyte/macrophage-like cells *RAW 264.7* [324] and monkey kidney epithelial cells [31], and Tn-5B1-4 insect cells [112].

The treatment of the human embryonic lung fibroblast cell line (HFL-I) with the MRJP mixture was confirmed to promote proliferation and reduce senescence [111]. Moreover, cells that were grown in MRJPs-containing medium had longer telomeres compared to cells grown in media without MRJPs. The molecular mechanisms underlying the anti-senescence effect of MRJPs were associated with the upregulation of *SOD1* and the downregulation of *mTOR*, catenin beta like-1 (*CTNNB*), and *TP53* at the gene level [111]. A similar effect was observed for recombinant MRJPs 1–7 which increased the viability of NIH-3T3 cells (murine fibroblasts) by protecting them against oxidative stress-induced apoptosis [29]. It is interesting that oligomeric MRJP1 stimulated the proliferation of human monocytes (U-937 and HB4C5 cell lines), whereas the monomeric form (royalactin) failed to stimulate the proliferation of these cells. Oligomeric MRJP1 also stimulated the growth of Jurkat and IEC-6 cells, while monomeric MRJP1 promoted the proliferation of human lymphoid cell lines, such as U-937, THP-1, U-M, HB4C5, and HF10B4 [31,332]. Furthermore, the monomeric MRJP1 may act as a pluripotency factor and activate the pluripotent gene regulatory network that enables the self-renewal of mouse embryonic stem cells [44]. MRJP2, MRJP3, and MRJP7 have the potential to promote wound healing by inducing the proliferation and migration of human epidermal keratinocytes [26]. The carboxyl-terminal penta-peptide repeats (TPRs) of MRJP3 stimulated the growth and wound healing activity of THP-1 and monkey kidney epithelial cells (Vero) [31].

5.14. Antiallergic Effect of Royal Jelly

An antiallergic effect of RJ has been confirmed in the mice model [37]. The antiallergic activity of RJ was attributed to MRJP3 which inhibited the production of IL-4 in mice splenocytes immunized with ovalbumin. MRJP3 not only inhibited IL-4, the key factor in immunoglobulin class switching to IgE in B cells, but also inhibited the production of IL-2 and IFN-γ by T cells and inhibited the proliferation of T cells. The potent immunoregulatory effect of MRJP3 regarding the inhibition of IgE and IgG1 production in immunized mice could be of clinical significance in designing MRJP3-based peptides with antiallergic properties.

In contrast to MRJP3, MRJP1 and MRJP2 can cause allergic reactions. They interacted with immunoglobulin E (IgE) of sera from patients exhibiting an RJ allergy [31,37]. IgE-binding was dependent on the glycosylation degree of MRJP1 and MRJP2.

Oka et al. [333] suggested that the suppression of an allergic reaction by RJ is related to the maintenance of macrophage function and the increased Th1/Th2 response. They have found that RJ maintains the GSH levels, increases the production of IL-12 p40 mRNA and NO expression, and reduces the production of E2 prostaglandin in the macrophage cells of mice immunized with 2, 4-dinitrophenylated keyhole limpet hemocyanin (DNP-KLH). Therefore, they concluded that RJ suppresses the production of allergen-specific IgE antibodies and histamine release, restores the macrophage function, and improves the Th1/Th2 cell response. The GSH levels may affect the response of the Th cells. The GSH increase in macrophages is a key factor for increasing the IL-12 levels and streamlining the Th1 response, which further favors a decrease in prostaglandin E2. It has been shown that prostaglandin E2 increases the suppression Th1 response and increases IgE production. In addition, it has been reported that increased NO levels suppress the degranulation of mast cells. Taken together, these findings indicate that RJ can protect from allergies or alleviate the symptoms of allergy.

RJ also reduced the development of skin lesions similar to atopic dermatitis in NC/Nga mice treated with picryl chloride [334]. The oral administration of RJ decreased the total skin weight, reduced the hypertrophy and hyperkeratosis of the epidermis, and inhibited the infiltration of inflammatory cells. The main mechanism of these effects was based on the reduced production of trinitrophenyl-conjugated keyhole limpet hemocyanin (TNP-KLH) TNP-specific IFN-γ and enhanced iNOS expression [334]. In another study, the oral intake of RJ reduced the number of splenic autoreactive B cells, serum IL-10 levels, and anti ssDNA, dsDNA, and erythrocyte autoantibodies in systemic lupus erythematosus (SLE)-prone New Zealand Black $\times$ New Zealand White F1 mice [335]. The positive effect of RJ on SLE was also confirmed in children taking 2 g of RJ for 3 months. The improvement of the disease severity was evident through the increased number of CD4+ and CD8+ regulatory T cells and a reduced number of apoptotic CD4+ T cells [336]. A potential immunoregulatory effect of RJ against Graves' disease was also demonstrated. Lymphocytes obtained from the patients with Graves' disease were incubated with RJ. This treatment reduced the level of TNF-α and increased the levels of IFN-γ, and shifted the Th1/Th2 cytokine ratios towards Th1 dominance [337].

Guendouz et al. [338] have demonstrated that RJ may help in the prevention of systemic and anaphylactic responses in a murine model of a cow's milk allergy. RJ was applied at doses of 0.5, 1, and 1.5 g/kg during seven days and significantly inhibited the production of serum IgG (31.15–43.78%) and IgE (64.28–66.6%) against β-lactoglobulin and reduced the plasma histamine level after the β-lactoglobulin challenge (66.62–67.36%). In addition, RJ reduced intestinal dysfunction by abolishing the sensitization-induced secretory response (70.73–72.23%). It also prevented tissue damage and increased the length of jejunal villi by 44.32–59.01%. These effects may be related to its inhibitory effects on the degranulation of mast cells [338].

It is also interesting to note that protease-treated RJ can promote an antigen-specific mucosal IgA response by enhancing the uptake of antigens by M cells, increasing the efficacy of the immune response of the intestinal mucosa [339].

5.15. Allergic Reactions as Side Effects of RJ Application

RJ is broadly used as a dietary supplement and for cosmetic purposes, and is generally considered as relatively safe. However, various proteins present in RJ can cause side effects such as allergic reactions. A mild-to-severe allergic reactions may include skin rashes, eczema, contact dermatitis, allergic rhinitis, conjunctivitis, minor gastrointestinal problems, hemorrhagic colitis, acute asthma, bronchospasm, anaphylactic shock, and in some cases, even death [340]. Considering the possibility of unwanted effects, the consumption of RJ is not recommended for expectant mothers, lactating women, and individuals prone to allergic reactions. Allergic reactions may occur after the first intake of RJ, suggesting the cross-reactivity with other allergens, especially mite and arthropod allergens. According to Hata et al. [340], for those with a history of allergic diseases, such as atopic dermatitis, asthma, and allergic rhinitis, caution is needed when consuming RJ products because of the potential cross-reactivity. In patients with atopic dermatitis who had never consumed RJ, RJ-binding IgE antibodies have been found. The cross-reactivity with RJ has been demonstrated for the European and American house dust mite, snow crab, edible crab, German cockroach, and honeybee venom. Most RJ proteins (app. 90%) are members of the MRJPs, and MRJP1, MRJP2, and MRJP3 are identified as allergens [340–343]. Li et al. [344] suggested that MRJP3 is the main cause of anaphylaxis and cross-reactivity with honeycomb, and that patients with an allergic reaction to RJ should avoid other bee products.

6. Scientific Claims about Effectiveness of RJ to Human Health According to PASSCLAIM Classification

The main objectives of the PASSCLAIM project (Process for the Assessment of Scientific Support for Claims on Foods) were to define the group of widely applicable criteria for the scientific explanation of health claims about the effectiveness of food. These criteria are considered powerful indicators for the assessment of the quality of data that support claims on health benefits of foods. According to EU Regulation No 1924/2006, different health claims about the benefits of RJ can be derived. According to the PASSCLAIM project classification of the International Life Science Institute (ILSI), the claims are grouped into the following themed areas:

(1) Diet and cardiovascular diseases,
(2) Bone health and osteoporosis,
(3) Physical strength and fitness,
(4) The regulation of body mass, insulin sensitivity, and risk of diabetes,
(5) Diet and cancer,
(6) Mental health and effectiveness,
(7) Bowel health, digestion, and immunity.

The health claims of RJ are supported for categories of diet and cardiovascular diseases, physical strength and fitness, diet and cancer, and mental health and effectiveness. In particular, a preventive intake of RJ at doses of 100 to 200 mg daily may enhance the health of the cardiovascular system by decreasing blood fats and cholesterol, the main cardiovascular risk factors [345]. RJ should be taken for 30 days and followed by 2-to-3-week break. After a break, it is recommended to restart with lower doses. Regarding physical strength, the intake of RJ may increase physical strength, fitness, and work ability, especially in the elderly (anti-age effect). Taking RJ also may decrease one's risk of cancer and enhance their mental status and physical effectiveness [177,191,197,346,347]. Again, these effects are particularly important in the elderly. Some of the above-mentioned effects are shown in Tables 3 and 4.

Table 3. Overview of biological and pharmacological effects of royal jelly shown in cell cultures and animal models.

Effect	References
Antibacterial, antiviral, antiparasitic effect (model—microrganisms)	
Antibacterial	[48,294,300–302]
Antifungal (fungicidal)	[3,7,48,57,295,304]
Antiviral	[293,305–311]
Activity against different parasites of family *Trypanosomidae*	[306]

Table 3. *Cont.*

Effect	References
Bio-stimulatory effect and anti-ageing effect (model cell culture and laboratory animals)	
Estrogenic and gonadotropic effects confirmed on cells and in rats	[28,86,207]
Increase in growth and animal weight	[52,108–110,291,345]
Anticancer effects, increases immune cells' activity and stress resistance	[36,37,226–230,232,243,246,254]
Increases reproduction capacity in rats and sheep	[121,209,211–214]
In vitro increases oxygen consumption in tissues, antihypoxic effect	[180,191,250]
Against male rabbits' infertility, increases sexual effectiveness in rats and hamsters	[55,59,212]
Prolongs lifespan in rats and hamsters	[39,104–107,129]
Immunomodulating effects: anticancer, antiallergic, and anti-inflammatory (model—laboratory animals and humans)	
Immunostimulant activity, increase in number of leukocytes	[68,77,125,230,246,268]
Anticancer effects	[34–40,42,44,49,50]
Prevents autoimmunity in mice	[335–337]
Anti-inflammatory effects	[7,13,36,68–70,127,137,262,271,304,334]
Heart and circulatory system effects (model—laboratory animals and humans)	
Decreases increased blood pressure, hypotensive effect, vasodilatation	[53–56,58,59,177,187,190,191,193–197]
Antiatherosclerotic effect: decreases cholesterol and triglyceride concentration in blood, increases HDL, decreases fibrinogen in plasma and thrombosis	[27,28,127,143,150,172–174,187,203,308]
Cardio-protective effect, prevents myocarditis	[58,77–80,92,93,100–103,172,173,178,202,345]
Increases thyroxin levels, albumin/globulin ratio in blood, and decreases serum proteins after oral application in rats	[75,76,113]
Effects on central and vegetative nervous system (model—laboratory animals)	
Effects on central nervous activity—protection and activation	[28,29]
Increases brain cell differentiation	[154,156,157]
Improves memory and learning through upregulation of neurotrophic factor synthesis such as that of GDNF and other neurotrophins	[137,139,156,157,176]
Acetyl-choline-like effects on bowels and smooth muscles nerves	[137,154,156,176,177,197]
Calming effects (rat)	[112,157]
Antioxidative, hepatoprotective and radio protective effects (model—laboratory animals)	
Antioxidative effect	[52,58,62,64,67,83,103,108,127,147]
Liver protection	[81–83,92,100,240,263,269,290]
Reducing stress and teratogen effects, lung edema, and liver or kidney damage after mycotoxine intake in rats	[67,98–102,107]
Stimulates DNA synthesis in hepatocytes and protects cells from apoptosis and mitogen effect, prolongs cell proliferation, and increases albumin production	[26,113]
Radiation protective effect in animal experiments	[247,249,250,278–283]
Other effects (model—laboratory animals and humans)	
Prevents osteoporosis and promotes bone formation	[87,127,204–220]
Skin protection: promotes collagen build-up	[114,117–120,131,304,318,325,334]
Hyperglycemic effect, prevents insulin resistance, antidiabetic effect	[166,167,169,174,184]
Decreases experimental colitis in rats	[61,62]
Antiallergic activity, decreases development of atopic dermatitis as skin lesions in rats	[334,340]

Table 4. Medical effects of royal jelly in humans.

Usage	References
Pediatrics:	
Pre-term babies or inadequate food intake: improves overall condition, increase in weight, appetite, red blood cells, and hemoglobin	[6,112]
Geriatrics:	
Increase in overall well-being and recuperation from fatigue and menopausal problems	[90,121,202,211,223,224]
Against stenocardia and after heart attack; arteriosclerosis and atherosclerosis; hypertension	[187,188,190,195,197,202–204]
Against respiratory system diseases, asthma	[333,338,339]
Against diseases of the eye, e.g., blepharitis, conjunctivitis and retina burns, circulatory disorders in the eye	[97,126,161]
Bio-stimulating effect, increases physical endurance and work ability and increases resistance to hypoxia	[52,124,125,152]
Increase memory, neuro-vegetative activation	[137,138,141,145,147,154,157]
Anti diabetes 1	[162–168,173,174]
Anticancer effects	[77,89]
Prevention of stomach and duodenum ulcer, stomach problems	[175–177]
Promote skin regeneration and skin lesion healing	[114,117,131,304,318,334]
Prevent degenerative processes and rheumatism	[85,88]
Prevent warts, acne, ulcers, seborea, neurodermatitis	[280,284,334]
Prevent kidney dysfunction	[264,265,269,288]

7. Need for Standardization of Important Biologically Active Compounds and Determination of Validity and Quality of Products with RJ

RJ has been used for a long time. The first recommendation for its use in human therapy dates from 1922 in France. Since then, RJ has become the subject of numerous studies. In many European and world countries, the medicinal use of RJ is monitored by the relevant ministries of health and regulatory bodies. In an effort to ensure the safe usage of RJ as a medicinal product, it is important to guarantee the presence of specific compounds important for its health benefits and to ensure quality production. Hence, the chemical composition and quality of RJ should be analyzed continuously. The basic nutritional requirements of RJ that must be ensured include water (min 62.0%–max 68.5%), lipids (min 2%–max 8%), 10-HDA (min 1.4%), proteins (min 11%–max 18%), total carbohydrates (min 7%–max 18%), and individual carbohydrates [fructose (2.3–7.6%), glucose, (2.9–8.1%), sucrose (<0.1–2.1%), maltose, and maltotriose (0.0–1.0%)] [7].

Various factors may affect the production and chemical composition of RJ, including the post-grafting period, harvest time, diet of the bee colonies, and seasonal variations [20,348]. Regarding the yield and nutritional composition, the optimal time to harvest RJ is after 72 h of grafting. On the contrary, the minimum yield is observed after 24 h. The lowest moisture and the highest content of crude proteins, ash, fructose, and glucose were obtained 72 h after harvesting. However, RJ collected after 24 h contained the highest lipid concentration. The content of 10-HDA in RJ also varies. It is dependent on the season of harvesting. In one study, the amount of 10-HDA was monitored from April to August. The highest concentration of 10-HDA was measured in June (1.84%), whereas the lowest amount was found in April (1.03%) [349]. Furthermore, a change of acidity was observed over time. These findings indicate the complexity of the RJ content. Accordingly, a comprehensive understanding is needed to produce RJ as a medical product with a defined chemical composition [350]. Furthermore, it is hard to gather data obtained in different studies due to the lack of homogeneity of the original materials with different sampling methods and production conditions. Additional sources of variability are various experimental conditions as well as the diversity of the analytical methods applied. Of note, it has been reported that pesticides may affect the quality and quantity of RJ. Milone et al. [351] observed differences in the metabolome, proteome, and phytosterol profile of RJ produced by colonies exposed to the multi-pesticide pollen. Some of the essential nutrients, such as 24-methylenecholesterol, MRJPs, and 10-HDA, were significantly reduced. Additionally, the quantity of RJ provided per queen was lower in colonies exposed to pesticides. According to the United States Environmental Protection Agency (USEPA) risk assessment guidelines, exposure to pesticides is app. 100 times lower in RJ compared to pollen and nectar (USEPA, 2014).

Milone et al. [351] also observed a reduction in the average RJ per cell between control and pesticide-exposed colonies (283 mg vs. 198 mg, respectively), but the difference was not statistically significant. The complete knowledge of the RJ components is essential for defining the standard composition and assessment of the quality of marketed products containing RJ [349–353]. Some countries, like Switzerland, Bulgaria, Brazil, and Uruguay, have defined national standards for RJ. Also, the difference between fresh RJ and lyophilized samples needs to be clearly stated. In general, the lyophilized RJ contains <5% water, 27–41% proteins, 22–31% carbohydrates, and 15–30% fat [353–355]. The analytical data indicate that the exposure to the temperature of 4 °C does not change its composition. In addition, the storage of frozen RJ prevents the decomposition of biologically active proteins. Hence, RJ needs to be frozen immediately after collection to preserve the bioactive compounds [352]. Some important differences in RJ composition are shown in Table 1.

The main nutritional value of dietary proteins, as well as RJ, is determined by the amino acid composition. Therefore, monitoring changes in the amino acid composition can be an effective method of assessing the quality of RJ. One of the most powerful tools for analyzing amino acid composition in RJ is ultra-performance liquid chromatography (UPLC). By using UPLC, it was determined that the average levels of free amino acids (FAAs) and total amino acids (TAA) in fresh RJ were 9.21 and 111.27 mg/g, respectively. The most abundant FAAs in RJ are proline, glutamine, lysine, and glutamic acid, whereas the most common TAAs are asparagine, glutamine, leucine, and lysine. Although the concentrations of the majority of the FAAs and TAAs did not change significantly during the storage, the amount of total methionine and free glutamine decreased over time. Hence, the authors suggested that the levels of total methionine and free glutamine may be considered as a marker of RJ quality. In another study, the concentrations of proline and lysine increased during the first three months, and then decreased after 6–10 months, indicating proteolytic activity over time.

Besides proteins, 10-HDA and 10-HDAA are specific components of RJ [5–7,13,14,353,356]. HDA is considered as the best marker of RJ quality. Moreover, it may be used as an indicator of forgery. Based on the standards of the International Organization for Standardization (ISO), the total amount of 10-HDA should be more than 1.4% to meet the quality control parameters (ISO, 2016). However, the composition of RJ and amounts of 10-HDA may vary widely. In two RJ samples of different origins (France and Thailand) stored at room temperature for one year, a reduction of 0.4% and 0.6% of 10-HDA was observed. In addition, 10-HDA is difficult to use as a measure of freshness as its values differ in fresh RJ. In general, the RJ of a European origin contains lower levels of 10-HDA. Hence, it is considered that the total concentration of fatty acids is a better indicator of freshness than 10-HDA itself [353,356]. Although the specification of RJ products requires the content of 10-HDA, which is chemically stable and unique to RJ, a potential limitation of using 10-HDA is that its levels in RJ decline during the production process. Furthermore, there is a possibility of manipulation by adding RJ rich in 10-HDA. On the contrary, amounts of apisin are fairly constant among different RJ samples. Therefore, it is likely that apisin could be used as an indicator for the evaluation of RJ quality. MRJP1, the main constituent of apisin, plays an essential role not only in the assessment of RJ quality, but also in the determination of RJ freshness [349–353]. However, properties of MRJP1 are dependent on storage conditions. Storage above 4 °C induces the degradation of MRJP1 due to its lytic activity. Furthermore, Mureşan and Buttstedt [357] investigated the stability of MRJPs in different pH environments and found a direct correlation between the pH levels and protein stability. In addition, carbohydrates from RJ, including trehalose, maltose, erlose, melibiose, ribose, gentiobiose, isomaltose, raffinose, and melezitose, are important for bee products' authenticity. The carbohydrate analysis also may help in the detection of forged RJ [353,354,358,359]. The ISO recommendation for the determination of the carbohydrate constituent is liquid chromatographic analysis (the reference method), titration method gas chromatographic analysis, and the Hydrophilic Interaction Liquid Chromatography–tandem Mass Spectrometry (HILIC-MS/MS) method [13,358–360]. Furthermore, the authenticity of RJ production can be determined by measuring the ratio of stable C and N isotopes. Geographical authenticity can be determined by pollen analysis [348,350]. In particular, the 87Sr/86Sr ratio indicates the geographic origin [361,362]. The levels of ADP, ATP, and AMP are used as indicators of the freshness of RJ as their levels are high in fresh samples. Taken together, the key parameters in the estimation of RJ quality are organoleptic, physical, and chemical properties and its composition as follows: (i) the water content in fresh and frozen samples of RJ; (ii) the concentration of total proteins and free amino acids; (iii) the concentration of carbohydrates; (iv) the concentration of lipids; total fatty acids and free acids; (v) 10-HDA; (vi) minerals; (vii) acidity; (viii) sediment analysis; (ix) furosine; and (xj) potential contamination. In addition, the freshness of RJ or its products may be estimated by measuring the activity of glucose oxidase, furosine, or superoxide dismutase [353–356]. Therefore, RJ and RJ-containing products need to be prepared according to detailed sanitary and hygienic protocols and monitored by trained experts to maintain the beneficial effects.

8. Closing Remarks

The biological characteristics of RJ, serving as the base for its potential use, are the following: its biostimulatory effect—the ability to increase tissue respiration, oxidative phosphorylation, exchange of matter, energy and fitness, increased resistance to stress and illnesses, the maintenance and strengthening of the hair, skin, and nails, the regeneration of cells and tissues, decrease in cholesterol levels, positive effect on the vascular system, stabilization of blood pressure, increase in memory (acetyl choline neurotransmitter), stimulation of the immune system, increased appetite, digestion regulation, hormonal balance maintenance, ease of menstrual symptoms, help with impotence and frigidity, fatigue and tiredness relief, positive effect on arthritis, anemia, muscle dystrophy, and neurodegenerative diseases, and pro-regenerative, anti-inflammatory, antiviral, and antibiotic effects (Tables 3 and 4).

It is interesting that exosome-like extracellular vesicles (EVs) found in honey from *Apis mellifera* contain MRJP1, defensin-1, and jellein-3 as intravesicular cargo, which indicates that honey-derived EVs could represent innovative approaches for preventing dental caries. RJ also contains a considerable number of extracellular vesicles (EVs). The molecular analysis of RJEV confirmed the presence of exosomal markers such as CD63 and syntenin, and cargo molecules MRJP1, defensin-1, and jellein-3. RJEV can modulate the differentiation and secretome of mesenchymal stem cells (MSCs), as well as reduce LPS-induced inflammation in macrophages by blocking the MAPK pathway. The most interesting for wound healing is the secretory profile of MSCs, which secrete various proteins, especially increasing the level of IGF, HGF, and VEGF, but not FGF acting on pro-angiogenic and promigratory effects in wound healing, while having minor effects on scars and fibrosis. Overall, RJEV exhibits a significant antibacterial effect and promotes wound healing by modulating underlying cellular responses. The antibacterial and antifungal activities of MRJPs and jelleines are achieved through the interactions of positively charged amino acids with the hydrophobic residues in bacterial cell membranes. Furthermore, it is important to highlight that RJ and its proteins prevent the replication of the SARS-CoV-2 virus and severe complications of the disease. It is possible that isolating EVs from raw RJ will reduce the high complexity of RJ components, enable standardization and quality control, and thus bring the application of natural nano-therapy closer to the clinic.

Regarding potential side effects, RJ can cause contact dermatitis and anaphylaxis in some people due to the presence of many proteins. The usage of RJ is limited in diseases such as bronchial asthma exacerbations (RJ is astringent and can lead to bronchiectasis), Addison disease, adrenal gland diseases, and tumors in the acute phase. The estrogenic and proliferative activities of RJ have been shown in MCF-7. However, the procarcinogenic and estrogenic effects of RJ on other tumors have not been confirmed. On the other hand, RJ is effective against anti-cancer agent-induced toxicities, such as mucositis, fibrosis, cardiotoxicity, intestinal damage, and renal and hepatic dysfunction. In addition, the modulatory effect of RJ on various biological activities, including cell survival, inflammation, and oxidative stress, is closely associated with its effects (Tables 3 and 4). An overview of the molecular and cellular mechanisms of RJ is shown in Table 5, while the doses of RJ used in some clinical trials are shown in Table 6.

Based on the above-mentioned characteristics of RJ and its effect on human health and quality of life, appropriate methods should be used for the standardization of RJ and RJ-containing products, especially regarding biologically active compounds, to ensure maximal effectiveness for human health. Knowledge about the main biological compounds and their seasonal and geographical variability, variability over time, proper ways of storage, as well as the determination of the safe therapeutic dose, are important factors in the prevention and protection from disease. Finally, knowledge about the medicinal effects of RJ will enable its wider use and will promote RJ production.

Table 5. Overview of the molecular and cellular effects of RJ and its biologically active components.

Biological Activity	Active Component	Molecular and Cellular Effect of RJ	References
Cellular senescence			
Immune system			
	RJ and its components	– stimulate immune surveillance and phagocytic potential – stimulate stress-induced replication – increase response of effector cells (T, B, macrophages, NK) – decrease risk of chronic, autoimmune diseases and cancer – increase number of hematopoietic stem cells in peripheral blood	[124,125] [98,132–134] [101,102]
Nervous system			
	RJ and its components	– decrease senescence in glial cells (microglia and astrocytes) – reduce neurotoxicity and accumulation of senescent microglial cells – decrease risk of neurodegenerative diseases	[52,110]
Cardiovascular system			
	RJ and its components	– decrease number of senescent cells – prevent changes of cellular signaling and maintain homeostasis in stressful conditions – reduce SASP induction – decrease risk of CVD	[98,132–134]
Genes expresion and pathways involved in senescence			
	MRP1	– prevents disruption of tumor suppressors (p53, p16, RB, PTEN) – regulates activation of cell cycle effectors (cyclins, CDKs) – regulates DNA damage response (ATR, ATM, Chk1) – acts on epigenetic changes and epigenetics regulators – upregulates SOD1 and downregulates mTOR, CTNNB1, and TP53, and has a stimulatory effect on DNA and protein syntheses – inhibits SASP pro-inflammatory factors, mostly NF-kB-dependent factors such as IL-6, IL-8, IL-1β, MCP-1, MCP-2 and MCP-4, HGF, FGF, and MMPs – upregulates S6K1, MAPK, and EGFR in the EGFR-mediated signaling – activates the Nrf2–HO-1 pathway – reduces expression of the proinflammatory cytokines (IL-1, IL-6, COX-2, and MCP-1) – reduces activation of NF-κB and c-Jun N-terminal kinase (JNK) pathways	[98,102,110] [111] [115] [129–132] [43,44,105–107] [132–134] [109,110,117–121]

Table 5. *Cont.*

Biological Activity	Active Component	Molecular and Cellular Effect of RJ	References
Cognition and AD-related pathology			
	RJ and its lipids	– alleviate Aβ pathology (reduce Aβ influx through the BBB via RAGE inhibition) – prevent cleavage of APP into Aβ by inhibiting BACE1 – facilitate degradation and clearance of Aβ by IDE, NEP, and LRP1 – activate AMPK and inhibits mTOR pathway, and promote autophagy and antioxidant production – suppress microglial inflammation by inhibiting various oxidative, inflammatory, and apoptotic pathways, e.g., iNOS and NF-κB – enhance production of neurotrophins such as NGF and BDNF by binding to estrogen receptors β and α – promote ACh production, neurogenesis, and synaptogenesis	[58,139,147] [58,135–137,139,140] [145,150] [58,145,146] [58] [146,155] [58,138–152,156] [147,154,156] [154,156]
	MRJPs	– improve brain metabolism by increasing levels of glucose and phosphoenolpyruvic acid – increase the level of nicotinic acid mononucleotide (NaMN), a precursor of NAD+, and xanthosine, which sustains the nucleic acid metabolism and supports DNA repair in aged rats – stimulate production of neuroprotective molecules in aged rats, mainly of cysteic acid – enhance memory	[139,159]
Aging and longetivity			
	MRJPs	– upregulate S6K1, MAPK, and EGFR in the EGFR-mediated signaling – increase telomere length, decrease senescence, and stimulate proliferation in human embryonic lung fibroblasts (HFL1 cell line) by downregulating p53, catenin beta like-1, and mTOR pathways – increase SOD1 gene expression and decrease levels of malonaldehyde, an oxidative stress marker	[11,111] [101,102,123] [110]
Anti-diabetic			

Table 5. *Cont.*

Biological Activity	Active Component	Molecular and Cellular Effect of RJ	References
	RJ	– increases insulin concentration and levels of albumin and total proteins in type 2 diabetes – increases serum apolipoproteins A-I (Apo-A-I), changes levels of apolipoproteins B and ratio of Apo-B and Apo-A-I – reduces FBS, HbA1c, and HOMA-IR – improves serum levels of triglycerides, cholesterol, HDL, LDL, VLDL, and Apo-A1 – reduces oxidative stress – increases antioxidant enzymes and total antioxidant capacity – regulates glycemic parameters (fasting blood glucose and glucose clearance as the most affected parameters) – reduces AST, ALT, ALP – maintains homeostasis by decreasing insulin resistance – decreases mRNA expression of glucose-6-phosphatase during long-term application – increases expression of adiponectin and adiponectin receptor 1 mRNA and pAMPK protein – improves hyperglycemia and insulin resistance by activating the expression of PGC-1α – improves hyperglycemia and partially reduces body weight in obese/diabetic KK-Ay mice – promotes expression of peroxisome proliferator-activated receptor-α (PPARα) and peroxisome proliferator-activated receptor-γ coactivator-1α (Pgc-1α) which improves lipid utilization and reduces body weight in KK-Ay mice – facilitates and enhances GLUT4 translocation	[170,171] [167,172] [28,127,172–174,203] [173] [167–169] [188] [183,189] [84,188,189] [181] [183] [184] [168]
Obesity			
	HDAA HDEA	– decrease obesity – decrease body fat accumulation – decrease total cholesterol – decrease insulin resistance – decreas C-reactive protein – increases adiponectin, total antioxidant capacity, endogenous antioxidants, bilirubin, and leptin – improve thermogenesis in brown adipose tissue (BAT) – increases UCP1 – reduce hyperglycemia and liver steatosis – increases irisin and metabolic thermogenesis in brown adipose tissues	[182–186] [184] [189] [182] [186] [185]

Table 5. *Cont.*

Biological Activity	Active Component	Molecular and Cellular Effect of RJ	References
Hypotensive and hypolipidemic activity			
	MRJP1, MRJP2, and MRJP3	– interact with bile acids, enhance the excretion of fecal bile acids, increase fecal excretion of cholesterol, and increase the hepatic cholesterol catabolism – show hypotensive effect acting on VSMCs, which regulate blood pressure – peptides derived from MRJP1 after gastrointestinal digestion show ACE inhibitory activity – RJ proteins, including royalisin and degradation products of MRJP1 and MRJP3 inhibit macrophage proliferation in atherosclerotic plaques	[187,188,197] [197,198] [190,196,200] [199]
	Peptides (Ile-Tyr, Val-Tyr, and Ile-Val-Tyr) formed by hydrolysis of RJ by protease N	– inhibit ACE activity – have anti-hypertensive effects by decreasing systolic blood pressure	[190]
	Peptides derived from MRJP1	– have strong ACE inhibitory activity – degradation products of MRJP1 and MRJP3 bind LDL-C and oxidized LDL-C components reducing atherosclerotic lesions – promote regression of atherosclerotic plaque by lowering plaque inflammation	[357] [28] [199,202–204]
Anti-inflammatory			
	MRJP1 MRJP2, MRJP3, 10-HDA	– increase macrophage stimulation – inhibit activation of p38 and JNK/AP-1 signaling pathways – decrease production of IgE and IgG1 – decrease levels of MMP-1, MMP-3, and p38 – inhibit lipolysaccharide (LPS)-induced production of inhibitor of kappa-B-zeta (IkB-z) and IL-6 – inhibit NF-κB and JNK pathways – inhibit production of TNF-α, IL-1β, IL-8, and NF-κB – reduce expression of the proinflammatory cytokines (IL-1, IL-6, COX-2, and MCP-1) – 10-HDA acts as histone deacetylase inhibitor (HDACI) and inhibits proliferation of FLS cells induced by RA	[62,63,68,75] [85] [13,69] [85,88]

Table 5. *Cont.*

Biological Activity	Active Component	Molecular and Cellular Effect of RJ	References
Inflammatory bowel diseases	RJ	– improves the colonic mucosal barrier and intestinal gut microbiota – reduces number of CD3+, CD5+, CD8+, and CD45+ T cells; secretion of pro-inflammatory cytokines IL-1β, TNF-α, COX-2, and NF-κB in TNBS-induced rat colitis model – alleviates the ulcerative erosion of colon tissue and number of colonic CD3+, CD45+ T cells, and mast cells in acetic-acid-induced colitis model – increases production of anti-inflammatory cytokine IL-10 and GPx activity – decreases intestinal permeability by increasing the expression of tight-junction proteins, goblet cells, and mucin MUC2 levels in DSS-induced ulcerative colitis model – reduces expression of proinflammatory cytokine IL-6 and increases expression of anti-inflammatory cytokine IL-10 and sIgA – increases immunity and antioxidant activity, and regulates composition and structure of the gut microbiota – improves gut dysbiosis and inflammation of the intestinal mucosa, regulates expression of nutrient absorption-related genes in the small intestine, increases excretion of saturated fatty acids in feces, and increases SCFA-producing intestinal bacteria – acts on the suppression of the secretion of pro-inflammatory cytokines such as IL1, TNF-α, and IL12, which affect number of innate lymphoid cells (ILC1 and ILC3) and their cytokines production (TNF-α, IFN-γ, IL-17, and IL-22)	[72–74] [77–89] [77,78]
	MRJP1, MRJP2, and MRJP3	– stimulate mouse macrophages and promote the immune response – improve the quantity of peripheral blood leukocytes, immunoglobulin content, immune factor levels, and the proliferation ability of spleen lymphocytes	[76]
Non-alcoholic fatty liver disease (NAFLD) and non-alcoholic steatohepatitis (NASH)	RJ and its 10-HDA, 10-HDAA, 2-DA, and SA	– improve adverse effects of estrogen deficiency, including body and liver weight gain, mental disorders, serum lipid profile abnormalities, liver lipid deposition, lipid peroxidation, and circadian gene expression disorders – decrease body and liver weights, improve cholesterol levels, downregulate ALT and AST levels, and combat NAFLD in OVX rats – attenuate the hepatic steatosis and liver injury – demonstrate strong anti-oxidative activity and capacity to ameliorate the disturbances of the circadian genes, *Per1* and *Per2*, provide quick energy to the liver, which reduces TC deposition and dyslipidemia – regulate activation of ERβ – decrease TC and LDL-C levels and increase HDL-C	[80–85] [82] [35]

Table 5. *Cont.*

Biological Activity	Active Component	Molecular and Cellular Effect of RJ	References
Rheumatoid arthritis (RA)	10-HDA	– inhibits activity of MMP-1, MMP-3, and p38 and JNK–AP-1 signaling pathways – inhibits TNF-α-induced expression of inflammatory cytokines and ECM-degrading enzymes – prevents cell proliferation of fibroblast-like synoviocytes by inhibiting target genes of PI3K–AKT pathway and genes of cytokine–cytokine receptor interactions – enhances Nrf2 translocation to the nucleus, activating the gene expression of the antioxidant and detoxifying enzymes	[86] [89]
Multiple sclerosis	RJ and 10-HDA	– reduce demyelination, modulate the inflammatory response by acting on the polarization of Th17 and Th1 cells, and reduce the infiltration of inflammatory cells in the CNS	[90,91]
Herpes stromal keratitis (HSK)	RJ and MRJP3 or its C-terminal tandem pentapeptide repeats (TPRs) sequence	– inhibit production of pro-inflammatory cytokines TNF-α, IL-1β, IL-2, IL-6, and IL-33	[92,93,363]
Anti-cancer			
	MRJPs MRJP-1 10-HDA	– decrease activity of MMP-9, AKT, and MAPK – increase levels of caspase 3 and 9, and Bax – inhibit metabolism of 2-aminofluorene (2-AF) metabolites in a human liver tumor cell line and decrease the 2-AF in J5 cells – inhibit tumor-induced angiogenesis and/or the activation of immune function – inhibit proliferation of B16F1 melanoma cells by inhibiting the expression of microphthalmia-associated transcription factor, tyrosinase-related protein 1 (TRP-1) and TRP-2, and inhibit melanin production, then inhibit skin pigmentation in mice – induce apoptosis of A549 human lung cancer cells through the ROS-ERK-p38 and CHOP pathways – inhibit production of TNF-α, IL-1β, IL-8, and NF-κB in WiDr cells – reduce Bcl-2 and Ki-67 expression, enhance p53 and caspase 3/7 – inhibit the expression of Bcl-2 and p53 in HepG2 cells – reduce the paraneoplastic syndrome in RCC patients by decreasing concentration of TNF-α and TGF-β – acts as a potent HDAC inhibitor	[232,252] [242,243] [240] [232] [233] [234,235] [68] [275] [241] [252] [47,88]
Anti-oxidative			

Table 5. *Cont.*

Biological Activity	Active Component	Molecular and Cellular Effect of RJ	References
	MRJP-2 dipeptides Free amino acids	– increase SOD, CAT, GR, and GPx activities and GSH levels – decrease levels of ROS – decrease MMPs, MDA, and NO – upregulate Nrf2 pathway – enhance HO-1 expression	[62–68] [85] [67,88] [67]
	4-hydroperoxy-2-decenoic acid ethyl ester (HPO-DAEE), and RJ fatty acid derivative	– increases the expression of HO-1 mRNA by activating Nrf2 signaling pathway in human neuroblastoma SH-SY5Y cells – promotes phosphorylation of eukaryotic initiation factor 2α (eIF2α) and nuclear accumulation of the activating transcription factor-4 (ATF4) – suppresses UVA-induced expression of MMP-1 and MMP-3 by inhibiting the activation of JNK and p38-MAPK pathways in human dermal fibroblasts – suppresses the expression of tyrosinase-related protein (TRP)-1 and TRP-2, which are oxidases and rate-limiting enzymes that regulate melanin production	[67,68] [237,238] [98] [117,224] [233]
Immunoregulatory activity			
	RJ and 10-HDA	– directly activate the immune functions of macrophages, T lymphocytes, B lymphocytes, and natural killer cells – promote macrophage recovery, their number, and activity – modulate innate immunity through IIS/DAF-16, p38 MAPK, and Wnt signaling pathways – stimulate production of cytokines, enabling regulation of the immune response – restore the proliferation of thymus and spleen cells – stimulate the hematopoietic function of the spleen and the survival of mice by reducing the level of prostaglandin which regulates the proliferation of lymphocytes and inhibits the tumoricidal activity of normal macrophages – increase plaque-forming splenocytes, antibody production, and immunocompetent cell proliferation – modulate immune responses via downregulation of NLRP1 – induce maturation of immune cells, stimulate innate and adaptive immune responses	[226] [36,226–230,246] [125] [246] [229,243–245] [230] [13] [76,238,243,246, 250] [267,268]
	MRP3	– suppresses production of IL-4, inhibits serum levels of anti-OVA IgE and IgG1	[37]
	MRJPs	– increase immunoglobulin content, immune factors levels, and proliferation of spleen lymphocytes	[74,77,246]

Table 5. *Cont.*

Biological Activity	Active Component	Molecular and Cellular Effect of RJ	References
Anti-allergic effect			
	RJ	– inhibits mast cell degranulation, suppresses cysteinyl-leukotriene release, reduces serum histamine, IgG, and IgE levels in various allergic conditions by suppressing expression of histamine H1 receptor – restores the macrophage function and improves Th1/Th2 cell response – enhances antigen-specific mucosal IgA response	[37,333–338] [333] [339]
Osteoporosis			
	10-HDA	– inhibits osteoclast differentiation and function by suppression of the NF-kB signaling pathway and its downstream molecules including NFATc1, CtsK, TRAP, V-ATPase D2, and MMP9, via FFAR4 – decreases RANK, RANKL, NF-κB, IL-1β,TNF-α, caspase 3, MMP9 and CTX-1, and number of mature osteoclast – increases ALP, RUNX2, OSX, collagen type 1, OPG – increases proliferation, osteoblast differentiation, and bone mineralization – increases bone strength	[206] [206,222] [206,220,221] [37,66,86,121,223–225]
	RJ and RJP	– enhance intestinal calcium absorption – RJP prevents bone abnormality caused by sex hormone deficiency – Inhibit RANKL-induced osteoclastogenesis	[220,221]
Estrogen effect			
	RJ and 10-HDA	– improves regularity of the estrus cycle, ovarian histology and function, and level of reproductive hormones (LH, T, FSH, E2) – improves ovarian oxidant–antioxidant status (MDA, TAC, GPx) – increases reproductive potential, follicular growth, and estradiol secretion	[121,211–214] [212,213] [208–211]
Spematogenesis			

Table 5. *Cont.*

Biological Activity	Active Component	Molecular and Cellular Effect of RJ	References
	RJ	– increases cellular antioxidant activity and levels of detoxifying molecules, including GSH, GPx, GR, SOD, CAT, and Nrf2 – preserves percentage of viable spermatozoa and glutathione levels during exposure to toxic metals and pro-oxidants – regulates levels of FSH, LH, TSH, T4, T3, and testosterone – protects testicular structure from the damaging effect of diabetic oxidative stress and preserve male fertility through its antioxidant effect	[215,216] [217] [217–219]
Growth-promoting and wound healing activities			
	RJ MRJP1	– stimulate growth of human lymphoid cell lines (U-937, THP-1, U-M, HB4C5, HF10B4) – RJ induces proliferation of human cell lines and partially replaces FBS – upregulates SOD1, mTOR, and catenin beta like-1, and downregulates p53 – promote wound repair – inhibit production of proinflammatory cytokine and NO – show scavenging activity – reduce MPO activity – posseses a healing effect against the chemotherapy- and radiotherapy-induced oral mucositis	[21,26,33,111,246, 332] [36,313–325] [111] [313–315] [313,314,327,329, 330] [326–331]
	SA, 10-HDA, and 10-HDAA	– have anti-inflammatory activity	[53]
	Royalactin, royalisin, 10-HDA	– show regenerative ability	[44,105,313–325]
	MRJP mixture (MRP1-MRP7)	– increases proliferation, minimizes senescence, and elongates telomeres – increases viability by protecting NIH-3T3 cells against oxidative stress-induced cell apoptosis – activates a pluripotency gene network that enables self-renewal in mouse embryonic stem cells (mESC) – promotes wound healing by inducing proliferation and migration of human epidermal keratinocytes – contribute to tissue regeneration and wound closure	[26,111,313–325] [29] [44] [26] [313–315]
Antimicrobial activity			

Table 5. *Cont.*

Biological Activity	Active Component	Molecular and Cellular Effect of RJ	References
	cysteine-rich AMPs and royalisin Jelleine-I-IV Chlorine-jelleine-I (Cl-J-I), bromine-jelleine-I (Br-J-I), and iodine-jelleine-I (I-J-I), MRJP1	– interact with membrane enzymes and proteins and cause an opposite flow of protons, affect cellular activity including energy production (membrane-coupled), membrane transport, metabolic regulatory functions, and synthesis of DNA and RNA, prevent protein translation, and suppress microbial virulence factors – participate in membrane permeabilization of the bacterial cell – increase total antibody and isotypes of antibodies such as IgM, IgG1, IgG2a, and IgG2b	[48,63,68,292–300] [301,304,305] [307]
	glucose oxidase enzyme (GOx)	– catalyzes oxidation of glucose to hydrogen peroxide which shows prominent antibacterial effect	[292,298,299]
Antiviral activity		-	
	10-HDA	– promotes human monocyte-derived dendritic cells to produce Th1 cytokine pattern – stimulates B lymphocytes to produce antibodies against HCV and HIV	[48,63,68,292–295] [307]
	MRJPs MRJP2 and MRJP2 X1 MRJP1	– exert an inhibitory influence, via different mechanisms, for SARS-CoV-2 non-structural proteins (main and papain proteases, RNA replicase, RNA-dependent RNA polymerase, and methyltransferase). – can bind to most of the oxy- and deoxyhemoglobin-binding sites or cofactor-binding site residues on the viral nsp3, nsp5, nsp9, nsp12, and nsp16 and prevent their hemoglobin attack – promote Th1 immune polarization (IFN-γ activates TCD8+ and TCD4+ lymphocytes against viral infections to eliminate infected cells)	[305–311] [308] [307]
	RJ	– reduces oxidative stress and levels of IL-6, IL-8, and TNF-α	[292,298,299,327–331]

Note: Aβ, amyloid beta; ACE, angiotensin-converting enzyme; Ach, acetylcholine; Akt, protein kinase B; ALP, alkaline phosphatase; ALT, alanin-aminotransferase; AMPK, AMP-activated protein kinase; anti-OVA, antibodies that detect ovalbumin; AP-1, Activator protein 1; ApoA-I, apolipoprotein A-I; Apo-B, apolipoprotein B; APP, amyloid precursor protein; ARE, antioxidant response element; AST, aspartate aminotransferase; ATF4, activating transcription factor-4; ATM, ataxia telangiectasia-mutated; ATR, ataxia telangiectasia-mutated and Rad3-related; BACE1, beta-site APP cleaving enzyme 1; BAT, brown adipose tissue; Bax, Bcl-2-associated X protein; BBB, blood–brain barrier; Bcl-2, B-cell lymphoma-2; BDNF, brain-derived neurotrophic factor; BMD, bone mineral density; CAT, catalase; CDKs, cyclin-dependent kinases; C/EBP, CCAAT/enhancer-binding protein; Chk1, checkpoint kinase 1; CHOP, C/EBP homologous protein; CNS, central nervous system; COX-2, Cyclooxygenase-2; CTNNB1, Catenin beta-1; CTSK, cathepsin K; CTX, C-terminal telopeptide; CVDs, cardiovascular diseases; DAF-16/FoxO, DAF-16, forkhead box o; DSS, dextran sulfate sodium; E2, estradiol; ECM, extracellular matrix; EGFR, epidermal growth factor receptor; eIF2α, eukaryotic initiation factor 2α; ERα, estrogen receptors alpha; ERβ, estrogen receptor beta; ERK, extracellular signal-regulated kinase; FBS, fetal bovine serum; FFAR4, free fatty acid receptor 4; FGF, fibroblast growth factor; FLS, fibroblast-like synoviocytes; FSH, follicle-stimulating hormone; GLUT-4, glucose transporter 4; GPx, glutathione peroxidase; GR, glutathione reductase; GSH, glutathione; HGF, human growth factor; HbA1c, glycated hemoglobin; HCV, hepatitis C virus; HDACI, histone deacetylase inhibitor; HDL-C, high-density lipoprotein cholesterol; HIV, human immunodeficiency virus; HO-1, heme oxygenase 1; HOMA-IR, Homeostatic Model Assessment for Insulin Resistance; IDE, insulin-degrading enzyme; IgE, immunoglobulin E; IgG1, immunoglobulin G1; IGH, insulin-like growth factor; IκB-ζ, induced inhibitor of kappa-B-zeta; IL-1β interleukin 1 beta; ILC1, innate lymphoid cells 1; ILC3, innate lymphoid cells 3; iNOS, Inducible nitric oxide synthase; IRS, insulin receptor substrate; JNK, c-Jun N-terminal kinase; LDL-C, low-density lipoprotein cholesterol; LH, luteinizing hormone; LPS, lipopolysaccharide; LEP-1, low-density lipoprotein receptor-related protein 1; MAPK, mitogen-activated protein kinase; MCP-1, monocyte chemoattractant protein-1; MCP-2, monocyte chemoattractant protein-2; MCP-4, monocyte chemoattractant protein-4; MDA, malondialdehyde; mESCs, mouse embryonic stem cells; MMP-1, matrix metalloproteinase 1; MMP-3, matrix metalloproteinase 3; MMP-9, matrix metalloproteinase 9; MMPs, matrix metalloproteinases; MPO, myeloperoxidase; mTOR, mammalian target of rapamycin; MUC2, mucin; NaMN, nicotinic acid mononucleotide; NEP, neprilysin; NFAT c1, nuclear factor of activated T cell; NF-κB, nuclear factor kappa-light-chain-enhancer of activated B cells; NGF, nerve growth factor; NLRP1, NOD-like receptor (NLR) family pyrin domain-containing 1; NO, nitric oxide; Nrf2, nuclear factor E2-related factor 2; OPG, osteoprotegerin; Osx, Osterix; OVX, ovariectomy; PGC-1α, peroxisome proliferator-activated receptor-γ coactivator-1 alpha; PI3K, phosphatidylinositol 3-kinase; PPAR-γ, peroxisome proliferator-activated receptor gamma; PTEN, phosphatase and tensin homolog; RAGE, receptor for advanced glycation end products; RANK, receptor activator of nuclear factor-κB; RANKL, receptor activator of NF-κB ligand; *RB*, retinoblastoma gene; RCC, renal cell carcinoma; ROS, reactive oxygen species; RUNX2, runt-related transcription factor 2; S6K1, S6 kinase 1; SASP, senescence-associated secretory phenotype; SCFAs, short-chain fatty acids; SOD, superoxide dismutase; T, Testosterone; T3, triiodothyronine; T4, thyroxine; TC, total cholesterol; TGF-β, transforming growth factor-beta; TNF-α, Tumor Necrosis Factor alpha; TNBS, 2, 4,6-trinitrobenzene sulfonic acid; TRP-1, tyrosinase-related protein 1; TRP-2, tyrosinase-related protein 2; TSH, thyroid stimulating hormone; UCP1, uncoupling protein 1; VLDL-C, very-low-density lipoprotein cholesterol; VSMCs, vascular smooth muscle cells.

Table 6. Dosage of Royal Jelly for human use—clinical trials.

Application	Dose/Period of Treatment	Conditions/Diseases	References
Infants:	0.5 g/day for 2–12 months	– growth and development – strengthen immunity and nervous system	[6]
For premature babies	50 mg to 1 g per day	– growth and development – strengthen immunity and nervous system	[6]
Children: Children aged 1–5 yrs old Children aged 5–12 yrs old	0.5 g/day 0.5–1 g/day different period, condition-depedent	– low immune system – nervous system impairment (foetal suffering, delivery complication when born) – weakness, loss of appetite, anorexia, – anemia, etc.	[6]
Children aged 1–5 yrs old Children aged 5–12 yrs old	2.5 g/day, 1–3 days 5 g/day, 1–3 days	– acute infection and colds	[6]
Children	2 g, 3 months	– reduces the consequences of SLE	[336]

Table 6. *Cont.*

Application	Dose/Period of Treatment	Conditions/Diseases	References
Adults:	1 to 2 g/day	– immunity – insomnia – skin disorders, rejuvenation – for maintenance of skin, hair, nails, bones, joints – anemia – low libido, sexual vitality – hormonal imbalance, wounds – premenstrual syndrome, menopause, osteoporosis, etc. – mental condition, memory, depression	[6,29,36]
	3–5 g/day	– diabetes – depression, Hashimoto's disease, – arthritis	[6]
	3000 mg, 6 months	– Osteoporosis, improved BMD, and strength in postmenopausal women	[223]
	Up to 10 g/day for 1–3 days	– in the beginning of colds	[6]
	10 g/day for 1–3 days 5–10 g/day up to 3–5 days	– in acute infections – to accelerate post-operative healing	[6]
	1000 mg, 8 weeks	– Menopausal symptoms	[91,211,224,225]
	5000, 8 weeks	– Sub-fertility	[6,364]
	1000 mg, 8 weeks	– Type 2 diabetes mellitus – high blood pressure	[365]
	3600 mg, 24 months	– Hemodialysis	[366]

Table 6. *Cont.*

Application	Dose/Period of Treatment	Conditions/Diseases	References
	500 mg, 3 weeks	– Multiple sclerosis	[90]
	10–15 g/day, long-term	– Neurodegenerative diseases, multiple sclerosis, Parkins, anti-depressive, anti-anxiety	[6,36]
	800 mg, 12 weeks	– Dry mouth sensations	[367]
	3000 mg, 2 weeks	– Traumatic brain injury	[368]
	100 mg, 8 weeks	– Infertility, impotence, hormonal regulator	[369]
	1000 mg, 8 weeks	– Genitourinary syndrome	[91,92]
	900 mg, 13 weeks	– Metastatic renal cell carcinoma	[252]
	3000 mg, 6–8 weeks	– Side effects of chemotherapy and radiotherapy such as paresthesia, pain or burning, sensation of fingers, imbalance during walking, the sensation of weakness in the legs – chronic fatigue – recovery from disease – immunological system stimulation	[252,264,281]

Author Contributions: Conceptualization, N.O.; writing—original draft preparation, N.O.; writing—review and editing, N.O. and M.J.J.; visualization, N.O. and M.J.J. All authors have read and agreed to the published version of the manuscript.

Funding: This research received no external funding.

Conflicts of Interest: The authors declare no conflicts of interest.

References

1. Tsopmo, A.; Hosseinian, F. Antioxidants in functional foods. *J. Food. Biochem.* **2022**, *46*, e14167. [CrossRef]
2. Popescu, O.; Mărghitaş, L.A.; Dezmirean, D.S. A study about physicochemical composition of fresh and lyophilized royal jelly. *Zooteh. Si Biotehnol.* **2008**, *41*, 328–332.
3. Collazo, N.; Carpena, M.; Nuñez-Estevez, B.; Otero, P.; Simal-Gandara, J.; Prieto, M.A. Health Promoting Properties of Bee Royal Jelly: Food of the Queens. *Nutrients* **2021**, *13*, 543. [CrossRef]
4. Oršolić, N.; Jazvinšćak Jembrek, M. Molecular and Cellular Mechanisms of Propolis and Its Polyphenolic Compounds against Cancer. *Int. J. Mol. Sci.* **2022**, *23*, 10479. [CrossRef] [PubMed]
5. Ahmad, S.; Campos, M.G.; Fratini, F.; Altaye, S.Z.; Li, J. New Insights into the Biological and Pharmaceutical Properties of Royal Jelly. *Int. J. Mol. Sci.* **2020**, *21*, 382. [CrossRef]
6. Strant, M.; Yücel, B.; Topal, E.; Puscasu, A.M.; Margaoan, R.; Varadi, A. Use of Royal Jelly as Functional Food on Human and Animal Health. *Hayvansal Üretim* **2019**, *60*, 131–144. [CrossRef]
7. Botezan, S.; Baci, G.-M.; Bagameri, L.; Paşca, C.; Dezmirean, D.S. Current Status of the Bioactive Properties of Royal Jelly: A Comprehensive Review with a Focus on Its Anticancer, Anti-Inflammatory, and Antioxidant Effects. *Molecules* **2023**, *28*, 1510. [CrossRef]
8. Xue, X.; Wu, L.; Wang, K. Chemical composition of royal jelly. In *Bee Products-Chemical and Biological Properties*; Alvarez-Suarez, J.M., Ed.; Springer International Publishing: Cham, Switzerland, 2017; pp. 181–190.
9. Buttstedt, A. The role of 10-hydroxy-Δ^2-decenoic acid in the formation of fibrils of the major royal jelly protein 1/apisimin/24-methylenecholesterol complex isolated from honey bee (*Apis mellifera*) royal jelly. *Eur. J. Entomol.* **2022**, *119*, 448–453. [CrossRef]
10. Furusawa, T.; Arai, Y.; Kato, K.; Ichihara, K. Quantitative Analysis of Apisin, a Major Protein Unique to Royal Jelly. *Evid. Based Complement. Altern. Med.* **2016**, *2016*, 5040528. [CrossRef] [PubMed]
11. Fang, Y.; Feng, M.; Ma, C.; Rueppell, O.; Li, J. Major royal jelly proteins influence the neurobiological regulation of the division of labor among honey bee workers. *Int. J. Biol. Macromol.* **2023**, *225*, 848–860. [CrossRef]
12. Ramanathan, A.N.K.G.; Nair, A.J.; Sugunan, V.S. A review on Royal Jelly proteins and peptides. *J. Funct. Foods* **2018**, *44*, 255–264. [CrossRef]
13. Bagameri, L.; Botezan, S.; Bobis, O.; Bonta, V.; Dezmirean, D.S. Molecular Insights into Royal Jelly Anti-Inflammatory Properties and Related Diseases. *Life* **2023**, *13*, 1573. [CrossRef] [PubMed]
14. Mureşan, C.I.; Dezmirean, D.S.; Marc, B.D.; Suharoschi, R.; Pop, O.L.; Buttstedt, A. Biological properties and activities of major royal jelly proteins and their derived peptides. *J. Funct. Foods* **2022**, *98*, 105286. [CrossRef]
15. Wang, X.; Dong, J.; Qiao, J.; Zhang, G.; Zhang, H. Purification and characteristics of individual major royal jelly protein 1–3. *J. Apic. Res.* **2020**, *59*, 1049–1060. [CrossRef]
16. Tian, W.; Li, M.; Guo, H.; Peng, W.; Xue, X.; Hu, Y.; Liu, Y.; Zhao, Y.; Fang, X.; Wang, K.; et al. Architecture of the native major royal jelly protein 1 oligomer. *Nat. Commun.* **2018**, *9*, 3373. [CrossRef] [PubMed]
17. Li, S.; Tao, L.; Yu, X.; Zheng, H.; Wu, J.; Hu, F. Royal Jelly Proteins and Their Derived Peptides: Preparation, Properties, and Biological Activities. *J. Agric. Food Chem.* **2021**, *69*, 14415–14427. [CrossRef] [PubMed]
18. Albert, S.; Klaudiny, J. The MRJP/YELLOW protein family of *Apis mellifera*: Identification of new members in the EST library. *J. Insect Physiol.* **2004**, *50*, 51–59. [CrossRef] [PubMed]
19. Drapeau, M.D.; Albert, S.; Kucharski, R.; Prusko, C.; Maleszka, R. Evolution of the Yellow/Major Royal Jelly Protein family and the emergence of social behavior in honey bees. *Genome Res.* **2006**, *16*, 1385–1394. [CrossRef] [PubMed]
20. Ward, R.; Coffey, M.; Kavanagh, K. Proteomic analysis of summer and winter *Apis mellifera* workers shows reduced protein abundance in winter samples. *J. Insect Physiol.* **2022**, *139*, 104397. [CrossRef]
21. Kimura, M.; Kimura, Y.; Tsumura, K.; Okihara, K.; Sugimoto, H.; Yamada, H.; Yonekura, M. 350-kDa royal jelly glycoprotein (apisin), which stimulates proliferation of human monocytes, bears the beta1-3galactosylated N-glycan: Analysis of the N-glycosylation site. *Biosci. Biotechnol. Biochem.* **2003**, *67*, 2055–2058. [CrossRef]
22. Li, J.; Wang, T.; Zhang, Z.; Pan, Y. Proteomic analysis of royal jelly from three strains of western honeybees (*Apis mellifera*). *J. Agric. Food Chem.* **2007**, *55*, 8411–8422. [CrossRef] [PubMed]
23. Ramadan, M.F.; Al-Ghamdi, A. Bioactive compounds and health-promoting properties of royal jelly: A review. *J. Funct. Foods* **2012**, *4*, 39–52. [CrossRef]
24. Nazemi-Rafie, J.; Fatehi, F.; Hasrak, S. A comparative transcriptome analysis of the head of 1 and 9 days old worker honeybees (*Apis mellifera*). *Bull. Entomol. Res.* **2023**, *113*, 253–270. [CrossRef] [PubMed]
25. Andyshe, R.; Nazemi-Rafie, J.; Maleki, M.; Fatehi, F. Comparative proteomics analysis of the head proteins of worker honey bees (*Apis mellifera*) in production stage of royal jelly. *J. Apic. Res.* **2022**, 1–15. [CrossRef]

26. Lin, Y.; Shao, Q.; Zhang, M.; Lu, C.; Fleming, J.; Su, S. Royal jelly-derived proteins enhance proliferation and migration of human epidermal keratinocytes in an in vitro scratch wound model. *BMC Complement. Altern. Med.* **2019**, *19*, 175. [CrossRef] [PubMed]
27. Kamakura, M.; Moriyama, T.; Sakaki, T. Changes in hepatic gene expression associated with the hypocholesterolaemic activity of royal jelly. *J. Pharm. Pharmacol.* **2006**, *58*, 1683–1689. [CrossRef] [PubMed]
28. Mishima, S.; Suzuki, K.M.; Isohama, Y.; Kuratsu, N.; Araki, Y.; Inoue, M.; Miyata, T. Royal jelly has estrogenic effects in vitro and in vivo. *J. Ethnopharmacol.* **2005**, *101*, 215–220. [CrossRef] [PubMed]
29. Park, M.J.; Kim, B.Y.; Deng, Y.; Park, H.G.; Choi, Y.S.; Lee, K.S.; Jin, B.R. Antioxidant capacity of major royal jelly proteins of honeybee (*Apis mellifera*) royal jelly. *J. Asia. Pac. Entomol.* **2020**, *23*, 445–448. [CrossRef]
30. Wan, D.C.; Morgan, S.L.; Spencley, A.L.; Mariano, N.; Chang, E.Y.; Shankar, G.; Luo, Y.; Li, T.H.; Huh, D.; Huynh, S.K.; et al. Honey bee Royalactin unlocks conserved pluripotency pathway in mammals. *Nat. Commun.* **2018**, *9*, 5078. [CrossRef]
31. Minegaki, N.; Koshizuka, T.; Nishina, S.; Kondo, H.; Takahashi, K.; Sugiyama, T.; Inoue, N. The carboxyl-terminal penta-peptide repeats of major royal jelly protein 3 enhance cell proliferation. *Biol. Pharm. Bull.* **2020**, *43*, 1911–1916. [CrossRef]
32. Narita, Y.; Ohta, S.; Suzuki, K.M.; Nemoto, T.; Abe, K.; Mishima, S. Effects of long-term administration of royal jelly on pituitary weight and gene expression in middle-aged female rats. *Biosci. Biotechnol. Biochem.* **2009**, *73*, 431–433. [CrossRef] [PubMed]
33. Watanabe, K.; Shinmoto, H.; Kobori, M.; Tsushida, T.; Shinohara, K.; Kanaeda, J.; Yonekura, M. Stimulation of cell growth in the U-937 human myeloid cell line by honey royal jelly protein. *Cytotechnology* **1998**, *26*, 23–27. [CrossRef] [PubMed]
34. Nakaya, M.; Onda, H.; Sasaki, K.; Yukiyoshi, A.; Tachibana, H.; Yamada, K. Effect of royal jelly on bisphenol A-induced proliferation of human breast cancer cells. *BioSci. Biotechnol. Biochem.* **2007**, *71*, 253–255. [CrossRef] [PubMed]
35. Simúth, J.; Bíliková, K.; Kovácová, E.; Kuzmová, Z.; Schroder, W. Immunochemical approach to detection of adulteration in honey: Physiologically active royal jelly protein stimulating TNF-alpha release is a regular component of honey. *J. Agric. Food Chem.* **2004**, *52*, 2154–2158. [CrossRef] [PubMed]
36. Kohno, K.; Okamoto, I.; Sano, O.; Arai, N.; Iwaki, K.; Ikeda, M.; Kurimoto, M. Royal jelly inhibits the production of proinflammatory cytokines by activated macrophages. *Biosci. Biotechnol. Biochem.* **2004**, *68*, 138–145. [CrossRef] [PubMed]
37. Okamoto, I.; Taniguchi, Y.; Kunikata, T.; Kohno, K.; Iwaki, K.; Ikeda, M.; Kurimoto, M. Major royal jelly protein 3 modulates immune responses in vitro and in vivo. *Life Sci.* **2003**, *73*, 2029–2045. [CrossRef] [PubMed]
38. Kim, B.Y.; Jin, B.R. Antimicrobial activity of the C-terminal of the major royal jelly protein 4 in a honeybee (*Apis cerana*). *J. Asia Pac. Entomol.* **2019**, *22*, 561–564. [CrossRef]
39. Ferioli, F.; Marcazzan, G.L.; Caboni, M.F. Determination of (E)-10-hydroxy-2-decenoic acid content in pure royal jelly: A comparison between a new CZE method and HPLC. *J. Sep. Sci.* **2007**, *30*, 1061–1069. [CrossRef]
40. Uversky, V.N.; Albar, A.H.; Khan, R.H.; Redwan, E.M. Multifunctionality and intrinsic disorder of royal jelly proteome. *Proteomics* **2021**, *21*, e2000237. [CrossRef]
41. Buttstedt, A.; Mureşan, C.I.; Lilie, H.; Hause, G.; Ihling, C.H.; Schulze, S.H.; Pietzsch, M.; Moritz, R.F.A. How Honeybees Defy Gravity with Royal Jelly to Raise Queens. *Curr. Biol.* **2018**, *28*, 1095–1100.e3. [CrossRef]
42. Kanelis, D.; Tananaki, C.; Liolios, V.; Dimou, M.; Goras, G.; Rodopoulou, M.A.; Karazafiris, E.; Thrasyvoulou, A. A suggestion for royal jelly specifications. *Arh. Hig. Rada Toksikol.* **2015**, *66*, 275–284. [CrossRef] [PubMed]
43. Kamakura, M. Royalactin induces queen differentiation in honeybees. *Nature* **2011**, *473*, 478–483. [CrossRef] [PubMed]
44. Renard, T.; Gueydan, C.; Aron, S. DNA methylation and expression of the egfr gene are associated with worker size in monomorphic ants. *Sci. Rep.* **2022**, *12*, 21228. [CrossRef] [PubMed]
45. Matsuyama, S.; Nagao, T.; Sasaki, K. Consumption of tyrosine in royal jelly increases brain levels of dopamine and tyramine and promotes transition from normal to reproductive workers in queenless honey bee colonies. *Gen. Comp. Endocrinol.* **2015**, *211*, 1–8. [CrossRef] [PubMed]
46. Pyrzanowska, J.; Piechal, A.; Blecharz-Klin, K.; Joniec-Maciejak, I.; Graikou, K.; Chinou, I.; Widy-Tyszkiewicz, E. Long-term administration of Greek royal jelly improves spatial memory and influences the concentration of brain neurotransmitters in naturally aged Wistar male rats. *J. Ethnopharmacol.* **2014**, *155*, 343–351. [CrossRef] [PubMed]
47. Alhosin, M. Epigenetics Mechanisms of Honeybees: Secrets of Royal Jelly. *Epigenet. Insights.* **2023**, *16*, 25168657231213717. [CrossRef] [PubMed]
48. Bagameri, L.; Baci, G.-M.; Dezmirean, D.S. Royal Jelly as a Nutraceutical Natural Product with a Focus on Its Antibacterial Activity. *Pharmaceutics* **2022**, *14*, 1142. [CrossRef] [PubMed]
49. Mumoki, F.N.; Crewe, R.M. Pheromone communication in honey bees (*Apis mellifera*). In *Insect Pheromone Biochemistry and Molecular Biology*, 2nd ed.; Blomquist, G.J., Vogt, R.G., Eds.; Academic Press: Cambridge, MA, USA; Elsevier: Cambridge, MA, USA, 2021; pp. 183–204. [CrossRef]
50. Polsinelli, G.A.; Yu, H.D. Regulation of histone deacetylase 3 by metal cations and 10-hydroxy-2E-decenoic acid: Possible epigenetic mechanisms of queen-worker bee differentiation. *PLoS ONE* **2018**, *13*, e0204538. [CrossRef] [PubMed]
51. Buttstedt, A.; Ihling, C.H.; Pietzsch, M.; Moritz, R.F.A. Royalactin is not a royal making of a queen. *Nature* **2016**, *537*, E10–E12. [CrossRef]
52. Moraru, D.; Alexa, E.; Cocan, I.; Obistioiu, D.; Radulov, I.; Simiz, E.; Berbecea, A.; Grozea, A.; Dragomirescu, M.; Vintila, T.; et al. Chemical Characterization and Antioxidant Activity of Apilarnil, Royal Jelly, and Propolis Collected in Banat Region, Romania. *Appl. Sci.* **2024**, *14*, 1242. [CrossRef]

53. Kunugi, H.; Mohammed Ali, A. Royal Jelly and Its Components Promote Healthy Aging and Longevity: From Animal Models to Humans. *Int. J. Mol. Sci.* **2019**, *20*, 4662. [CrossRef] [PubMed]
54. Terker, A.S.; Zhang, C.; McCormick, J.A.; Lazelle, R.A.; Zhang, C.; Meermeier, N.P.; Siler, D.A.; Park, H.J.; Fu, Y.; Cohen, D.M.; et al. Potassium modulates electrolyte balance and blood pressure through effects on distal cell voltage and chloride. *Cell Metab.* **2015**, *21*, 39–50. [CrossRef] [PubMed]
55. Jomova, K.; Makova, M.; Alomar, S.Y.; Alwasel, S.H.; Nepovimova, E.; Kuca, K.; Rhodes, C.J.; Valko, M. Essential metals in health and disease. *Chem. Biol. Interact.* **2022**, *367*, 110173. [CrossRef] [PubMed]
56. Cormick, G.; Betran, A.P.; Romero, I.B.; Cormick, M.S.; Belizán, J.M.; Bardach, A.; Ciapponi, A. Effect of Calcium Fortified Foods on Health Outcomes: A Systematic Review and Meta-Analysis. *Nutrients* **2021**, *13*, 316. [CrossRef] [PubMed]
57. Yuan, S.; Yu, L.; Gou, W.; Wang, L.; Sun, J.; Li, D.; Lu, Y.; Cai, X.; Yu, H.; Yuan, C.; et al. Health effects of high serum calcium levels: Updated phenome-wide Mendelian randomisation investigation and review of Mendelian randomisation studies. *eBioMedicine* **2022**, *76*, 103865. [CrossRef] [PubMed]
58. Mureşan, C.I.; Schierhorn, A.; Buttstedt, A. The Fate of Major Royal Jelly Proteins during Proteolytic Digestion in the Human Gastrointestinal Tract. *J. Agric. Food Chem.* **2018**, *66*, 4164–4170. [CrossRef] [PubMed]
59. Ali, A.M.; Kunugi, H. Royal Jelly as an Intelligent Anti-Aging Agent—A Focus on Cognitive Aging and Alzheimer's Disease: A Review. *Antioxidants* **2020**, *9*, 937. [CrossRef] [PubMed]
60. Khazaei, M.; Ansarian, A.; Ghanbari, E. New Findings on Biological Actions and Clinical Applications of Royal Jelly: A Review. *J. Diet Suppl.* **2018**, *15*, 757–775. [CrossRef] [PubMed]
61. Hassan, A.A.M.; Elenany, Y.E.; Nassrallah, A.; Cheng, W.; Abd El-Maksoud, A.A. Royal Jelly Improves the Physicochemical Properties and Biological Activities of Fermented Milk with Enhanced Probiotic Viability. *Lebensm. Wiss. Technol.* **2022**, *155*, 112912. [CrossRef]
62. Nabas, Z.; Haddadin, M.S.Y.; Haddadin, J.; Nazer, I.K. Chemical composition of royal jelly and effects of synbiotic with two different locally isolated probiotic strains on antioxidant activities. *Pol. J. Food Nutr. Sci.* **2014**, *64*, 171–180. [CrossRef]
63. Kocot, J.; Kiełczykowska, M.; Luchowska-Kocot, D.; Kurzepa, J.; Musik, I. Antioxidant Potential of Propolis, Bee Pollen, and Royal Jelly: Possible Medical Application. *Oxidative Med. Cell. Longev.* **2018**, *2018*, 7074209. [CrossRef] [PubMed]
64. Li, Q.; Zhang, W.; Zhou, E.; Tao, Y.; Wang, M.; Qi, S.; Zhao, L.; Tan, Y.; Wu, L. Integrated microbiomic and metabolomic analyses reveal the mechanisms by which bee pollen and royal jelly lipid extracts ameliorate colitis in mice. *Food Res. Int.* **2023**, *171*, 113069. [CrossRef] [PubMed]
65. Guo, H.; Kouzuma, Y.; Yonekura, M. Structures and properties of antioxidative peptides derived from royal jelly protein. *Food Chem.* **2009**, *113*, 238–245. [CrossRef]
66. Martinello, M.; Mutinelli, F. Antioxidant Activity in Bee Products: A Review. *Antioxidants* **2021**, *10*, 71. [CrossRef] [PubMed]
67. Chi, X.; Liu, Z.; Wang, H.; Wang, Y.; Wei, W.; Xu, B. Royal jelly enhanced the antioxidant activities and modulated the gut microbiota in healthy mice. *J. Food Biochem.* **2021**, *45*, e13701. [CrossRef] [PubMed]
68. Yang, Y.C.; Chou, W.M.; Widowati, D.A.; Lin, I.P.; Peng, C.C. 10-hydroxy-2-decenoic acid of royal jelly exhibits bactericide and anti-inflammatory activity in human colon cancer cells. *BMC Complement. Med. Ther.* **2018**, *18*, 202. [CrossRef] [PubMed]
69. El-Seedi, H.R.; Eid, N.; Abd El-Wahed, A.A.; Rateb, M.E.; Afifi, H.S.; Algethami, A.F.; Zhao, C.; Al Naggar, Y.; Alsharif, S.M.; Tahir, H.E.; et al. Honey Bee Products: Preclinical and Clinical Studies of Their Anti-inflammatory and Immunomodulatory Properties. *Front. Nutr.* **2022**, *8*, 761267. [CrossRef]
70. Aslan, Z.; Aksoy, L. Anti-inflammatory effects of royal jelly on ethylene glycol induced renal inflammation in rats. *Int. Braz. J. Urol.* **2015**, *41*, 1008–1013. [CrossRef] [PubMed]
71. Qu, N.; Jiang, J.; Sun, L.; Lai, C.; Sun, L.; Wu, X. Proteomic characterization of royal jelly proteins in Chinese (*Apis cerana*) and European (*Apis mellifera*) honeybees. *Biochemistry* **2008**, *73*, 676–680. [CrossRef]
72. Guo, J.; Ma, B.; Wang, Z.; Chen, Y.; Tian, W.; Dong, Y. Royal Jelly Protected against Dextran-Sulfate-Sodium-Induced Colitis by Improving the Colonic Mucosal Barrier and Gut Microbiota. *Nutrients* **2022**, *14*, 2069. [CrossRef]
73. Wu, H.; Zhou, S.; Ning, W.; Wu, X.; Xu, X.; Liu, Z.; Liu, W.; Liu, K.; Shen, L.; Wang, J. Major royal-jelly proteins intake modulates immune functions and gut microbiota in mice. *Food Sci. Hum. Wellness* **2024**, *13*, 444–453. [CrossRef]
74. Miyauchi-Wakuda, S.; Kagota, S.; Maruyama-Fumoto, K.; Wakuda, H.; Yamada, S.; Shinozuka, K. Effect of Royal Jelly on Mouse Isolated Ileum and Gastrointestinal Motility. *J. Med. Food* **2019**, *22*, 789–796. [CrossRef] [PubMed]
75. Bron, P.A.; Kleerebezem, M.; Brummer, R.-J.; Cani, P.D.; Mercenier, A.; MacDonald, T.T.; Garcia-Rodenas, C.L.; Wells, J.M. Can probiotics modulate human disease by impacting intestinal barrier function? *Br. J. Nutr.* **2017**, *117*, 93–107. [CrossRef] [PubMed]
76. Wang, W.; Li, X.; Li, D.; Pan, F.; Fang, X.; Peng, W.; Tian, W. Effects of Major Royal Jelly Proteins on the Immune Response and Gut Microbiota Composition in Cyclophosphamide-Treated Mice. *Nutrients* **2023**, *15*, 974. [CrossRef] [PubMed]
77. Alvarez-Curto, E.; Milligan, G. Metabolism Meets Immunity: The Role of Free Fatty Acid Receptors in the Immune System. *Biochem. Pharmacol.* **2016**, *114*, 3–13. [CrossRef] [PubMed]
78. Koch, P.D.; Pittet, M.J.; Weissleder, R. The Chemical Biology of IL-12 Production: Via the Non-Canonical NFkB Pathway. *RSC Chem. Biol.* **2020**, *1*, 166–176. [CrossRef] [PubMed]
79. Zinatizadeh, M.R.; Schock, B.; Chalbatani, G.M.; Zarandi, P.K.; Jalali, S.A.; Miri, S.R. The Nuclear Factor Kappa B (NF-KB) Signaling in Cancer Development and Immune Diseases. *Genes Dis.* **2021**, *8*, 287–297. [CrossRef] [PubMed]

80. Kobayashi, G.; Okamura, T.; Majima, S.; Senmaru, T.; Okada, H.; Ushigome, E.; Nakanishi, N.; Nishimoto, Y.; Yamada, T.; Okamoto, H.; et al. Effects of Royal Jelly on Gut Dysbiosis and NAFLD in *db/db* Mice. *Nutrients* **2023**, *15*, 2580. [CrossRef] [PubMed]
81. Mazzoccoli, G.; Vinciguerra, M.; Oben, J.; Tarquini, R.; De Cosmo, S. Non-alcoholic fatty liver disease: The role of nuclear receptors and circadian rhythmicity. *Liver Int.* **2014**, *34*, 1133–1152. [CrossRef]
82. You, M.M.; Liu, Y.C.; Chen, Y.F.; Pan, Y.M.; Miao, Z.N.; Shi, Y.Z.; Si, J.J.; Chen, M.L.; Hu, F.L. Royal jelly attenuates nonalcoholic fatty liver disease by inhibiting oxidative stress and regulating the expression of circadian genes in ovariectomized rats. *J. Food Biochem.* **2020**, *44*, e13138. [CrossRef]
83. Zhu, Y.Y.; Meng, X.C.; Zhou, Y.J.; Zhu, J.X.; Chang, Y.N. Major royal jelly proteins alleviate non-alcoholic fatty liver disease in mice model by regulating disordered metabolic pathways. *J. Food Biochem.* **2022**, *46*, e14214. [CrossRef] [PubMed]
84. Felemban, A.H.; Alshammari, G.M.; Yagoub, A.E.A.; Al-Harbi, L.N.; Alhussain, M.H.; Yahya, M.A. Activation of AMPK Entails the Protective Effect of Royal Jelly against High-Fat-Diet-Induced Hyperglycemia, Hyperlipidemia, and Non-Alcoholic Fatty Liver Disease in Rats. *Nutrients* **2023**, *15*, 1471. [CrossRef] [PubMed]
85. Yang, X.Y.; Yang, D.S.; Wang, J.M.; Li, C.Y.; Lei, K.F.; Chen, X.F.; Shen, N.H.; Jin, L.Q.; Wang, J.G. 10-Hydroxy-2-decenoic acid from Royal jelly: A potential medicine for RA. *J. Ethnopharmacol.* **2010**, *128*, 314–321. [CrossRef] [PubMed]
86. Ishida, K.; Matsumaru, D.; Shimizu, S.; Hiromori, Y.; Nagase, H.; Nakanishi, T. Evaluation of the Estrogenic Action Potential of Royal Jelly by Genomic Signaling Pathway In Vitro and In Vivo. *Biol. Pharm. Bull.* **2022**, *45*, 1510–1517. [CrossRef] [PubMed]
87. Hanai, R.; Matsushita, H.; Minami, A.; Abe, Y.; Tachibana, R.; Watanabe, K.; Takeuchi, H.; Wakatsuki, A. Effects of 10-Hydroxy-2-decenoic Acid and 10-Hydroxydecanoic Acid in Royal Jelly on Bone Metabolism in Ovariectomized Rats: A Pilot Study. *J. Clin. Med.* **2023**, *12*, 5309. [CrossRef] [PubMed]
88. Wang, J.; Zhang, W.; Zou, H.; Lin, Y.; Lin, K.; Zhou, Z.; Qiang, J.; Lin, J.; Chuka, C.M.; Ge, R.; et al. 10-Hydroxy-2-decenoic acid inhibiting the proliferation of fibroblast-like synoviocytes by PI3K-AKT pathway. *Int. Immunopharmacol.* **2015**, *28*, 97–104. [CrossRef] [PubMed]
89. Oshvandi, K.; Aghamohammadi, M.; Kazemi, F.; Masoumi, S.Z.; Mazdeh, M.; Molavi Vardanjani, M. Effect of royal jelly capsule on quality of life of patients with multiple sclerosis: A double-blind randomized controlled clinical trial. *Iran. Red. Crescent. Med. J.* **2020**, *22*, e74. [CrossRef]
90. Seyyedi, F.; Kopaei, M.R.; Miraj, S. Comparison between vaginal royal jelly and vaginal estrogen effects on quality of life and vaginal atrophy in postmenopausal women: A clinical trial study. *Electron Phys.* **2016**, *8*, 3184–3192. [CrossRef] [PubMed]
91. Vahid, M.; Fatemeh, D. Royal jelly for genitourinary syndrome of menopause: A randomized controlled trial. *Gyn. Obst. Clin. Med.* **2021**, *1*, 211–215. [CrossRef]
92. Pourmobini, H.; Kazemi Arababadi, M.; Salahshoor, M.R.; Roshankhah, S.; Taghavi, M.M.; Taghipour, Z.; Shabanizadeh, A. The effect of royal jelly and silver nanoparticles on liver and kidney inflammation. *Avicenna J. Phytomed.* **2021**, *11*, 218–223.
93. Salahshoor, M.R.; Jalili, C.; Roshankhah, S. Can royal jelly protect against renal ischemia/reperfusion injury in rats? *Chin. J. Physiol.* **2019**, *62*, 131–137. [CrossRef]
94. Elmallah, M.I.Y.; Elkhadragy, M.F.; Al-Olayan, E.M.; Abdel Moneim, A.E. Protective Effect of *Fragaria ananassa* Crude Extract on Cadmium-Induced Lipid Peroxidation, Antioxidant Enzymes Suppression, and Apoptosis in Rat Testes. *Int. J. Mol. Sci.* **2017**, *18*, 957. [CrossRef] [PubMed]
95. Almeer, R.S.; Soliman, D.; Kassab, R.B.; AlBasher, G.I.; Alarifi, S.; Alkahtani, S.; Ali, D.; Metwally, D.; Abdel Moneim, A.E. Royal Jelly Abrogates Cadmium-Induced Oxidative Challenge in Mouse Testes: Involvement of the Nrf2 Pathway. *Int. J. Mol. Sci.* **2018**, *19*, 3979. [CrossRef] [PubMed]
96. Jenkhetkana, W.; Thitiorulb, S.; Jansomc, C.; Ratanavalachai, T. Genoprotective effects of that royal jelly against doxorubicin in human lymphocytes in vitro. *Nat. Prod. Commun.* **2018**, *13*, 79–84. [CrossRef]
97. Inoue, Y.; Hara, H.; Mitsugi, Y.; Yamaguchi, E.; Kamiya, T.; Itoh, A.; Adachi, T. 4-Hydroperoxy-2-decenoic acid ethyl ester protects against 6-hydroxydopamine-induced cell death via activation of Nrf2-ARE and eIF2α-ATF4 pathways. *Neurochem. Int.* **2018**, *112*, 288–296. [CrossRef] [PubMed]
98. Kumari, R.; Jat, P. Mechanisms of Cellular Senescence: Cell Cycle Arrest and Senescence Associated Secretory Phenotype. *Front. Cell Dev. Biol.* **2021**, *9*, 645593. [CrossRef]
99. McHugh, D.; Gil, J. Senescence and aging: Causes, consequences, and therapeutic avenues. *J. Cell Biol.* **2018**, *217*, 65–77. [CrossRef]
100. Pedroza-Diaz, J.; Arroyave-Ospina, J.C.; Serna Salas, S.; Moshage, H. Modulation of Oxidative Stress-Induced Senescence during Non-Alcoholic Fatty Liver Disease. *Antioxidants* **2022**, *11*, 975. [CrossRef]
101. Calder, P.C.; Carr, A.C.; Gombart, A.F.; Eggersdorfer, M. Optimal Nutritional Status for a Well-Functioning Immune System Is an Important Factor to Protect against Viral Infections. *Nutrients* **2020**, *12*, 1181. [CrossRef]
102. Aiello, A.; Farzaneh, F.; Candore, G.; Caruso, C.; Davinelli, S.; Gambino, C.M.; Ligotti, M.E.; Zareian, N.; Accardi, G. Immunosenescence and Its Hallmarks: How to Oppose Aging Strategically? A Review of Potential Options for Therapeutic Intervention. *Front. Immunol.* **2019**, *10*, 2247. [CrossRef]
103. Ali, A.M.; Kunugi, H. Bee honey protects astrocytes against oxidative stress: A preliminary in vitro investigation. *Neuropsychopharmacol. Rep.* **2019**, *39*, 312–314. [CrossRef] [PubMed]

104. Xin, X.X.; Chen, Y.; Chen, D.; Xiao, F.; Parnell, L.D.; Zhao, J.; Liu, L.; Ordovas, J.M.; Lai, C.Q.; Shen, L.R. Supplementation with Major Royal-Jelly Proteins Increases Lifespan, Feeding, and Fecundity in Drosophila. *J. Agric. Food Chem.* **2016**, *64*, 5803–5812. [CrossRef] [PubMed]
105. Detienne, G.; De Haes, W.; Ernst, U.R.; Schoofs, L.; Temmerman, L. Royalactin extends lifespan of *Caenorhabditis elegans* through epidermal growth factor signaling. *Exp. Gerontol.* **2014**, *60*, 129–135. [CrossRef] [PubMed]
106. Wang, X.; Cook, L.F.; Grasso, L.M.; Cao, M.; Dong, Y. Royal Jelly-Mediated Prolongevity and Stress Resistance in *Caenorhabditis elegans* Is Possibly Modulated by the Interplays of DAF-16, SIR-2.1, HCF-1, and 14-3-3 Proteins. *J. Gerontol. A Biol. Sci. Med. Sci.* **2015**, *70*, 827–838. [CrossRef] [PubMed]
107. Honda, Y.; Araki, Y.; Hata, T.; Ichihara, K.; Ito, M.; Tanaka, M.; Honda, S. 10-Hydroxy-2-decenoic Acid, the Major Lipid Component of Royal Jelly, Extends the Lifespan of *Caenorhabditis elegans* through Dietary Restriction and Target of Rapamycin Signaling. *J. Aging Res.* **2015**, *2015*, 425261. [CrossRef] [PubMed]
108. Ali, A.M.; Kunugi, H. Apitherapy for Age-Related Skeletal Muscle Dysfunction (Sarcopenia): A Review on the Effects of Royal Jelly, Propolis, and Bee Pollen. *Foods* **2020**, *9*, 1362. [CrossRef] [PubMed]
109. Sahin, H. Royal jelly: Healthy aging and longevity. In *Bee Products and Their Applications in the Food and Pharmaceutical Industries*; Boyacioglu, D., Ed.; Academic Press: Cambridge, MA, USA, 2022; pp. 245–260. [CrossRef]
110. Ji, W.Z.; Zhang, C.P.; Wei, W.T.; Hu, F.L. The in vivo antiaging effect of enzymatic hydrolysate from royal jelly in d-galactose induced aging mouse. *J. Chin. Inst. Food Sci. Technol.* **2016**, *16*, 18–25. [CrossRef]
111. Jiang, C.M.; Liu, X.; Li, C.X.; Qian, H.C.; Chen, D.; Lai, C.Q.; Shen, L.R. Anti-senescence effect and molecular mechanism of the major royal jelly proteins on human embryonic lung fibroblast (HFL-I) cell line. *J. Zhejiang Univ. Sci. B.* **2018**, *19*, 960–972. [CrossRef] [PubMed]
112. Salazar-Olivo, L.A.; Paz-Gonzalez, V. Screening of biological activities present in honeybee (*Apis mellifera*) royal jelly. *Toxicol. Vitr.* **2005**, *19*, 645–651. [CrossRef]
113. Kamakura, M.; Suenobu, N.; Fukushima, M. Fifty-seven-kDa protein in royal jelly enhances proliferation of primary cultured rat hepatocytes and increases albumin production in the absence of serum. *Biochem. Biophys Res. Commun.* **2001**, *282*, 865–874. [CrossRef]
114. Kawano, Y.; Makino, K.; Jinnin, M.; Sawamura, S.; Shimada, S.; Fukushima, S.; Ihn, H. Royal jelly regulates the proliferation of human dermal microvascular endothelial cells through the down-regulation of a photoaging-related microRNA. *Drug Discov. Ther.* **2019**, *13*, 268–273. [CrossRef] [PubMed]
115. Oršolić, N. Allergic Inflammation: Effect of Propolis and Its Flavonoids. *Molecules* **2022**, *27*, 6694. [CrossRef] [PubMed]
116. Park, H.M.; Hwang, E.; Lee, K.G.; Han, S.M.; Cho, Y.; Kim, S.Y. Royal jelly protects against ultraviolet B-induced photoaging in human skin fibroblasts via enhancing collagen production. *J. Med. Food* **2011**, *14*, 899–906. [CrossRef] [PubMed]
117. Qiu, W.; Chen, X.; Tian, Y.; Wu, D.; Du, M.; Wang, S. Protection against oxidative stress and anti-aging effect in Drosophila of royal jelly-collagen peptide. *Food Chem. Toxicol.* **2020**, *135*, 110881. [CrossRef] [PubMed]
118. Al-U'datt, D.G.F.; Alu'datt, M.H.; Tranchant, C.C.; Al-Dwairi, A.; Al-Shboul, O.; Almajwal, A.; Elsalem, L.; Jaradat, S.; Alzoubi, K.H.; Faleh, B.G.; et al. Royal jelly mediates fibrotic signaling, collagen cross-linking and cell proliferation in cardiac fibroblasts. *Biomed. Pharmacother.* **2023**, *164*, 114922. [CrossRef] [PubMed]
119. Koya-Miyata, S.; Okamoto, I.; Ushio, S.; Iwaki, K.; Ikeda, M.; Kurimoto, M. Identification of a collagen production-promoting factor from an extract of royal jelly and its possible mechanism. *Biosci. Biotechnol. Biochem.* **2004**, *68*, 767–773. [CrossRef] [PubMed]
120. Bălan, A.; Moga, M.A.; Dima, L.; Toma, S.; Elena Neculau, A.; Anastasiu, C.V. Royal Jelly—A Traditional and Natural Remedy for Postmenopausal Symptoms and Aging-Related Pathologies. *Molecules* **2020**, *25*, 3291. [CrossRef] [PubMed]
121. Khani-Eshratabadi, M.; Talebpour, A.; Bagherzadeh, A.; Mehranfar, P.; Motallebzadeh Khanmiri, J.; Ghorbani, M.; Abtahi-Eivary, S.H. Potential Anti-Apoptotic Impacts and Telomerase Activity of Royal Jelly on Different Tissues of Rats. *Arch. Med. Lab. Sci.* **2022**, *8*, 1–10.e3. [CrossRef]
122. Liu, Z.; Liang, Q.; Ren, Y.; Guo, C.; Ge, X.; Wang, L.; Cheng, Q.; Luo, P.; Zhang, Y.; Han, X. Immunosenescence: Molecular mechanisms and diseases. *Sig. Transduct. Target. Ther.* **2023**, *8*, 200. [CrossRef]
123. Bouamama, S.; Merzouk, H.; Latrech, H.; Charif, N.; Bouamama, A. Royal jelly alleviates the detrimental effects of aging on immune functions by enhancing the in vitro cellular proliferation, cytokines, and nitric oxide release in aged human PBMCS. *J. Food Biochem.* **2021**, *45*, e13619. [CrossRef]
124. Natarajan, O.; Angeloni, J.T.; Bilodeau, M.F.; Russi, K.E.; Dong, Y.; Cao, M. The Immunomodulatory Effects of Royal Jelly on Defending against Bacterial Infections in the *Caenorhabditis elegans* Model. *J. Med. Food* **2021**, *24*, 358–369. [CrossRef] [PubMed]
125. Ito, T.; Rojasawasthien, T.; Takeuchi, S.Y.; Okamoto, H.; Okumura, N.; Shirakawa, T.; Matsubara, T.; Kawamoto, T.; Kokabu, S. Royal Jelly Enhances the Ability of Myoblast C_2C_{12} Cells to Differentiate into Multilineage Cells. *Molecules* **2024**, *29*, 1449. [CrossRef] [PubMed]
126. Inoue, S.; Koya-Miyata, S.; Ushio, S.; Iwaki, K.; Ikeda, M.; Kurimoto, M. Royal Jelly prolongs the life span of C_3H/HeJ mice: Correlation with reduced DNA damage. *Exp. Gerontol.* **2003**, *38*, 965–969. [CrossRef] [PubMed]
127. Oršolić, N.; Nemrava, J.; Jeleč, Ž.; Kukolj, M.; Odeh, D.; Jakopović, B.; Jazvinšćak Jembrek, M.; Bagatin, T.; Fureš, R.; Bagatin, D. Antioxidative and Anti-Inflammatory Activities of Chrysin and Naringenin in a Drug-Induced Bone Loss Model in Rats. *Int. J. Mol. Sci.* **2022**, *23*, 2872. [CrossRef] [PubMed]

128. Jazvinšćak Jembrek, M.; Oršolić, N.; Karlović, D.; Peitl, V. Flavonols in Action: Targeting Oxidative Stress and Neuroinflammation in Major Depressive Disorder. *Int. J. Mol. Sci.* **2023**, *24*, 6888. [CrossRef] [PubMed]
129. Macedo, F.; Romanatto, T.; Gomes de Assis, C.; Buis, A.; Kowaltowski, A.J.; Aguilaniu, H.; Marques da Cunha, F. Lifespan-extending interventions enhance lipid-supported mitochondrial respiration in *Caenorhabditis elegans*. *FASEB J.* **2020**, *34*, 9972–9981. [CrossRef] [PubMed]
130. Çiçek, G.; Öz Bağcı, F. Effects of royal jelly on the antisenescence, mitochondrial viability and osteogenic differentiation capacity of umbilical cord-derived mesenchymal stem cells. *Histochem. Cell Biol.* **2023**, *161*, 183–193. [CrossRef] [PubMed]
131. Kurek-Górecka, A.; Górecki, M.; Rzepecka-Stojko, A.; Balwierz, R.; Stojko, J. Bee Products in Dermatology and Skin Care. *Molecules* **2020**, *25*, 556. [CrossRef] [PubMed]
132. Haston, S.; Gonzalez-Gualda, E.; Morsli, S.; Ge, J.; Reen, V.; Calderwood, A.; Moutsopoulos, I.; Panousopoulos, L.; Deletic, P.; Carreno, G.; et al. Clearance of senescent macrophages ameliorates tumorigenesis in KRAS-driven lung cancer. *Cancer Cell* **2023**, *41*, 1242–1260.e6. [CrossRef]
133. Zhou, L.; Ruscetti, M. Senescent macrophages: A new "old" player in lung cancer development. *Cancer Cell* **2023**, *41*, 1201–1203. [CrossRef]
134. Reynolds, L.E.; Maallin, S.; Haston, S.; Martinez-Barbera, J.P.; Hodivala-Dilke, K.M.; Pedrosa, A.R. Effects of senescence on the tumour microenvironment and response to therapy. *FEBS J.* 2023; *ahead of print*. [CrossRef]
135. Li, J.; Sun, M.; Cui, X.; Li, C. Protective Effects of Flavonoids against Alzheimer's Disease: Pathological Hypothesis, Potential Targets, and Structure-Activity Relationship. *Int. J. Mol. Sci.* **2022**, *23*, 10020. [CrossRef]
136. Zubčić, K.; Hof, P.R.; Šimić, G.; Jazvinšćak Jembrek, M. The Role of Copper in Tau-Related Pathology in Alzheimer's Disease. *Front. Mol. Neurosci.* **2020**, *13*, 572308. [CrossRef] [PubMed]
137. Charlton, T.; Prowse, N.; McFee, A.; Heiratifar, N.; Fortin, T.; Paquette, C.; Hayley, S. Brain-derived neurotrophic factor (BDNF) has direct anti-inflammatory effects on microglia. *Front. Cell. Neurosci.* **2023**, *7*, 1188672. [CrossRef]
138. Raoufi, S.; Salavati, Z.; Komaki, A.; Shahidi, S.; Zarei, M. Royal jelly improves learning and memory deficits in an amyloid β-induced model of Alzheimer's disease in male rats: Involvement of oxidative stress. *Metab. Brain Dis.* **2023**, *38*, 1239–1248. [CrossRef]
139. Zhang, X.; Yu, Y.; Sun, P.; Fan, Z.; Zhang, W.; Feng, C. Royal jelly peptides: Potential inhibitors of β-secretase in N2a/APP695swe cells. *Sci. Rep.* **2019**, *9*, 168. [CrossRef] [PubMed]
140. Nisa, N.; Rasmita, B.; Arati, C.; Uditraj, C.; Siddhartha, R.; Dinata, R.; Bhanushree, B.; Bidanchi, R.M.; Manikandan, B.; Laskar, S.A.; et al. Repurposing of phyto-ligand molecules from the honey bee products for Alzheimer's disease as novel inhibitors of BACE-1: Small molecule bioinformatics strategies as amyloid-based therapy. *Environ. Sci. Pollut. Res. Int.* **2023**, *30*, 51143–51169. [CrossRef]
141. Gong, Y.; Luo, H.; Li, Z.; Feng, Y.; Liu, Z.; Chang, J. Metabolic Profile of Alzheimer's Disease: Is 10-Hydroxy-2-decenoic Acid a Pertinent Metabolic Adjuster? *Metabolites* **2023**, *13*, 954. [CrossRef] [PubMed]
142. Ge, Z.; Liu, J.-C.; Sun, J.-A.; Mao, X.-Z. Tyrosinase Inhibitory Peptides from Enzyme Hydrolyzed Royal Jelly: Production, Separation, Identification and Docking Analysis. *Foods* **2023**, *12*, 2240. [CrossRef]
143. Pan, Y.; Xu, J.; Jin, P.; Yang, Q.; Zhu, K.; You, M.; Hu, F.; Chen, M. Royal Jelly Ameliorates Behavioral Deficits, Cholinergic System Deficiency, and Autonomic Nervous Dysfunction in Ovariectomized Cholesterol-Fed Rabbits. *Molecules* **2019**, *24*, 1149. [CrossRef]
144. Sirinupong, N.; Chansuwan, W.; Kaewkaen, P. Hydrolase-Treated Royal Jelly Attenuates H_2O_2- and Glutamate-Induced SH-SY5Y Cell Damage and Promotes Cognitive Enhancement in a Rat Model of Vascular Dementia. *Int. J. Food Sci.* **2021**, *2021*, 2213814. [CrossRef]
145. You, M.; Pan, Y.; Liu, Y.; Chen, Y.; Wu, Y.; Si, J.; Wang, K.; Hu, F. Royal Jelly Alleviates Cognitive Deficits and β-Amyloid Accumulation in APP/PS1 Mouse Model Via Activation of the cAMP/PKA/CREB/BDNF Pathway and Inhibition of Neuronal Apoptosis. *Front. Aging Neurosci.* **2019**, *10*, 428. [CrossRef]
146. You, M.; Miao, Z.; Sienkiewicz, O.; Jiang, X.; Zhao, X.; Hu, F. 10-Hydroxydecanoic acid inhibits LPS-induced inflammation by targeting p53 in microglial cells. *Int. Immunopharmacol.* **2020**, *84*, 106501. [CrossRef]
147. Ali, A.M.; Hendawy, A.O. Royal jelly acid, 10-hydroxy-trans-2-decenoic acid, for psychiatric and neurological disorders: How helpful could it be?! *Edelweiss Food Sci. Technol.* **2019**, *1*, 1–4. [CrossRef]
148. Wang, X.; Cao, M.; Dong, Y. Royal jelly promotes DAF-16-mediated proteostasis to tolerate β-amyloid toxicity in *C. elegans* model of Alzheimer's disease. *Oncotarget* **2016**, *7*, 54183–54193. [CrossRef] [PubMed]
149. You, M.; Wang, K.; Pan, Y.; Tao, L.; Ma, Q.; Zhang, G.; Hu, F. Combined royal jelly 10-hydroxydecanoic acid and aspirin has a synergistic effect against memory deficit and neuroinflammation. *Food Funct.* **2022**, *13*, 2336–2353. [CrossRef] [PubMed]
150. Pan, Y.; Xu, J.; Chen, C.; Chen, F.; Jin, P.; Zhu, K.; Hu, C.W.; You, M.; Chen, M.; Hu, F. Royal Jelly Reduces Cholesterol Levels, Ameliorates Aβ Pathology and Enhances Neuronal Metabolic Activities in a Rabbit Model of Alzheimer's Disease. *Front. Aging Neurosci.* **2018**, *10*, 50. [CrossRef]
151. de Souza E Silva, T.G.; do Val de Paulo, M.E.F.; da Silva, J.R.M.; da Silva Alves, A.; Britto, L.R.G.; Xavier, G.F.; Lopes Sandoval, M.R. Oral treatment with royal jelly improves memory and presents neuroprotective effects on icv-STZ rat model of sporadic Alzheimer's disease. *Heliyon* **2020**, *6*, e03281. [CrossRef]
152. Karimi, E.; Arab, A.; Sepidarkish, M.; Khorvash, F.; Saadatnia, M.; Amani, R. Effects of the royal jelly consumption on post-stroke complications in patients with ischemic stroke: Results of a randomized controlled trial. *Front. Nutr.* **2024**, *10*, 1227414. [CrossRef]

153. Hashimoto, M.; Kanda, M.; Ikeno, K.; Hayashi, Y.; Nakamura, T.; Ogawa, Y.; Fukumitsu, H.; Nomoto, H.; Furukawa, S. Oral administration of royal jelly facilitates mRNA expression of glial cell line-derived neurotrophic factor and neurofilament H in the hippocampus of the adult mouse brain. *Biosci. Biotechnol. Biochem.* **2005**, *69*, 800–805. [CrossRef]
154. Hattori, N.; Ohta, S.; Sakamoto, T.; Mishima, S.; Furukawa, S. Royal jelly facilitates restoration of the cognitive ability in trimethyltin-intoxicated mice. *Evid. Based Complement. Alternat. Med.* **2011**, *2011*, 165968. [CrossRef]
155. You, M.M.; Chen, Y.F.; Pan, Y.M.; Liu, Y.C.; Tu, J.; Wang, K.; Hu, F.L. Royal jelly attenuates LPS-induced inflammation in BV-2 microglial cells through modulating NF-kappaB and p38/JNK signaling pathways. *Mediat. Inflamm.* **2018**, *2018*, 7834381. [CrossRef] [PubMed]
156. Hattori, N.; Nomoto, H.; Fukumitsu, H.; Mishima, S.; Furukawa, S. Royal jelly and its unique fatty acid, 10-hydroxy-trans-2-decenoic acid, promote neurogenesis by neural stem/progenitor cells in vitro. *Biomed. Res.* **2007**, *28*, 261–266. [CrossRef] [PubMed]
157. Hattori, N.; Nomoto, H.; Fukumitsu, H.; Mishima, S.; Furukawa, S. AMP N(1)-oxide, a unique compound of royal jelly, induces neurite outgrowth from PC12 cells via signaling by protein kinase A independent of that by mitogen-activated protein kinase. *Evid. Based Complement. Alternat. Med.* **2011**, *7*, 63–68. [CrossRef] [PubMed]
158. Aslan, A.; Beyaz, S.; Gok, O.; Parlak, G.; Can, M.I.; Agca, C.A.; Ozercan, I.H.; Parlak, A.E. Royal jelly protects brain tissue against fluoride-induced damage by activating Bcl-2/NF-κB/caspase-3/caspase-6/Bax and Erk signaling pathways in rats. *Environ. Sci. Pollut. Res. Int.* **2023**, *30*, 49014–49025. [CrossRef] [PubMed]
159. Chen, D.; Liu, F.; Wan, J.-B.; Lai, C.Q.; Shen, L. Effect of Major Royal Jelly Proteins on Spatial Memory in Aged Rats: Metabolomics Analysis in Urine. *J. Agric. Food Chem.* **2017**, *65*, 3151–3159. [CrossRef] [PubMed]
160. Pourfard, H.; Ahmadi, A.; Habibi, Z.; Asadi-Samani, M.; Shahinfard, N.; Soleimani, A. The Effect of Tang Forte (Royal Jelly) Capsule on Hypoglycemia and Clinical Course in COVID-19 Patients Under Corticosteroid Therapy. *J. Evid. Based Integr. Med.* **2023**, *28*, 2515690X231165333. [CrossRef] [PubMed]
161. Al Nohair, S.F.; Ahmed, S.S.; Ismail, M.S.; El Maadawy, A.A.; Albatanony, M.A.; Rasheed, Z. Potential of honey against the onset of autoimmune diabetes and its associated nephropathy, pancreatitis, and retinopathy in type 1 diabetic animal model. *Open Life Sci.* **2022**, *17*, 351–361. [CrossRef] [PubMed]
162. Maleki, V.; Jafari-Vayghan, H.; Saleh-Ghadimi, S.; Adibian, M.; Kheirouri, S.; Alizadeh, M. Effects of Royal jelly on metabolic variables in diabetes mellitus: A systematic review. *Complement. Ther. Med.* **2019**, *43*, 20–27. [CrossRef] [PubMed]
163. Horvat, A.; Vlašić, I.; Štefulj, J.; Oršolić, N.; Jazvinšćak Jembrek, M. Flavonols as a Potential Pharmacological Intervention for Alleviating Cognitive Decline in Diabetes: Evidence from Preclinical Studies. *Life* **2023**, *13*, 2291. [CrossRef]
164. El-Seedi, H.R.; Salama, S.; El-Wahed, A.A.A.; Guo, Z.; Di Minno, A.; Daglia, M.; Li, C.; Guan, X.; Buccato, D.G.; Khalifa, S.A.M.; et al. Exploring the Therapeutic Potential of Royal Jelly in Metabolic Disorders and Gastrointestinal Diseases. *Nutrients* **2024**, *16*, 393. [CrossRef]
165. Ghanbari, E.; Nejati, V.; Khazaei, M. Antioxidant and protective effects of Royal jelly on histopathological changes in testis of diabetic rats. *Int. J. Reprod. Biomed.* **2016**, *14*, 519–526. [CrossRef] [PubMed]
166. Nomura, M.; Maruo, N.; Zamami, Y.; Takatori, S.; Doi, S.; Kawasaki, H. Effect of long-term treatment with royal jelly on insulin resistance in Otsuka Long-Evans Tokushima Fatty (OLETF) rats. *Yakugaku Zasshi* **2007**, *127*, 1877–1882. [CrossRef] [PubMed]
167. Zamami, Y.; Takatori, S.; Goda, M.; Koyama, T.; Iwatani, Y.; Jin, X.; Takai-Doi, S.; Kawasaki, H. Royal jelly ameliorates insulin resistance in fructose-drinking rats. *Biol. Pharm. Bull.* **2008**, *31*, 2103–2107. [CrossRef] [PubMed]
168. Omer, K.; Gelkopf, M.J.; Newton, G. Effectiveness of royal jelly supplementation in glycemic regulation: A systematic review. *World J. Diabetes* **2019**, *10*, 96–113. [CrossRef] [PubMed]
169. Gohari, I.; Khajehlandi, A.; Mohammadi, A. Effect of High-intensity Interval Training with Royal Jelly Consumption on Serum Levels of Glucose, Insulin, and Insulin Resistance Index of Overweight and Obese Middle-aged Men: A Quasi-experimental Study. *Jundishapur J. Chronic Dis. Care* **2022**, *11*, e123363. [CrossRef]
170. Münstedt, K.; Bargello, M.; Hauenschild, A. Royal jelly reduces the serum glucose levels in healthy subjects. *J. Med. Food* **2009**, *12*, 1170–1172. [CrossRef] [PubMed]
171. Khoshpey, B.; Djazayeri, S.; Amiri, F.; Malek, M.; Hosseini, A.F.; Hosseini, S.; Shidfar, S.; Shidfar, F. Effect of Royal Jelly Intake on Serum Glucose, Apolipoprotein A-I (ApoA-I), Apolipoprotein B (ApoB) and ApoB/ApoA-I Ratios in Patients with Type 2 Diabetes: A Randomized, Double-Blind Clinical Trial Study. *Can. J. Diabetes* **2016**, *40*, 324–328. [CrossRef] [PubMed]
172. Nohair, S.F.A. Antidiabetic efficacy of a honey-royal jelly mixture: Biochemical study in rats. *Int. J. Health Sci.* **2021**, *15*, 4–9.
173. Pourmoradian, S.; Mahdavi, R.; Mobasseri, M.; Faramarzi, E.; Mobasseri, M. Effects of royal jelly supplementation on glycemic control and oxidative stress factors in type 2 diabetic female: A randomized clinical trial. *Chin. J. Integr. Med.* **2014**, *20*, 347–352. [CrossRef]
174. Shidfar, F.; Jazayeri, S.; Mousavi, S.N.; Malek, M.; Hosseini, A.F.; Khoshpey, B. Does Supplementation with Royal Jelly Improve Oxidative Stress and Insulin Resistance in Type 2 Diabetic Patients? *Iran. J. Public Health* **2015**, *44*, 797–803.
175. Siavash, M.; Shokri, S.; Haghighi, S.; Shahtalebi, M.A.; Farajzadehgan, Z. The efficacy of topical royal jelly on healing of diabetic foot ulcers: A double-blind placebo-controlled clinical trial. *Int. Wound J.* **2015**, *12*, 137–142. [CrossRef] [PubMed]
176. Yakoot, M.; Abdelatif, M.; Helmy, S. Efficacy of a new local limb salvage treatment for limb-threatening diabetic foot wounds—A randomized controlled study. *Diabetes Metab. Syndr. Obes.* **2019**, *12*, 1659–1665. [CrossRef] [PubMed]

177. Liang, Y.; Kagota, S.; Maruyama, K.; Oonishi, Y.; Miyauchi-Wakuda, S.; Ito, Y.; Yamada, S.; Shinozuka, K. Royal jelly increases peripheral circulation by inducing vasorelaxation through nitric oxide production under healthy conditions. *Biomed. Pharmacother.* **2018**, *106*, 1210–1219. [CrossRef] [PubMed]
178. Oršolić, N.; Sirovina, D.; Odeh, D.; Gajski, G.; Balta, V.; Šver, L.; Jazvinšćak Jembrek, M. Efficacy of Caffeic Acid on Diabetes and Its Complications in the Mouse. *Molecules* **2021**, *26*, 3262. [CrossRef] [PubMed]
179. Ilić, I.; Oršolić, N.; Rođak, E.; Odeh, D.; Lovrić, M.; Mujkić, R.; Delaš Aždajić, M.; Grgić, A.; Tolušić Levak, M.; Vargek, M.; et al. The effect of high-fat diet and 13-cis retinoic acid application on lipid profile, glycemic response and oxidative stress in female Lewis rats. *PLoS ONE* **2020**, *15*, e0238600. [CrossRef] [PubMed]
180. Vajdi, M.; Musazadeh, V.; Khajeh, M.; Safaei, E.; Darzi, M.; Noshadi, N.; Bazyar, H.; Askari, G. The effects of royal jelly supplementation on anthropometric indices: A GRADE-assessed systematic review and dose-response meta-analysis of randomized controlled trials. *Front. Nutr.* **2023**, *10*, 1196258. [CrossRef] [PubMed]
181. Yoneshiro, T.; Kaede, R.; Nagaya, K.; Aoyama, J.; Saito, M.; Okamatsu-Ogura, Y.; Kimura, K.; Terao, A. Royal jelly ameliorates diet-induced obesity and glucose intolerance by promoting brown adipose tissue thermogenesis in mice. *Obes. Res. Clin. Pract.* **2016**, *12* (Suppl. S2), 127–137. [CrossRef] [PubMed]
182. Mesri Alamdari, N.; Irandoost, P.; Roshanravan, N.; Vafa, M.; Asghari Jafarabadi, M.; Alipour, S.; Roshangar, L.; Alivand, M.; Farsi, F.; Shidfar, F. Effects of Royal Jelly and Tocotrienol Rich Fraction in obesity treatment of calorie-restricted obese rats: A focus on white fat browning properties and thermogenic capacity. *Nutr. Metab.* **2020**, *17*, 42. [CrossRef] [PubMed]
183. Yoshida, M.; Hayashi, K.; Watadani, R.; Okano, Y.; Tanimura, K.; Kotoh, J.; Sasaki, D.; Matsumoto, K.; Maeda, A. Royal jelly improves hyperglycemia in obese/diabetic KK-Ay mice. *J. Vet. Med. Sci.* **2017**, *79*, 299–307. [CrossRef]
184. Watadani, R.; Kotoh, J.; Sasaki, D.; Someya, A.; Matsumoto, K.; Maeda, A. Hydroxy-2-decenoic acid, a natural product, improves hyperglycemia and insulin resistance in obese/diabetic KK-Ay mice, but does not prevent obesity. *J. Vet. Med. Sci.* **2017**, *79*, 1596–1602. [CrossRef]
185. Çakir, S. The Effect of Royal Jelly on Irisin in Experimentally Diabetic Rats. *SAUJS* **2023**, *27*, 912–919. [CrossRef]
186. Irandoost, P.; Mesri Alamdari, N.; Saidpour, A.; Shidfar, F.; Farsi, F.; Asghari Jafarabadi, M.; Alivand, M.R.; Vafa, M. The effect of royal jelly and tocotrienol-rich fraction along with calorie restriction on hypothalamic endoplasmic reticulum stress and adipose tissue inflammation in diet-induced obese rats. *BMC Res. Notes* **2020**, *13*, 409. [CrossRef] [PubMed]
187. Kashima, Y.; Kanematsu, S.; Asai, S.; Kusada, M.; Watanabe, S.; Kawashima, T.; Nakamura, T.; Shimada, M.; Goto, T.; Nagaoka, S. Identification of a novel hypocholesterolemic protein, major royal jelly protein 1, derived from royal jelly. *PLoS ONE* **2014**, *9*, e105073. [CrossRef] [PubMed]
188. Petelin, A.; Kenig, S.; Kopinč, R.; Deželak, M.; Černelič Bizjak, M.; Jenko Pražnikar, Z. Effects of Royal Jelly Administration on Lipid Profile, Satiety, Inflammation, and Antioxidant Capacity in Asymptomatic Overweight Adults. *Evid. Based Complement. Alternat. Med.* **2019**, *2019*, 4969720. [CrossRef] [PubMed]
189. Pandeya, P.R.; Lamichhane, R.; Lee, K.H.; Kim, S.G.; Lee, D.H.; Lee, H.K.; Jung, H.J. Bioassay-guided isolation of active anti-adipogenic compound from royal jelly and the study of possible mechanisms. *BMC Complement. Altern. Med.* **2019**, *19*, 33. [CrossRef] [PubMed]
190. Tahir, R.A.; Bashir, A.; Yousaf, M.N.; Ahmed, A.; Dali, Y.; Khan, S.; Sehgal, S.A. In Silico identification of angiotensin-converting enzyme inhibitory peptides from MRJP1. *PLoS ONE* **2020**, *15*, e0228265. [CrossRef] [PubMed]
191. Matsui, T.; Yukiyoshi, A.; Doi, S.; Sugimoto, H.; Yamada, H.; Matsumoto, K. Gastrointestinal enzyme production of bioactive peptides from royal jelly protein and their antihypertensive ability in SHR. *J. Nutr. Biochem.* **2002**, *13*, 80–86. [CrossRef] [PubMed]
192. Tokunaga, K.H.; Yoshida, C.; Suzuki, K.M.; Maruyama, H.; Futamura, Y.; Araki, Y.; Mishima, S. Antihypertensive effect of peptides from royal jelly in spontaneously hypertensive rats. *Biol. Pharm. Bull.* **2004**, *27*, 189–192. [CrossRef] [PubMed]
193. Morita, H.; Ikeda, T.; Kajita, K.; Fujioka, K.; Mori, I.; Okada, H.; Uno, Y.; Ishizuka, T. Effect of royal jelly ingestion for six months on healthy volunteers. *Nutr. J.* **2012**, *11*, 77. [CrossRef]
194. Guo, H.; Saiga, A.; Sato, M.; Miyazawa, I.; Shibata, M.; Takahata, Y.; Morimatsu, F. Royal jelly supplementation improves lipoprotein metabolism in humans. *J. Nutr. Sci. Vitaminol.* **2007**, *53*, 345–348. [CrossRef]
195. Vittek, J. Effect of royal jelly on serum lipids in experimental animals and humans with atherosclerosis. *Experientia* **1995**, *51*, 927–935. [CrossRef] [PubMed]
196. Takaki-Doi, S.; Hashimoto, K.; Yamamura, M.; Kamei, C. Antihypertensive activities of royal jelly protein hydrolysate and its fractions in spontaneously hypertensive rats. *Acta Med. Okayama* **2009**, *63*, 57–64. [CrossRef] [PubMed]
197. Pan, Y.; Rong, Y.; You, M.; Ma, Q.; Chen, M.; Hu, F. Royal jelly causes hypotension and vasodilation induced by increasing nitric oxide production. *Food Sci. Nutr.* **2019**, *7*, 1361–1370. [CrossRef] [PubMed]
198. Lee, H.C.; Akhmedov, A.; Chen, C.H. Spotlight on very-low-density lipoprotein as a driver of cardiometabolic disorders: Implications for disease progression and mechanistic insights. *Front. Cardiovasc. Med.* **2022**, *9*, 993633. [CrossRef] [PubMed]
199. Sato, A.; Unuma, H.; Ebina, K. Royal Jelly Proteins Inhibit Macrophage Proliferation: Interactions with Native- and Oxidized-Low Density Lipoprotein. *Protein J.* **2021**, *40*, 699–708. [CrossRef] [PubMed]
200. Chiang, S.-H.; Yang, K.-M.; Sheu, S.-C.; Chen, C.-W. The Bioactive Compound Contents and Potential Protective Effects of Royal Jelly Protein Hydrolysates against DNA Oxidative Damage and LDL Oxidation. *Antioxidants* **2021**, *10*, 580. [CrossRef] [PubMed]

201. Hu, X.; Liu, Z.; Lu, Y.; Chi, X.; Han, K.; Wang, H.; Wang, Y.; Ma, L.; Xu, B. Glucose metabolism enhancement by 10-hydroxy-2-decenoic acid via the PI3K/AKT signaling pathway in high-fat-diet/streptozotocin induced type 2 diabetic mice. *Food Funct.* **2022**, *13*, 9931–9946. [CrossRef] [PubMed]
202. Lambrinoudaki, I.; Augoulea, A.; Rizos, D.; Politi, M.; Tsoltos, N.; Moros, M.; Chinou, I.; Graikou, K.; Kouskouni, E.; Kambani, S.; et al. Greek-origin royal jelly improves the lipid profile of postmenopausal women. *Gynecol. Endocrinol.* **2016**, *32*, 835–839. [CrossRef]
203. Moutsatsou, P.; Papoutsi, Z.; Kassi, E.; Heldring, N.; Zhao, C.; Tsiapara, A.; Melliou, E.; Chrousos, G.P.; Chinou, I.; Karshikoff, A.; et al. Fatty acids derived from royal jelly are modulators of estrogen receptor functions. *PLoS ONE* **2010**, *5*, e15594. [CrossRef]
204. Oršolić, N.; Nemrava, J.; Jeleč, Ž.; Kukolj, M.; Odeh, D.; Terzić, S.; Fureš, R.; Bagatin, T.; Bagatin, D. The Beneficial Effect of Proanthocyanidins and Icariin on Biochemical Markers of Bone Turnover in Rats. *Int. J. Mol. Sci.* **2018**, *19*, 2746. [CrossRef]
205. Siddiqui, S.; Mahdi, A.A.; Arshad, M. Genistein contributes to cell cycle progression and regulates oxidative stress in primary culture of osteoblasts along with osteoclasts attenuation. *BMC Complement. Med. Ther.* **2020**, *20*, 277. [CrossRef] [PubMed]
206. Tsuchiya, Y.; Hayashi, M.; Nagamatsu, K.; Ono, T.; Kamakura, M.; Iwata, T.; Nakashima, T. The key royal jelly component 10-hydroxy-2-decenoic acid protects against bone loss by inhibiting NF-κB signaling downstream of FFAR4. *J. Biol. Chem.* **2020**, *295*, 12224–12232. [CrossRef] [PubMed]
207. Suzuki, K.M.; Isohama, Y.; Maruyama, H.; Yamada, Y.; Narita, Y.; Ohta, S.; Araki, Y.; Miyata, T.; Mishima, S. Estrogenic activities of fatty acids and a sterol isolated from royal jelly. *Evid. Complement. Alternat. Med.* **2008**, *5*, 295–302. [CrossRef] [PubMed]
208. Husein, M.Q.; Kridli, R.T. Reproductive responses following royal jelly treatment administered orally or intramuscularly into progesterone-treated Awassi ewes. *Anim. Reprod. Sci.* **2002**, *74*, 45–53. [CrossRef] [PubMed]
209. Husein, M.Q.; Haddad, S.G. A new approach to enhance reproductive performance in sheep using royal jelly in comparison with equine chorionic gonadotropin. *Anim. Reprod. Sci.* **2006**, *93*, 24–33. [CrossRef] [PubMed]
210. El-Tarabany, M.S.; Nassan, M.A.; Salah, A.S. Royal Jelly Improves the Morphology of the Reproductive Tract, Internal Egg Quality, and Blood Biochemical Parameters in Laying Hens at the Late Stage of Production. *Animals* **2021**, *11*, 1861. [CrossRef] [PubMed]
211. Sharif, S.N.; Darsareh, F. Effect of royal jelly on menopausal symptoms: A randomized placebo-controlled clinical trial. *Complement. Ther. Clin. Pract.* **2019**, *37*, 47–50. [CrossRef]
212. Ab Hamid, N.; Abu Bakar, A.B.; Mat Zain, A.A.; Nik Hussain, N.H.; Othman, Z.A.; Zakaria, Z.; Mohamed, M. Composition of Royal Jelly (RJ) and Its Anti-Androgenic Effect on Reproductive Parameters in a Polycystic Ovarian Syndrome (PCOS) Animal Model. *Antioxidants* **2020**, *9*, 499. [CrossRef]
213. Ghanbari, E.; Khazaei, M.R.; Khazaei, M.; Nejati, V. Royal jelly promotes ovarian follicles growth and increases steroid hormones in immature rats. *Int. J. Fertil. Steril.* **2018**, *11*, 263–269. [CrossRef]
214. Liu, X.; Jiang, C.; Chen, Y.; Shi, F.; Lai, C.; Shen, L. Major royal jelly proteins accelerate onset of puberty and promote ovarian follicular development in immature female mice. *Food Sci. Hum. Wellness.* **2020**, *9*, 338–345. [CrossRef]
215. Shahzad, Q.; Mehmood, M.U.; Khan, H.; ul Husna, A.; Qadeer, S.; Azam, A.; Naseer, Z.; Ahmad, E.; Safdar, M.; Ahmad, M. Royal jelly supplementation in semen extender enhances post-thaw quality and fertility of Nili-Ravi buffalo bull sperm. *Anim. Reprod. Sci.* **2016**, *167*, 83–88. [CrossRef] [PubMed]
216. El-Hanoun, A.M.; Elkomy, A.E.; Fares, W.A.; Shahien, E.H. Impact of royal jelly to improve reproductive performance of male rabbits under hot summer conditions. *World Rabbit Sci.* **2014**, *22*, 241–248. [CrossRef]
217. Al-Nahari, H.; Al Eisa, R. Effect of turmeric (*Curcuma longa*) on some pituitary, thyroid and testosterone hormone against aluminum chloride ($AlCl_3$) induced toxicity in rat. *Adv. Environ. Biol.* **2016**, *10*, 250–261.
218. El Helew, E.A.; Hamed, W.S.; Moustafa, A.M.; Sakkara, Z.A. Structural changes in testes of Streptozotocin induced diabetic rats and possible protective effect of royal jelly: Light and electron microscopic study. *Ultrastruct. Pathol.* **2024**, *48*, 1–15. [CrossRef] [PubMed]
219. Shi, Z.; Enayatullah, H.; Lv, Z.; Dai, H.; Wei, Q.; Shen, L.; Karwand, B.; Shi, F. Freeze-Dried Royal Jelly Proteins Enhanced the Testicular Development and Spermatogenesis in Pubescent Male Mice. *Animals* **2019**, *9*, 977. [CrossRef] [PubMed]
220. Kafadar, I.H.; Güney, A.; Türk, C.Y.; Oner, M.; Silici, S. Royal jelly and bee pollen decrease bone loss due to osteoporosis in an oophorectomized rat model. *Eklem Hastalik Cerrahisi* **2012**, *23*, 100–105. [PubMed]
221. Hattori, S.; Omi, N. The effects of royal jelly protein on bone mineral density and strength in ovariectomized female rats. *Phys. Act. Nutr.* **2021**, *25*, 33–37. [CrossRef] [PubMed]
222. Shimizu, S.; Matsushita, H.; Minami, A.; Kanazawa, H.; Suzuki, T.; Watanabe, K.; Wakatsuki, A. Royal jelly does not prevent bone loss but improves bone strength in ovariectomized rats. *Climacteric* **2018**, *21*, 601–606. [CrossRef]
223. Matsushita, H.; Shimizu, S.; Morita, N.; Watanabe, K.; Wakatsuki, A. Effects of royal jelly on bone metabolism in postmenopausal women: A randomized, controlled study. *Climacteric* **2021**, *24*, 164–170. [CrossRef]
224. Münstedt, K.; Männle, H. Apitherapy for menopausal problems. *Arch. Gynecol. Obstet.* **2020**, *302*, 1495–1502. [CrossRef]
225. Aydin, B.; Müge Atar, M.; Pirgon, Ö. The effect of royal jelly supplementation for three months on bone markers in postmenopausal osteoporotic women. *Mellifera* **2021**, *21*, 59–68.
226. Attia, W.; Gabry, M.; Othman, G. Immunostimulatory effect of royal jelly and its relation with host resistance against tumor in mice. *Egypt. J. Exp. Biol.* **2007**, *3*, 241–250.
227. Orsolić, N.; Knezević, A.; Sver, L.; Terzić, S.; Hackenberger, B.K.; Basić, I. Influence of honey bee products on transplantable murine tumors. *Vet. Comp. Oncol.* **2003**, *1*, 216–226. [CrossRef] [PubMed]

228. Oršolić, N.; Sacases, F.; Percie Du Sert, P.; Bašić, I. Antimetastatic ability of honey bee products. *Period. Biol.* **2007**, *109*, 173–180.
229. Oršolić, N.; Terzić, S.; Šver, L.; Bašić, I. Honey-bee products in preventive and/or terapy of murine transplantable tumours. *J. Sci. Food Agr.* **2005**, *85*, 363–370. [CrossRef]
230. Sver, L.; Orsolić, N.; Tadić, Z.; Njari, B.; Valpotić, I.; Basić, I. A royal jelly a new potential immunomodulator in rats and mice. *Comp. Immun. Microbiol. Infect. Dis.* **1996**, *19*, 31–38. [CrossRef]
231. Kimura, Y. Antitumor and antimetastatic actions of various natural products. *Stud. Nat. Prod. Chem.* **2008**, *34*, 35–76. [CrossRef]
232. Vucevic, D.; Melliou, E.; Vasilijic, S.; Gasic, S.; Ivanovski, P.; Chinou, I.; Colic, M. Fatty acids isolated from royal jelly modulate dendritic cell-mediated immune response in vitro. *Int. Immunopharmacol.* **2007**, *7*, 1211–1220. [CrossRef] [PubMed]
233. Peng, C.C.; Sun, H.T.; Lin, I.P.; Kuo, P.C.; Li, J.C. The functional property of royal jelly 10-hydroxy-2-decenoic acid as a melanogenesis inhibitor. *BMC Complement. Altern. Med.* **2017**, *17*, 392. [CrossRef] [PubMed]
234. Lin, X.M.; Liu, S.B.; Luo, Y.H.; Xu, W.T.; Zhang, Y.; Zhang, T.; Xue, H.; Zuo, W.B.; Li, Y.N.; Lu, B.X.; et al. 10-HDA Induces ROS-Mediated Apoptosis in A549 Human Lung Cancer Cells by Regulating the MAPK, STAT3, NF-κB, and TGF-β1 Signaling Pathways. *Biomed. Res. Int.* **2020**, *2020*, 3042636. [CrossRef]
235. Kamiya, T.; Watanabe, M.; Hara, H.; Mitsugi, Y.; Yamaguchi, E.; Itoh, A.; Adachi, T. Induction of Human-Lung-Cancer-A549-Cell Apoptosis by 4-Hydroperoxy-2-decenoic Acid Ethyl Ester through Intracellular ROS Accumulation and the Induction of Proapoptotic CHOP Expression. *J. Agric. Food Chem.* **2018**, *66*, 10741–10747. [CrossRef] [PubMed]
236. Shakib Khoob, M.; Hosseini, S.M.; Kazemi, S. In Vitro and In Vivo Antioxidant and Anticancer Potentials of Royal Jelly for Dimethylhydrazine-Induced Colorectal Cancer in Wistar Rats. *Oxid. Med. Cell. Longev.* **2022**, *2022*, 9506026. [CrossRef] [PubMed]
237. Gismondi, A.; Trionfera, E.; Canuti, L.; Di Marco, G.; Canini, A. Royal jelly lipophilic fraction induces antiproliferative effects on SH-SY5Y human neuroblastoma cells. *Oncol. Rep.* **2017**, *38*, 1833–1844. [CrossRef] [PubMed]
238. Simsek Ozek, N. Exploring the in vitro potential of royal jelly against glioblastoma and neuroblastoma: Impact on cell proliferation, apoptosis, cell cycle, and the biomolecular content. *Analyst* **2024**, *149*, 1872–1884. [CrossRef] [PubMed]
239. Makino, J.; Ogasawara, R.; Kamiya, T.; Hara, H.; Mitsugi, Y.; Yamaguchi, E.; Itoh, A.; Adachi, T. Royal Jelly Constituents Increase the Expression of Extracellular Superoxide Dismutase through Histone Acetylation in Monocytic THP-1 Cells. *J. Nat. Prod.* **2016**, *79*, 1137–1143. [CrossRef] [PubMed]
240. Yu, C.S.; Yeh, F.T.; Yu, F.S.; Cheng, K.C.; Chung, J.G. Royal jelly inhibited N-acetylation and metabolism of 2-aminofluorene in human liver tumor cells (J5). *Toxicol. Environ. Chem.* **2005**, *87*, 83–90. [CrossRef]
241. Abu-Serie, M.M.; Habashy, N.H. Two purified proteins from royal jelly with in vitro dual anti-hepatic damage potency: Major royal jelly protein 2 and its novel isoform X1. *Int. J. Biol. Macromol.* **2019**, *128*, 782–795. [CrossRef] [PubMed]
242. Albalawi, A.E.; Althobaiti, N.A.; Alrdahe, S.S.; Alhasani, R.H.; Alaryani, F.S.; BinMowyna, M.N. Antitumor Activity of Royal Jelly and Its Cellular Mechanisms against Ehrlich Solid Tumor in Mice. *Biomed. Res. Int.* **2022**, *2022*, 7233997. [CrossRef] [PubMed]
243. Bincoletto, C.; Eberlin, S.; Figueiredo, C.A.; Luengo, M.B.; Queiroz, M.L. Effects produced by Royal Jelly on haematopoiesis: Relation with host resistance against Ehrlich ascites tumour challenge. *Int. Immunopharmacol.* **2005**, *5*, 679–688. [CrossRef]
244. Zang, S.; Ma, X.; Wu, Y.; Liu, W.; Cheng, H.; Li, J.; Liu, J.; Huang, A. PGE_2 synthesis and signaling in malignant transformation and progression of human hepatocellular carcinoma. *Hum. Pathol.* **2017**, *63*, 120–127. [CrossRef]
245. Xie, C.; Xu, X.; Wang, X.; Wei, S.; Shao, L.; Chen, J.; Cai, J.; Jia, L. Cyclooxygenase-2 induces angiogenesis in pancreatic cancer mediated by prostaglandin E_2. *Oncol. Lett.* **2018**, *16*, 940–948. [CrossRef] [PubMed]
246. Wang, S.Y.; Chen, C.W. Effects of royal jelly extracts on growth inhibition, differentiation human leukemic U937 cells and its immunomodulatory activity. *Biocell* **2019**, *43*, 29–41.
247. Cihan, Y.; Deniz, K. The effects of royal jelly against radiation-induced acute oral mucositis. *Int. J. Hematol. Oncol.* **2014**, *24*, 45–53. [CrossRef]
248. Rafat, N.; Monfared, A.S.; Shahidi, M.; Pourfallah, T.A. The modulating effect of royal jelly consumption against radiation-induced apoptosis in human peripheral blood leukocytes. *J. Med. Phys.* **2016**, *41*, 52–57. [CrossRef] [PubMed]
249. Cihan, Y.; Ozturk, A.; Gokalp, S.S. Protective role of royal jelly against radiation-induced oxidative stress in rats. *Int. J. Hematol. Oncol.* **2013**, *23*, 79–87. [CrossRef]
250. Azab, K.S.; Bashandy, M.; Salem, M.; Ahmed, O.; Tawfik, Z.; Helal, H. Royal jelly modulates oxidative stress and tissue injury in gamma irradiated male Wister Albino rats. *N. Am. J. Med. Sci.* **2011**, *3*, 268–276. [CrossRef]
251. Kwon, Y. Potential Pro-Tumorigenic Effect of Bisphenol A in Breast Cancer via Altering the Tumor Microenvironment. *Cancers* **2022**, *14*, 3021. [CrossRef] [PubMed]
252. Miyata, Y.; Sakai, H. Anti-Cancer and Protective Effects of Royal Jelly for Therapy-Induced Toxicities in Malignancies. *Int. J. Mol. Sci.* **2018**, *19*, 3270. [CrossRef] [PubMed]
253. Salama, S.; Shou, Q.; Abd El-Wahed, A.A.; Elias, N.; Xiao, J.; Swillam, A.; Umair, M.; Guo, Z.; Daglia, M.; Wang, K.; et al. Royal Jelly: Beneficial Properties and Synergistic Effects with Chemotherapeutic Drugs with Particular Emphasis in Anticancer Strategies. *Nutrients* **2022**, *14*, 4166. [CrossRef]
254. Roohi, M.A.; Langroudi, L.; Nosratabadi, R.; Ranjbar, M.; Khajepour, F.; Zangouyee, M.R. Royal Jelly Nanoparticle Alleviates Experimental Model of Breast Cancer Through Suppressing Regulatory T Cells and Upregulating TH1 Cells. *Clin. Lab.* **2023**, *69*, 1–5. [CrossRef]
255. Xu, H.; Li, L.; Wang, S.; Wang, Z.; Qu, L.; Wang, C.; Xu, K. Royal jelly acid suppresses hepatocellular carcinoma tumorigenicity by inhibiting H3 histone lactylation at H3K9la and H3K14la sites. *Phytomedicine* **2023**, *118*, 154940. [CrossRef] [PubMed]

256. Zhang, S.; Shao, Q.; Geng, H.; Su, S. The effect of royal jelly on the growth of breast cancer in mice. *Oncol. Lett.* **2017**, *14*, 7615–7621. [CrossRef] [PubMed]
257. Oršolić, N.; Horvat-Knežević, A.; Benković, V.; Bašić, I. Benefits of use of propolis and related flavonoids against the toxicity of chemotherapeutic agents. In *Scientific Evidence of the Use of Propolis in Ehtnomedicine*; Ethnopharmacology—Review Book; Oršolić, N., Bašić, I., Eds.; Transworld Research Network: Trivandrum, India, 2008; pp. 195–222.
258. Oršolić, N.; Bevanda, M.; Bendelja, K.; Horvat-Knežević, A.; Benković, V.; Bašić, I. Propolis and related polyphenolic compounds; their relevance on host resistance and interaction with chemotherapy. In *Scientific Evidence of the Use of Propolis in Ethnomedicine*; Ethnopharmacology—Review Book; Oršolić, N., Bašić, I., Eds.; Transworld Research Network: Trivandrum, India, 2008; pp. 223–250.
259. Kučan, D.; Oršolić, N.; Odeh, D.; Ramić, S.; Jakopović, B.; Knežević, J.; Jazvinšćak Jembrek, M. The Role of Hyperthermia in Potentiation of Anti-Angiogenic Effect of Cisplatin and Resveratrol in Mice Bearing Solid Form of Ehrlich Ascites Tumour. *Int. J. Mol. Sci.* **2023**, *24*, 11073. [CrossRef] [PubMed]
260. Abandansari, R.M.; Parsian, H.; Kazerouni, F.; Porbagher, R.; Zabihi, E.; Rahimipour, A. Effect of Simultaneous Treatment with Royal Jelly and Doxorubicin on the Survival of the Prostate Cancer Cell Line (PC3): An In Vitro Study. *Int. J. Cancer Manag.* **2018**, *11*, e13780. [CrossRef]
261. Safaei Pourzamani, M.; Oryan, S.; Yaghmaei, P.; Jalili, C.; Ghanbari, A. Royal jelly alleviates side effects of Doxorubicin on male reproductive system: A mouse model simulated human chemotherapy cycles. *Res. J. Pharmacogn.* **2022**, *9*, 77–87. [CrossRef]
262. Mohamed, H.K.; Mobasher, M.A.; Ebiya, R.A.; Hassen, M.T.; Hagag, H.M.; El-Sayed, R.; Abdel-Ghany, S.; Said, M.M.; Awad, N.S. Anti-Inflammatory, Anti-Apoptotic, and Antioxidant Roles of Honey, Royal Jelly, and Propolis in Suppressing Nephrotoxicity Induced by Doxorubicin in Male Albino Rats. *Antioxidants* **2022**, *11*, 1029. [CrossRef] [PubMed]
263. Bhalchandra, W.; Alqadhi, Y.A. Administration of Honey and Royal Jelly Ameliorate Cisplatin Induced Changes in Liver and Kidney Function in Rat. *Biomed. Pharmacol. J.* **2018**, *11*, 2191–2199. [CrossRef]
264. Osama, H.; Abdullah, A.; Gamal, B.; Emad, D.; Sayed, D.; Hussein, E.; Mahfouz, E.; Tharwat, J.; Sayed, S.; Medhat, S.; et al. Effect of Honey and Royal Jelly against Cisplatin-Induced Nephrotoxicity in Patients with Cancer. *J. Am. Coll. Nutr.* **2017**, *36*, 342–346. [CrossRef]
265. Abdel-Hafez, S.M.N.; Rifaai, R.A.; Abdelzaher, W.Y. Possible protective effect of royal jelly against cyclophosphamide induced prostatic damage in male albino rats; a biochemical, histological and immuno-histo-chemical study. *Biomed. Pharmacother.* **2017**, *90*, 15–23. [CrossRef]
266. Albalawi, A.E.; Althobaiti, N.A.; Alrdahe, S.S.; Alhasani, R.H.; Alaryani, F.S.; BinMowyna, M.N. Anti-Tumor Effects of Queen Bee Acid (10-Hydroxy-2-Decenoic Acid) Alone and in Combination with Cyclophosphamide and Its Cellular Mechanisms against Ehrlich Solid Tumor in Mice. *Molecules* **2021**, *26*, 7021. [CrossRef]
267. Khazaei, F.; Ghanbari, E.; Khazaei, M. Protective Effect of Royal Jelly against Cyclophosphamide-Induced Thrombocytopenia and Spleen and Bone Marrow Damages in Rats. *Cell J.* **2020**, *22*, 302–309. [CrossRef] [PubMed]
268. Fan, P.; Han, B.; Hu, H.; Wei, Q.; Zhang, X.; Meng, L.; Nie, J.; Tang, X.; Tian, X.; Zhang, L.; et al. Proteome of thymus and spleen reveals that 10-hydroxydec-2-enoic acid could enhance immunity in mice. *Expert Opin. Ther. Targets* **2020**, *24*, 267–279. [CrossRef] [PubMed]
269. Karadeniz, A.; Simsek, N.; Karakus, E.; Yildirim, S.; Kara, A.; Can, I.; Kisa, F.; Emre, H.; Turkeli, M. Royal jelly modulates oxidative stress and apoptosis in liver and kidneys of rats treated with cisplatin. *Oxid. Med. Cell. Longev.* **2011**, *2011*, 981793. [CrossRef] [PubMed]
270. Hamza, R.Z.; Al-Eisa, R.A.; El-Shenawy, N.S. Possible Ameliorative Effects of the Royal Jelly on Hepatotoxicity and Oxidative Stress Induced by Molybdenum Nanoparticles and/or Cadmium Chloride in Male Rats. *Biology* **2022**, *11*, 450. [CrossRef] [PubMed]
271. Tohamy, H.G.; El-Neweshy, M.S.; Soliman, M.M.; Sayed, S.; Shukry, M.; Ghamry, H.I.; Abd-Ellatieff, H. Protective potential of royal jelly against hydroxyurea -induced hepatic injury in rats via antioxidant, anti-inflammatory, and anti-apoptosis properties. *PLoS ONE* **2022**, *17*, e0265261. [CrossRef] [PubMed]
272. Zargar, H.R.; Hemmati, A.A.; Ghafourian, M.; Arzi, A.; Rezaie, A.; Javad-Moosavi, S.A. Long-term treatment with royal jelly improves bleomycin-induced pulmonary fibrosis in rats. *Can. J. Physiol. Pharmacol.* **2017**, *95*, 23–31. [CrossRef] [PubMed]
273. Moskwa, J.; Naliwajko, S.K.; Dobiecka, D.; Socha, K. Bee Products and Colorectal Cancer—Active Components and Mechanism of Action. *Nutrients* **2023**, *15*, 1614. [CrossRef] [PubMed]
274. Kurdi, L.; Alhusayni, F. Cytotoxicity effect of 5-fluorouracil and bee products on the HTC-116 human colon cancer cell line. *Life Sci. J.* **2019**, *16*, 56–61. [CrossRef]
275. Moubarak, M.M.; Chanouha, N.; Abou Ibrahim, N.; Khalife, H.; Gali-Muhtasib, H. Thymoquinone anticancer activity is enhanced when combined with royal jelly in human breast cancer. *World J. Clin. Oncol.* **2021**, *12*, 342–354. [CrossRef]
276. Filipič, B.; Gradišnik, L.; Rihar, K.; Šooš, E.; Pereyra, A.; Potokar, J. The influence of royal jelly and human interferon-alpha (HuIFN-αN3) on proliferation, glutathione level and lipid peroxidation in human colorectal adenocarcinoma cells in vitro. *Arh. Hig. Rada Toxicol.* **2015**, *66*, 269–274. [CrossRef]
277. Okic-Djordjevic, I.; Trivanovic, D.; Krstic, J.; Jaukovic, A.; Mojsilovic, S.; Santibanez, J.F.; Terzic, M.; Vesovic, D.; Bugarski, D. GE132+Natural: Novel promising dietetic supplement with antiproliferative influence on prostate, colon, and breast cancer cells. *J. BUON.* **2013**, *18*, 504–510. [PubMed]

278. Damiani, A.P.; Magenis, M.L.; Dagostin, L.S.; Beretta, Â.C.D.L.; Sarter, R.J.; Longaretti, L.M.; Monteiro, I.O.; Andrade, V.M. Royal jelly reduce DNA damage induced by alkylating agent in mice. *Mutat Res.* **2022**, *825*, 111796. [CrossRef]
279. Sarhan, H.; Naoum, L. Protective Role of Royal Jelly Against Gamma Radiation Induced Oxidative Stress, Cardio-Toxicity and Organ Dysfunctions in Male Rats. *Egypt J. Hosp. Med.* **2020**, *78*, 62–67. [CrossRef]
280. Erdem, O.; Güngörmüş, Z. The effect of royal jelly on oral mucositis in patients undergoing radiotherapy and chemotherapy. *Holist. Nurs. Pract.* **2014**, *28*, 242–246. [CrossRef]
281. Campos, M.G.; Anjos, O.; Ahmad, S. Prevention of side effects from chemoradiotherapy and antitumor potential of royal jelly and its components: A systematic review. In *Bee Products and Their Applications in the Food and Pharmaceutical Industries*; Boyacioglu, D., Ed.; Academic Press: Cambridge, MA, USA, 2022; pp. 221–244. [CrossRef]
282. El-Fiky, S.A.; Othman, O.E.; Balabel, E.A.; Abd-Elbaset, S.A. The protective role of royal jelly against mutagenic effect of adriamycin and gamma radiation separately and in combination. *Trends Appl. Sci. Res.* **2008**, *3*, 303–318.
283. Fatmawati, F.; Erizka, E.; Hidayat, R. Royal Jelly (Bee Product) Decreases Inflammatory Response in Wistar Rats Induced with Ultraviolet Radiation. *Open Access Maced. J. Med. Sci.* **2019**, *7*, 2723–2727. [CrossRef]
284. Okumura, N.; Ito, T.; Degawa, T.; Moriyama, M.; Moriyama, H. Royal Jelly Protects against Epidermal Stress through Upregulation of the NQO1 Expression. *Int. J. Mol. Sci.* **2021**, *22*, 12973. [CrossRef] [PubMed]
285. Almeer, R.S.; Alarifi, S.; Alkahtani, S.; Ibrahim, S.R.; Ali, D.; Moneim, A. The potential hepatoprotective effect of royal jelly against cadmium chloride-induced hepatotoxicity in mice is mediated by suppression of oxidative stress and upregulation of Nrf2 expression. *Biomed. Pharmacother.* **2018**, *106*, 1490–1498. [CrossRef]
286. Almeer, R.S.; AlBasher, G.I.; Alarifi, S.; Alkahtani, S.; Ali, D.; Abdel Moneim, A.E. Royal jelly attenuates cadmium-induced nephrotoxicity in male mice. *Sci. Rep.* **2019**, *9*, 5825. [CrossRef]
287. Focak, M.; Suljevic, D. Ameliorative Effects of Propolis and Royal Jelly against CCl_4 -Induced Hepatotoxicity and Nephrotoxicity in Wistar Rats. *Chem. Biodivers.* **2023**, *20*, e202200948. [CrossRef]
288. Khalifa, H.A.M.I.; Eleiwa, N.Z.H.; Nazim, H.A. Royal Jelly, A Super Food, Protects Against Celecoxib-Induced Renal Toxicity in Adult Male Albino Rats. *Can. J. Kidney Health Dis.* **2024**, *11*, 20543581241235526. [CrossRef]
289. Dkhil, M.A.; Abdel Moneim, A.E.; Hafez, T.A.; Mubaraki, M.A.; Mohamed, W.F.; Thagfan, F.A.; Al-Quraishy, S. *Myristica fragrans* Kernels Prevent Paracetamol-Induced Hepatotoxicity by Inducing Anti-Apoptotic Genes and Nrf2/HO-1 Pathway. *Int. J. Mol. Sci.* **2019**, *20*, 993. [CrossRef]
290. Nejati, V.; Zahmatkesh, E.; Babaei, M. Protective Effects of Royal Jelly on Oxymetholone-Induced Liver Injury in Mice. *Iran. Biomed. J.* **2016**, *20*, 229–234. [CrossRef]
291. Qu, L.; Wang, L.; Ji, H.; Fang, Y.; Lei, P.; Zhang, X.; Jin, L.; Sun, D.; Dong, H. Toxic Mechanism and Biological Detoxification of Fumonisins. *Toxins* **2022**, *14*, 182. [CrossRef] [PubMed]
292. Lima, W.G.; Brito, J.C.M.; Verly, R.M.; Lima, M.E. Jelleine, a Family of Peptides Isolated from the Royal Jelly of the Honey Bees (*Apis mellifera*), as a Promising Prototype for New Medicines: A Narrative Review. *Toxins* **2024**, *16*, 24. [CrossRef]
293. Wu, Q.; Patočka, J.; Kuča, K. Insect Antimicrobial Peptides, a Mini Review. *Toxins* **2018**, *10*, 461. [CrossRef] [PubMed]
294. Fujiwara, S.; Imai, J.; Fujiwara, M.; Yaeshima, T.; Kawashima, T.; Kobayashi, K. A potent antibacterial protein in royal jelly. Purification and determination of the primary structure of royalisin. *J. Biol. Chem.* **1990**, *265*, 11333–11337. [CrossRef]
295. Bílikova, K.; Huang, S.C.; Lin, I.P.; Šimuth, J.; Peng, C.C. Structure and antimicrobial activity relationship of royalisin, an antimicrobial peptide from royal jelly of *Apis mellifera*. *Peptides* **2015**, *68*, 190–196. [CrossRef] [PubMed]
296. Fontana, R.; Mendes, M.A.; de Souza, B.M.; Konno, K.; César, L.M.; Malaspina, O.; Palma, M.S. Jelleines: A family of antimicrobial peptides from the Royal Jelly of honeybees (*Apis mellifera*). *Peptides* **2004**, *25*, 919–928. [CrossRef]
297. Han, B.; Fang, Y.; Feng, M.; Lu, X.; Huo, X.; Meng, L.; Wu, B.; Li, J. In-depth phosphoproteomic analysis of royal jelly derived from western and eastern honeybee species. *J. Proteome Res.* **2014**, *13*, 5928–5943. [CrossRef]
298. Zhou, J.; Zhang, L.; He, Y.; Liu, K.; Zhang, F.; Zhang, H.; Lu, Y.; Yang, C.; Wang, Z.; Fareed, M.S.; et al. An optimized analog of antimicrobial peptide Jelleine-1 shows enhanced antimicrobial activity against multidrug resistant P. aeruginosa and negligible toxicity in vitro and in vivo. *Eur. J. Med. Chem.* **2021**, *219*, 113433. [CrossRef] [PubMed]
299. Jia, F.; Yu, Q.; Wang, R.; Zhao, L.; Yuan, F.; Guo, H.; Shen, Y.; He, F. Optimized Antimicrobial Peptide Jelleine-I Derivative Br-J-I Inhibits Fusobacterium Nucleatum to Suppress Colorectal Cancer Progression. *Int. J. Mol. Sci.* **2023**, *24*, 1469. [CrossRef] [PubMed]
300. Fratini, F.; Cilia, G.; Mancini, S.; Felicioli, A. Royal Jelly: An ancient remedy with remarkable antibacterial properties. *Microbiol. Res.* **2016**, *192*, 130–141. [CrossRef] [PubMed]
301. Brudzynski, K.; Sjaarda, C.; Lannigan, R. MRJP1-containing glycoproteins isolated from honey, a novel antibacterial drug candidate with broad spectrum activity against multi-drug resistant clinical isolates. *Front. Microbiol.* **2015**, *6*, 711. [CrossRef] [PubMed]
302. Leiva-Sabadini, C.; Alvarez, S.; Barrera, N.P.; Schuh, C.M.A.P.; Aguayo, S. Antibacterial Effect of Honey-Derived Exosomes Containing Antimicrobial Peptides against Oral Streptococci. *Int. J. Nanomed.* **2021**, *16*, 4891–4900. [CrossRef] [PubMed]
303. Álvarez, S.; Contreras-Kallens, P.; Aguayo, S.; Ramírez, O.; Vallejos, C.; Ruiz, J.; Carrasco-Gallardo, E.; Troncoso-Vera, S.; Morales, B.; Schuh, C.M.A.P. Royal jelly extracellular vesicles promote wound healing by modulating underlying cellular responses. *Mol. Ther. Nucleic Acids* **2023**, *31*, 541–552. [CrossRef] [PubMed]

304. Uthaibutra, V.; Kaewkod, T.; Prapawilai, P.; Pandith, H.; Tragoolpua, Y. Inhibition of Skin Pathogenic Bacteria, Antioxidant and Anti-Inflammatory Activity of Royal Jelly from Northern Thailand. *Molecules* **2023**, *28*, 996. [CrossRef]
305. Naghib, M.; Kariminik, A.; Arababadi, M.K.; Rokhbakhsh-Zamin, F.; Mollaei, H.R. Effect of Royal Jelly on Gene Expression of Toll-like Receptors 1–9 in Patients with Hepatitis, B. *Clin Lab.* **2023**, *69*, 77. [CrossRef] [PubMed]
306. Alkhaibari, A.M.; Alanazi, A.D. Insecticidal, Antimalarial, and Antileishmanial Effects of Royal Jelly and Its Three Main Fatty Acids, *trans*-10-Hydroxy-2-decenoic Acid, 10-Hydroxydecanoic Acid, and Sebacic Acid. *Evid. Based. Complement. Alternat. Med.* **2022**, *2022*, 7425322. [CrossRef]
307. Mahdavi, M.; Cheragh, M.; Bagheri, K.P.; Adibzadeh, M.M.; Tajik, A.H.; Memariani, H.; Savoji, M.A.; MahdiGhahari, S.M.; Shahbazzadeh, D. Adjuvant Effect of Royal Jelly on HIV-1 Multi-Epitope Vaccine Candidate: Induction of Th1 Cytokine Pattern. *MOJ Immunol.* **2017**, *5*, 43–48. [CrossRef]
308. Habashy, N.H.; Abu-Serie, M.M. The potential antiviral effect of major royal jelly protein2 and its isoform X1 against severe acute respiratory syndrome coronavirus 2 (SARS-CoV-2): Insight on their sialidase activity and molecular docking. *J. Funct. Foods* **2020**, *75*, 104282. [CrossRef] [PubMed]
309. Habashy, N.H.; Hamouda, A.F.; Abu Serie, M.M. Identification of effective anti-HCV and anti-HIV royal jelly constituents and their acute toxicity evaluation in Albino rats. *Food Chem Toxicol.* **2023**, *182*, 114170. [CrossRef] [PubMed]
310. Abu-Serie, M.M.; Habashy, N.H. Major royal jelly proteins elicited suppression of SARS-CoV-2 entry and replication with halting lung injury. *Int. J. Biol. Macromol.* **2023**, *228*, 715–731. [CrossRef] [PubMed]
311. Elfiky, A.A. Ribavirin, Remdesivir, Sofosbuvir, Galidesivir, and Tenofovir against SARS-CoV-2 RNA dependent RNA polymerase (RdRp): A molecular docking study. *Life Sci.* **2020**, *253*, 117592. [CrossRef] [PubMed]
312. Ozgok Kangal, M.K.; Regan, J.P. Wound Healing. In *StatPearls*; StatPearls Publishing: St. Petersburg, FL, USA, 2023.
313. Majd, S.A.; Rabbani Khorasgani, M.; Zaker, S.R.; Khezri, M.; Aliasghari Veshareh, A. Comparative Efficacy Study of N-Chromosome Royal Jelly Versus Semelil (ANGIPARS) on Wound Healing of Diabetic Rats. *Int. J. Diabetes Obes.* **2022**, *14*, 223–230. [CrossRef]
314. El-Gayar, M.H.; Ishak, R.A.H.; Esmat, A.; Aboulwafa, M.M.; Aboshanab, K.M. Evaluation of lyophilized royal jelly and garlic extract emulgels using a murine model infected with methicillin-resistant Staphylococcus aureus. *AMB Express* **2022**, *12*, 37. [CrossRef] [PubMed]
315. Lin, Y.; Zhang, M.; Wang, L.; Lin, T.; Wang, G.; Peng, J.; Su, S. The in vitro and in vivo wound-healing effects of royal jelly derived from *Apis mellifera* L. during blossom seasons of *Castanea mollissima* Bl. and *Brassica napus* L. in South China exhibited distinct patterns. *BMC Complement. Med. Ther.* **2020**, *20*, 357. [CrossRef] [PubMed]
316. Jovanović, M.M.; Šeklić, D.S.; Rakobradović, J.D.; Planojević, N.S.; Vuković, N.L.; Vukić, M.D.; Marković, S.D. Royal Jelly and *trans*-10-Hydroxy-2-Decenoic Acid Inhibit Migration and Invasion of Colorectal Carcinoma Cells. *Food Technol. Biotechnol.* **2022**, *60*, 213–224. [CrossRef] [PubMed]
317. Bokhari, N.; Ali, A.; Yasmeen, A.; Khalid, H.; Safi, S.Z.; Sharif, F. Fabrication of green composite hand knitted silk mesh reinforced with silk hydrogel. *Int. J. Biol. Macromol.* **2023**, *253*, 127284. [CrossRef]
318. Parhizkari, N.; Eidi, M.; Mahdavi-Ortakand, M.; Ebrahimi-Kia, Y.; Zarei, S.; Pazoki, Z. The effect of oral treatment of royal jelly on the expression of the PDGF-β gene in the skin wound of male mice. *J. Tissue Viab.* **2023**, *32*, 536–540. [CrossRef]
319. Ashrafi, B.; Chehelcheraghi, F.; Rashidipour, M.; Hadavand, S.; Beiranvand, B.; Taherikalani, M.; Soroush, S. Electrospun Nanofibrous Biocomposite of Royal Jelly/Chitosan/Polyvinyl Alcohol (RJ/CS/PVA) Gel as a Biological Dressing for *P. aeruginosa*-Infected Burn Wound. *Appl. Biochem. Biotechnol.* 2023; *ahead of print*. [CrossRef]
320. Saadeldin, I.M.; Tanga, B.M.; Bang, S.; Maigoro, A.Y.; Kang, H.; Cha, D.; Lee, S.; Lee, S.; Cho, J. MicroRNA profiling of royal jelly extracellular vesicles and their potential role in cell viability and reversing cell apoptosis. *Funct. Integr. Genomics* **2023**, *23*, 200. [CrossRef] [PubMed]
321. Kudłacik-Kramarczyk, S.; Krzan, M.; Jamroży, M.; Przybyłowicz, A.; Drabczyk, A. Exploring the Potential of Royal-Jelly-Incorporated Hydrogel Dressings as Innovative Wound Care Materials. *Int. J. Mol. Sci.* **2023**, *24*, 8738. [CrossRef] [PubMed]
322. Tan, D.; Zhu, W.; Liu, L.; Pan, Y.; Xu, Y.; Huang, Q.; Li, L.; Rao, L. In situ formed scaffold with royal jelly-derived extracellular vesicles for wound healing. *Theranostics* **2023**, *13*, 2811–2824. [CrossRef] [PubMed]
323. Zheng, Y.; Pan, C.; Xu, P.; Liu, K. Hydrogel-mediated extracellular vesicles for enhanced wound healing: The latest progress, and their prospects for 3D bioprinting. *J. Nanobiotechnol.* **2024**, *22*, 57. [CrossRef] [PubMed]
324. Kowalska, G.; Rosicka-Kaczmarek, J.; Miśkiewicz, K.; Zakłos-Szyda, M.; Rohn, S.; Kanzler, C.; Wiktorska, M.; Niewiarowska, J. Arabinoxylan-Based Microcapsules Being Loaded with Bee Products as Bioactive Food Components Are Able to Modulate the Cell Migration and Inflammatory Response—In Vitro Study. *Nutrients* **2022**, *14*, 2529. [CrossRef] [PubMed]
325. Ramírez, O.J.; Alvarez, S.; Contreras-Kallens, P.; Barrera, N.P.; Aguayo, S.; Schuh, C.M.A.P. Type I collagen hydrogels as a delivery matrix for royal jelly derived extracellular vesicles. *Drug Deliv.* **2020**, *27*, 1308–1318. [CrossRef] [PubMed]
326. Yamauchi, K.; Kogashiwa, Y.; Moro, Y.; Kohno, N. The effect of topical application of royal jelly on chemoradiotherapy-induced mucositis in head and neck cancer: A preliminary study. *Int. J. Otolaryngol.* **2014**, *2014*, 974967. [CrossRef] [PubMed]
327. Suemaru, K.; Cui, R.; Li, B.; Watanabe, S.; Okihara, K.; Hashimoto, K.; Yamada, H.; Araki, H. Topical application of royal jelly has a healing effect for 5-fluorouracil-induced experimental oral mucositis in hamsters. *Methods Find. Exp. Clin. Pharmacol.* **2008**, *30*, 103–106. [CrossRef]

328. Wang, X.; Zeng, L.; Feng, X.; Zhao, N.; Feng, N.; Du, X. Did you choose appropriate mouthwash for managing chemoradiotherapy-induced oral mucositis? The therapeutic effect compared by a Bayesian network meta-analysis. *Front Oral Health* **2023**, 3, 977830. [CrossRef] [PubMed] [PubMed Central]
329. Severo, M.L.B.; Thieme, S.; Silveira, F.M.; Tavares, R.P.M.; Gonzaga, A.K.G.; Zucolotto, S.M.; de Araújo, A.A.; Martins, M.A.T.; Martins, M.D.; da Silveira, É.J.D. Comparative study of royal jelly, propolis, and photobiomodulation therapies in 5-fluorouracil-related oral mucositis in rats. *Support. Care Cancer* **2022**, *30*, 2723–2734. [CrossRef]
330. Watanabe, S.; Suemaru, K.; Takechi, K.; Kaji, H.; Imai, K.; Araki, H. Oral mucosal adhesive films containing royal jelly accelerate recovery from 5-fluorouracil-induced oral mucositis. *J. Pharmacol. Sci.* **2013**, *121*, 110–118. [CrossRef] [PubMed]
331. Daugėlaitė, G.; Užkuraitytė, K.; Jagelavičienė, E.; Filipauskas, A. Prevention and Treatment of Chemotherapy and Radiotherapy Induced Oral Mucositis. *Medicina* **2019**, *55*, 25. [CrossRef] [PubMed]
332. Chen, D.; Xin, X.X.; Qian, H.C.; Yu, Z.Y.; Shen, L.R. Evaluation of the major royal jelly proteins as an alternative to fetal bovine serum in culturing human cell lines. *J. Zhejiang Univ. Sci. B* **2016**, *17*, 476–483. [CrossRef] [PubMed]
333. Oka, H.; Emori, Y.; Kobayashi, N.; Hayashi, Y.; Nomoto, K. Suppression of allergic reactions by royal jelly in association with the restoration of macrophage function and the improvement of Th1/Th2 cell responses. *Int. Immunopharmacol.* **2001**, *1*, 521–532. [CrossRef] [PubMed]
334. Taniguchi, Y.; Kohno, K.; Inoue, S.; Koya-Miyata, S.; Okamoto, I.; Arai, N.; Iwaki, K.; Ikeda, M.; Kurimoto, M. Oral administration of royal jelly inhibits the development of atopic dermatitis-like skin lesions in NC/Nga mice. *Int. Immunopharmacol.* **2003**, *3*, 1313–1324. [CrossRef]
335. Mannoor, M.K.; Shimabukuro, I.; Tsukamotoa, M.; Watanabe, H.; Yamaguchi, K.; Sato, Y. Honeybee royal jelly inhibits autoimmunity in SLE-prone NZB × NZW F1 mice. *Lupus* **2009**, *18*, 44–52. [CrossRef]
336. Zahran, A.M.; Elsayh, K.I.; Saad, K.; Eloseily, E.M.; Osman, N.S.; Alblihed, M.A.; Badr, G.; Mahmoud, M.H. Effects of royal jelly supplementation on regulatory T cells in children with SLE. *Food Nutr. Res.* **2016**, *60*, 32963. [CrossRef]
337. Erem, C.; Deger, O.; Ovali, E.; Barlak, Y. The effects of royal jelly on autoimmunity in Graves' disease. *Endocrine* **2006**, *30*, 175–183. [CrossRef] [PubMed]
338. Guendouz, M.; Haddi, A.; Grar, H.; Kheroua, O.; Saidi, D.; Kaddouri, H. Preventive effects of royal jelly against anaphylactic response in a murine model of cow's milk allergy. *Pharm. Biol.* **2017**, *55*, 2145–2152. [CrossRef]
339. Kai, H.; Motomura, Y.; Saito, S.; Hashimoto, K.; Tatefuji, T.; Takamune, N.; Misumi, S. Royal jelly enhances antigen-specific mucosal IgA response. *Food Sci. Nutr.* **2013**, *1*, 222–227. [CrossRef]
340. Hata, T.; Furusawa-Horie, T.; Arai, Y.; Takahashi, T.; Seishima, M.; Ichihara, K. Studies of royal jelly and associated cross-reactive allergens in atopic dermatitis patients. *PLoS ONE* **2020**, *15*, e0233707. [CrossRef] [PubMed]
341. Mizutani, Y.; Shibuya, Y.; Takahashi, T.; Tsunoda, T.; Moriyama, T.; Seishima, M. Major royal jelly protein 3 as a possible allergen in royal jelly-induced anaphylaxis. *J. Dermatol.* **2011**, *38*, 1079–1081. [CrossRef] [PubMed]
342. Furusawa, T.; Rakwal, R.; Nam, H.W.; Shibato, J.; Agrawal, G.K.; Kim, Y.S.; Ogawa, Y.; Yoshida, Y.; Kouzuma, Y.; Masuo, Y.; et al. Comprehensive royal jelly (RJ) proteomics using one- and two-dimensional proteomics platforms reveals novel RJ proteins and potential phospho/glycoproteins. *J. Proteome Res.* **2008**, *7*, 3194–3229. [CrossRef] [PubMed]
343. Rosmilah, M.; Shahnaz, M.; Patel, G.; Lock, J.; Rahman, D.; Masita, A.; Noormalin, A. Characterization of major allergens of royal jelly *Apis mellifera*. *Trop. Biomed.* **2008**, *25*, 243–251. [PubMed]
344. Li, J.D.; Cui, L.; Xu, Y.Y.; Guan, K. A Case of Anaphylaxis Caused by Major Royal Jelly Protein 3 of Royal Jelly and Its Cross-Reactivity with Honeycomb. *J. Asthma Allergy* **2021**, *14*, 1555–1557. [CrossRef] [PubMed]
345. El-Nekeety, A.A.; El-Kholy, W.; Abbas, N.F.; Ebaid, A.; Amra, H.A.; Abdel-Wahhab, M.A. Efficacy of royal jelly against the oxidative stress of fumonisin in rats. *Toxicon* **2007**, *50*, 256–269. [CrossRef] [PubMed]
346. Fan, P.; Han, B.; Feng, M.; Fang, Y.; Zhang, L.; Hu, H.; Hao, Y.; Qi, Y.; Zhang, X.; Li, J. Functional and Proteomic Investigations Reveal Major Royal Jelly Protein 1 Associated with Anti-Hypertension Activity in Mouse Vascular Smooth Muscle Cells. *Sci. Rep.* **2016**, *6*, 30230. [CrossRef] [PubMed]
347. Escamilla, K.I.A.; Ordóñez, Y.B.M.; Sandoval-Peraza, V.M.; Fernández, J.J.A.; Ancona, D.A.B. Anti-Hypertensive Activity In Vitro and In Vivo on Royal Jelly Produced by Different Diets. *Emir. J. Food Agric.* **2022**, *34*, 9–15. [CrossRef]
348. Mazzei, P.; Piccolo, A.; Brescia, M.; Caprio, E. Assessment of geographical origin and production period of royal jelly by NMR metabolomics. *Chem. Biol. Technol. Agric.* **2020**, *7*, 24. [CrossRef]
349. Emir, M. Effect of harvesting period on chemical and bioactive properties of royal jelly from Turkey. *Eur. Food Sci. Eng.* **2020**, *1*, 9–12.
350. Ghosh, S.; Jung, C. Chemical Composition and Nutritional Value of Royal Jelly Samples Obtained from Honey Bee (*Apis mellifera*) Hives Fed on Oak and Rapeseed Pollen Patties. *Insects* **2024**, *15*, 141. [CrossRef] [PubMed]
351. Milone, J.P.; Chakrabarti, P.; Sagili, R.R.; Tarpy, D.R. Colony-level pesticide exposure affects honey bee (*Apis mellifera* L.) royal jelly production and nutritional composition. *Chemosphere* **2021**, *263*, 128183. [CrossRef] [PubMed]
352. Sagona, S.; Coppola, F.; Giannaccini, G.; Betti, L.; Palego, L.; Tafi, E.; Casini, L.; Piana, L.; Dall'Olio, R.; Felicioli, A. Impact of Different Storage Temperature on the Enzymatic Activity of *Apis mellifera* Royal Jelly. *Foods* **2022**, *11*, 3165. [CrossRef] [PubMed]
353. Arfa, A.; Reyad, Y.M.; Nikeety, M.E. Quality Parameters of Royal Jelly in national and international standards: Specifications, differences and suggestions. *Ann. Rom. Soc. Cell Biol.* **2021**, *25*, 7977–7997.

354. Chen, D.; Guo, C.; Lu, W.; Zhang, C.; Xiao, C. Rapid quantification of royal jelly quality by mid-infrared spectroscopy coupled with backpropagation neural network. *Food Chem.* **2023**, *418*, 135996. [CrossRef] [PubMed]
355. Oršolić, N. Učinkovitost biološki aktivnih sastavnica matične mliječi: Analiza i standardizacija. *Arh. Hig. Rada Toksikol.* **2013**, *64*, 445–460. [CrossRef] [PubMed]
356. Spanidi, E.; Athanasopoulou, S.; Liakopoulou, A.; Chaidou, A.; Hatziantoniou, S.; Gardikis, K. Royal Jelly Components Encapsulation in a Controlled Release System-Skin Functionality, and Biochemical Activity for Skin Applications. *Pharmaceuticals* **2022**, *15*, 907. [CrossRef] [PubMed]
357. Mureşan, C.I.; Buttstedt, A. pH-dependent stability of honey bee (*Apis mellifera*) major royal jelly proteins. *Sci. Rep.* **2019**, *9*, 9014. [CrossRef] [PubMed]
358. Daniele, G.; Casabianca, H. Sugar composition of French Royal Jelly for comparison with commercial and artificial sugar samples. *Food Chem.* **2012**, *134*, 1025–1029. [CrossRef]
359. Virgiliou, C.; Kanelis, D.; Pina, A.; Gika, H.; Tananaki, C.; Zotou, A.; Theodoridis, G. A targeted approach for studying the effect of sugar bee feeding on the metabolic profile of Royal Jelly. *J. Chromatogr. A.* **2020**, *1616*, 460783. [CrossRef]
360. Fuente-Ballesteros, A.; Jano, A.; Bernal, J.; Ares, A.M. Development and validation of an analytical methodology based on solvent extraction and gas chromatography for determining pesticides in royal jelly and propolis. *Food Chem.* **2024**, *437*, 137911. [CrossRef] [PubMed]
361. Stocker, A. Isolation and Characterisation of Substances from Royal Jelly. Ph.D. Thesis, Universite´ d'Orle´ans, Orle´ans, France, 2003.
362. Wang, Z.; Ren, P.; Wu, Y.; He, Q. Recent advances in analytical techniques for the detection of adulteration and authenticity of bee products—A review. *Food Addit. Contam. Part A Chem. Anal. Control. Expo. Risk. Assess.* **2021**, *38*, 533–549. [CrossRef] [PubMed]
363. Minegaki, N.; Koshizuka, T.; Hatasa, K.; Kondo, H.; Kato, H.; Tannaka, M.; Takahashi, K.; Tsuji, M.; Inoue, N. The C-Terminal Penta-Peptide Repeats of Major Royal Jelly Protein 3 Ameliorate the Progression of Inflammation In Vivo and In Vitro. *Biol Pharm Bull.* **2022**, *45*, 583–589. [CrossRef] [PubMed]
364. Tahereh, F.N.; Nayereh, K.; Narjes, B.; Mojtaba, M.; Shirin, S.; Sareh, D. The Fertility Outcome of Royal Jelly versus Intra Uterine Insemination: A Pilot Randomized Controlled Trial Study, Jundishapur. *J. Nat. Prod.* **2021**, *16*, e107420.
365. Basmeh, K.; Farzad, S.; Shima, J.; Mojtaba, M.A.; Fatemeh, H. Effect of royal jelly intake on serum glucose, HbA1c, and total antioxidant capacity (TAC) in type 2 diabetic patients: A randomized, double blind clinical trial study. *Red Jacket Middle Sch.* **2013**, *19*, 33–40.
366. Ohba, K.; Miyata, Y.; Shinzato, T.; Funakoshi, S.; Maeda, K.; Matsuo, T.; Mitsunari, K.; Mochizuki, Y.; Nishino, T.; Sakai, H. Effect of oral intake of royal jelly on endothelium function in hemodialysis patients: Study protocol for multicenter, double-blind, randomized control trial. *Trials* **2022**, *22*, 950. [CrossRef] [PubMed]
367. Yumi, M.; Fumihiko, T.; Yuji, K.; Hiroyuki, H. The Effects of The Royal Jelly on Dry Mouth Sensation with Normal Saliva Function: A Double-Blind, Placebo-Controlled, Cross-Over Trial Clinical Study. *JCDR* **2023**, *17*, KC01–KC04. [CrossRef]
368. Shafiee, Z.; Hanifi, N.; Rashtchi, V. The effect ofroyal jelly on the level of consciousness in patients with traumatic brain injury: A double-blind randomized clinical trial. *Nurs. Midwifery Stud.* **2022**, *11*, 96–102. [CrossRef]
369. Peivandi, S.; Khalili, S.S.; Abbasi, Z.; Zamaniyan, M.; Gordani, N.; Moradi, S. Effect of Royal Jelly on Sperm Parameters and Testosterone Levels in Infertile Men. *J. Maz. Univ. Med. Sci.* **2022**, *31*, 43–52.

International Journal of
Molecular Sciences

MDPI

Review

Antioxidant Enzymes and Their Potential Use in Breast Cancer Treatment

María Magdalena Vilchis-Landeros [1], Héctor Vázquez-Meza [1], Melissa Vázquez-Carrada [2], Daniel Uribe-Ramírez [3] and Deyamira Matuz-Mares [1,*]

[1] Departamento de Bioquímica, Facultad de Medicina, Universidad Nacional Autónoma de México, Avenida Universidad 3000, Cd. Universitaria, Mexico City C.P. 04510, Mexico; vilchisl@unam.mx (M.M.V.-L.); hvazquez@bq.unam.mx (H.V.-M.)

[2] Institute of Microbiology, Cluster of Excellence on Plant Sciences, Heinrich Heine University Düsseldorf, 40225 Düsseldorf, Germany; m.vazquez-carrada@hhu.de

[3] Departamento de Ingeniería Bioquímica, Escuela Nacional de Ciencias Biológicas, Instituto Politécnico Nacional, Av. Wilfrido Massieu 399, Nueva Industrial Vallejo, Gustavo A. Madero, Mexico City C.P. 07738, Mexico; daniel.uriberam@gmail.com

* Correspondence: deya@bq.unam.mx; Tel.: +52-55-5623-2168

Abstract: According to the World Health Organization (WHO), breast cancer (BC) is the deadliest and the most common type of cancer worldwide in women. Several factors associated with BC exert their effects by modulating the state of stress. They can induce genetic mutations or alterations in cell growth, encouraging neoplastic development and the production of reactive oxygen species (ROS). ROS are able to activate many signal transduction pathways, producing an inflammatory environment that leads to the suppression of programmed cell death and the promotion of tumor proliferation, angiogenesis, and metastasis; these effects promote the development and progression of malignant neoplasms. However, cells have both non-enzymatic and enzymatic antioxidant systems that protect them by neutralizing the harmful effects of ROS. In this sense, antioxidant enzymes such as superoxide dismutase (SOD), catalase (CAT), glutathione peroxidase (GPx), glutathione reductase (GR), thioredoxin reductase (TrxR), and peroxiredoxin (Prx) protect the body from diseases caused by oxidative damage. In this review, we will discuss mechanisms through which some enzymatic antioxidants inhibit or promote carcinogenesis, as well as the new therapeutic proposals developed to complement traditional treatments.

Keywords: antioxidant; breast cancer; superoxide dismutase; catalase; glutathione peroxidase; glutathione reductase; thioredoxin reductase; peroxiredoxin

1. Introduction

Cancer is one of the leading causes of death worldwide and is a crucial factor reducing life expectancy. In 2022, 19.96 million new cases and almost 10 million deaths caused by cancer were recorded [1]. Currently, the World Health Organization (WHO) recognizes breast cancer (BC) as the most common type of cancer on a global scale [2]. In 2022, according to the United Nations, BC was reported as the cancer with the highest incidence, with 2.29 million new cases, representing 11.5% of all cancer diagnoses worldwide [3,4].

In Latin America, BC is the most common and the deadliest cancer in women as well. In 2022, the recorded incidence was 114,900 diagnoses, coupled with a mortality rate of 13.2 per 100,000 inhabitants [3]. The high mortality in this region could be attributed to several factors, such as late-stage diagnosis, lack of access to specialized cancer hospitals, and limited health insurance coverage for high-cost medications [4].

In Mexico, during 2020, malignant tumors accounted for the death of 97,323 people. Among them, 8% were attributed to BC, causing the death of 7821 women and 58 men. The highest rate of female deaths caused by BC is recorded in the 60-year-old and older age group (49,08 per 100,000 women in this age group) [5]. BC is a multifactorial disease and depending on its etiology, it can be classified as sporadic or hereditary. Sporadic BC represents around 90% of cases, while hereditary BC corresponds to 10–15% of malignant breast tumors.

Several factors associated with BC exert their effects through the modulation of the oxidative stress state in cells [6,7]. This stress can cause genetic mutations or alterations in cell growth, favoring neoplastic development and generating reactive oxygen species (ROS) from endogenous sources (intracellular elements such as peroxisomes, mitochondria, cytochrome P450, and extracellular elements such as inflammatory cells) and exogenous sources (xenobiotics, metals, pathogens, drugs, and radiation) [8–10]. The generated ROS can activate many signal transduction pathways factors such as vascular endothelial growth factor (VEGF), hypoxia-inducible factor 1 alpha subunit (HIF1α), nuclear factor erythroid 2 (Nrf2), activator protein 1 (AP-1) and nuclear factor kappa light chain gene enhancer in activated B cells (NF-kB). These factors transcribe cell growth regulatory genes [11,12] and they can also trigger the activation of kinases such as mitogen-activated protein kinase (MAPK), extracellular-regulated kinase (Erk), c-jun NH-2 terminal kinase (JNK), and p38 MAPK, which are involved in cell migration and invasion [13]. These signaling cascades generate an inflammatory environment that leads to different events such as the suppression of programmed cell death, tumor proliferation, angiogenesis, and metastasis; all of these favor the development and progression of malignant neoplasms [14].

On the other hand, chemical carcinogens have been shown to abrogate cellular antioxidant systems and/or DNA repair systems [15]. Oxidative stress arises due to an imbalance between the production and the elimination of ROS and performs a fundamental role in the pathogenesis of various disorders and pathophysiological processes such as BC [6,16,17].

In this regard, it is known that the increment of the oxidative stress markers and the decrement of the antioxidant defense system are considered factors that correlate with the appearance and progression of BC [18]. The DNA of BC cells contains many base modifications and shows oxidation products, such as 8-hydroxydeoxyguanosine (8-OHdG), an element that appears to play a significant role in the progression of this disease [19]. Elevated levels of urinary 8-OHdG have been detected in women with BC, and this value becomes more significant in the late stage of cancer, a fact that suggests that ROS might play a role in early carcinogenesis [20]. ROS also appear to participate in the architecture distortion of the mammary epithelium, inducing fibroblast proliferation, epithelial hyperplasia, cellular atypia, and BC [21].

The function of both non-enzymatic and enzymatic antioxidant systems is to protect cells from oxidative stress and neutralize the damaging effects of ROS [11]. According to this, antioxidant enzymes such as superoxide dismutase (SOD), catalase (CAT), glutathione peroxidase (GPx), glutathione reductase (GR), thioredoxin reductase (TrxR), and peroxiredoxin (Prx) protect the body from diseases caused by oxidative damage. In this review, we will discuss various mechanisms through which some enzymatic antioxidants can either inhibit or promote carcinogenesis, as well as the new therapeutic proposals developed to complement traditional treatments.

2. Oxidative Stress

During cellular metabolism, many short- and long-lived ROS are generated: superoxide ($O_2^{\cdot-}$), hydroxyl radical ($OH^{\cdot}$), and hydrogen peroxide (H_2O_2). Depending on their concentration, location, and intracellular conditions, ROS can cause toxicity or act as signaling molecules [22]. This ROS dual role is supported by growing evidence that has shown they act within cells, either as second messengers in intracellular signaling cascades or by inducing and maintaining the oncogenic phenotype of cancer cells. On the other hand, ROS can also play a role in cellular senescence and apoptosis, functioning as antitumor species [23,24]. In cancer cells, ROS production is elevated due to an increased metabolic rate and relative hypoxia, resulting in the induction of genetic mutations and changes in transcriptional processes and ultimately, in the development of cancer [25]. Furthermore, cancer cells adapt to elevated ROS levels by activating antioxidant pathways, resulting in increased ROS scavenging [26].

3. Antioxidant Systems

The cellular levels of ROS are controlled by two well-established mechanisms: (i) non-enzymatic antioxidant systems, such as glutathione, thioredoxin, and vitamins like C and E; and (ii) enzymatic antioxidant systems (Figure 1). This battery of enzymes, involved in the control of ROS, includes SOD, CAT, GPx, GR, TrxR, and Prx [27,28].

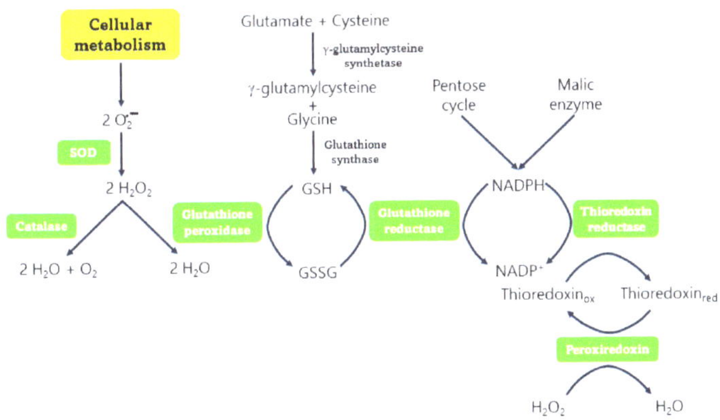

Figure 1. The antioxidant enzymatic system is made up of six enzymes: superoxide dismutase (SOD), catalase (CAT), glutathione peroxidase (GPx), glutathione reductase (GR), thioredoxin reductase (TrxR), and peroxiredoxin (Prx). SOD eliminates the 2 $O_2^{\cdot-}$, generating two H_2O_2 molecules and CAT destroys them, producing H_2O and O_2. GPx, GR, TrxR, and Prx remove H_2O_2 by regulating the redox conditions of glutathione, thioredoxin, and NADPH.

3.1. Non-Enzymatic Antioxidant Systems

Non-enzymatic antioxidant barriers are a set of compounds that are obtained from the diet [29] and they work together with antioxidant enzymes [27]. These are also known as scavenger antioxidants since they counteract the beginning of the oxidation chain and interrupt its propagation reactions, thus neutralizing ROS by donating electrons to them [30,31]. Some non-enzymatic antioxidants are glutathione; thioredoxin; lipoic acid; bilirubin; ubiquinones; flavonoids; vitamins A, C, and E; and carotenoids [27,29]. The minerals selenium, copper, zinc and magnesium are part of the molecular structure of some of the antioxidant enzymes [32].

3.2. Enzymatic Antioxidant Systems

3.2.1. Superoxide Dismutase (SOD)

The function of SOD is to convert $O_2^{\cdot-}$ anions into H_2O_2 and oxygen (O_2), while other enzymes, such as peroxidases and CAT, convert H_2O_2 into water [33]. SODs are the first line of defense against ROS-mediated injuries. The SOD family includes copper and zinc-dependent SOD (Cu/ZnSOD or SOD1), manganese-dependent SOD (MnSOD or SOD2), iron-dependent SOD, and extracellular superoxide dismutase (FeSOD or SOD3 or EcSOD) [34], and all of these play a crucial role in the removal of $O_2^{\cdot-}$ [22]. SODs are involved in the regulation of oxidative stress, lipid metabolism, inflammation, and oxidation in cells. Furthermore, they can prevent lipid peroxidation, oxidation of low-density lipoproteins in macrophages, formation of lipid droplets, and adhesion of inflammatory cells to endothelial monolayers [35]. Additionally, it has been reported that there is a significant decrease in the activity of Cu/ZnSOD and MnSOD in cancer cells (Table 1) [35–37].

Table 1. Antioxidant enzymes that participate in the regulation of breast cancer: location and function.

Enzyme	Type	Tissue Expression	Cellular Localization	Pathological Function	Therapeutical Use	Sample Type	References
Catalase	Typical	Highest enzyme activity in liver and erythrocytes, high activity in kidney and adipose tissue, intermediate in lung and pancreas, and very low in heart and brain	Peroxisomes	Dichotomous role: Protection from tumor formation and progression; however, it is also necessary for tumor progression and metastasis. It is frequently decreased in breast tumors and blood of patients with BC and BC cell cultures	Increasing CAT levels in breast tumors decreases hypoxia and attenuates the tumoral microenvironment immunosuppression condition through tumor-associated macrophages reprogramming from M2 (pro-tumoral) to M1 (anti-tumoral) due to increased O_2 in the tumor, reversing hypoxia-induced chemotherapy resistance	Serum and tissue samples from BC patients and human BC MCF-7 cell line	[38–44]
SOD1	CuZn-SOD	Pons, substantia nigra pars compacta, dorsal root ganglion, lateral nuclear group of the thalamus	Cytosol, nucleus, and mitochondria	Reduced expression and activity, generating an increase in oxidative stress within the cell	In BC cells, the decrease in NAD-dependent deacetylase sirtuin-3 (SIRT3) expression can be counteracted by an upregulation of SOD1. As a result, the total level of ROS in the mitochondria is maintained within a window compatible with cell survival. In addition, it was reported that, using a panel of mammary cell lines, SOD1 is overexpressed and SIRT3 is decreased	MCF-10A, MCF-7, MDA-MB-231, and MDA-MB-157	[45,46]

Table 1. *Cont.*

Enzyme	Type	Tissue Expression	Cellular Localization	Pathological Function	Therapeutical Use	Sample Type	References
SOD2	Mn-SOD	Lungs, placenta, kidney, pancreas and uterus, cartilage, skeletal muscle, brain, and eye	Mitochondrial matrix	Reduced expression and activity, generating an increase in oxidative stress within the cell and mitochondria	Almost all tumors have reduced Mn-SOD activity. Extensive epidemiological studies have mainly focused on the Ala16Val dimorphism of Mn-SOD as a risk factor for BC. Ambrosone and his colleagues were the first to report Ala16-MnSOD as a risk factor for BC	Data were collected in a case–control study of diet and BC in western New York from 1986 to 1991. Caucasian women with incident, primary, histologically confirmed BC were frequency-matched by age and county of residence to community controls. Blood specimens were collected and processed from a subset of participants in the study (266 cases and 295 controls)	[37,47,48]
SOD3	Ec-SOD	Cardiovascular endothelium, lungs, and placenta. Displays moderate activity within the kidney, pancreas, uterus, cartilage, skeletal muscle, adipose tissue, brain, and eye	Extracellular	Reduced activity, $OH^{\cdot}$ levels are increased through the Fenton and Harber–Weiss reactions. In addition, the oxidation of $NO^{\bullet}$ mediated by superoxide is increased, generating high concentrations of peroxynitrite ($ONOO^{-}$)	Ec-SOD overexpression inhibited in vitro proliferation, clonogenic survival, and invasion of a triple-negative breast cancer cell (TNCB) line, in part by suppressing heparanase-mediated cleavage of cell surface proteoglycans and by reducing the bioavailability of VEGFA (vascular endothelial growth factor A). Ec-SOD overexpression also significantly inhibited tumor metastasis in both an experimental lung and a mouse model of spontaneous metastasis	Non-malignant, post-stasis human mammary epithelial cells extracted from reduction mammoplasty, human mammary epithelial cells (HMEC) immortalized, non-malignant breast epithelial MCF-10A cells, human mammary adenocarcinoma cell lines, MCF-7 cells, MDA-MB-231 cells, and MDA-MB-435 cells	[48–51]

Table 1. *Cont.*

Enzyme	Type	Tissue Expression	Cellular Localization	Pathological Function	Therapeutical Use	Sample Type	References
GPx1	Selenium-dependent	Red blood cells, liver, lung, and kidney	Cytosol, nucleus, and mitochondria	Acts as a tumor promoter by regulating the proliferation, invasion, migration, apoptosis, immune response, and drug sensitivity of tumor cells	Enzyme glutamate dehydrogenase 1 (GDH1) controlling the intracellular levels of alpha-ketoglutarate (α-KG) and subsequent metabolite fumarate. Fumarate binds to and activates GPx1, leading to attenuated cancer, cell proliferation, and tumor growth (cell culture) (decreased GPx1 expression in tumorous breast tissue) (in human BC cell lines, GPx1 is downregulated)	BC cell line MDA-MB-231. Tissue samples from human patients aged 44–82 years with BC and MCF-7 human carcinoma cells. Human BC MCF-7 and MDA-MB-231 cell lines compared with healthy breast MCF-10A cells	[52–55]
GPx2	Selenium-dependent	Gastrointestinal tract, breast	Cytosol and nucleus	It is upregulated in a variety of tumor cells and is associated with tumor cell proliferation and a poor prognosis of patients. It causes vascular malfunction and hypoxia	Once a cell has been programmed to proliferate in an uncontrolled way, GPx2 supports the growth of cells by inhibiting apoptosis. GPx2 loss stimulates malignant progression due to reactive oxygen species/hypoxia inducible factor-α (HIF1α)/VEGFA signaling, causing poor perfusion and hypoxia (in human BC cell lines, GPx2 is upregulated)	MCF-7 and MDA-MB-231 cell lines compared with healthy breast MCF-10A cells	[7,52,54,56]
GPx3	Selenium-dependent	Kidney, lung, epididymis, breast, heart, and muscle	Plasma and mitochondria	Reduced expression can promote the proliferation, motility, and invasion of melanoma cells	GPx3 directly targets the ERα gene in white adipose tissue, for which it was proposed as an important mediator of the estrogen effects in association with fat mass. Considering the link between visceral fat and BC initiation and progression, it is reasonable to observe an overexpression of GPx3 in BC cells (in human BC cell lines, GPx2 is upregulated)	MCF-7 and MDA-MB-231 cell lines compared with healthy breast MCF-10A cells	[7,57]

Table 1. *Cont.*

Enzyme	Type	Tissue Expression	Cellular Localization	Pathological Function	Therapeutical Use	Sample Type	References
GPx4	Selenium-dependent	Thyroid gland, bronchus, duodenum, lung, breast, heart, and muscle	Nucleus, cytosol, and mitochondria	Increased expression may promote the malignant progression of BC	It is an inducer of ferroptosis and apoptosis through ubiquitination of GPx4 (GPx4 is downregulated, with reduced expression in several cell lines, including human BC)	MCF-7 and MDA-MB-231 cell lines compared with healthy breast MCF-10A cells	[7,54,58,59]
GPx5	Non-Selenium-dependent	Epididymis	Extracellular	Downregulated	In human BC cell lines, GPx5 is downregulated	MCF-7 and MDA-MB-231 cell lines compared with healthy breast MCF-10A cells	[7]
GPx6	Selenium-dependent	Olfactory epithelium	Epithelium	No data	No data	No data	[52]
GPx7	Non-Selenium-dependent	Preadipocytes	Lumen of the endoplasmic reticulum.	Downregulated	In human breast cancer cell lines, GPx7 is downregulated	MCF-7 and MDA-MB2-31 cell lines compared with healthy breast MCF-10A cells	[7,52]
GPx8	Non-Selenium-dependent	Lung	Transmembrane of the endoplasmic reticulum	Expression is upregulated	In human BC cell lines, GPx8 is upregulated. If GPx8 is suppressed in these cells, they express a non-functional IL-6 receptor, which does not interact with IL-6. This altered binding hinders the activation of the JAK/STAT3 signaling pathway, thus inhibiting the transition of cancer cells to an aggressive phenotype	Human breast cancer cell line MDA-MB-231	[54,60]
GR	Selenoprotein	Pylorus, islet of Langerhans, epithelium of nasopharynx	Mitochondria, nucleus, and cytoplasm	Protects cancer cells against increased oxidative stress and provides a survival advantage	Increased GR activity in tumor cells and in the blood of BC patients. Therefore, inhibition of glutathione reductase in BC cells causes increased oxidative stress in the cell, which stops the growth of the cancer cell	The studies have been carried out on tissue samples from human patients with BC, aged 20 to 65 years; some were taken from ductal carcinoma; in the case of human BC cell lines, T-47D and MCF-7, D492 have been used	[61–64]

Table 1. *Cont.*

Enzyme	Type	Tissue Expression	Cellular Localization	Pathological Function	Therapeutical Use	Sample Type	References
PrxI	2-Cysteine peroxidase	Thyroid gland, nasal cavity epithelium, olfactory segment of nasal mucosa, palpebral conjunctiva	Cytoplasm, melanosome, nucleus	Overexpressed in BC tissue. Correlated with shortened patient survival	Inhibition of PrxI gene upregulation may cause disadvantage to the survival and proliferation of tumor cells	Tissue from BC (type I to IV stage) patients	[65–69]
PrxII	2-Cysteine peroxidase	Thalamus, trabecular bone tissue, substantia nigra pars compacta, substantia nigra pars reticulata	Cytoplasm, nucleus	Overexpressed in BC tissue. Induces carcinogenic changes, maintains cancer stem cells phenotype and stemness properties	Inhibition of PrxII with siRNA partially reverses the radioresistant phenotype in radiation-resistant BC cells	Tissue from BC (type I to IV stage) patients	[67,69,70]
PrxIII	2-Cysteine peroxidase	Adrenal tissue, adrenal gland cortex, heart right ventricle, biceps brachii	Mitochondrion, cytoplasm, early endosome	Overexpressed in BC tissue. Related to tumorigenesis	Potential proliferation marker. Related to a better prognosis	Human BC MCF-7 and MDA-MB-231 cell lines. Tissue from BC patients	[68,69,71–73]
PrxIV	2-Cysteine peroxidase	Pancreas, tibia, adrenal tissue	Cytoplasm, endoplasmic reticulum	Overexpressed in progesterone receptor positive cases. Promoted migration and invasion of cancer cells	Promising therapeutic target for inflammatory diseases and cancer. Related to a better prognosis	Tissue from BC patients	[73–76]
PrxV	2-Cysteine peroxidase	Bronchial epithelial cell, epithelium of nasopharynx, palpebral conjunctiva, fallopian tube (uterine tube)	Mitochondria, cytoplasm, peroxisome matrix	Overexpression of PrxV gene is correlated with a larger tumor size, positive lymph node status, and shorter survival. Deficiency induced M2 macrophage polarization	PrxV is a putative therapeutic target and clinical strategy in breast, bladder, lung, cervical, ovarian, prostate, esophageal, and hepatocellular tumors	Human BC MCF-7 cell line	[68,73,77–80]

Table 1. *Cont.*

Enzyme	Type	Tissue Expression	Cellular Localization	Pathological Function	Therapeutical Use	Sample Type	References
PrxVI	1-Cysteine peroxidase (GSHs reductant)	Corpus epididymis, gastrocnemius, mucosa of stomach, amniotic fluid	Cytoplasm, lysosome, lamellar bodies, nucleus	Upregulated in progesterone receptor positive cases. Overexpression of PrxVI leads to a more invasive phenotype and metastatic potential in BC. Increased in most metastatic cell lines	Prx6 stable knockdown xenografts exhibited decreased tumor growth and metastasis	BC cell lines, xenograft tumor model in athymic mice	[81,82]
TrxR1	Selenocysteine-containing protein	Ovary, spleen, heart, liver, kidney, and pancreas	Cytoplasm	TrxR overexpression has been correlated with aggressive tumor growth, worse prognosis, and decreased patient survival.	Inhibition of TrxR causes malignant cells to become more susceptible to cytotoxicity, cytostasis, and cell death.	Human BC MDA-MB-435 S, MDA-MB-231, BT-549, and MCF-10A cell lines	[83–86]
TrxR2	Selenocysteine-containing protein	Pharyngeal and body wall muscles	Mitochondria	Overexpressed in cancer cells, conferring apoptosis resistance.	Increases the mitochondrial concentration of reactive oxygen species and shifts the thiol redox state toward a more oxidized condition	Human BC MCF-7 cell line	[87,88]
TrxR3	Selenocysteine-containing protein	Testis	No data	No data	No data	No data	[89]

Consult Supplementary Table S1 to check the characteristics of the mentioned cell lines.

3.2.2. Catalase (CAT)

CATs are enzymes that break down H_2O_2 into O_2 and H_2O [90]. They have a key role in the defense of cells against oxidative stress and their overexpression modulates the H_2O_2 levels and inflammation processes [91]. Catalase expression is altered in cancer cells, a fact that plays an important dichotomous role [40]. These enzymes are classified into three types: typical, peroxidases, and with manganese. The first two types of enzymes contain a heme group, while the third type contains a non-heme manganese group. Typical CATs are commonly isolated from aerobic organisms, including animals, plants, fungi, and bacteria. CAT-peroxidases have been isolated from fungi, eubacteria, and archaea, while non-heme CATs have been found exclusively in bacteria [92]. Human CAT belongs to the group of typical CATs [90] (Table 1).

In BC, blood samples have shown an increase of ROS production, a decreased CAT activity, as well as a low concentration of reduced glutathione (GSH). Those results support the hypothesis of oxidative stress in carcinogenesis [43]. In some studies, it has been observed that mammography density in benign tissue is influenced by markers of oxidative stress and the menopausal status of the patient [93]. Furthermore, CAT activity decreases with the progression of the pathology according to the Breast Imaging Reporting and Data System (BIRADS). Randecovic et al. in 2013 showed how the levels of CAT change in tumor tissue from patients with BC with respect to mammographic studies. Patients with BIRADS 5 had significantly lower levels of CAT activity compared to patients with BIRADS 4c, 4b, or 4a mammography. So, patients with BIRADS 4c had significantly lower CAT activity compared to patients with BIRADS 4a or 4b on mammography. Therefore, they concluded that the CAT activity in the BC decreased significantly with the increase in the BIRADS category [94]. This work is in agreement with other studies published for BC, which show a decrease in CAT activity associated with an aggressive phenotype [95].

Moreover, in acute myeloid leukemia it has been observed that cells from patients who remain in complete remission for longer periods have higher levels of CAT than patients who exhibit resistance to treatment; this suggests that the acquisition of cellular resistance to drugs is associated with higher levels of ROS [96]. In MCF-7 cancer cells (human adenocarcinoma cells), the overexpression of CAT affects their proliferation and migration, leading to a less aggressive phenotype and an altered response to chemotherapy, since they are more sensitive to paclitaxel, etoposide, and arsenic trioxide and more resistant to redox-based drugs [97]. Ruqayah et al. in 2020 showed decreased CAT activity and glutathione concentration levels in women patients with BC and they concluded that the biochemical changes in CAT and GSH levels can be viewed as biomarkers for the early detection of recurrent disease as well as for tracking the patients' response to therapy during follow-up [98]. Zinczuk et al. found that the activity of SOD was significantly higher whereas the activity of CAT, GPx and GR was considerably lower in colorectal cancer (CRC) patients compared to the control group ($p < 0.0001$). They concluded that redox biomarkers can be potential diagnostic indicators of CRC advancement [99]. In addition, Glorieux et al. showed that CAT overexpression in mammary cancer cells leads to a less aggressive phenotype and an altered response to chemotherapy. The proliferation and migration capacities of MCF-7 cells were impaired by the overexpression of CAT as compared to parental cells. Regarding their sensitivity to anticancer treatments, they observed that cells overexpressing CAT were more sensitive to paclitaxel, etoposide and arsenic trioxide. However, no effect was observed in the cytotoxic response to ionizing radiation, 5-fluorouracil, cisplatin or doxorubicin. Finally, they observed that CAT overexpression protects cancer cells against the pro-oxidant combination of ascorbate and menadione, suggesting that changes in the expression of antioxidant enzymes could be a mechanism of resistance of cancer cells toward redox-based chemotherapeutic drugs [97].

These findings show that CAT can be a biomarker for the early detection, prognosis, and treatment of BC and cancer in general.

3.2.3. Glutathione Peroxidase (GPx)

The main defense systems against the damage caused by H_2O_2 and lipid hydroperoxides are glutathione, thioredoxin, and CAT [100]. GPxs are a group of enzymes that use glutathione as a donor of reduced equivalents [101,102]. They convert H_2O_2 into H_2O by oxidizing the glutathione (GSSG), which returns to its reduced form (GSH) through the action of the NADPH-dependent GR enzyme [102]. These enzymes are characterized by having selenium–cysteine in their active site and can reduce organic and inorganic hydroperoxides [100]. So far, based on their structural similarities, eight GPxs have been identified in mammalian cells [55,103,104] and their expression levels are altered in BC (Table 1).

GPx1 has been implicated in the development and prevention of numerous cardiovascular diseases and cancer [55,104]. In the case of cancer, it is known that in cell culture both GPx1 and GPx2 can prevent oxidative DNA mutations and counteract the production of proinflammatory mediators derived from cyclooxygenase (COX)/lipoxygenase (LOX), such as prostaglandins and leukotrienes. This capacity allows the prevention of carcinogenesis at least in the initial phase [105]. GPx4 regulates ferroptosis, which is an iron-mediated cell death mechanism. This pathway has been studied in several in vitro models and is under investigation as a potential therapeutic target for many types of cancer, including breast, ovarian, liver, and prostate cancer [59].

3.2.4. Glutathione Reductase (GR)

GR is responsible for maintaining adequate concentrations of glutathione by converting GSSG into GSH; for that reason, its activity is relevant to maintaining the redox state of cells [106]. It has been determined that the levels of "activity and/or expression" of GR are increased in cancer cells, especially breast, lung, colorectal, and prostate cancer, thus affecting the concentration of GSSG in the cell and responses to treatment [106–108]. In addition, it has been found that in cell lines A-431, MCF-7, NCI-H226, and OVCAR-3, an increase in GR activity has been associated with resistance to radiotherapy treatments [108,109]. On the other hand, GR inhibition leads to an accumulation of GSSG, making cells more susceptible to ROS damage [110].

The use of coordinated therapies to inhibit BC growth has been proposed, such as chemotherapies and the use of inhibitors that affect the activity of antioxidant enzymes, such as GR [111]. An example of this is the inhibition of GR and TrxR enzymes, producing a decrease in GSH and Trx levels in BC (Table 1). This can be considered an effective strategy to combat tumor cells by disrupting their ability to eliminate ROS and cope with oxidative damage [112]. Studies that have observed the inhibition of cells indicate that their antitumor activity could be attributed to the inhibition of GR and TrxR activities [113].

3.2.5. Thioredoxin Reductase (TrxR)

TrxR catalyzes the NADPH-dependent reduction of Trx [114,115]. By preserving protein thiols in a reduced state, Trx and TrxR help maintain a reduced cellular environment and keep transcription factors active [116]. These enzymes are a family of selenium-containing pyridine nucleotide-disulfide oxidoreductases [117]. There are three isoforms of TrxR (Table 1): TrxR1 located in the cytosol, TrxR2 located in the mitochondria, and TrxR3 or thioredoxin glutathione reductase, which is located mainly in the testes, where it participates in the maturation of the sperm [89,118].

TrxR1 is an oxidoreductase that has an active site with a dithiol disulfide, which in turn reduces oxidized cysteine residues in cellular proteins. This cytosolic enzyme is overexpressed in many types of human cancers, including BC, which is the reason for its usage as a biomarker [118,119]. Regarding TrxR2, it has been suggested that it has a protective role in cells during exogenous attacks such as radiation and certain anticancer drugs. It has been suggested that along with Prx, it regulates the release of cytochrome c, protecting cells from cancerous apoptotic processes [120].

3.2.6. Peroxiredoxin (Prx)

Prxs are a family of peroxidases that are divided into six groups (Prx I–VI), and all of them can reduce H_2O_2 through Trx or other oxidative substrates [67]. They play a role as H_2O_2 sensors in cell signaling and differentiation systems, apoptosis, and redox homeostasis [73,121]. Human Prxs are expressed in different subcellular compartments [82] and the specific function of each isoform is related to their oligomeric and redox states [122]. Those oligomeric states could be influenced by ionic strength, pH, or protein concentration [123]. Moreover, they can be inhibited by tyrosine or threonine phosphorylation, and also by hyperoxidation [82]. These enzymes are also known as redox relays, yet they can transfer disulfide groups through proteins for redox signaling [124].

Prxs are overexpressed in many cancer tissues, suggesting that their proliferative effect could be related to the development or progression of the disease [67]. Mammalian tumors show high levels of Prx expression, indicating that antioxidant defenses provide a survival advantage for tumor development (Table 1). Consequently, Prx inhibitors are being explored as therapeutic agents in different cancer models and this enzyme is proposed as a potential biomarker in cancer due to the overexpression profiles found in malignant mammalian cells associated with survival [125].

4. Dichotomy of Some Antioxidant Enzymes

There is a "dichotomy" regarding the role of some antioxidant enzymes in cancer [126,127]. An example of this phenomenon is observed in the case of CAT, where a decrease in the activity of this enzyme is observed in BC; however, its activity has been positively correlated with advanced invasive and metastatic phenotypes in vivo in BC [94,127]. This enzyme is also frequently found to be decreased in acute myeloid leukemia (AML) and colorectal, pancreatic, and prostate cancers [40].

On the other hand, there is sufficient evidence from experimental and clinical studies regarding high levels and activity of SOD in tumor tissues [128]. In the most recent study on SOD dichotomy, researchers evaluated the levels of Mn-SOD, CuZn-SOD, and other antioxidant enzymes such as CAT and GPx in both tumors and adjacent non-tumor tissue from colorectal cancer patients. That study found that tumors exhibited higher levels of Mn-SOD. Notably, this enzyme's level increased in stages II and III in comparison to stage I and the precancerous stage [129]. Moreover, some researchers claim that SOD2 undergoes a functional shift, transitioning from a tumor initiation suppressor to an actual tumor promoter, contributing to the progression toward more malignant phenotypes once the disease is established [130]. These observations are further supported by highlighting the importance of aerobic glycolysis in the survival of tumor cells [130]. Increased Mn-SOD suppresses mitochondrial oxidative phosphorylation and leads to the activation of MAPK where glucose is metabolized through glycolysis [128]. The change in the glycolytic phenotype of malignant cells is considered an adaptative advantage that reduces their dependence on mitochondrial respiration and allows them to proliferate and invade normal peritumoral tissue [131].

In humans, most Prxs show an increase in their expression levels during BC development [67,73]. Altered expression levels of CAT and Prx2 enzymes have been identified in nipple secretions [132], as well as the Prx2 and Prx6 in the serum of BC patients [133]. Furthermore, the detection of elevated levels of Prx1 in biopsies is associated with a better prognosis in estrogen receptor-positive BC [134]. Although its mechanism to protect cancer cells remains unclear, Prx is also known for participating in signaling pathways such as cell proliferation and death [121].

The functions of GPx change depending on the type of cancer and the type of study. GPx1 can reduce tumor growth, indicating its inhibitory effect on tumorigenesis [135]. GPx1 expression is decreased in BC [136], while in colorectal cancer, GPx2 expression is increased [137]. Conversely, in prostate intraepithelial neoplasia, its expression is decreased [138], which suggests that GPx2 shows diverse and complex functions in tumorigenesis. Furthermore, GPx3 is considered a tumor suppressing protein [139], and its expression is decreased in patients with Barrett's esophagus [140], endometrial adenocarcinoma [141], and breast and prostate cancers [142]. GPx4 is also considered a tumor suppressor [135,139]. On the other hand, GPx7 has potential tumor suppressive effects in gastric and esophageal adenocarcinoma [143]. The roles of GPx5, GPx6, and GPx8 in tumorigenesis are still unclear [54].

Despite the large amount of information found in the literature on GR and TrxR, insufficient data have been found to support their possible dichotomous role in cancer.

5. Ferroptosis

In the treatment of BC, resistance to apoptosis has been observed. Consequently, new procedures or therapies aimed at inhibiting its progression have been sought [59]. In this sense, ferroptosis, a type of cell death that is characterized by an excess of lipid peroxidation induced by ROS, might represent an effective treatment against aggressive tumors resistant to traditional drugs [54,59,144]. In BC, the modulators associated with ferroptosis are glutathione, GPx4, Prxs, iron, Nrf2, SOD, lipoxygenase, and coenzyme Q (Figure 2) [145].

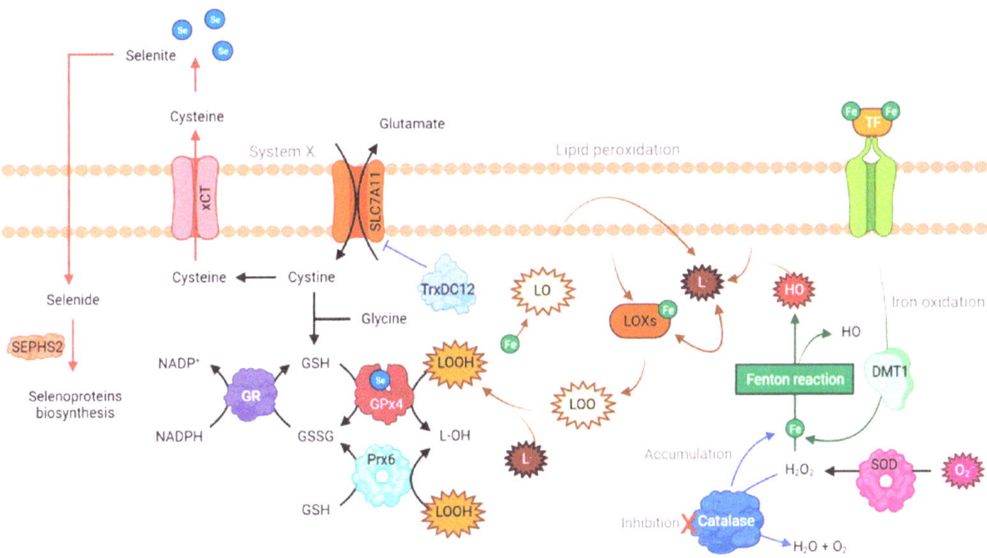

Figure 2. Relationship between antioxidant enzymes and ferroptosis. GPx4, Prx6, and GR act as negative regulators of iron-mediated death. GPx4 and Prx6 use GSH as a reducer and by inhibiting them it is possible to activate ferroptosis. Similarly, the concentration of these selenoproteins can be reduced by inhibition of selenophosphate synthetase 2 (SEPHS2), which is necessary for cancer cells to detoxify the selenide that enters through SLC7A11 and is useful in its biosynthesis. Furthermore, the GSH content can also decrease due to the activation of SOD and the modulation of the cystine-glutamate antiporter (SLC7A11) by TrdxDC12. Also, the inhibition of CAT causes the accumulation of Fe^{2+}, favoring the Fenton reaction and, in turn, ferroptosis.

In the case of GPx4, it has been shown that its inactivation results in an effective eradication of cancer cells by inducing cell death through ferroptosis [59,146]. As a result of this discovery, several pharmacological therapies have been developed to activate ferroptotic cell death by targeting GPx4. These therapies act on the biosynthesis, activity, or degradation of this enzyme [147–149].

Regarding CAT, it has been observed that thiosemicarbazone (BT-Br), a benzaldehyde derivative and an effective inhibitor of this enzyme, increases ROS levels in DU145 castration-resistant prostate cancer (CRPC) cells. BT-Br can induce endoplasmic reticulum stress and subsequent autophagy in these cells, causing the degradation of ferritin heavy peptide 1 (FTH1) and the accumulation of Fe^{2+}. Consequently, these effects promote the Fenton reaction and •OH is produced, inducing ferroptosis in DU145 cells and eventually reducing CRPC tumors. Overall, CAT inhibition has the potential to be a novel strategy to induce ferroptosis of cancer cells through the dual regulation of ROS levels and iron ions [150].

Moreover, GR is inversely related to ferroptosis because when it is overexpressed in cancer cells it regulates GSH homeostasis, rendering the cells insensitive to this process [151]. Concerning Prxs, Prx6 has been described as a negative regulator of cell death via ferroptosis, and it is suggested that through its Ca^{2+}-independent phospholipase A2 inhibitory activity it eliminates the fatty acid hydroperoxide (LOOH), which protects cells against iron death. Therefore, its deletion results in a potential target for cancer therapy by inducing ferroptosis [152].

Regarding the role of the Trx/TrxR system in the regeneration of GSH, which protects against ferroptosis, TrxR should participate along with GPx4 in antiferroptotic activity. However, this is not the case, as the loss of TrxR1 protects pancreatic cancer cells from ferroptosis by inhibiting GPx4. The authors found that the loss of TrxR generates an increase in GPx4 protein levels by increasing the cellular pool of selenocysteine. Selenocysteine is an amino acid found in low intracellular concentrations, yet it is essential for the structure and function of both polypeptides. Hence, the disappearance of one induces the biogenesis of the second [153]. Certain drugs have been created to interfere in the redox homeostasis through the inhibition of TrxR and by inducing the death process through ferroptosis, which allows tumor cells to be sensitized to radiotherapy treatments [154].

However, despite how promising the induction of ferroptosis seems to be in the treatment of BC, further tests and a thorough examination of its safety and adverse effects in vivo must be carried out since preliminary studies have not reached clinical trials in human cancer therapy. Furthermore, it is necessary to consider that inhibiting CAT, GPx4, Prxs, TrxR, and other antioxidant enzymes can cause adverse reactions in other organs and tissues, which hinders their widespread application in human cancer. For these reasons, the development of inhibitors and more effective and specific targeting methods are needed to achieve optimal effects in the selective elimination of resistant human cancers, as well as the reduction of the potential adverse effects associated with ferroptosis.

6. Nanotechnology Applied to the Clinic

Nanotechnology has emerged as a valuable tool that can be used to address the problem of cancer. Compared to conventional medicine, nanoparticles (NPs) offer advantages such as biocompatibility and affinity, lower immunogenicity [155], higher half-time life of attached drugs in blood circulation, specific accumulation in cancer tissues for a longer and more accurate effect [156], metastasis prevention [157], cell cycle arrest [158], and metabolic stress due to the low glycolysis level. Additionally, leveraging these characteristics, NPs can function as imaging agents for tumor monitoring and as a way to remodel the microenvironment with minimal to no toxic side effects on the patients [159]. Figure 3 and Table 2 show some of the compounds that have been employed in the treatment of BC using nanotechnology and antioxidant enzymes.

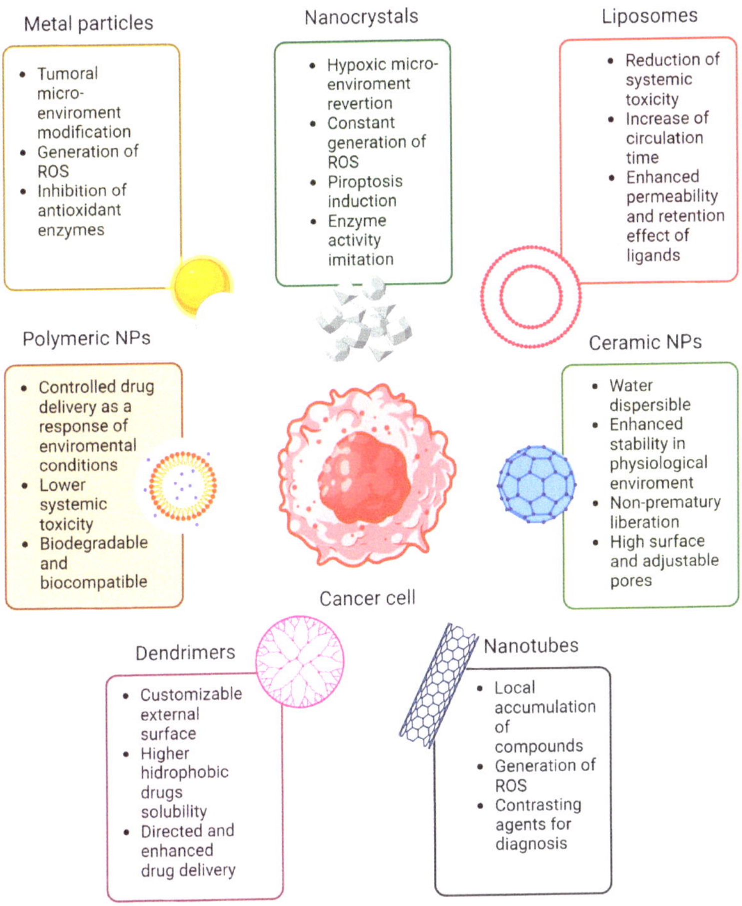

Figure 3. Characteristics of some nanoparticles used in nanomedicine in the treatment of BC.

Table 2. Nanotechnology targeting antioxidant enzymes in BC treatment.

Target Antioxidant Enzyme	Compound	Action Mode	References
SOD	PSE-PCF-NPs: Shell poly (lactic acid-co-glycolic) (PLGA)-NPs coated with folic acid (FA)-chitosan (PCF-NPs) loaded with *Peganum harmala* smoke extract (PSE)	The combination of chitosan and PGLA increases the bioavailability, toxicity, and release of the drug. In addition, the use of folic acid on the surface of the NPs is one of the most effective strategies to internalize into cancer cells through receptor-mediated endocytosis and the administration of anticancer agents. As a result, an increase in ROS and a decrease in the SOD enzyme was obtained in MCF-7 cells treated with PSE-PCF-NP.	[160]
	Fe_3O_4@mSiO_2-DSF@PEI-FA, mMDPF: Disulfiram (DSF) loading, encapsulated folic acid (FA) conjugated polyethyleneimine magnetic mesoporous silica (Fe_3O_4@mSiO_2) NPs	Disulfiram is a SOD inhibitor due to its affinity for sulfhydryl groups and the ability to bind to the copper and zinc of SOD. Inhibition of SOD can cause superoxide accumulation in cells inducing oxidative stress, apoptosis, and cell cycle arrest; it also reduces cancer cell proliferation, angiogenesis, tumor metastasis, and multidrug resistance. Fe_3O_4@mSiO_2 is a drug carrier system based on magnetic mesoporous silica NPs and folic acid, and it is used to increase both its solubility in water and its specificity for cancer cells. Finally, the addition of Cu^{2+} increases the therapeutic effect of DSF in different types of cancer cells.	[161]
	PC + $C_{22}PEG_{900}$GlcNAc: Diethyldithiocarbamate (DETC), zinc phthalocyanine (ZnPc) loaded in liposomes	The encapsulation of photosensitizers with liposomes improves their therapeutic activity while preserving their photophysical properties, in addition to reducing their toxic effect. The principle of photodynamic therapy (PDT) involves the production of high levels of ROS photosensitizing molecules, which when exposed to visible light can kill nearby cells. ZnPc is a second-generation photosensitizer used in PDT to produce singlet oxygen, while DETC is a hydrophilic metal chelating agent and a known SOD inhibitor. Thus, the inhibition of SOD increases the ROS generated by PDT, causing an increase in the death of tumor cells.	[162]
CAT	PMO-Ce6@Catalase: Mesoporous organosilica (PMO) coupled with chlorine e6 (Ce6) and CAT	PMO-Ce6@Catalase is selectively absorbed and stored by tumor tissue. Then, after local irradiation with light of appropriate wavelength, the photosensitizer (Ce6@) is activated to produce a photosensitizing effect to generate high levels of ROS. CAT increases the concentration of oxygen around the cells and solves the problem of hypoxia in the tumor, in addition to enhancing the effects of Ce6@.	[163]
	CAT@PDL1-SSLs: CAT-loaded and PDL1 (programmed death-ligand 1) monoclonal antibody modified immunoliposomes	PDL1 monoclonal antibodies are used as immune checkpoint blockers (ICBs) to significantly improve the efficacy of tumor immunotherapy by blocking the PD-1/PD-L1 inhibitory pathway. CAT helps the system overcome hypoxia, which is a limitation for PDL1. The results of this nanoparticle are activating and increasing the infiltration of CD8+ T cells at the tumor site and inhibiting tumor growth with low systemic toxicity.	[164]

Table 2. *Cont.*

Target Antioxidant Enzyme	Compound	Action Mode	References
CAT	FA-L@MBDP@CAT: Lyso-targeted NIR photosensitizer (MBDP), CAT and doxorubicin (Dox) encapsulated within folic acid (FA) modified liposomes	Increased M1-MQ polarization; increased recruitment of CD8+ T cells. Photosensitizer (MBDP) has deep tissue penetration and high phototoxicity toward cancer cells. Doxorubicin has a good therapeutic effect on BC and metastatic tumors by inducing DNA damage and inhibiting the progression of topoisomerase II enzyme. For these liposomes, folate increases active targeting and prevents them from being recognized and phagocytosed by the reticuloendothelial system (RES) due to the existence of the PEG framework. The released CAT catalyzes overexpressed hydrogen peroxide to increase tumor oxygenation, providing sufficient oxygen for PDT and reversing the immunosuppressive TME by modulating immune cytokines to favor antitumor immunities, enhancing tumor inhibition in vivo.	[165]
	CAT@Pt(IV)-liposome: CAT-loaded cisplatin constructed liposome	CAT is encapsulated together with cisplatin (IV), forming a CAT@Pt(IV) liposome to improve cancer chemoradiotherapy. After loading into the liposomes, the CAT within the CAT@Pt(IV) liposome shows retained and well-protected enzymatic activity and is capable of triggering the breakdown of H_2O_2 produced by tumor cells, to produce additional oxygen for relieve hypoxia. As a result, CAT@Pt(IV) liposome treatment induces the highest level of DNA damage in cancer cells after X-ray irradiation.	[166]
	CAT-TCPP/FCS: Assembled FCS (fluorinated chitosan) with meso-tetra(4-carboxyphenyl) porphyrin (TCPP) conjugated CAT	These NPs exhibit greatly improved transmucosal adsorption and intratumoral penetration, due to their abilities to reversibly modulate transepithelial electrical resistance (TEER) and open tight junctions of the bladder epithelium. Such actions, together with the in situ O_2 generation triggered by the CAT-catalyzed decomposition of the endogenous H_2O_2 of the tumor, would contribute to drastically improve the efficacy of sonodynamic therapy to destroy orthotopic bladder tumors.	[167]
	ZCM nanocapsule: CAT and methylene blue co-loaded into mesoporous of zeolite nanocarriers	Free CAT efficiently modulates tumor hypoxia and enhances intratumoral contrast through sustained decomposition of endogenous H_2O_2 and in situ production of O_2 gas bubbles. Meanwhile, loading methylene blue into zeolite matrices prevents rapid leaching of photosensitizer in tumor tissue, achieving well-sustained release effect of photosensitizer. According to synchronous mechanisms, after near-infrared laser irradiation, local pancreatic cancer cells die completely, and no therapy-induced toxicity or recurrence is observed.	[168]
	PLGA-R837@CAT: CAT and R837 co-loaded in core/shell poli (lactic acid-co-glycolic) (PLGA) NPs platform	Reduced tumor metastasis; increased M1-MQ polarization; enhanced immunological cell death. The formed PLGA-R837@CAT nanoparticles can greatly improve the efficacy of radiotherapy by alleviating tumor hypoxia and modulating the immunosuppressive tumor microenvironment. Antigens with R837 will induce strong antitumor immune responses, which together with the blockade of the cytotoxic T lymphocyte-associated protein 4 (CTLA-4) checkpoint will be able to effectively inhibit tumor metastases through a strong abscopal effect (the reduction or disappearance of tumors in parts of the body that were not the direct target of local therapy, such as radiotherapy.	[169]

Table 2. *Cont.*

Target Antioxidant Enzyme	Compound	Action Mode	References
GPx4	FCSP@DOX MOF: Fe and Cu ions bridged by disulfide bonds with PEGylation (FCSP MOFs) loaded with doxorubicin (Dox)	FCSP@DOX MOFs are structures activated by the redox environment of the tumor, which causes the release of Fe^{2+}/Cu^{+} ions to produce ROS through the Fenton reaction, triggering the depletion of GSH levels and the inhibition of GPx4, which causes an elevation of lipid peroxidation and the onset of ferroptosis. Additionally, better tumor therapeutic efficiency is achieved by loading DOX, since it can not only cause apoptosis, but also indirectly produces H_2O_2 to amplify the Fenton reaction, which allows the notable antitumor effect of FCSP@DOX MOFs.	[170]
	ChA CQDs: Carbon quantum dots (CQDs) prepared into nanozymes from chlorogenic acid (ChA)	CQDs have GSH oxidase-like activity by catalyzing the conversion of GSH to GSSG. Due to this, ChACQDs induce ferroptosis by promoting an unbalanced redox reaction due to the depletion of GSH and the inactivation of GPx4, with the consequent accumulation of ROS and lipid peroxidation.	[171]
	HMTBF: Metal-polyphenol network coated Prussian blue NPs	The HMTBF nanocomplex promotes ferroptosis/apoptosis synergism. During the intracellular degradation of this nanocomplex, the Fe^{3+}/Fe^{2+} conversion mediated by tannic acid (TA) is favored, initiating the Fenton reaction and increasing the level of ROS, subsequent lipid peroxidation and, therefore, causing ferroptotic cell death. Furthermore, the degradation of HMTBF allows the release of the compound ML210, which inhibits the activity of GPx4 to activate the ferroptosis pathway.	[172]
	DBCO-RSL3-DHA: Dibenzocyclooctyne-modified disulfide-bridged nanoassemblies loaded with RSL3 and dihydroartemisinin	DBCO-RSL3-DHA nanoassemblies are loaded with the ferroptosis inducer RSL3 and the ferritinophagy initiator dihydroartemisinin (DHA). DHA induces ferritinophagy to release iron in the form of Fe^{2+}. The cellular abundance of Fe^{2+} is the driving force of lipid peroxidation, together with the inhibition of GPx4 caused by RSL3, which triggers iron-dependent cell death (ferroptosis).	[173]
	Cu-TCPP(Fe): Metal-organic framework (MOF) incorporated with gold NPs and RSL3	Cu^{2+} ions immobilized on Cu-TCPP(Fe) nanosheets rapidly oxidize GSH to GSSG, potentially depleting GPx4 cofactors to inactivate its antiferroptotic functions. Furthermore, the nanosheet system can release the attached RSL3, which binds to the catalytic selenocysteine residue of GPx4. Overall, the multienzyme reactivity can simultaneously inhibit the GPx4 and ferroptosis suppressor protein 1 (FSP1) pathways that catalyze the recycling of coenzyme Q10 to ubiquinol, both ferroptosis-suppressing mechanisms.	[174]
	(RSL3@COF-Fc): Ferrocene-functionalized covalent organic framework loaded with RSL3	The RSL3@COF-Fc nanodrug carries a GPx4 inhibitor and RSL3. This nanodrug promotes in situ reactions similar to the Fenton reaction, triggering the production of hydroxyl radicals (·OH) by increasing the level of ROS in cells and irreversible covalent inhibition of GPx4, resulting in massive lipid peroxide accumulation, cellular damage, and ultimately, ferroptosis.	[175]
	Mn12-heparin: Manganese cluster NPs (Mn12) encapsulated with heparin	Manganese (Mn12) NPs encapsulated with heparin (Mn12-heparin) are a chemodynamic therapeutic agent that mediates the increase in ROS levels since manganese reacts with H_2O_2 to generate ·OH through a pathway similar to the reaction of Fenton. Increased ROS and depletion of endogenous GSH indirectly leads to GPx4 inhibition, consequently increasing the level of lipid peroxidation to cause ferroptosis.	[176]

Table 2. *Cont.*

Target Antioxidant Enzyme	Compound	Action Mode	References
GPx4	PFP@Fe/Cu-SS MOF: Phloroglucinol, iron (Fe^{3+}), and copper (Cu^{2+}) are the corresponding coordination metals. Perfluoropentane (PFP) was loaded into MOF	The high concentration of GSH present in tumor cells will accelerate the breakdown of the PFP@Fe/Cu-SS MOF nanocarrier structure, producing the release of Fe^{2+}/Cu^{2+} ions that react with H_2O_2, producing ·OH through the Fenton reaction, causing the depletion of GSH levels and inhibition of GPx4. In turn, this causes the accumulation of intracellular lipid peroxides to eventually induce ferroptosis.	[177]
GR	HSpyN: pyrimidine-2 thiol	Phosphine-gold(I) thiolate complexes are promising anticancer agents for antiproliferative activities in vitro and in vivo. The ability of HSpyN to inhibit the proliferation of human BC cells, MCF-7, was evaluated by measuring cell death through the induction of apoptosis. In addition, this compound is a potent inhibitor of GR.	[178]
Prx1	Auf-Asc-Men: Auronofin (Auf) treatment in combination with ascorbate (Asc) and menadione (Men)	Prx1 can protect TNBC cells from the effects of prooxidant compounds, while Asc and Men treatment increases H_2O_2 levels. When Auf is added, Prx1 is inhibited, so the effects of H_2O_2 cause rapid toxicity, irreversible cell damage, and as a consequence, cell death instead of adaptation or survival.	[179]
TrxR	Auf-MI-463: Auronofin plus MI-463	Menin-MLL inhibitors have been shown to be effective against BC. MI-463 unexpectedly induced ferroptotic cell death. In addition, heme oxygenase-1 (HO-1) was inhibited, which increased the effect of MI-463 plus Auf.	[180]
	Auf-anti-PD-L1: Auronofin plus anti-PD-L1 antibody	Auf treatment acts as a TrxR inhibitor, causing specific cell death and affects cell growth. Auf increased tumor infiltration of CD8 + Ve T cells in vivo and amplified the expression of the immune checkpoint PD-L1 in an ERK1/2-MYC-dependent manner. Furthermore, the combination of Auf with anti-PD-L1 antibody synergistically impaired the growth of 4T1.2 TNBC primary tumors.	[64]
	Auf-Vitamin C: Auronofin plus vitamin C	Auf simultaneously targeted the antioxidant systems thioredoxin and glutathione, causing cell death. AUF/VC combinations exerted synergistic H_2O_2-mediated cytotoxicity on BC cell lines.	[181]

Within the NPs, nanozymes (artificial enzymes) have been developed to combine the characteristics of nanomaterials and enzymes. Natural enzymes often entail high production costs, susceptibility to denaturation and inactivation, and low yields, which make their application in different procedures difficult. However, nanozymes have high catalytic activities and share properties with nanomaterials, which could improve natural enzyme deficiencies. Nanozymes have been developed for CAT, SOD, oxidase, and peroxidase [182].

On the other hand, many drugs used in BC treatment increase the ROS levels to induce cell damage but the cytoprotective effect of antioxidant enzymes allows the cells to adapt to the new conditions and then survive. In this case, the metal particles coupled in NPs can directly inhibit antioxidant enzymes, and the carried chemical compounds' action is effectively enhanced [179].

For example, the use of manganese dioxide (MnO_2) and gold–platinum (Au-Pt) NPs helps to modify the tumor immunosuppressor microenvironment because they act as generators of radioactive nano-oxygen (nanobubbles composed of gas such as oxygen), improving the infiltration of cytotoxic T cells, affecting the cancer cells' metabolism and reducing their proliferation by downregulating the expression of hypoxia-inducible factor 1α (HIF-1α) and C-MYC [183], and consequently, tumor progression [184,185].

In addition to this, the use of $LaFeO_3$ perovskite nanocrystals–enzymes, which present enzyme-mimicking activities, including oxidase, peroxidase, GPx, and CAT activities, reverse the hypoxic microenvironment and the depletion of endogenous glutathione and promote the continuous production of ROS and the process of pyroptosis, presenting an alternative in the treatment of BC [186].

Moreover, nanozymes can be coupled to carbon nanotubules; for instance, a peroxidase activity nanozyme comprising a 1D ferriporphyrin covalent organic framework coated on a carbon nanotube (COF-CNT) with a conductor hydrogel can be injected into tumor tissues to generate ROS. Its use in the treatment of 4T1 BC, in mice, demonstrated that carcinoma was significantly suppressed [187].

It is known that NPs diminish the adverse effects of common cancer therapies [188] but their self-side effects are not well-documented yet and some of them can cause toxicity via cellular function disruption and initiate cell degradation through autophagy (e.g., gold, titanium dioxide or zinc oxide particles) [156]. Therefore, NPs must fulfill specific characteristics for clinical usage: 1. They need to be made of biocompatible and nontoxic elements, 2. their size should be small (10–200 nm), 3. more than 50% of the chemical compound is required to be encapsulated within the particle, 4. NPs should be stable in the physiological environment to prevent sequestration or agglomeration in undesirable sites, 5. they must have a reasonable circulation time, 6. they should target specifically the selected tissue or cell type, 7. the release of the attached compounds needs to be biological or extrinsically controlled, and finally, 8. the clearance of the particle needs to be ensured to prevent cumulative or long-term effects [188]. The developed NPs do not meet most and certainly not all of these characteristics, but with the required studies (absorption, metabolism, excretion, etc.) their application would improve the future of BC treatments.

The use of various types of NPs (liposomes, polymeric compounds, micelles, dendrimers, carbon nanotubes, etc.) has achieved significant advances in BC treatment due to their advantages compared to conventional therapies, such as reduced pharmaceutical toxicity and overcoming the chemoresistance of chemotherapy [189]. However, there are still several problems that remain to be addressed, so it is necessary to develop safer and more efficient BC treatments based on nanotechnology combined with the classical biochemical and immunological tools that have shown good results.

Many drugs used in the treatment of BC increase ROS levels to induce cellular damage, but the cytoprotective effect of antioxidant enzymes allows cells to adapt to the new conditions and then survive. In this case, metal particles coupled in NPs can directly inhibit antioxidant enzymes, and the action of the transported chemical compounds is effectively enhanced [179].

BC can be classified into three main groups based on their molecular and histological differences: BC expressing hormone receptors [estrogen receptor (ER^+) or progesterone receptor (PR^+)], BC expressing human epidermal receptor 2 ($HER2^+$), and triple negative breast cancer (TNBC) (ER^-, PR^-, $HER2^-$) [190,191]. In addition, TNBC is divided into six categories: basal-like 1 (BL-1), basal-like 2 (BL-2), immunomodulatory (IM), mesenchymal (M), mesenchymal stem cell-like (MSL), and luminal androgen receptor (LAR) [190], which makes the treatment protocol more complex. Therapy must be based on the molecular and histological characteristics of the type of BC.

Different investigations have been conducted to determine the efficiency of NPs on different types of cancer; among them, the incorporation of hormonal agents into NPs coated with polyethylene glycol to enter BC cells are working [192]. Furthermore, Gao et al. incorporated the TYKERB, lapatinib, into lipid NPs to improve their blood circulation time and bioavailability [193,194]. Other studies have indicated that BC cells could easily take up lipid NPs, thereby reducing tumor growth in mice. One of the key limitations of the clinical use of RNA is its rapid intravascular degradation. According to the findings of Wang et al. [194] in this regard, RNA loading onto lipid NPs caused an increase in intracellular siRNA uptake by MDA-MB-468 TNBC cells in vitro. In photothermal ablation (PTA), NPs (especially metallic NPs such as gold and silver) could produce heat at temperatures above 50 °C in BC tissues by absorbing and transforming energy from near-infrared waves, which results in the disruption of the cancerous tumors through necrosis.

Finally, the continuous development of NPs technology allows them to act on different types of BC. This generates greater efficiency in the death of cancer cells, which considerably reduces the toxic effects of traditional treatments (e.g., chemotherapy). In addition, the pharmacological effect becomes more effective and long-lasting, so healthy tissues are not affected. Hence, future research in this regard is expected to be directed toward the use of specific NPs at human clinical levels with minimal damage to surrounding healthy cells [156].

7. Conclusions

BC has a very high incidence worldwide, particularly in Latin America. Public health systems in this part of the world are seriously lagging in terms of prevention, a timely diagnosis and adequate guidance for patients with BC. This delay increases the mortality rate due to the poor availability of medications, long waiting lists for screening and clinical diagnosis, a low number of centers specialized in cancer care, a lack of trained personnel, centralization of health services, social inequality, and a deficiency of campaigns that encourage self-examination, among others. For these reasons, it is necessary to improve public health policies to strengthen research, development and the implementation of new oncological treatments, complementary to existing ones, to benefit a greater number of patients. Furthermore, it is necessary to implement new therapeutic targets, using antioxidant enzymes and biotechnological strategies such as ferroptosis and NPs, which will allow patients to be offered a more efficient treatment with fewer side effects, providing a better quality of life.

Supplementary Materials: The following supporting information can be downloaded at: https://www.mdpi.com/article/10.3390/ijms25115675/s1. References [195,196] are mentioned in Supplementary Materials.

Author Contributions: Conceptualization, H.V.-M., M.M.V.-L. and D.M.-M.; funding acquisition M.M.V.-L.; writing—original draft preparation, H.V.-M., M.M.V.-L., M.V.-C., D.U.-R. and D.M.-M.; writing—review, H.V.-M., M.M.V.-L., M.V.-C., D.U.-R. and D.M.-M.; editing, H.V.-M., M.V.-C. and D.M.-M. All authors have read and agreed to the published version of the manuscript.

Funding: This research was funded by UNAM-PAPIIT grant IN-218821 to M.M.V.-L. and the Research Division of the Medical School, and a UNAM grant to D.M.-M.

Acknowledgments: We thank Brenda Sandoval Meza from the Research Division of the Faculty of Medicine (UNAM) for the style correction and language review.

Conflicts of Interest: The authors declare no conflicts of interest.

References

1. Sung, H.; Ferlay, J.; Siegel, R.L.; Laversanne, M.; Soerjomataram, I.; Jemal, A.; Bray, F. Global Cancer Statistics 2020: GLOBOCAN Estimates of Incidence and Mortality Worldwide for 36 Cancers in 185 Countries. *CA Cancer J. Clin.* **2021**, *71*, 209–249. [CrossRef] [PubMed]
2. World Health Organization. *Breast Cancer*; World Health Organization: Geneva, Switzerland, 2021.
3. International Agency for Research on Cancer. Available online: https://gco.iarc.fr/ (accessed on 10 May 2024).
4. Pinto, J.A.; Pinillos, L.; Villarreal-Garza, C.; Morante, Z.; Villaran, M.V.; Mejia, G.; Caglevic, C.; Aguilar, A.; Fajardo, W.; Usuga, F.; et al. Barriers in Latin America for the management of locally advanced breast cancer. *Ecancermedicalscience* **2019**, *13*, 897. [CrossRef] [PubMed]
5. INEGI. *Estadisticas a Proposito del día Mundial de la Lucha Contra el Cáncer de Mama. Comunicado de Prensa*; INEGI: Aguascalientes, Mexico, 2021; p. 5.
6. Nourazarian, A.R.; Kangari, P.; Salmaninejad, A. Roles of oxidative stress in the development and progression of breast cancer. *Asian Pac. J. Cancer Prev.* **2014**, *15*, 4745–4751. [CrossRef] [PubMed]
7. Rusolo, F.; Capone, F.; Pasquale, R.; Angiolillo, A.; Colonna, G.; Castello, G.; Costantini, M.; Costantini, S. Comparison of the seleno-transcriptome expression between human non-cancerous mammary epithelial cells and two human breast cancer cell lines. *Oncol. Lett.* **2017**, *13*, 2411–2417. [CrossRef] [PubMed]
8. Majumder, D.; Nath, P.; Debnath, R.; Maiti, D. Understanding the complicated relationship between antioxidants and carcinogenesis. *J. Biochem. Mol. Toxicol.* **2021**, *35*, e22643. [CrossRef]
9. Panth, N.; Paudel, K.R.; Parajuli, K. Reactive Oxygen Species: A Key Hallmark of Cardiovascular Disease. *Adv. Med.* **2016**, *2016*, 9152732. [CrossRef]
10. Snezhkina, A.V.; Kudryavtseva, A.V.; Kardymon, O.L.; Savvateeva, M.V.; Melnikova, N.V.; Krasnov, G.S.; Dmitriev, A.A. ROS Generation and Antioxidant Defense Systems in Normal and Malignant Cells. *Oxidative Med. Cell. Longev.* **2019**, *2019*, 6175804. [CrossRef]
11. Hawk, M.A.; McCallister, C.; Schafer, Z.T. Antioxidant Activity during Tumor Progression: A Necessity for the Survival of Cancer Cells? *Cancers* **2016**, *8*, 92. [CrossRef]
12. Reuter, S.; Gupta, S.C.; Chaturvedi, M.M.; Aggarwal, B.B. Oxidative stress, inflammation, and cancer: How are they linked? *Free Radic. Biol. Med.* **2010**, *49*, 1603–1616. [CrossRef]
13. Tochhawng, L.; Deng, S.; Pervaiz, S.; Yap, C.T. Redox regulation of cancer cell migration and invasion. *Mitochondrion* **2013**, *13*, 246–253. [CrossRef]
14. Aggarwal, V.; Tuli, H.S.; Varol, A.; Thakral, F.; Yerer, M.B.; Sak, K.; Varol, M.; Jain, A.; Khan, M.A.; Sethi, G. Role of Reactive Oxygen Species in Cancer Progression: Molecular Mechanisms and Recent Advancements. *Biomolecules* **2019**, *9*, 735. [CrossRef] [PubMed]
15. Klaunig, J.E.; Zemin, W. Oxidative stress in carcinogenesis. *Curr. Opin. Toxicol.* **2018**, *7*, 116–121. [CrossRef]
16. Lushchak, V.I. Free radicals, reactive oxygen species, oxidative stress and its classification. *Chem. Biol. Interact.* **2014**, *224*, 164–175. [CrossRef]
17. Slimen, I.B.; Najar, T.; Ghram, A.; Dabbebi, H.; Ben Mrad, M.; Abdrabbah, M. Reactive oxygen species, heat stress and oxidative-induced mitochondrial damage. A review. *Int. J. Hyperth.* **2014**, *30*, 513–523. [CrossRef] [PubMed]
18. Hewala, T.I.; Elsoud, M.R.A. The clinical significance of serum oxidative stress biomarkers in breast cancer females. *Med. Res. J.* **2019**, *4*, 1–7. [CrossRef]
19. Bjelland, S.; Seeberg, E. Mutagenicity, toxicity and repair of DNA base damage induced by oxidation. *Mutat. Res.* **2003**, *531*, 37–80. [CrossRef] [PubMed]
20. Yamamoto, T.; Hosokawa, K.; Tamura, T.; Kanno, H.; Urabe, M.; Honjo, H. Urinary 8-hydroxy-2′-deoxyguanosine (8-OHdG) levels in women with or without gynecologic cancer. *J. Obstet. Gynaecol. Res.* **1996**, *22*, 359–363. [CrossRef]
21. Murrell, T.G. Epidemiological and biochemical support for a theory on the cause and prevention of breast cancer. *Med. Hypotheses* **1991**, *36*, 389–396. [CrossRef]
22. Miao, L.; St Clair, D.K. Regulation of superoxide dismutase genes: Implications in disease. *Free Radic. Biol. Med.* **2009**, *47*, 344–356. [CrossRef]
23. Gorrini, C.; Harris, I.S.; Mak, T.W. Modulation of oxidative stress as an anticancer strategy. *Nat. Rev. Drug Discov.* **2013**, *12*, 931–947. [CrossRef]
24. Valko, M.; Rhodes, C.J.; Moncol, J.; Izakovic, M.; Mazur, M. Free radicals, metals and antioxidants in oxidative stress-induced cancer. *Chem. Biol. Interact.* **2006**, *160*, 1–40. [CrossRef] [PubMed]
25. Perillo, B.; Di Donato, M.; Pezone, A.; Di Zazzo, E.; Giovannelli, P.; Galasso, G.; Castoria, G.; Migliaccio, A. ROS in cancer therapy: The bright side of the moon. *Exp. Mol. Med.* **2020**, *52*, 192–203. [CrossRef] [PubMed]
26. Schafer, Z.T.; Grassian, A.R.; Song, L.; Jiang, Z.; Gerhart-Hines, Z.; Irie, H.Y.; Gao, S.; Puigserver, P.; Brugge, J.S. Antioxidant and oncogene rescue of metabolic defects caused by loss of matrix attachment. *Nature* **2009**, *461*, 109–113. [CrossRef] [PubMed]
27. He, L.; He, T.; Farrar, S.; Ji, L.; Liu, T.; Ma, X. Antioxidants Maintain Cellular Redox Homeostasis by Elimination of Reactive Oxygen Species. *Cell. Physiol. Biochem.* **2017**, *44*, 532–553. [CrossRef] [PubMed]

28. Jakubczyk, K.; Dec, K.; Kaldunska, J.; Kawczuga, D.; Kochman, J.; Janda, K. Reactive oxygen species—Sources, functions, oxidative damage. *Pol. Merkur. Lek.* **2020**, *48*, 124–127.
29. Jakubczyk, K.; Kaldunska, J.; Dec, K.; Kawczuga, D.; Janda, K. Antioxidant properties of small-molecule non-enzymatic compounds. *Pol. Merkur. Lek.* **2020**, *48*, 128–132.
30. Sharma, S.K.; Singh, D.; Pandey, H.; Jatav, R.B.; Singh, V.; Pandey, D. An Overview of Roles of Enzymatic and Nonenzymatic Antioxidants in Plant. In *Antioxidant Defense in Plants*; Aftab, T., Hakeem, K.R., Eds.; Springer: Singapore, 2022. [CrossRef]
31. Zhang, L.; Wang, X.; Cueto, R.; Effi, C.; Zhang, Y.; Tan, H.; Qin, X.; Ji, Y.; Yang, X.; Wang, H. Biochemical basis and metabolic interplay of redox regulation. *Redox Biol.* **2019**, *26*, 101284. [CrossRef] [PubMed]
32. Hariharan, S.; Dharmaraj, S. Selenium and selenoproteins: It's role in regulation of inflammation. *Inflammopharmacology* **2020**, *28*, 667–695. [CrossRef]
33. McCord, J.M.; Fridovich, I. Superoxide dismutase. An enzymic function for erythrocuprein (hemocuprein). *J. Biol. Chem.* **1969**, *244*, 6049–6055. [CrossRef]
34. Younus, H. Therapeutic potentials of superoxide dismutase. *Int. J. Health Sci.* **2018**, *12*, 88–93.
35. Islam, M.N.; Rauf, A.; Fahad, F.I.; Emran, T.B.; Mitra, S.; Olatunde, A.; Shariati, M.A.; Rebezov, M.; Rengasamy, K.R.R.; Mubarak, M.S. Superoxide dismutase: An updated review on its health benefits and industrial applications. *Crit. Rev. Food Sci. Nutr.* **2022**, *62*, 7282–7300. [CrossRef] [PubMed]
36. Bafana, A.; Dutt, S.; Kumar, S.; Ahuja, P.S. Superoxide dismutase: An industrial perspective. *Crit. Rev. Biotechnol.* **2011**, *31*, 65–76. [CrossRef] [PubMed]
37. Oberley, L.W. Mechanism of the tumor suppressive effect of MnSOD overexpression. *BioMed. Pharmacother.* **2005**, *59*, 143–148. [CrossRef] [PubMed]
38. Bohm, B.; Heinzelmann, S.; Motz, M.; Bauer, G. Extracellular localization of catalase is associated with the transformed state of malignant cells. *Biol. Chem.* **2015**, *396*, 1339–1356. [CrossRef]
39. Chance, B.; Sies, H.; Boveris, A. Hydroperoxide metabolism in mammalian organs. *Physiol. Rev.* **1979**, *59*, 527–605. [CrossRef]
40. Galasso, M.; Gambino, S.; Romanelli, M.G.; Donadelli, M.; Scupoli, M.T. Browsing the oldest antioxidant enzyme: Catalase and its multiple regulation in cancer. *Free Radic. Biol. Med.* **2021**, *172*, 264–272. [CrossRef] [PubMed]
41. Glorieux, C.; Sandoval, J.M.; Dejeans, N.; Nonckreman, S.; Bahloula, K.; Poirel, H.A.; Calderon, P.B. Evaluation of Potential Mechanisms Controlling the Catalase Expression in Breast Cancer Cells. *Oxidative Med. Cell. Longev.* **2018**, *2018*, 5351967. [CrossRef] [PubMed]
42. Najafi, A.; Keykhaee, M.; Khorramdelazad, H.; Karimi, M.Y.; Nejatbakhsh Samimi, L.; Aghamohamadi, N.; Karimi, M.; Falak, R.; Khoobi, M. Catalase application in cancer therapy: Simultaneous focusing on hypoxia attenuation and macrophage reprogramming. *BioMed. Pharmacother.* **2022**, *153*, 113483. [CrossRef] [PubMed]
43. Negahdar, M.; Jalali, M.; Abtahi, H.; Sadeghi, M.R.; Javadi, E.; Aghvami, T.; Layegh, H. Blood superoxide dismutase and catalase activities in women affected with breast cancer. *Iran J. Public Health* **2005**, *34*, 39–43.
44. Sahu, A.; Varma, M.; Kachhawa, K. A prognostic study of MDA, SOD and catalase in breast Cancer patients. *Int. J. Sci. Res.* **2015**, *4*, 157–159.
45. Finley, L.W.; Carracedo, A.; Lee, J.; Souza, A.; Egia, A.; Zhang, J.; Teruya-Feldstein, J.; Moreira, P.I.; Cardoso, S.M.; Clish, C.B.; et al. SIRT3 opposes reprogramming of cancer cell metabolism through HIF1alpha destabilization. *Cancer Cell* **2011**, *19*, 416–428. [CrossRef] [PubMed]
46. Papa, L.; Hahn, M.; Marsh, E.L.; Evans, B.S.; Germain, D. SOD2 to SOD1 switch in breast cancer. *J. Biol. Chem.* **2014**, *289*, 5412–5416. [CrossRef]
47. Ambrosone, C.B.; Freudenheim, J.L.; Thompson, P.A.; Bowman, E.; Vena, J.E.; Marshall, J.R.; Graham, S.; Laughlin, R.; Nemoto, T.; Shields, P.G. Manganese superoxide dismutase (MnSOD) genetic polymorphisms, dietary antioxidants, and risk of breast cancer. *Cancer Res.* **1999**, *59*, 602–606.
48. Griess, B.; Tom, E.; Domann, F.; Teoh-Fitzgerald, M. Extracellular superoxide dismutase and its role in cancer. *Free Radic. Biol. Med.* **2017**, *112*, 464–479. [CrossRef] [PubMed]
49. Marklund, S.L. Extracellular superoxide dismutase in human tissues and human cell lines. *J. Clin. Investig.* **1984**, *74*, 1398–1403. [CrossRef]
50. Teoh, M.L.; Fitzgerald, M.P.; Oberley, L.W.; Domann, F.E. Overexpression of extracellular superoxide dismutase attenuates heparanase expression and inhibits breast carcinoma cell growth and invasion. *Cancer Res.* **2009**, *69*, 6355–6363. [CrossRef]
51. Teoh-Fitzgerald, M.L.; Fitzgerald, M.P.; Zhong, W.; Askeland, R.W.; Domann, F.E. Epigenetic reprogramming governs EcSOD expression during human mammary epithelial cell differentiation, tumorigenesis and metastasis. *Oncogene* **2014**, *33*, 358–368. [CrossRef]
52. Brigelius-Flohe, R.; Maiorino, M. Glutathione peroxidases. *Biochim. Biophys. Acta* **2013**, *1830*, 3289–3303. [CrossRef]
53. Jin, L.; Li, D.; Alesi, G.N.; Fan, J.; Kang, H.B.; Lu, Z.; Boggon, T.J.; Jin, P.; Yi, H.; Wright, E.R.; et al. Glutamate dehydrogenase 1 signals through antioxidant glutathione peroxidase 1 to regulate redox homeostasis and tumor growth. *Cancer Cell* **2015**, *27*, 257–270. [CrossRef] [PubMed]
54. Zhang, M.L.; Wu, H.T.; Chen, W.J.; Xu, Y.; Ye, Q.Q.; Shen, J.X.; Liu, J. Involvement of glutathione peroxidases in the occurrence and development of breast cancers. *J. Transl. Med.* **2020**, *18*, 247. [CrossRef]

55. Zhao, Y.; Wang, H.; Zhou, J.; Shao, Q. Glutathione Peroxidase GPX1 and Its Dichotomous Roles in Cancer. *Cancers* **2022**, *14*, 2560. [CrossRef] [PubMed]
56. Ren, Z.; Liang, H.; Galbo, P.M., Jr.; Dharmaratne, M.; Kulkarni, A.S.; Fard, A.T.; Aoun, M.L.; Martinez-Lopez, N.; Suyama, K.; Benard, O.; et al. Redox signaling by glutathione peroxidase 2 links vascular modulation to metabolic plasticity of breast cancer. *Proc. Natl. Acad. Sci. USA* **2022**, *119*, e2107266119. [CrossRef] [PubMed]
57. Saelee, P.; Pongtheerat, T.; Sophonnithiprasert, T. Reduced Expression of GPX3 in Breast Cancer Patients in Correlation with Clinical Significance. *Glob. Med. Genet.* **2020**, *7*, 87–91. [CrossRef]
58. Ding, Y.; Chen, X.; Liu, C.; Ge, W.; Wang, Q.; Hao, X.; Wang, M.; Chen, Y.; Zhang, Q. Identification of a small molecule as inducer of ferroptosis and apoptosis through ubiquitination of GPX4 in triple negative breast cancer cells. *J. Hematol. Oncol.* **2021**, *14*, 19. [CrossRef]
59. Lee, J.; Roh, J.L. Targeting GPX4 in human cancer: Implications of ferroptosis induction for tackling cancer resilience. *Cancer Lett.* **2023**, *559*, 216119. [CrossRef]
60. Khatib, A.; Solaimuthu, B.; Ben Yosef, M.; Abu Rmaileh, A.; Tanna, M.; Oren, G.; Schlesinger Frisch, M.; Axelrod, J.H.; Lichtenstein, M.; Shaul, Y.D. The glutathione peroxidase 8 (GPX8)/IL-6/STAT3 axis is essential in maintaining an aggressive breast cancer phenotype. *Proc. Natl. Acad. Sci. USA* **2020**, *117*, 21420–21431. [CrossRef] [PubMed]
61. Abboud, M.M.; Al Awaida, W.; Alkhateeb, H.H.; Abu-Ayyad, A.N. Antitumor Action of Amygdalin on Human Breast Cancer Cells by Selective Sensitization to Oxidative Stress. *Nutr. Cancer* **2019**, *71*, 483–490. [CrossRef]
62. di Ilio, C.; Sacchetta, P.; del Boccio, G.; la Rovere, G.; Federici, G. Glutathione peroxidase, glutathione S-transferase and glutathione reductase activities in normal and neoplastic human breast tissue. *Cancer Lett.* **1985**, *29*, 37–42. [CrossRef]
63. el-Sharabasy, M.M.; el-Dosoky, I.; Horria, H.; Khalaf, A.H. Elevation of glutathione, glutathione-reductase and nucleic acids in both normal tissues and tumour of breast cancer patients. *Cancer Lett.* **1993**, *72*, 11–15. [CrossRef]
64. Raninga, P.V.; Lee, A.C.; Sinha, D.; Shih, Y.Y.; Mittal, D.; Makhale, A.; Bain, A.L.; Nanayakarra, D.; Tonissen, K.F.; Kalimutho, M.; et al. Therapeutic cooperation between auranofin, a thioredoxin reductase inhibitor and anti-PD-L1 antibody for treatment of triple-negative breast cancer. *Int. J. Cancer* **2020**, *146*, 123–136. [CrossRef]
65. Dahou, H.; Minati, M.A.; Jacquemin, P.; Assi, M. Genetic Inactivation of Peroxiredoxin-I Impairs the Growth of Human Pancreatic Cancer Cells. *Antioxidants* **2021**, *10*, 570. [CrossRef] [PubMed]
66. Kang, S.W.; Chae, H.Z.; Seo, M.S.; Kim, K.; Baines, I.C.; Rhee, S.G. Mammalian peroxiredoxin isoforms can reduce hydrogen peroxide generated in response to growth factors and tumor necrosis factor-alpha. *J. Biol. Chem.* **1998**, *273*, 6297–6302. [CrossRef]
67. Noh, D.Y.; Ahn, S.J.; Lee, R.A.; Kim, S.W.; Park, I.A.; Chae, H.Z. Overexpression of peroxiredoxin in human breast cancer. *Anticancer Res.* **2001**, *21*, 2085–2090. [PubMed]
68. Park, J.H.; Kim, Y.S.; Lee, H.L.; Shim, J.Y.; Lee, K.S.; Oh, Y.J.; Shin, S.S.; Choi, Y.H.; Park, K.J.; Park, R.W.; et al. Expression of peroxiredoxin and thioredoxin in human lung cancer and paired normal lung. *Respirology* **2006**, *11*, 269–275. [CrossRef] [PubMed]
69. Song, I.S.; Jeong, Y.J.; Jung, Y.; Park, Y.H.; Shim, S.; Kim, S.J.; Eom, D.W.; Hong, S.M.; Lee, P.C.W.; Kim, S.U.; et al. The sulfiredoxin-peroxiredoxin redox system regulates the stemness and survival of colon cancer stem cells. *Redox Biol.* **2021**, *48*, 102190. [CrossRef] [PubMed]
70. Wang, T.; Diaz, A.J.; Yen, Y. The role of peroxiredoxin II in chemoresistance of breast cancer cells. *Breast Cancer Targets Ther.* **2014**, *6*, 73–80. [CrossRef]
71. Chandimali, N.; Jeong, D.K.; Kwon, T. Peroxiredoxin II Regulates Cancer Stem Cells and Stemness-Associated Properties of Cancers. *Cancers* **2018**, *10*, 305. [CrossRef]
72. Chua, P.J.; Lee, E.H.; Yu, Y.; Yip, G.W.; Tan, P.H.; Bay, B.H. Silencing the Peroxiredoxin III gene inhibits cell proliferation in breast cancer. *Int. J. Oncol.* **2010**, *36*, 359–364.
73. Karihtala, P.; Mantyniemi, A.; Kang, S.W.; Kinnula, V.L.; Soini, Y. Peroxiredoxins in breast carcinoma. *Clin. Cancer Res.* **2003**, *9*, 3418–3424.
74. Jin, D.Y.; Chae, H.Z.; Rhee, S.G.; Jeang, K.T. Regulatory role for a novel human thioredoxin peroxidase in NF-kappaB activation. *J. Biol. Chem.* **1997**, *272*, 30952–30961. [CrossRef]
75. Park, S.Y.; Lee, Y.J.; Park, J.; Kim, T.H.; Hong, S.C.; Jung, E.J.; Ju, Y.T.; Jeong, C.Y.; Park, H.J.; Ko, G.H.; et al. PRDX4 overexpression is associated with poor prognosis in gastric cancer. *Oncol. Lett.* **2020**, *19*, 3522–3530. [CrossRef]
76. Thapa, P.; Ding, N.; Hao, Y.; Alshahrani, A.; Jiang, H.; Wei, Q. Essential Roles of Peroxiredoxin IV in Inflammation and Cancer. *Molecules* **2022**, *27*, 6513. [CrossRef] [PubMed]
77. Ismail, T.; Kim, Y.; Lee, H.; Lee, D.S.; Lee, H.S. Interplay Between Mitochondrial Peroxiredoxins and ROS in Cancer Development and Progression. *Int. J. Mol. Sci.* **2019**, *20*, 4407. [CrossRef] [PubMed]
78. Kim, B.; Kim, Y.S.; Ahn, H.M.; Lee, H.J.; Jung, M.K.; Jeong, H.Y.; Choi, D.K.; Lee, J.H.; Lee, S.R.; Kim, J.M.; et al. Peroxiredoxin 5 overexpression enhances tumorigenicity and correlates with poor prognosis in gastric cancer. *Int. J. Oncol.* **2017**, *51*, 298–306. [CrossRef]
79. Seong, J.B.; Kim, B.; Kim, S.; Kim, M.H.; Park, Y.H.; Lee, Y.; Lee, H.J.; Hong, C.W.; Lee, D.S. Macrophage peroxiredoxin 5 deficiency promotes lung cancer progression via ROS-dependent M2-like polarization. *Free Radic. Biol. Med.* **2021**, *176*, 322–334. [CrossRef]
80. Sjoblom, T.; Jones, S.; Wood, L.D.; Parsons, D.W.; Lin, J.; Barber, T.D.; Mandelker, D.; Leary, R.J.; Ptak, J.; Silliman, N.; et al. The consensus coding sequences of human breast and colorectal cancers. *Science* **2006**, *314*, 268–274. [CrossRef]

81. Chang, X.Z.; Li, D.Q.; Hou, Y.F.; Wu, J.; Lu, J.S.; Di, G.H.; Jin, W.; Ou, Z.L.; Shen, Z.Z.; Shao, Z.M. Identification of the functional role of peroxiredoxin 6 in the progression of breast cancer. *Breast Cancer Res.* **2007**, *9*, R76. [CrossRef] [PubMed]
82. Forshaw, T.E.; Holmila, R.; Nelson, K.J.; Lewis, J.E.; Kemp, M.L.; Tsang, A.W.; Poole, L.B.; Lowther, W.T.; Furdui, C.M. Peroxiredoxins in Cancer and Response to Radiation Therapies. *Antioxidants* **2019**, *8*, 11. [CrossRef]
83. Nguyen, P.; Awwad, R.T.; Smart, D.D.; Spitz, D.R.; Gius, D. Thioredoxin reductase as a novel molecular target for cancer therapy. *Cancer Lett.* **2006**, *236*, 164–174. [CrossRef]
84. Rackham, O.; Shearwood, A.M.; Thyer, R.; McNamara, E.; Davies, S.M.; Callus, B.A.; Miranda-Vizuete, A.; Berners-Price, S.J.; Cheng, Q.; Arner, E.S.; et al. Substrate and inhibitor specificities differ between human cytosolic and mitochondrial thioredoxin reductases: Implications for development of specific inhibitors. *Free Radic. Biol. Med.* **2011**, *50*, 689–699. [CrossRef]
85. Rodriguez-Fanjul, V.; Lopez-Torres, E.; Mendiola, M.A.; Pizarro, A.M. Gold(III) bis(thiosemicarbazonate) compounds in breast cancer cells: Cytotoxicity and thioredoxin reductase targeting. *Eur. J. Med. Chem.* **2018**, *148*, 372–383. [CrossRef]
86. Seo, M.J.; Kim, I.Y.; Lee, D.M.; Park, Y.J.; Cho, M.Y.; Jin, H.J.; Choi, K.S. Dual inhibition of thioredoxin reductase and proteasome is required for auranofin-induced paraptosis in breast cancer cells. *Cell Death Dis.* **2023**, *14*, 42. [CrossRef]
87. Galassi, R.; Burini, A.; Ricci, S.; Pellei, M.; Rigobello, M.P.; Citta, A.; Dolmella, A.; Gandin, V.; Marzano, C. Synthesis and characterization of azolate gold(I) phosphane complexes as thioredoxin reductase inhibiting antitumor agents. *Dalton Trans.* **2012**, *41*, 5307–5318. [CrossRef] [PubMed]
88. Li, W.; Bandyopadhyay, J.; Hwaang, H.S.; Park, B.J.; Cho, J.H.; Lee, J.I.; Ahnn, J.; Lee, S.K. Two thioredoxin reductases, trxr-1 and trxr-2, have differential physiological roles in Caenorhabditis elegans. *Mol. Cells* **2012**, *34*, 209–218. [CrossRef] [PubMed]
89. Holmgren, A.; Lu, J. Thioredoxin and thioredoxin reductase: Current research with special reference to human disease. *Biochem. Biophys. Res. Commun.* **2010**, *396*, 120–124. [CrossRef]
90. Nandi, A.; Yan, L.J.; Jana, C.K.; Das, N. Role of Catalase in Oxidative Stress- and Age-Associated Degenerative Diseases. *Oxidative Med. Cell. Longev.* **2019**, *2019*, 9613090. [CrossRef] [PubMed]
91. Han, W.; Fessel, J.P.; Sherrill, T.; Kocurek, E.G.; Yull, F.E.; Blackwell, T.S. Enhanced Expression of Catalase in Mitochondria Modulates NF-kappaB-Dependent Lung Inflammation through Alteration of Metabolic Activity in Macrophages. *J. Immunol.* **2020**, *205*, 1125–1134. [CrossRef] [PubMed]
92. Zamocky, M.; Koller, F. Understanding the structure and function of catalases: Clues from molecular evolution and in vitro mutagenesis. *Prog. Biophys. Mol. Biol.* **1999**, *72*, 19–66. [CrossRef] [PubMed]
93. Hong, C.C.; Tang, B.K.; Rao, V.; Agarwal, S.; Martin, L.; Tritchler, D.; Yaffe, M.; Boyd, N.F. Cytochrome P450 1A2 (CYP1A2) activity, mammographic density, and oxidative stress: A cross-sectional study. *Breast Cancer Res.* **2004**, *6*, R338–R351. [CrossRef]
94. Radenkovic, S.; Milosevic, Z.; Konjevic, G.; Karadzic, K.; Rovcanin, B.; Buta, M.; Gopcevic, K.; Jurisic, V. Lactate dehydrogenase, catalase, and superoxide dismutase in tumor tissue of breast cancer patients in respect to mammographic findings. *Cell Biochem. Biophys.* **2013**, *66*, 287–295. [CrossRef]
95. Kattan, Z.; Minig, V.; Leroy, P.; Dauca, M.; Becuwe, P. Role of manganese superoxide dismutase on growth and invasive properties of human estrogen-independent breast cancer cells. *Breast Cancer Res. Treat.* **2008**, *108*, 203–215. [CrossRef]
96. Handschuh, L.; Kazmierczak, M.; Milewski, M.C.; Goralski, M.; Luczak, M.; Wojtaszewska, M.; Uszczynska-Ratajczak, B.; Lewandowski, K.; Komarnicki, M.; Figlerowicz, M. Gene expression profiling of acute myeloid leukemia samples from adult patients with AML-M1 and -M2 through boutique microarrays, real-time PCR and droplet digital PCR. *Int. J. Oncol.* **2018**, *52*, 656–678. [CrossRef]
97. Glorieux, C.; Dejeans, N.; Sid, B.; Beck, R.; Calderon, P.B.; Verrax, J. Catalase overexpression in mammary cancer cells leads to a less aggressive phenotype and an altered response to chemotherapy. *Biochem. Pharmacol.* **2011**, *82*, 1384–1390. [CrossRef]
98. Ruqayah Ali, O.F A -R, Decreased catalase activity and glutathione concentration levels in women patients with breast cancer. *Ann. Trop. Med. Public Health* **2020**, *23*, SP231371. [CrossRef]
99. Zinczuk, J.; Maciejczyk, M.; Zareba, K.; Romaniuk, W.; Markowski, A.; Kedra, B.; Zalewska, A.; Pryczynicz, A.; Matowicka-Karna, J.; Guzinska-Ustymowicz, K. Antioxidant Barrier, Redox Status, and Oxidative Damage to Biomolecules in Patients with Colorectal Cancer. Can Malondialdehyde and Catalase Be Markers of Colorectal Cancer Advancement? *Biomolecules* **2019**, *9*, 637. [CrossRef]
100. Birben, E.; Sahiner, U.M.; Sackesen, C.; Erzurum, S.; Kalayci, O. Oxidative stress and antioxidant defense. *World Allergy Organ. J.* **2012**, *5*, 9–19. [CrossRef]
101. Adamiec, M.; Skonieczna, M. UV radiation in HCT 116 cells influences intracellular H2O2 and glutathione levels, antioxidant expression, and protein glutathionylation. *Acta Biochim. Pol.* **2019**, *66*, 605–610. [CrossRef]
102. Tan, B.L.; Norhaizan, M.E.; Liew, W.P.; Sulaiman Rahman, H. Antioxidant and Oxidative Stress: A Mutual Interplay in Age-Related Diseases. *Front. Pharmacol.* **2018**, *9*, 1162. [CrossRef]
103. Espinosa-Diez, C.; Miguel, V.; Mennerich, D.; Kietzmann, T.; Sanchez-Perez, P.; Cadenas, S.; Lamas, S. Antioxidant responses and cellular adjustments to oxidative stress. *Redox Biol.* **2015**, *6*, 183–197. [CrossRef] [PubMed]
104. OA, I.O.a.A. First line defence antioxidants-superoxide dismutase (SOD), catalase (CAT) and glutathione peroxidase (GPX): Their fundamental role in theentire antioxidant defence grid. *Alex. J. Med.* **2018**, *54*, 287–290. [CrossRef]
105. Koeberle, S.C.; Gollowitzer, A.; Laoukili, J.; Kranenburg, O.; Werz, O.; Koeberle, A.; Kipp, A.P. Distinct and overlapping functions of glutathione peroxidases 1 and 2 in limiting NF-kappaB-driven inflammation through redox-active mechanisms. *Redox Biol.* **2020**, *28*, 101388. [CrossRef] [PubMed]

106. Asaduzzaman Khan, M.; Tania, M.; Zhang, D. Antioxidant enzymes and cancer. *Cancer Res.* **2010**, *22*, 87–92. [CrossRef]
107. Cecerska-Heryc, E.; Surowska, O.; Heryc, R.; Serwin, N.; Napiontek-Balinska, S.; Dolegowska, B. Are antioxidant enzymes essential markers in the diagnosis and monitoring of cancer patients—A review. *Clin. Biochem.* **2021**, *93*, 1–8. [CrossRef]
108. Lorestani, S.; Hashemy, S.I.; Mojarad, M.; Keyvanloo Shahrestanaki, M.; Bahari, A.; Asadi, M.; Zahedi Avval, F. Increased Glutathione Reductase Expression and Activity in Colorectal Cancer Tissue Samples: An Investigational Study in Mashhad, Iran. *Middle East J. Cancer* **2018**, *9*, 99–104. [CrossRef]
109. Zhao, Y.; Seefeldt, T.; Chen, W.; Carlson, L.; Stoebner, A.; Hanson, S.; Foll, R.; Matthees, D.P.; Palakurthi, S.; Guan, X. Increase in thiol oxidative stress via glutathione reductase inhibition as a novel approach to enhance cancer sensitivity to X-ray irradiation. *Free Radic. Biol. Med.* **2009**, *47*, 176–183. [CrossRef]
110. Niu, B.; Liao, K.; Zhou, Y.; Wen, T.; Quan, G.; Pan, X.; Wu, C. Application of glutathione depletion in cancer therapy: Enhanced ROS-based therapy, ferroptosis, and chemotherapy. *Biomaterials* **2021**, *277*, 121110. [CrossRef]
111. Weydert, C.J.; Zhang, Y.; Sun, W.; Waugh, T.A.; Teoh, M.L.; Andringa, K.K.; Aykin-Burns, N.; Spitz, D.R.; Smith, B.J.; Oberley, L.W. Increased oxidative stress created by adenoviral MnSOD or CuZnSOD plus BCNU (1,3-bis(2-chloroethyl)-1-nitrosourea) inhibits breast cancer cell growth. *Free Radic. Biol. Med.* **2008**, *44*, 856–867. [CrossRef] [PubMed]
112. Bouchmaa, N.; Ben Mrid, R.; Boukharsa, Y.; Nhiri, M.; Ait Mouse, H.; Taoufik, J.; Ansar, M.; Zyad, A. Cytotoxicity of new pyridazin-3(2H)-one derivatives orchestrating oxidative stress in human triple-negative breast cancer (MDA-MB-468). *Arch. Pharm.* **2018**, *351*, e1800128. [CrossRef]
113. Bouchmaa, N.; Ben Mrid, R.; Bouargalne, Y.; Ajouaoi, S.; Cacciola, F.; El Fatimy, R.; Nhiri, M.; Zyad, A. In vitro evaluation of dioscin and protodioscin against ER-positive and triple-negative breast cancer. *PLoS ONE* **2023**, *18*, e0272781. [CrossRef]
114. Arner, E.S.; Holmgren, A. Physiological functions of thioredoxin and thioredoxin reductase. *Eur. J. Biochem.* **2000**, *267*, 6102–6109. [CrossRef]
115. Mustacich, D.; Powis, G. Thioredoxin reductase. *Biochem. J.* **2000**, *346 Pt 1*, 1–8. [CrossRef]
116. Arner, E.S.; Holmgren, A. The thioredoxin system in cancer. *Semin. Cancer Biol.* **2006**, *16*, 420–426. [CrossRef]
117. Gandin, V.; Fernandes, A.P. Metal- and Semimetal-Containing Inhibitors of Thioredoxin Reductase as Anticancer Agents. *Molecules* **2015**, *20*, 12732–12756. [CrossRef]
118. Gencheva, R.; Cheng, Q.; Arner, E.S.J. Thioredoxin reductase selenoproteins from different organisms as potential drug targets for treatment of human diseases. *Free Radic. Biol. Med.* **2022**, *190*, 320–338. [CrossRef]
119. Kalin, S.N.; Altay, A.; Budak, H. Inhibition of thioredoxin reductase 1 by vulpinic acid suppresses the proliferation and migration of human breast carcinoma. *Life Sci.* **2022**, *310*, 121093. [CrossRef]
120. Penney, R.B.; Roy, D. Thioredoxin-mediated redox regulation of resistance to endocrine therapy in breast cancer. *Biochim. Biophys. Acta* **2013**, *1836*, 60–79. [CrossRef]
121. Hampton, M.B.; O'Connor, K.M. Peroxiredoxins and the Regulation of Cell Death. *Mol. Cells* **2016**, *39*, 72–76. [CrossRef]
122. Hall, A.; Nelson, K.; Poole, L.B.; Karplus, P.A. Structure-based insights into the catalytic power and conformational dexterity of peroxiredoxins. *Antioxid. Redox Signal.* **2011**, *15*, 795–815. [CrossRef]
123. Morais, M.A.; Giuseppe, P.O.; Souza, T.A.; Alegria, T.G.; Oliveira, M.A.; Netto, L.E.; Murakami, M.T. How pH modulates the dimer-decamer interconversion of 2-Cys peroxiredoxins from the Prx1 subfamily. *J. Biol. Chem.* **2015**, *290*, 8582–8590. [CrossRef]
124. Stocker, S.; Van Laer, K.; Mijuskovic, A.; Dick, T.P. The Conundrum of Hydrogen Peroxide Signaling and the Emerging Role of Peroxiredoxins as Redox Relay Hubs. *Antioxid. Redox Signal.* **2018**, *28*, 558–573. [CrossRef]
125. Hampton, M.B.; Vick, K.A.; Skoko, J.J.; Neumann, C.A. Peroxiredoxin Involvement in the Initiation and Progression of Human Cancer. *Antioxid. Redox Signal.* **2018**, *28*, 591–608. [CrossRef] [PubMed]
126. Kim, Y.S.; Gupta Vallur, P.; Phaeton, R.; Mythreye, K.; Hempel, N. Insights into the Dichotomous Regulation of SOD2 in Cancer. *Antioxidants* **2017**, *6*, 86. [CrossRef] [PubMed]
127. Zahra, K.F.; Lefter, R.; Ali, A.; Abdellah, E.C.; Trus, C.; Ciobica, A.; Timofte, D. The Involvement of the Oxidative Stress Status in Cancer Pathology: A Double View on the Role of the Antioxidants. *Oxidative Med. Cell. Longev.* **2021**, *2021*, 9965916. [CrossRef] [PubMed]
128. Dhar, S.K.; Tangpong, J.; Chaiswing, L.; Oberley, T.D.; St Clair, D.K. Manganese superoxide dismutase is a p53-regulated gene that switches cancers between early and advanced stages. *Cancer Res.* **2011**, *71*, 6684–6695. [CrossRef] [PubMed]
129. Gaya-Bover, A.; Hernandez-Lopez, R.; Alorda-Clara, M.; Ibarra de la Rosa, J.M.; Falco, E.; Fernandez, T.; Company, M.M.; Torrens-Mas, M.; Roca, P.; Oliver, J.; et al. Antioxidant enzymes change in different non-metastatic stages in tumoral and peritumoral tissues of colorectal cancer. *Int. J. Biochem. Cell Biol.* **2020**, *120*, 105698. [CrossRef] [PubMed]
130. Palma, F.R.; He, C.; Danes, J.M.; Paviani, V.; Coelho, D.R.; Gantner, B.N.; Bonini, M.G. Mitochondrial superoxide dismutase: What the established, the intriguing, and the novel reveal about a key cellular redox switch. *Antioxid. Redox Signal.* **2020**, *32*, 701–714. [CrossRef] [PubMed]
131. Gatenby, R.A.; Gawlinski, E.T. The glycolytic phenotype in carcinogenesis and tumor invasion: Insights through mathematical models. *Cancer Res.* **2003**, *63*, 3847–3854. [PubMed]
132. Kurono, S.; Kaneko, Y.; Matsuura, N.; Oishi, H.; Noguchi, S.; Kim, S.J.; Tamaki, Y.; Aikawa, T.; Kotsuma, Y.; Inaji, H.; et al. Identification of potential breast cancer markers in nipple discharge by protein profile analysis using two-dimensional nano-liquid chromatography/nanoelectrospray ionization-mass spectrometry. *Proteom. Clin. Appl.* **2016**, *10*, 605–613. [CrossRef] [PubMed]

133. Liu, F.J.; Wang, X.B.; Cao, A.G. Screening and functional analysis of a differential protein profile of human breast cancer. *Oncol. Lett.* **2014**, *7*, 1851–1856. [CrossRef]
134. O'Leary, P.C.; Terrile, M.; Bajor, M.; Gaj, P.; Hennessy, B.T.; Mills, G.B.; Zagozdzon, A.; O'Connor, D.P.; Brennan, D.J.; Connor, K.; et al. Peroxiredoxin-1 protects estrogen receptor alpha from oxidative stress-induced suppression and is a protein biomarker of favorable prognosis in breast cancer. *Breast Cancer Res.* **2014**, *16*, R79. [CrossRef]
135. Liu, J.; Du, J.; Zhang, Y.; Sun, W.; Smith, B.J.; Oberley, L.W.; Cullen, J.J. Suppression of the malignant phenotype in pancreatic cancer by overexpression of phospholipid hydroperoxide glutathione peroxidase. *Hum. Gene Ther.* **2006**, *17*, 105–116. [CrossRef]
136. Krol, M.B.; Galicki, M.; Gresner, P.; Wieczorek, E.; Jablonska, E.; Reszka, E.; Morawiec, Z.; Wasowicz, W.; Gromadzinska, J. The ESR1 and GPX1 gene expression level in human malignant and non-malignant breast tissues. *Acta. Biochim. Pol.* **2018**, *65*, 51–57. [CrossRef]
137. Al-Taie, O.H.; Uceyler, N.; Eubner, U.; Jakob, F.; Mork, H.; Scheurlen, M.; Brigelius-Flohe, R.; Schottker, K.; Abel, J.; Thalheimer, A.; et al. Expression profiling and genetic alterations of the selenoproteins GI-GPx and SePP in colorectal carcinogenesis. *Nutr. Cancer* **2004**, *48*, 6–14. [CrossRef]
138. Yang, M.; Zhu, X.; Shen, Y.; He, Q.; Qin, Y.; Shao, Y.; Yuan, L.; Ye, H. GPX2 predicts recurrence-free survival and triggers the Wnt/beta-catenin/EMT pathway in prostate cancer. *PeerJ* **2022**, *10*, e14263. [CrossRef]
139. Jiao, Y.; Wang, Y.; Guo, S.; Wang, G. Glutathione peroxidases as oncotargets. *Oncotarget* **2017**, *8*, 80093–80102. [CrossRef]
140. Lee, O.J.; Schneider-Stock, R.; McChesney, P.A.; Kuester, D.; Roessner, A.; Vieth, M.; Moskaluk, C.A.; El-Rifai, W. Hypermethylation and loss of expression of glutathione peroxidase-3 in Barrett's tumorigenesis. *Neoplasia* **2005**, *7*, 854–861. [CrossRef]
141. Falck, E.; Karlsson, S.; Carlsson, J.; Helenius, G.; Karlsson, M.; Klinga-Levan, K. Loss of glutathione peroxidase 3 expression is correlated with epigenetic mechanisms in endometrial adenocarcinoma. *Cancer Cell Int.* **2010**, *10*, 46. [CrossRef]
142. Yu, Y.P.; Yu, G.; Tseng, G.; Cieply, K.; Nelson, J.; Defrances, M.; Zarnegar, R.; Michalopoulos, G.; Luo, J.H. Glutathione peroxidase 3, deleted or methylated in prostate cancer, suppresses prostate cancer growth and metastasis. *Cancer Res.* **2007**, *67*, 8043–8050. [CrossRef]
143. Chen, Z.; Hu, T.; Zhu, S.; Mukaisho, K.; El-Rifai, W.; Peng, D.F. Glutathione peroxidase 7 suppresses cancer cell growth and is hypermethylated in gastric cancer. *Oncotarget* **2017**, *8*, 54345–54356. [CrossRef] [PubMed]
144. Koeberle, S.C.; Kipp, A.P.; Stuppner, H.; Koeberle, A. Ferroptosis-modulating small molecules for targeting drug-resistant cancer: Challenges and opportunities in manipulating redox signaling. *Med. Res. Rev.* **2023**, *43*, 614–682. [CrossRef] [PubMed]
145. Sui, S.; Xu, S.; Pang, D. Emerging role of ferroptosis in breast cancer: New dawn for overcoming tumor progression. *Pharmacol. Ther.* **2022**, *232*, 107992. [CrossRef]
146. Liu, H.; Schreiber, S.L.; Stockwell, B.R. Targeting Dependency on the GPX4 Lipid Peroxide Repair Pathway for Cancer Therapy. *Biochemistry* **2018**, *57*, 2059–2060. [CrossRef]
147. Chen, M.; Shi, Z.; Sun, Y.; Ning, H.; Gu, X.; Zhang, L. Prospects for Anti-Tumor Mechanism and Potential Clinical Application Based on Glutathione Peroxidase 4 Mediated Ferroptosis. *Int. J. Mol. Sci.* **2023**, *24*, 1607. [CrossRef]
148. Liu, H.; Forouhar, F.; Lin, A.J.; Wang, Q.; Polychronidou, V.; Soni, R.K.; Xia, X.; Stockwell, B.R. Small-molecule allosteric inhibitors of GPX4. *Cell Chem. Biol.* **2022**, *29*, 1680–1693.e9. [CrossRef]
149. Stockwell, B.R.; Jiang, X. The Chemistry and Biology of Ferroptosis. *Cell Chem. Biol.* **2020**, *27*, 365–375. [CrossRef]
150. Cao, Y.; Zhang, H.; Tang, J.; Wang, R. Ferulic Acid Mitigates Growth and Invasion of Esophageal Squamous Cell Carcinoma through Inducing Ferroptotic Cell Death. *Dis. Markers* **2022**, *2022*, 4607966. [CrossRef]
151. Xu, F.L.; Wu, X.H.; Chen, C.; Wang, K.; Huang, L.Y.; Xia, J.; Liu, Y.; Shan, X.F.; Tang, N. SLC27A5 promotes sorafenib-induced ferroptosis in hepatocellular carcinoma by downregulating glutathione reductase. *Cell Death Dis.* **2023**, *14*, 22. [CrossRef]
152. Lu, Y.; Zhang, X.S.; Zhou, X.M.; Gao, Y.Y.; Chen, C.L.; Liu, J.P.; Ye, Z.N.; Zhang, Z.H.; Wu, L.Y.; Li, W.; et al. Peroxiredoxin 1/2 protects brain against H(2)O(2)-induced apoptosis after subarachnoid hemorrhage. *FASEB J.* **2019**, *33*, 3051–3062. [CrossRef]
153. Vabulas, R.M. Ferroptosis-Related Flavoproteins: Their Function and Stability. *Int. J. Mol. Sci.* **2021**, *22*, 430. [CrossRef] [PubMed]
154. Yang, Z.; Huang, S.; Liu, Y.; Chang, X.; Liang, Y.; Li, X.; Xu, Z.; Wang, S.; Lu, Y.; Liu, Y.; et al. Biotin-Targeted Au(I) Radiosensitizer for Cancer Synergistic Therapy by Intervening with Redox Homeostasis and Inducing Ferroptosis. *J. Med. Chem.* **2022**, *65*, 8401–8415. [CrossRef] [PubMed]
155. Singh, R.; Lillard, J.W., Jr. Nanoparticle-based targeted drug delivery. *Exp. Mol. Pathol.* **2009**, *86*, 215–223. [CrossRef]
156. Tang, X.; Loc, W.S.; Dong, C.; Matters, G.L.; Butler, P.J.; Kester, M.; Meyers, C.; Jiang, Y.; Adair, J.H. The use of nanoparticulates to treat breast cancer. *Nanomedicine* **2017**, *12*, 2367–2388. [CrossRef]
157. Zhang, Z.; Yao, Y.; Yuan, Q.; Lu, C.; Zhang, X.; Yuan, J.; Hou, K.; Zhang, C.; Du, Z.; Gao, X.; et al. Gold clusters prevent breast cancer bone metastasis by suppressing tumor-induced osteoclastogenesis. *Theranostics* **2020**, *10*, 4042–4055. [CrossRef]
158. Zhou, J.; Li, K.; Zang, X.; Xie, Y.; Song, J.; Chen, X. ROS-responsive Galactosylated-nanoparticles with Doxorubicin Entrapment for Triple Negative Breast Cancer Therapy. *Int. J. Nanomed.* **2023**, *18*, 1381–1397. [CrossRef]
159. Hong, S.; Choi, D.W.; Kim, H.N.; Park, C.G.; Lee, W.; Park, H.H. Protein-Based Nanoparticles as Drug Delivery Systems. *Pharmaceutics* **2020**, *12*, 604. [CrossRef]
160. Homayouni Tabrizi, M. Fabrication of folic acid-conjugated chitosan-coated PLGA nanoparticles for targeted delivery ofPeganum harmalasmoke extract to breast cancer cells. *Nanotechnology* **2022**, *33*, 495101. [CrossRef]
161. Solak, K.; Mavi, A.; Yilmaz, B. Disulfiram-loaded functionalized magnetic nanoparticles combined with copper and sodium nitroprusside in breast cancer cells. *Mater. Sci. Eng. C Mater. Biol. Appl.* **2021**, *119*, 111452. [CrossRef] [PubMed]

162. Feuser, P.E.; Cordeiro, A.P.; de Bem Silveira, G.; Borges Correa, M.E.A.; Lock Silveira, P.C.; Sayer, C.; de Araujo, P.H.H.; Machado-de-Avila, R.A.; Dal Bo, A.G. Co-encapsulation of sodium diethyldithiocarbamate (DETC) and zinc phthalocyanine (ZnPc) in liposomes promotes increases phototoxic activity against (MDA-MB 231) human breast cancer cells. *Colloids Surf. B Biointerfaces* **2021**, *197*, 111434. [CrossRef]
163. Tian, W.; Wang, S.; Tian, Y.; Su, X.; Sun, H.; Tang, Y.; Lu, G.; Liu, S.; Shi, H. Periodic mesoporous organosilica coupled with chlorin e6 and catalase for enhanced photodynamic therapy to treat triple-negative breast cancer. *J. Colloid Interface Sci.* **2022**, *610*, 634–642. [CrossRef]
164. Hei, Y.; Teng, B.; Zeng, Z.; Zhang, S.; Li, Q.; Pan, J.; Luo, Z.; Xiong, C.; Wei, S. Multifunctional Immunoliposomes Combining Catalase and PD-L1 Antibodies Overcome Tumor Hypoxia and Enhance Immunotherapeutic Effects Against Melanoma. *Int. J. Nanomed.* **2020**, *15*, 1677–1691. [CrossRef] [PubMed]
165. Shi, C.; Li, M.; Zhang, Z.; Yao, Q.; Shao, K.; Xu, F.; Xu, N.; Li, H.; Fan, J.; Sun, W.; et al. Catalase-based liposomal for reversing immunosuppressive tumor microenvironment and enhanced cancer chemo-photodynamic therapy. *Biomaterials* **2020**, *233*, 119755. [CrossRef] [PubMed]
166. Zhang, R.; Song, X.; Liang, C.; Yi, X.; Song, G.; Chao, Y.; Yang, Y.; Yang, K.; Feng, L.; Liu, Z. Catalase-loaded cisplatin-prodrug-constructed liposomes to overcome tumor hypoxia for enhanced chemo-radiotherapy of cancer. *Biomaterials* **2017**, *138*, 13–21. [CrossRef]
167. Li, G.; Wang, S.; Deng, D.; Xiao, Z.; Dong, Z.; Wang, Z.; Lei, Q.; Gao, S.; Huang, G.; Zhang, E.; et al. Fluorinated Chitosan To Enhance Transmucosal Delivery of Sonosensitizer-Conjugated Catalase for Sonodynamic Bladder Cancer Treatment Post-intravesical Instillation. *ACS Nano* **2020**, *14*, 1586–1599. [CrossRef] [PubMed]
168. Hu, D.; Chen, Z.; Sheng, Z.; Gao, D.; Yan, F.; Ma, T.; Zheng, H.; Hong, M. A catalase-loaded hierarchical zeolite as an implantable nanocapsule for ultrasound-guided oxygen self-sufficient photodynamic therapy against pancreatic cancer. *Nanoscale* **2018**, *10*, 17283–17292. [CrossRef] [PubMed]
169. Chen, Q.; Chen, J.; Yang, Z.; Xu, J.; Xu, L.; Liang, C.; Han, X.; Liu, Z. Nanoparticle-Enhanced Radiotherapy to Trigger Robust Cancer Immunotherapy. *Adv. Mater.* **2019**, *31*, e1802228. [CrossRef] [PubMed]
170. Liang, Y.; Zhang, L.; Peng, C.; Zhang, S.; Chen, S.; Qian, X.; Luo, W.; Dan, Q.; Ren, Y.; Li, Y.; et al. Tumor microenvironments self-activated nanoscale metal-organic frameworks for ferroptosis based cancer chemodynamic/photothermal/chemo therapy. *Acta Pharm. Sin. B* **2021**, *11*, 3231–3243. [CrossRef]
171. Yao, L.; Zhao, M.M.; Luo, Q.W.; Zhang, Y.C.; Liu, T.T.; Yang, Z.; Liao, M.; Tu, P.; Zeng, K.W. Carbon Quantum Dots-Based Nanozyme from Coffee Induces Cancer Cell Ferroptosis to Activate Antitumor Immunity. *ACS Nano* **2022**, *16*, 9228–9239. [CrossRef] [PubMed]
172. Zhou, L.; Chen, J.; Li, R.; Wei, L.; Xiong, H.; Wang, C.; Chai, K.; Chen, M.; Zhu, Z.; Yao, T.; et al. Metal-Polyphenol-Network Coated Prussian Blue Nanoparticles for Synergistic Ferroptosis and Apoptosis via Triggered GPX4 Inhibition and Concurrent In Situ Bleomycin Toxification. *Small* **2021**, *17*, e2103919. [CrossRef] [PubMed]
173. Li, Y.; Li, M.; Liu, L.; Xue, C.; Fei, Y.; Wang, X.; Zhang, Y.; Cai, K.; Zhao, Y.; Luo, Z. Cell-Specific Metabolic Reprogramming of Tumors for Bioactivatable Ferroptosis Therapy. *ACS Nano* **2022**, *16*, 3965–3984. [CrossRef]
174. Li, K.; Lin, C.; Li, M.; Xu, K.; He, Y.; Mao, Y.; Lu, L.; Geng, W.; Li, X.; Luo, Z.; et al. Multienzyme-like Reactivity Cooperatively Impairs Glutathione Peroxidase 4 and Ferroptosis Suppressor Protein 1 Pathways in Triple-Negative Breast Cancer for Sensitized Ferroptosis Therapy. *ACS Nano* **2022**, *16*, 2381–2398. [CrossRef]
175. Zhou, L.L.; Guan, Q.; Li, W.Y.; Zhang, Z.; Li, Y.A.; Dong, Y.B. A Ferrocene-Functionalized Covalent Organic Framework for Enhancing Chemodynamic Therapy via Redox Dyshomeostasis. *Small* **2021**, *17*, e2101368. [CrossRef]
176. Chen, Y.; Chen, M.; Zhai, T.; Zhou, H.; Zhou, Z.; Liu, X.; Yang, S.; Yang, H. Glutathione-Responsive Chemodynamic Therapy of Manganese(III/IV) Cluster Nanoparticles Enhanced by Electrochemical Stimulation via Oxidative Stress Pathway. *Bioconjugate Chem.* **2022**, *33*, 152–163. [CrossRef]
177. He, H.; Du, L.; Guo, H.; An, Y.; Lu, L.; Chen, Y.; Wang, Y.; Zhong, H.; Shen, J.; Wu, J.; et al. Redox Responsive Metal Organic Framework Nanoparticles Induces Ferroptosis for Cancer Therapy. *Small* **2020**, *16*, e2001251. [CrossRef]
178. Fereidoonnezhad, M.; Ahmadi, M.; Abedanzadeh, S.; Yazdani, A.; Alamdarlou, A.; Babaghasabha, M.; Almansaf, Z.; Faghih, Z.; McConnell, Z.; Shahsavari, H.R.; et al. Synthesis and biological evaluation of thiolate gold(I) complexes as thioredoxin reductases (TrxRs) and glutathione reductase (GR) inhibitors. *New J. Chem.* **2019**, *43*, 13173–13182. [CrossRef]
179. Bajor, M.; Graczyk-Jarzynka, A.; Marhelava, K.; Kurkowiak, M.; Rahman, A.; Aura, C.; Russell, N.; Zych, A.O.; Firczuk, M.; Winiarska, M.; et al. Triple Combination of Ascorbate, Menadione and the Inhibition of Peroxiredoxin-1 Produces Synergistic Cytotoxic Effects in Triple-Negative Breast Cancer Cells. *Antioxidants* **2020**, *9*, 320. [CrossRef]
180. Kato, I.; Kasukabe, T.; Kumakura, S. Menin-MLL inhibitors induce ferroptosis and enhance the anti-proliferative activity of auranofin in several types of cancer cells. *Int. J. Oncol.* **2020**, *57*, 1057–1071. [CrossRef]
181. Hatem, E.; Azzi, S.; El Banna, N.; He, T.; Heneman-Masurel, A.; Vernis, L.; Baille, D.; Masson, V.; Dingli, F.; Loew, D.; et al. Auranofin/Vitamin C: A Novel Drug Combination Targeting Triple-Negative Breast Cancer. *J. Natl. Cancer Inst.* **2018**, *111*, 597–608. [CrossRef]
182. Zhang, X.; Chen, X.; Zhao, Y. Nanozymes: Versatile Platforms for Cancer Diagnosis and Therapy. *Nanomicro Lett.* **2022**, *14*, 95. [CrossRef]

183. Pei, P.; Shen, W.; Zhang, Y.; Zhang, Y.; Qi, Z.; Zhou, H.; Liu, T.; Sun, L.; Yang, K. Radioactive nano-oxygen generator enhance anti-tumor radio-immunotherapy by regulating tumor microenvironment and reducing proliferation. *Biomaterials* **2022**, *280*, 121326. [CrossRef] [PubMed]
184. Jiang, W.; Han, X.; Zhang, T.; Xie, D.; Zhang, H.; Hu, Y. An Oxygen Self-Evolving, Multistage Delivery System for Deeply Located Hypoxic Tumor Treatment. *Adv. Health Mater.* **2020**, *9*, e1901303. [CrossRef] [PubMed]
185. Kheshtchin, N.; Hadjati, J. Targeting hypoxia and hypoxia-inducible factor-1 in the tumor microenvironment for optimal cancer immunotherapy. *J. Cell. Physiol.* **2022**, *237*, 1285–1298. [CrossRef] [PubMed]
186. Chang, M.; Wang, Z.; Dong, C.; Zhou, R.; Chen, L.; Huang, H.; Feng, W.; Wang, Z.; Wang, Y.; Chen, Y. Ultrasound-Amplified Enzyodynamic Tumor Therapy by Perovskite Nanoenzyme-Enabled Cell Pyroptosis and Cascade Catalysis. *Adv. Mater.* **2023**, *35*, e2208817. [CrossRef] [PubMed]
187. Yao, S.; Zhao, X.; Wang, X.; Huang, T.; Ding, Y.; Zhang, J.; Zhang, Z.; Wang, Z.L.; Li, L. Bioinspired Electron Polarization of Nanozymes with a Human Self-Generated Electric Field for Cancer Catalytic Therapy. *Adv. Mater.* **2022**, *34*, e2109568. [CrossRef] [PubMed]
188. Adair, J.H.; Parette, M.P.; Altinoglu, E.I.; Kester, M. Nanoparticulate alternatives for drug delivery. *ACS Nano* **2010**, *4*, 4967–4970. [CrossRef] [PubMed]
189. Yang, F.; He, Q.; Dai, X.; Zhang, X.; Song, D. The potential role of nanomedicine in the treatment of breast cancer to overcome the obstacles of current therapies. *Front. Pharmacol.* **2023**, *14*, 1143102. [CrossRef] [PubMed]
190. Lehmann, B.D.; Bauer, J.A.; Chen, X.; Sanders, M.E.; Chakravarthy, A.B.; Shyr, Y.; Pietenpol, J.A. Identification of human triple-negative breast cancer subtypes and preclinical models for selection of targeted therapies. *J. Clin. Investig.* **2011**, *121*, 2750–2767. [CrossRef]
191. Liedtke, C.; Mazouni, C.; Hess, K.R.; Andre, F.; Tordai, A.; Mejia, J.A.; Symmans, W.F.; Gonzalez-Angulo, A.M.; Hennessy, B.; Green, M.; et al. Response to neoadjuvant therapy and long-term survival in patients with triple-negative breast cancer. *J. Clin. Oncol.* **2008**, *26*, 1275–1281. [CrossRef] [PubMed]
192. Hussain, Z.; Khan, J.A.; Murtaza, S. Nanotechnology: An Emerging Therapeutic Option for Breast Cancer. *Crit. Rev. Eukaryot. Gene Expr.* **2018**, *28*, 163–175. [CrossRef] [PubMed]
193. Gao, H.; Chen, C.; Xi, Z.; Chen, J.; Zhang, Q.; Cao, S.; Jiang, X. In vivo behavior and safety of lapatinib-incorporated lipid nanoparticles. *Curr. Pharm. Biotechnol.* **2014**, *14*, 1062–1071. [CrossRef] [PubMed]
194. Wang, X.; Yu, B.; Wu, Y.; Lee, R.J.; Lee, L.J. Efficient down-regulation of CDK4 by novel lipid nanoparticle-mediated siRNA delivery. *Anticancer Res.* **2011**, *31*, 1619–1626.
195. American Type Culture Collection. 2024. The Global Bioresource Center. Available online: https://www.atcc.org/ (accessed on 8 May 2024).
196. Briem, E.; Ingthorsson, S.; Traustadottir, G.A.; Hilmarsdottir, B.; Gudjonsson, T. Application of the D492 Cell Lines to Explore Breast Morphogenesis, EMT and Cancer Progression in 3D Culture. *J. Mammary Gland Biol. Neoplasia* **2019**, *24*, 139–147. [CrossRef] [PubMed]

International Journal of
Molecular Sciences

MDPI

Review

Antioxidant Enzymes in Cancer Cells: Their Role in Photodynamic Therapy Resistance and Potential as Targets for Improved Treatment Outcomes

Wachirawit Udomsak [1], Malgorzata Kucinska [1], Julia Pospieszna [1], Hanna Dams-Kozlowska [2,3], Waranya Chatuphonprasert [4] and Marek Murias [1,5,*]

1 Department of Toxicology, Poznan University of Medical Sciences, ul Rokietnicka 3, 60-608 Poznan, Poland; wachirawit5414@gmail.com (W.U.); kucinska@ump.edu.pl (M.K.); julia.pospieszna@gmail.com (J.P.)
2 Department of Cancer Immunology, Poznan University of Medical Sciences, ul. Garbary 15, 61-866 Poznan, Poland; hdamskozlowska@ump.edu.pl or hanna.dams-kozlowska@wco.pl
3 Department of Diagnostics and Cancer Immunology, Greater Poland Cancer Centre, ul.Garbary 15, 61-866 Poznan, Poland
4 Faculty of Medicine, Mahasarakham University, Maha Sarakham 44000, Thailand; waranya.c@msu.ac.th
5 Center for Advanced Technology, Adam Mickiewicz University, ul. Uniwersytetu Poznańskiego 10, 61-614 Poznan, Poland
* Correspondence: marek.murias@ump.edu.pl

Abstract: Photodynamic therapy (PDT) is a selective tumor treatment that consists of a photosensitive compound—a photosensitizer (PS), oxygen, and visible light. Although each component has no cytotoxic properties, their simultaneous use initiates photodynamic reactions (PDRs) and sequentially generates reactive oxygen species (ROS) and/or free radicals as cytotoxic mediators, leading to PDT-induced cell death. Nevertheless, tumor cells develop various cytoprotective mechanisms against PDT, particularly the adaptive mechanism of antioxidant status. This review integrates an in-depth analysis of the cytoprotective mechanism of detoxifying ROS enzymes that interfere with PDT-induced cell death, including superoxide dismutase (SOD), catalase, glutathione redox cycle, and heme oxygenase-1 (HO-1). Furthermore, this review includes the use of antioxidant enzymes inhibitors as a strategy in order to diminish the antioxidant activities of tumor cells and to improve the effectiveness of PDT. Conclusively, PDT is an effective tumor treatment of which its effectiveness can be improved when combined with a specific antioxidant inhibitor.

Keywords: photodynamic therapy; superoxide dismutase; catalase; glutathione redox cycle; heme oxygenase-1; antioxidant inhibitors; cancer

1. Introduction

Photodynamic therapy (PDT) is a selective tumor treatment that has been approved by the United States Food and Drug Administration (FDA) since the late 1990s [1–3]. PDT generates cytotoxic reactive oxygen species (ROS), including singlet oxygen ($^1O_2$), hydroxyl radicals ($HO^•$), and superoxide anions ($O_2^{•-}$), in the presence of oxygen, through various types of photodynamic reactions (PDRs). In order to initiate a PDR, a photosensitizer (PS) needs to be activated by visible light of a specific wavelength. The light excites the electron of the PS in the ground state into an excited singlet state. Then, the excited PS can return to its ground state, producing photon emission (fluorescence), or convert to a triplet state through intersystem crossing. Eventually, the excited triplet state PS transfers its electrons to the formation of free radical species (e.g., hydroxyl radicals and superoxide anions) and oxidizes the subcellular substrates as type I PDR electron transfer. In the meantime, the excited triplet state PS can transfer energy to oxygen molecules for the formation of singlet oxygen and can cause cell death via type II PDR energy transfer. It is important to note that both type I and II PDRs are oxygen-dependent reactions that can proceed simultaneously depending on PS properties and the cellular oxygen level [4–6]. Recently, PDRs have been additionally classified into types III and IV based on the direct activation of the PS. After activation, types III and IV PDRs can immediately exert cytotoxicity and require neither additional reactions nor oxygen molecules [7–10].

The anticancer effects of PDT-induced therapy are classified into three mechanisms depending on the properties of the PS, light dosage, and tumor environment, as follows: (1) irreversible direct cell killing—the cytotoxic ROS directly injures organelles of cancer cells, which results in the induction of several cell death pathways, including conventional (apoptosis, autophagy, and necrosis) and "non-conventional" pathways, such as ferroptosis, mitotic catastrophe, paraptosis, pyroptosis, parthanatos, necroptosis, and immunogenic cell death (ICD); (2) vasculature damage—the PS, localized in the endothelial cells, destroys blood vessel walls, resulting in blood supply interruption; and (3) inflammation and immune responses—PDT can trigger inflammatory and immune responses by recruiting inflammatory mediators, e.g., cytokines, leukotrienes, and tumor necrosis factors [5,11–16]. PDT surpasses conventional chemotherapy in various aspects, especially in specificity and efficacy. The enhanced permeability and retention (EPR) effect, resulting from the leaky tumor vasculature, combined with the overexpression of low-density lipoprotein receptors, enables the passive delivery of the PS to tumor sites [17]. As a result of PS exposure to visible light of a specific wavelength, precise radiation is delivered to the tumor niche. This, in turn, triggers a PDR, producing cancer cell-specific ROS. Moreover, PDT often shows minimal cross-resistance with chemoresistance, radioresistance, or other PSs [18]. Combining PDT with other therapeutic modalities, such as surgery, chemotherapy, radiotherapy, and immunotherapy, can synergistically improve treatment outcomes [19–22].

Although the first PS was clinically introduced in 1978, many aspects of PDT still need refinement, especially regarding the hypoxic conditions in the tumor environment and the specific wavelength required for the excitation of the PS [2,23]. Despite PDT having many advantages, some factors limit its widespread use in clinical practice. First and foremost, in the classical understanding of PDT, oxygen is necessary for the cytotoxic effect to occur during PDT. Tumor hypoxia is not only considered the cause of cell resistance against chemo- or radiotherapy but also lowers the effectiveness of PDT, whether in vitro, pre-clinical, or clinical. Hypoxia is a well-known tumor feature and many regions of the tumor show deficient oxygen levels (less than 5 mmHg partial pressure of oxygen (pO_2); 5 mmHg corresponds to approximately 0.7% O_2 in the gas phase or 7 μM in solution) [24]. The effectiveness of PDT, especially that which is mainly mediated by oxygen-dependent type II PDRs, is eventually diminished due to a lower ROS production in the hypoxic environment of tumor cells [20]. Moreover, the wavelength of visible light must be specific to the PS to initiate the PDR. Nonetheless, the optical window to penetrate the tissue in PDT has been limited to only between 600 and 800 nm (red to deep red). More than 800 nm of light does not provide enough energy to activate the PS and produce ROS. At the same time, up to 600 nm light could be absorbed by water, leading to the minimization of the penetration of irradiation through the tissue, causing ineffectiveness against deep tumor sites. The light of a wavelength between 700 and 800 nm can penetrate deep into the tissue, approximately 1 cm, whereas 600 nm is limited to only 0.5 cm [25]. The absorption spectra of significant chromophores in tissues, i.e., cytochromes, melanin, water, deoxyhemoglobin, and oxyhemoglobin, were reported by Plaetzer's group [26]. It is important to note that hemoglobin and oxyhemoglobin exhibit similar absorption wavelengths to some photosynthesizers used in PDT. Certain studies suggest that PDT may elevate the production of methemoglobin and deoxygenated hemoglobin, particularly under the conditions of hemolysis [27–30]. Consequently, there is no ideal visible light for all PDT indications. To select the optimal wavelength, one should consider the characteristics of the PS, such as its fluorescence excitation and action spectra, dosimetry factors like light dosage, exposure time, delivery mode, fluence rate, and disease attributes, including accessibility, location, size, and tissue specificity [19,31–34].

Another issue affecting PDT's efficacy is the compensatory pathways activated in cancer cells in response to treatment. Cancer cells deploy different cytoprotective mechanisms, including the control of (1) antioxidant molecules levels, (2) enzymes in ROS detoxification, and (3) expression of specific genes encoding proteins in response to PDT [35]. Typically, cells balance between cellular oxidants and antioxidants under physiological conditions through redox homeostasis, which the ROS control at sub-micromolar levels. Paradoxically, cancer cells produce elevated ROS levels as an adaptive mechanism, sustaining a consistently pro-oxidative state that promotes tumor initiation and progression [36]. However, if ROS levels are extremely high, they can lead to tumor cell death. Therefore, this adaptive mechanism develops antioxidant systems against excessive ROS and becomes redox resetting, contributing resistance to various ROS-mediated tumor therapies, including PDT (Figure 1) [37,38].

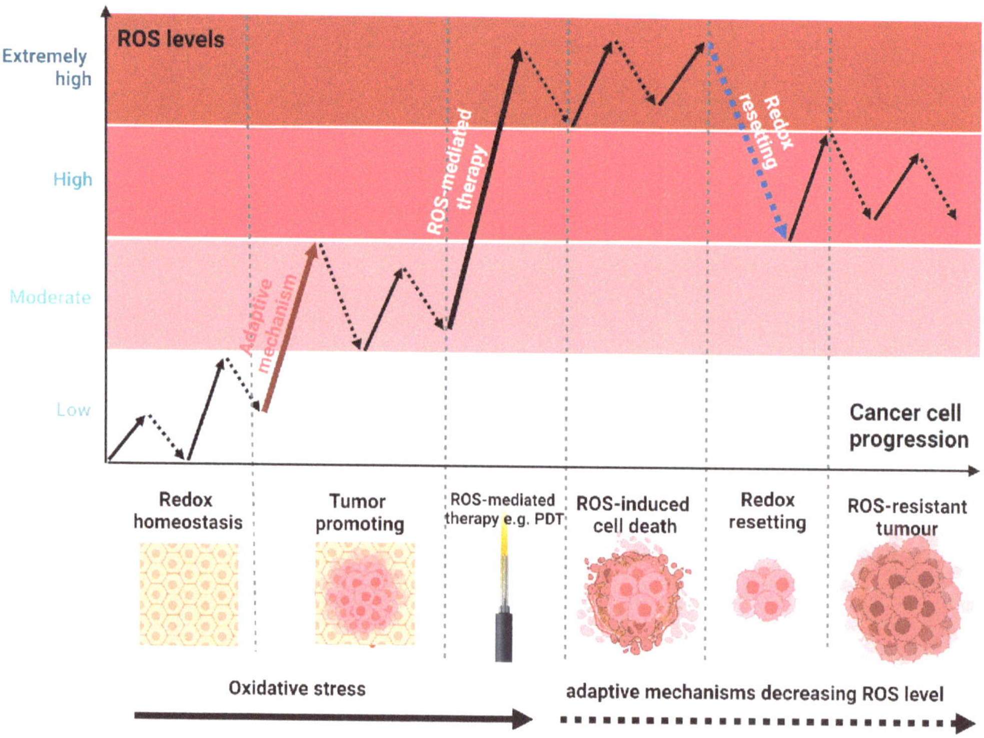

Figure 1. Relationship between reactive oxygen species (ROS) level and cancer cell progression. Modified from Liu et al., Gorrini et al., and Nakamura et al. [38–40]. Created with Biorender.com.

To date, targeting redox proteins has been proposed as a potential strategy to enhance the therapeutic efficacy of various anticancer modalities, such as chemotherapy, radiotherapy, and PDT. However, it should be emphasized that antioxidant therapeutic strategies in cancer are quite complex, as they may involve both the supplementation of and the reduction in antioxidant activity in cancer cells. The beneficial effects of antioxidants are linked to their ability to mitigate the side effects of excessive free radical formation during anticancer treatments. Additionally, free radicals/ROS play crucial roles in tumorigenesis and cancer development. However, in the context of ROS-mediated therapy, decreasing antioxidant activity is particularly interesting, and certain selected agents or naturally occurring compounds have also been tested. In this review, we provide an in-depth analysis of the cytoprotective mechanisms of detoxifying ROS enzymes, generally considered as antioxidant enzymes that interfere with PDT-induced cell death. This paper will focus on three main antioxidant enzymes, as follows: superoxide dismutase, catalase, and the glutathione redox cycle. The relationships between these enzymes are depicted in Figure 2. Moreover, in this review, we also focused on heme oxygenase, since several reports showed the promising results for combining its inhibitor with PDT.

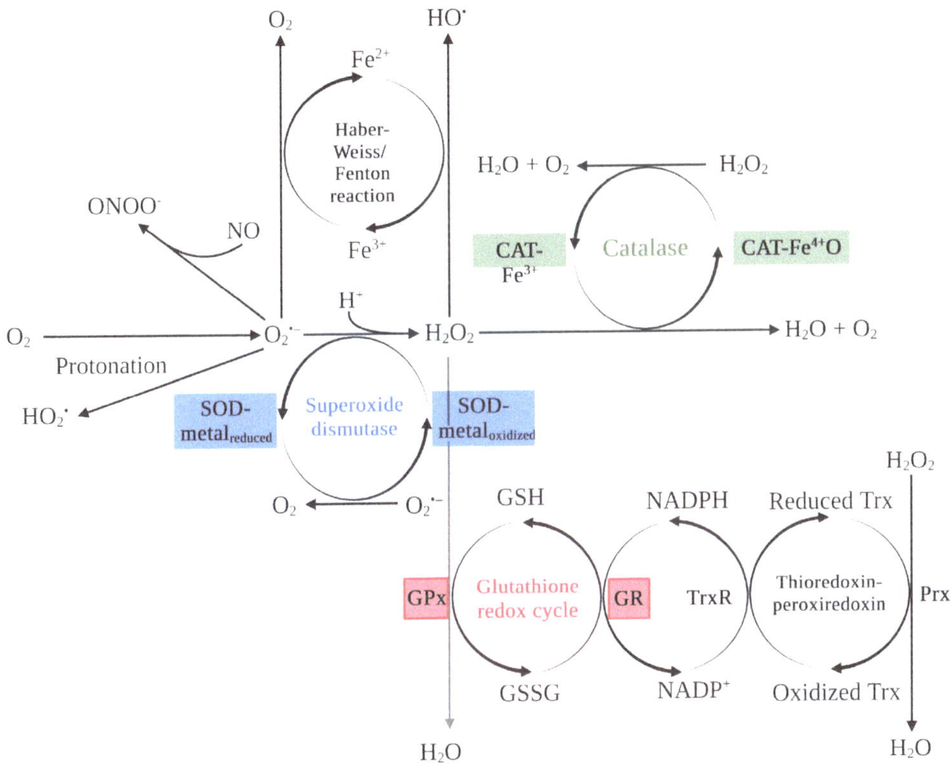

Figure 2. Antioxidant system: Superoxide Dismutase (SOD), Catalase (CAT), and Glutathione/Thioredoxin redox cycle enzymes. Abbreviations: CAT-Fe^{3+}, ferricatalase; CAT-Fe^{4+}O, compound I; GPx, glutathione peroxidase; GR, glutathione reductase; GSH, glutathione; GSSG, glutathione disulfide; H_2O_2, hydrogen peroxide; $HO^{\bullet}$, hydroxyl radical; $HO_2^{\bullet}$, hydroperoxyl radical; NADPH, nicotinamide adenine dinucleotide phosphate; NO, nitric oxide; $O_2^{\bullet-}$, superoxide anion; $ONOO^-$, peroxynitrite; Prx, peroxiredoxins; ROS, reactive oxygen species; Trx, thioredoxin; TrxR, thioredoxin reductase [41].

2. Antioxidant Enzymes Responsible for ROS-Mediated Treatment Resistance

2.1. Superoxide Dismutase (SOD)

Superoxide dismutases are the central antioxidant enzymes in the oxidoreductase group of the ROS defense system responsible for the dismutation of a rapidly reactive ROS, the superoxide anion (Figure 2) [42]. The superoxide anion is generated by various intracellular sources, including the mitochondrial electron transport chain (ETC), NADPH oxidase (NOX), nitric oxide synthase (NOS), lipoxygenase, xanthine oxidase (XO), cyclooxygenase (COX), cytosolic xanthine oxidase, cytochrome P450 mono-oxygenases, and mitochondrial enzymes (Mits) [40,43]. Under the pathological conditions of cardiovascular diseases, the superoxide anion causes oxidative stress and redox imbalance toward ROS/reactive nitrogen species (RNS)-related pathways. The simplest way is the protonation of the superoxide anion to a hydroperoxyl radical ($HO_2^{\bullet}$), a strong oxidant that can further trigger lipid peroxidation [44–46]. An antioxidant, nitric oxide (NO), rapidly reacts with the superoxide anion, producing the strong oxidant, peroxynitrite ($ONOO^-$), disrupting both endothelial and mitochondrial functions, leading to atherosclerosis, diabetes, hypercholesterolemia, hypertension, and aging [47,48]. The superoxide anion facilitates the generation of the highly toxic hydroxyl radical via reducing ferric iron (Fe^{3+}) to ferrous iron (Fe^{2+}) via the Haber–Weiss reaction, before reacting with H_2O_2 and turning back to Fe^{3+} via the Fenton reaction [46,49]. SODs are responsible for removing ROS via the catalysis of the superoxide anion to H_2O_2 involved with catalases, thioredoxin-peroxiredoxin, and glutathione. The scavenging mechanism of SODs has been called the "ping-pong" mechanism as it relates to both the reduction and the oxidation of catalytic metals, such as copper (Cu) or manganese (Mn) at the active site of the enzyme [42,50].

There are three distinct isoforms of SODs in mammals (Table 1). SOD1 (copper- and zinc-containing SOD) is localized in intracellular cytoplasmic compartments, including the cytoplasm, mitochondrial intermembrane space, lysosomes, peroxisomes, and nucleus. It regulates NOX2 activity, increasing endosome superoxide anions. Then, it catalyzes the dismutation of superoxide anions at the endosomal surface and produces localized hydrogen peroxide (H_2O_2), leading to the activation of the transcriptional factor NF-kB (nuclear factor kappa-light-chain-enhancer of activated B cells) [51]. However, SOD1 in the nucleus is essential for protecting against the oxidative DNA damage caused by H_2O_2. It acts as a transcriptional factor that regulates the expression of oxidative response genes, resulting in oxidative stress resistance [52]. SOD2 (manganese-containing SOD), specifically localized in the mitochondria matrix, generates H_2O_2 signaling inside the mitochondria, regulating blood vessel formation, cell differentiation, and pulmonary hypertension development [42,53]. SOD3 (copper- and zinc-containing SOD) is localized in the vascular extracellular space, extracellular matrix, cell surface, plasma, and extracellular fluids (i.e., lungs, blood vessels, kidneys, uterus, and heart). It plays a vital role in maintaining the redox homeostasis of the tissues from oxidative and inflammatory damage. It is also well known to possess anti-angiogenic, anti-inflammatory, antichemotactic, antiproliferative, and immunomodulatory properties [42,54–56].

In unhealthy cells, SODs impair the apoptosis induction of tumor cells by interrupting the hypochlorous acid (HOCl) and NO/peroxynitrite signaling pathways. Tumor cells require a high production rate of extracellular superoxide anions and H_2O_2 to maintain their development and progression [57–59]. On the other hand, H_2O_2 is a primary substrate for HOCl generation in the pathway of apoptosis-mediated PDT, namely HOCl signaling (Figure 3). HOCl is a potent oxidizing agent and, under physiological conditions, is mainly generated by the interaction between H_2O_2 and the chloride anion (Cl^-), catalyzed by peroxidases (PODs), such as myeloperoxidase (MPO) or the peroxidase domain of dual oxidase (DUOX) [60,61]. After interaction with extracellular superoxide anions in tumor cells, HOCl yields an apoptosis-induced hydroxyl radical, which results in selective anti-tumor activity. Hence, the anti-tumor activity of HOCl signaling correlates with the hydroxyl radical level, which depends on the superoxide anion and HOCl levels in tumor cells. Hydroxyl radicals can reach the cell membrane and trigger lipid peroxidation, specifically in the membrane of tumor cells. Then, apoptosis is activated in the mitochondrial pathway relating to caspase-9 and -3 activity [62–66]. Furthermore, HOCl modulates immune response through an accumulation of neutrophils and the induction of tumor necrotic factor α (TNFα) production in peripheral blood mononuclear cells, contributing to inflammatory responses [67,68].

Another trail of apoptosis-mediated PDT is the NO/peroxynitrite signaling pathway (Figure 3). NO plays a vital role in both metabolic and cardiovascular balance, boasting properties that promote vasodilation, combat inflammation, and prevent thrombosis, as well as acting as an antioxidant [69]. Yet, when NO swiftly interacts with superoxide anions, it results in the formation of a potent oxidant known as peroxynitrite. This formidable oxidant has the capacity to modify a range of molecules. Among its targets are the heme of soluble guanylate cyclase, various lipids, and the endothelial NOS cofactor BH4. Such interactions can result in mitochondrial dysfunction, escalated ROS production, and lipid peroxidation [42]. Furthermore, peroxynitrite can be protonated to peroxynitrous acid (ONOOH) before decomposing to nitrogen dioxide (NO_2) and the apoptosis-inducing hydroxyl radical. This protonation can specifically occur in the membrane of tumor cells, due to the acidic conditions in the presence of the proton pump of tumor cells. The in-depth mechanisms of HOCl and NO/peroxynitrite signaling have been thoroughly explained by Bauer and co-workers [70,71].

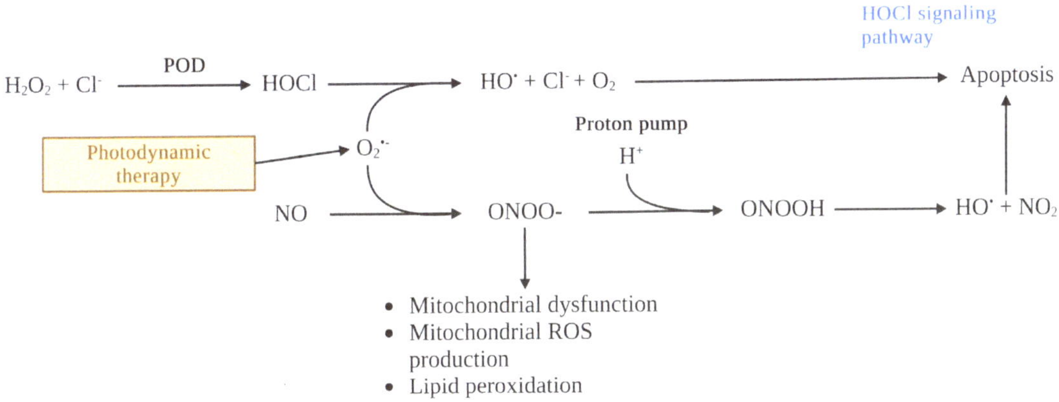

Figure 3. Apoptosis-inducing signaling through the hypochlorous acid (HOCl) and nitric oxide (NO)/peroxynitrite pathways [70,71].

All isoforms of SODs are responsible for scavenging extracellular superoxide anions and converting them into H_2O_2. Next, H_2O_2 can be converted to H_2O by catalase, peroxiredoxins (Prxs), or glutathione peroxidases (GPxs). Thus, they interfere with HOCl signaling by lowering the extracellular superoxide anion levels, leading to diminishing hydroxyl radical production and HOCl-mediated apoptosis induction (Figure 4) [71]. Likewise, NO/peroxynitrite signaling has been intercepted by SODs by preserving NO within the endothelium and preventing its interaction with superoxide anions, leading to a decrease in peroxynitrite formation. These mechanisms imply the evolution of free radical resistance within ROS/NOS apoptotic signaling pathways in tumor cells associated with SODs [42,72]. Bauer et al. reported that HOCl-mediated apoptosis induction was entirely inhibited by SOD2 treatment in gastric carcinoma MKN-45 cells [62]. They also confirmed that extracellular superoxide anion concentration in tumor cells could be increased by SOD inhibition. Likewise, pretreatment with a neutralizing antibody against SOD increased the cell sensitivity to HOCl-mediated apoptosis by increasing the HOCl concentration in a model of murine melanoma B16F10 cells. It suggested that SOD inhibition increased both the production of available superoxide anions and HOCl signaling [62]. Liu and co-workers discovered that the elevated protein level of SOD2 was associated with lymph node metastasis in a tongue squamous cell carcinoma (TSCC) model [73,74]. Among three TSCC cell lines, UM1 possessed the highest migration and invasion abilities correlated with the highest SOD2 protein level and activity. In addition, the H_2O_2 production and proliferation rate of UM1 cells were significantly higher than UM2 cells, another TSCC cell line with lower migration and invasion abilities. On the contrary, the aggressiveness of TSCC was reduced after knockdown of the expression of the SOD2 gene. UM1 transfected with SOD2 shRNA showed lower migration and invasion abilities, H_2O_2 production, and cell proliferation rate. Therefore, the migration and invasion abilities of TSCC were dependent on the production of H_2O_2 that was regulated by SOD2 [75].

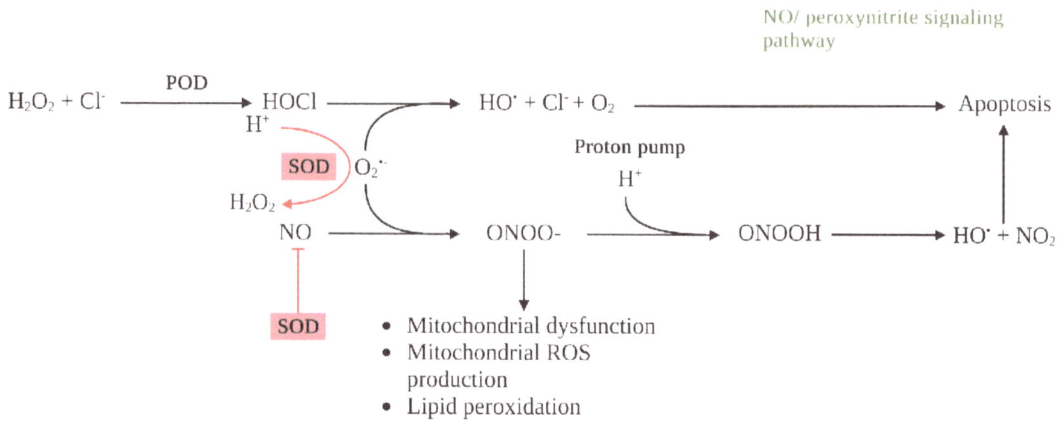

Figure 4. Cytoprotective mechanism of superoxide dismutase (SOD) through hypochlorous acid (HOCl) and nitric oxide (NO)/peroxynitrite signaling in tumor cells.

Various evidence indicates the impact of SODs on the effectiveness of PDT. An immortalized T lymphocyte cell line, Jurkat, characterized by an enhanced SOD2 activity due to transfection with a gene encoding wild-type SOD2, showed a significant decrease in the generation of superoxide, activation of caspase-3, and apoptosis-induced cell death after PDT treatment, silicon phthalocyanine Pc 4, when compared with cells transfected with the control vector [76]. In contrast to the cell expressing wild-type SOD2, the Jurkat cells expressing mutated SOD2 were characterized by enhanced apoptosis-induced cell death after Pc 4 treatment, due to an increased generation of superoxide, activation of caspase-3, and apoptosis-induced cell death. These results were subsequently confirmed by comparing the mouse embryonic fibroblasts (MEFs) derived from SOD2-knockdown (Sod2 −/−) and wild-type (Sod2+/+) mice. Pc 4-based PDT, apoptosis-induced cell death was enhanced in Sod2 −/− MEFs through the induction of caspase-3-like activity, nuclear apoptotic changes, and ceramide accumulation compared with Sod2+/+ MEFs [76]. The intravenous administration of SOD2 following PDT treatment meaningfully reduced the curative effect of Photofrin-based PDT in SCCVII (squamous carcinoma cells) and RIF-1 and FsaR (fibrosarcoma cells) implanted in syngeneic C3H/HeN and BALB/c mice, respectively [77]. These results indicated that SOD could attenuate the cytotoxic effects of the superoxide radical generated by PDT, which promotes oxidative stress at the endothelium and NO/peroxynitrite-mediated apoptosis [77].

Soares' group showed that SOD2 activity affected the cytotoxicity of PDT differently, depending on the main cytotoxic mediators of PDT [78]. Human lung adenocarcinoma A549 cells that exhibited lower SOD2 and catalase activities after PDT treatment were more sensitive to the cytotoxic superoxide anions and singlet oxygen produced by redaporfin-based PDT than mouse colon adenocarcinoma CT26 cells, but were resistant against the singlet oxygen produced after temoporfin-based PDT. In contrast to A549 cells, CT26 cells, which exhibited a higher activity of SOD2 and catalase after PDT treatment, were more resistant to superoxide radicals and singlet oxygen from redaporfin-based PDT, but were sensitive to the singlet oxygen from temoporfin-based PDT [78]. Consequently, SOD2 is one of the key enzymes in protecting tumor cells against cytotoxic superoxide anions mediated by PDT. Nonetheless, the SOD1 role against PDT was not prominent. Golab et al. showed that the addition of a cell-permeable SOD mimetic, MnTBAP, and the transient transgenic expression of SOD2 into urinary bladder cancer T24 cells significantly decreased cell susceptibility to the cytotoxicity of Photofrin-based PDT, compared with the control cells. On the other hand, T24 cells transfected only with the SOD1 expression plasmid did not show a modified cytotoxic effect from PDT [79]. In contrast, after knockdown of the

SOD1 gene by siRNA in human cervical HeLa and oral squamous cell carcinoma Cal27 cells, an increase in singlet oxygen levels was obtained, which enhanced the cytotoxicity of zinc phthalocyanine-based PDT loaded into orthogonal upconversion nanoparticles (UCNPs). Furthermore, SOD1, siRNA-containing UCNPs significantly reduced tumor growth in Balb/c nude mice xenografted with Cal27 tumors, compared with the control [80].

2.2. Catalase

Catalase is considered a crucial antioxidant enzyme in physiological conditions due to its catalyzing of the dismutation of H_2O_2 in a two-step reaction (Table 1). The first step is the oxidation of catalase, as follows: free catalase (ferricatalase; CAT-Fe^{3+}) is oxidized by H_2O_2 into an intermediate, compound I (CAT-$Fe^{4+}O$), and produces a water molecule (Figure 2). The second step is the reduction of compound I; compound I is reduced back to free catalase by another molecule of H_2O_2, producing one molecule each of water and oxygen. In total, catalase breaks down two molecules of H_2O_2 into two molecules of water and one molecule of oxygen [81,82]. Catalase is distributed throughout the body, particularly in the liver, kidneys, and erythrocytes. It sequentially protects healthy cells against ROS-mediated oxidative damage and tumor metastasis [83–85]. The importance of catalase has been demonstrated in numerous studies. For instance, catalase overexpression in mice mitochondria and heart extended their life span and reduced ischemia/reperfusion injury, respectively [86,87]. The administration of catalase conjugated with polyethylene glycol significantly inhibited hydrogen peroxide-induced lipid peroxidation in mice [88]. The gene mutation of catalase is related to diabetes, hypertension, vitiligo, or Alzheimer's disease [89,90]. Moreover, hereditary catalase deficiency, acatalasemia, and hypocatalasemia, which were characterized by less than 10% and 50% of regular catalase activity, respectively, caused oral gangrene ulceration in Japanese or hypertension patients [91–93]. It is important to note that the role and activity of catalase undergoes enormous changes during tumor development [94,95].

To avoid the apoptosis-induced effects from HOCl and NO/peroxynitrite signaling, tumor cells establish cytoprotective systems consisting of membrane-associated catalase as a chief enzyme. Catalase abrogates HOCl and NO/peroxynitrite signaling through the dismutation of H_2O_2, the oxidation of NO, and the decomposition of peroxynitrite, respectively (Figure 5) [96–99]. This results in a decrease in HOCl and the hydroxyl radical production generated by HOCl and NO/peroxynitrite signaling, leading to attenuated apoptosis-inducing signaling in tumor cells. Interestingly, although extracellular singlet oxygen generated by PDT can inactivate a few catalase molecules of the cancer cell membrane and cause apoptosis, catalase still interrupts apoptosis-inducing signaling and diminishes PDT-induced cell death [100]. On the other hand, the inactivation of catalase may potentiate PDT-induced cell death, generating extracellular singlet oxygen. H_2O_2 dismutation, NO oxidation, and peroxynitrite decomposition no longer occur without catalase activity, leading to the formation of hydroperoxide radicals that can react with superoxide anions and generate singlet oxygen [101]. These reactions are specific in cancer cells due to a complex interaction between H_2O_2 and peroxynitrite [70].

Although the level of catalase expression varies among different types of cancer, the depletion of catalase expression or the inhibition of its enzymatic activity reduces tumor resistance to oxidative damage due to ROS-mediated therapies, including PDT [102,103]. One of the mechanisms exhibited by ROS-resistant glioma cells is the production of antioxidant enzymes, particularly catalase. Smith and co-workers reported that rat glioma-derived cell lines (C6, 36B10, RG2, and RT2), and human glioma cell lines (SNB19, U251, and A172) which overexpressed catalase protein showed elevated catalase enzymatic activity [104]. Knockdown of the *Cat* gene in 36B10 rat glioma cells significantly increased intracellular and extracellular ROS production, improving sensitivity against radiation (137Cs γ-irradiator) and H_2O_2 treatment [104]. Moreover, a study by Kang et al. elucidated that the synergistic action of the tumor suppressor p53 and the pro-apoptotic protein, p53-inducible gene 3 (PIG3), led to a diminution of catalase activity during UV-induced apoptosis. The resulting increase in ROS production enhanced the apoptotic cell death of HCT116, a human colon carcinoma cell line [105]. A study by Zhao and co-workers indicated that among three tested human tumor cell lines, a human hepatoma cell line, HepG2 cells, showed the highest antioxidant activity regulated primarily by catalase [106]. Whilst the glutathione redox cycle mainly controlled the other two cell lines, i.e., human cervical HeLa and lung adenocarcinoma A549 cells. The cytotoxicity of an ROS-dependent apoptosis inducer, artesunate, was affected by neither a γ-glutamylcysteine synthetase (GCS) inhibitor, L-buthionine-sulfoximine (BSO), nor glutathione (GSH) treatment in HepG2 cells. Whereas, a catalase inhibitor, 3-aminotriazole (3-AT), and catalase silencing meaningfully promoted sensitivity to H_2O_2- and artesunate-induced cytotoxicity. It was concluded that a strong resistance against ROS in HepG2 cells was dominated by catalase activity, while A549 and Hela cells exhibited a weak resistance against ROS due to a low catalase activity [106].

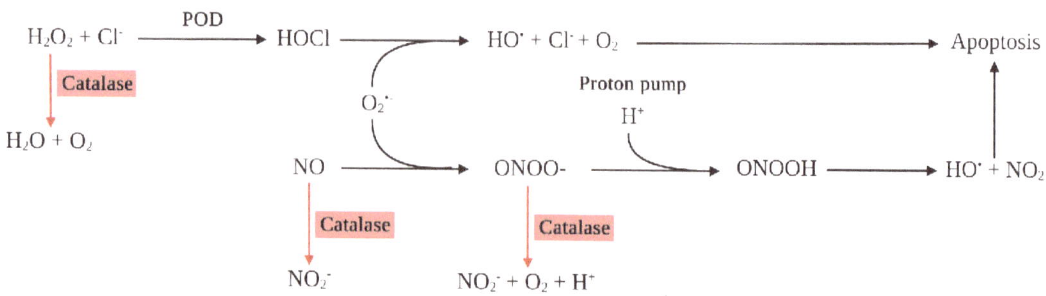

Figure 5. Cytoprotective mechanism of catalase through hypochlorous acid (HOCl) and nitric oxide (NO)/peroxynitrite signaling in tumor cells.

Klingelhoeffer and co-workers demonstrated that among 13 human cell lines, BT-20, a breast carcinoma, possessed the highest catalase protein level and activity, which led to cytotoxic resistance against the powerful pro-oxidant, H_2O_2, produced by ascorbic acid [103]. Notably, catalase-silenced BT-20 cells indicated a significant reduction in catalase protein level and its activity, which increased cell susceptibility against the ascorbic acid-mediated cytotoxic effect via elevating cell death and caspase-3/7 activity [103]. Glorieux et al. showed that human breast cancer cells, MCF-7, were sensitive to the combination of pro-oxidant drugs (ascorbate/menadione). Nevertheless, the elevation of the catalase protein level via treatment with 5-aza-2′-deoxycytidine, a DNA methyltransferase (DNMT) inhibitor, significantly developed a cell resistance phenomenon [102]. A decrease in catalase activity via treatment with 3-AT, a catalase inhibitor, meaningfully improved MCF-7 cell sensitivity to the combination of pro-oxidant drugs. Notably, the catalase overexpression in MCF-7 cells did not result in cell resistance against conventional chemotherapies such as cisplatin, 5-fluorouracil, doxorubicin, or paclitaxel. It suggested that altering antioxidant enzyme expression, including catalase, might cause a resistance mechanism only towards redox-based chemotherapeutic agents in tumor cells [107]. Among 32 patients suffering from mesothelioma, 24 (75%) cases indicated catalase expression in tumor cells. Additionally, a human mesothelioma cell line, M38K, showed a high catalase protein level and the catalase inhibition by 3-AT improved cells' sensitivity to epirubicin [108]. In the case of PDT, the exogenous addition of catalase potentially reduced the LD_{50} of hematoporphyrin-based PDT by 60% in Ehrlich ascites carcinoma (EAC) cells, suggesting that an increase in catalase can promote cell resistance against PDT-induced cytotoxicity [109].

2.3. Glutathione Redox Cycle

Not only is catalase responsible for removing H_2O_2, but is also responsible for the removal of nicotinamide adenine dinucleotide phosphate (NADPH)-dependent antioxidants; glutathione (GSH; L-γ-glutamyl-L-cysteinyl-glycine) and thioredoxin-peroxiredoxin redox systems facilitate elimination of H_2O_2 (Figure 2) [110,111]. GSH is an intracellular antioxidant molecule that plays a crucial role in maintaining redox status, xenobiotic metabolism, and regulation of gene expression and programmed cell death (Table 1). Two ATP-dependent enzymes regulate the synthesis of GSH, as follows: (1) glutamate–cysteine ligase (GCL) or γ-glutamylcysteine synthetase (GCS) that facilitates the formation of γ-glutamyl cysteine using glutamic acid and cysteine, and (2) GSH synthase (GS) that catalyzes the addition of glycine to the dipeptide (Figure 6). The γ-glutamyl bond makes glutathione more resistant to degradation by cellular proteases, which typically cleave α-peptide bonds. Additionally, the presence of the γ-glutamyl bond has implications for transporting glutathione and its precursor amino acids across cell membranes. Specific transporters in cell membranes recognize the γ-glutamyl moiety and facilitate the uptake of glutathione [112]. Under oxidizing conditions, GSH shows antioxidant activity via acting as a reducing agent or electron donor to reduce H_2O_2, lipid hydroperoxides (LOOHs), and peroxynitrite, before being converted to oxidized glutathione or glutathione disulfide (GSSG) by glutathione peroxidase (GPx), resulting in a decrease in the GSH/GSSG ratio. GSSG can be converted back to GSH using NADPH, catalyzed by glutathione reductase (GR) [113–115].

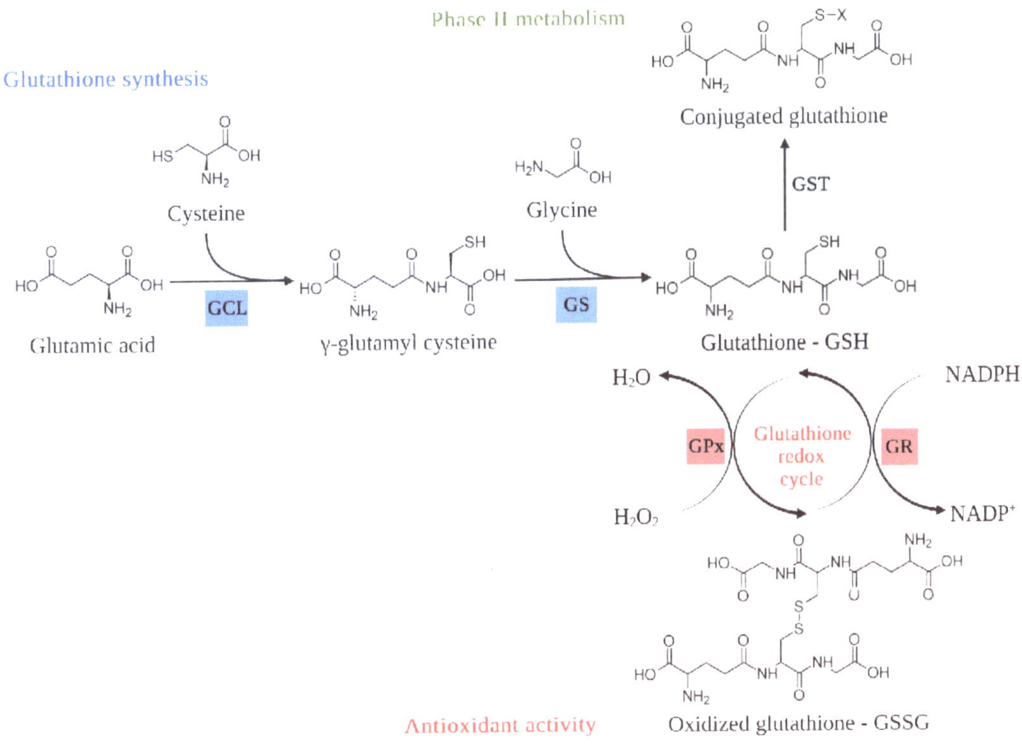

Figure 6. The glutathione synthesis pathway and its function as an antioxidant and detoxifying agent. Abbreviations: GCL, γ-glutamylcysteine synthetase; GS, glutathione synthetase; GR, glutathione reductase; GPx, glutathione peroxidase; GST, glutathione *S*-transferase; NADPH, nicotinamide adenine dinucleotide phosphate; X, xenobiotic.

Furthermore, glutathione *S*-transferase (GST), which is considered a xenobiotic-conjugating enzyme in phase II metabolism, can further maintain the cellular redox state and defense against cytotoxic ROS through a wide range of molecular mechanisms, such as the Jun N-terminal kinase, apoptosis signaling kinase 1, 4-hydroxy-2-transnonenal, and mitogen-activated protein kinase pathway [116–121].

The glutathione redox cycle is a crucial cytoprotective mechanism against cytotoxic ROS in tumor cells. Zhao et al. showed that the glutathione redox cycle potentially affected ROS-mediated anticancer therapies, H_2O_2, and artesunate-induced apoptosis in HeLa and A549 cells [106]. Treatment with a GCS inhibitor, buthionine sulfoximine (BSO) eliminated the cell resistance to H_2O_2 and enhanced the H_2O_2-induced cytotoxicity in HeLa and A549 cells, which were regulated by GPx and catalase activity. Moreover, the pretreatment of the cells with GSH abolished the cytotoxicity of artesunate. It is important to note that artesunate cytotoxicity was not affected by BSO or GSH treatment in HepG2 cells, which was mainly controlled by catalase [106]. The glutathione redox cycle plays an essential role in ROS cytotoxicity generated by PDT. Lee et al. showed a crucial role of GSH in the sensitivity of chlorin e6 (Ce6)-based PDT in two human cholangiocarcinoma cell lines, HuCC-T1 and SNU1196 [122]. SNU1196 cells possessed higher GSH basal levels, catalytic subunit GSC expression, and GPx and GR activity compared with HuCC-T1 cells. Thus, HuCC-T1 cells were more sensitive to Ce6-based PDT, exhibiting three and two times higher apoptotic and necrotic cell deaths, respectively, than SNU1196 cells. The addition of exogenous GSH to HuCC-T1 cells reduced the ROS generation and cytotoxicity of Ce6-based PDT. At the same time, a GPx inhibitor, mercaptosuccinic acid (MSA), displayed opposite effects in SNU1196 cells [122]. After the addition of an exogenous GSH, GSH monoethyl ester significantly abrogated ROS induction and apoptosis mediated by hypericin-based PDT in human colorectal cancer HCT8 and HCT116 cells [123]. Wang and co-workers reported that GPx protected MCF-7 cells against lipid peroxidation, leading to cell resistance against singlet oxygen-induced oxidative damage due to Photofrin-based PDT. GPx-overexpressed MCF-7 cells indicated a lower level of a lipid peroxidation marker, LOOH, suggesting that GPx could repair lipid peroxidation. GPx minimized membrane damage and singlet oxygen-induced apoptosis, increasing cell survival after PDT treatment [124]. Likewise, Dabrowski et al. reported that GST facilitated the resistance to PDT. The human kidney fibroblast K293 cell line was transfected with a plasmid-encoding green fluorescent protein and GSTP1-1 (pIRES-GFP-GSTP) to increase the expression of GSTP1-1. The GSTP1-1-overexpressed K293 cells showed resistance against PDT by reducing the hypericin-based PDT cytotoxicity [117]. Furthermore, in 2004, Lu and Atkins reported that the production of ROS induced by hypericin can be attenuated by the ligandin of GST [125]. Interestingly, hydrogen sulfide (H_2S) has been observed to diminish the activity of PDT-based therapy via ROS/RNS scavenging [126]. The cytotoxicity of 5-ALA was dramatically reduced following exposure to H_2S in the murine adenocarcinoma LM2 cell line. The outcomes were associated with an elevation of GSH levels and catalase activity, with a reduction in singlet oxygen level [127].

2.4. Heme Oxygenase-1 (HO-1)

Heme oxygenase (HO) is known as an enzyme that metabolizes pro-oxidant heme into the antioxidant biliverdin (which is converted to bilirubin), iron (Fe^{2+}), and carbon monoxide (CO) (Table 1) [128–130]. The heme catabolism pathway is presented in Figure 7. There are three isoforms of HO, HO-1, HO-2, and HO-3, encoded by separate genes [131–133]. Genes encode heme oxygenase-1 (*Hmox1*) and heme oxygenase-2 (*Hmox2*) that are located on chromosome 22 and 16, respectively [134–136]. HO-1 protein (32.8 kDa) is highly expressed in spleen, liver, bone marrow, and senescent red blood cells [134,137,138], while HO-2 protein (36 kDa) is expressed in brain, testis, and endothelial and smooth muscle cells from cerebral vessels [139–141]. HO-3 is thought to be a pseudogene derived from HO-2 transcripts and its function remains unknown [133].

HO-1 is known to have essential functions in heme catabolism. Moreover, it has anti-inflammatory, anti-apoptotic, and cytoprotective effects [142–146]. Its upregulation has been observed in response to various stressors, including oxidative stress, which may be induced by PDT [142–146]. HO-1 expression is also regulated by several transcription factors, such as Nrf2 (nuclear factor erythroid 2-related factor 2), AP-1 (activator protein-1), Bach1, and HIF (hypoxia-inducible factor) [143,144,147,148].

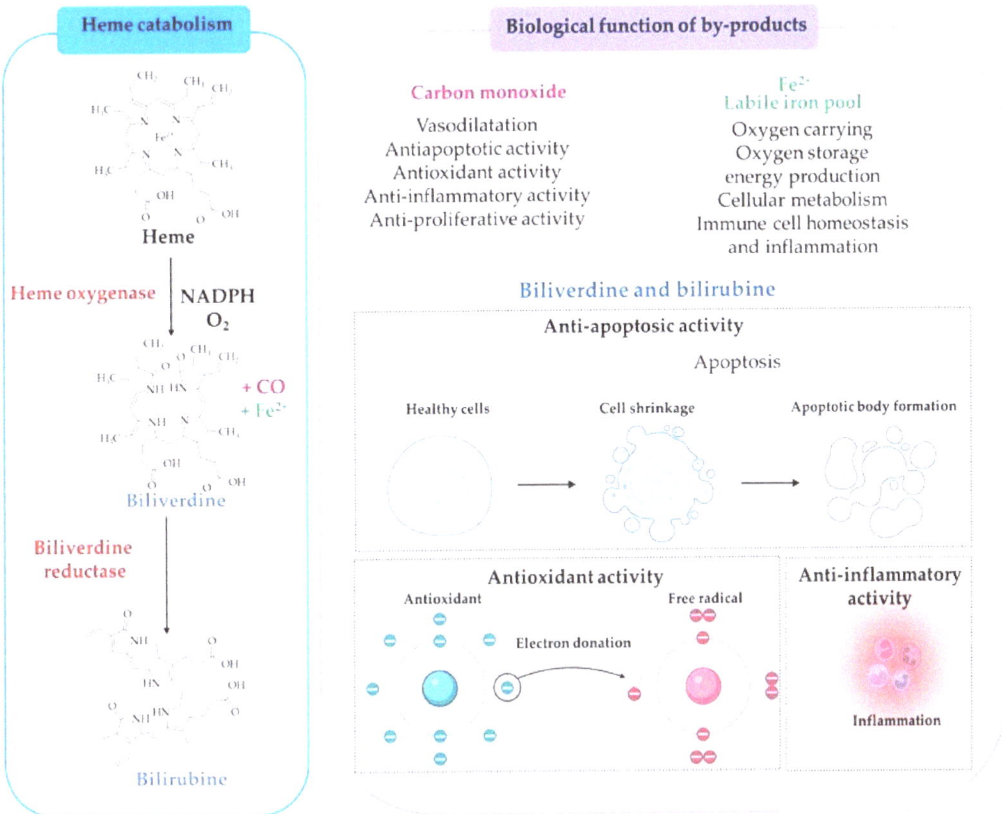

Figure 7. A scheme presenting the heme degradation pathway and role of heme oxygenase in producing the biologically active intermediates. Created with Biorender.com.

The degradation products of heme are essential biologically active compounds (Figure 7). Carbon monoxide (CO) is a toxic gas that can be deadly in high concentrations [149]. However, some studies have shown that low levels of CO generate cell-protective effects. Moreover, CO has anti-inflammatory and anti-apoptotic effects, which can protect cells from the damage caused by oxidative stress [150–153]. Biliverdin is a green pigment produced from the breakdown of heme via OH-1. Biliverdin is then converted into bilirubin via the enzyme biliverdin reductase. Biliverdin and bilirubin are powerful antioxidants that can scavenge peroxyl radicals and prevent lipid peroxidation. Bilirubin demonstrates scavenging abilities against superoxide, peroxyl radicals, and peroxynitrite [154–158].

The role of HO-1 in PDT resistance has been investigated in studies conducted on various cancer cell lines. Cytotoxicity analysis confirmed that HO-1 exhibits a cytoprotective effect on the cells attacked by ROS-based therapy, including PDT [142–145]. It was demonstrated that HO-1 protects tumor cells against PDT-mediated cytotoxicity by alleviating oxidative stress and promoting cell survival [142]. Furthermore, the induction of HO-1 in rat malignant meningioma cells subjected to talaporfin sodium-mediated PDT was explored, emphasizing the upregulation of HO-1 as a cellular response to oxidative stress induced by PDT [143,144]. Also, these findings were extended by highlighting the influence of HO-1 on the outcome of 5-aminolevulinic acid (5-ALA)-mediated PDT in melanoma cells [145]. Collectively, these investigations underscore the significance of HO-1 as a key player in the cellular defense against PDT-induced oxidative stress, providing valuable insights into the mechanisms underlying the cytoprotective effects observed in cells exposed to photodynamic treatment.

In addition, PDT induces the expression of *Hmox1* [142–144,146], which may contribute to the acquisition of resistance to PDT by cancer cells [143,144]. Several studies also suggest that inhibiting HO-1 activity or expression can sensitize cancer cells to PDT and enhance the therapeutic outcome of this treatment. Several studies have explored the use of HO-1 inhibitors to increase the effectiveness of PDT [142,145,159,160]. Cheng et al. reported that a natural antioxidant, alpha-lipoic acid (ALA), can increase cell resistance against oxidative stress. ALA administration significantly increased the expression and activity of HO-1 in rat aortic smooth muscle A10 cells, further reducing cytotoxicity after H_2O_2 treatment. Interestingly, the cytotoxicity of H_2O_2 can be reversed by treatment with an HO-1 inhibitor, Zn(II) protoporphyrin IX (ZnPPIX) [161]. In the study of the role of mitogen-activated protein kinase (p38MAPK) and phosphatidylinositol 3-kinase (PI3K) pathways in HO-1 induction, it was found that the application of p38MAPK and PI3K inhibitors, PD169316 and LY294002, respectively, significantly reduced HO-1 expression [146]. Inhibitor application enhanced the cytotoxicity of hypericin-based PDT in human urinary bladder carcinoma T24 cells. In addition, the transfection of T24 cells with an HO-1 siRNA significantly promoted apoptosis and increased the caspase-3 level after hypericin-based PDT treatment. It indicates that a reduction in HO-1 expression can enhance susceptibility to apoptosis-mediated PDT [146].

Activity of HO-1 in PDT can be reduced by using pharmacological agents, namely well-known and characterized metalloporphyrins (MPs) [159,162–165]. Metalloporphyrins are porphyrins in which the porphyrin macrocycle is chelated to a metal cation, acting as a tetradentate ligand [162]. MPs do not have oxygen-binding capacity and they are not subject to oxidative degradation. MPs also exhibit significantly greater binding affinity to HO isoforms compared to heme [163]. There are several studies which have confirmed that MPs cause a decrease in HO-1 activity. Nowis et al. showed that ZnPPIX increased the cytotoxic effect of PDT in colon and ovarian carcinoma cells [142]. Also ZnPPIX-mediated HO-1 inhibition increased the sensitivity of nasopharyngeal carcinoma cells to radiotherapy [164]. There are also studies showing that another MP, SnPPIX, enhanced the effect of PDT on melanoma tumors and reduced the growth of Kaposi sarcoma in vivo [159,165].

Overall, these findings suggest that HO-1 plays a critical role in PDT resistance and targeting this enzyme could be a promising approach to improve the efficacy of PDT in cancer treatment. However, further research is needed to determine the optimal strategy for targeting HO-1 in combination with PDT.

Table 1. Antioxidant enzymes in cancer treatment.

Antioxidant Enzymes	Target of Action	Location	Function	Therapeutic Effects on Cancers	Ref.
SOD	Superoxide anion	SOD1: Cytoplasmic compartments SOD2: Mitochondria SOD3: Extracellular space	Dismutation of superoxide anion	Anticancer agents • Tumor-growth suppressor • Apoptosis induction Chemo- and radioprotectors • Protection of normal cells against ionizing irradiation and chemotherapeutic agents SOD mimetics • Induction of SOD activity by mimetic molecules • Enhancement of anticancer agent activities in combination therapy • Protection of normal cells against chemotherapeutic agents Therapeutic targeting SOD • SOD2 promotes resistance to apoptotic cell death of cancer cells • SOD2 facilitates cancer cell growth	[42,56,166–169]
Catalase	H_2O_2	Peroxisomes	Dismutation of H_2O_2	Catalase mimetics • Induction of catalase activity by mimetic molecules • Enhancement of anticancer agent activities in combination therapy Therapeutic targeting catalase • Catalase prevents oxidative injury and apoptotic cell death of cancer cells	[85,95,169]
GCS	Glutamic acid and cysteine	Cytosol	Synthesis of glutathione	Anticancer agents t • Enhancement of anticancer agent activities in combination therapy	[170,171]

Table 1. *Cont.*

Antioxidant Enzymes	Target of Action	Location	Function	Therapeutic Effects on Cancers	Ref.
GR	GSSG	Cytosol	Conversion of GSSG to GSH	Therapeutic targeting GR • The accumulation of GSSG in the cell can exert a pro-oxidative effect, • Inhibiting its reduction may enhance the efficacy of some anticancer drugs.	[170]
GPx	H_2O_2	Cytosol and mitochondria	Reduction of H_2O_2	Therapeutic targeting GPx • Target of chemotherapy, hemodynamic therapy, and photodynamic therapy	[172]
GST	Xenobiotics	Microsome, mitochondria, and cytosol	Conjugation of xenobiotics with GSH	Therapeutic targeting GST • GSH conjugation with anticancer drugs catalyzed by GST protects cancer cells. • GST isoenzymes have become promising targets for therapy due to their overexpression in a wide range of tumors.	[115,120]
HO-1	Heme	Endoplasmic reticulum, mitochondria, the vacuole, nucleus, and plasma membrane	Metabolism of heme into biliverdin	Predictive marker • HO-1 expression is associated with cancer response rate	[130,173]

Note. GCS, γ-glutamylcysteine synthetase; GPx, glutathione peroxidase; GR, glutathione reductase; GSH, glutathione; GST, glutathione *S*-transferase; GSSG, oxidized glutathione; HO-1, heme oxygenase-1; SOD, superoxide dismutase.

3. The Inhibitors of Antioxidant Enzymes Used to Overcome Cancer Resistance to PDT

Alteration of the level of the antioxidant molecules in cancer cells is one of the essential cytoprotective mechanisms that occur during PDT. Below, we summarize the strategies based on the application of inhibitors against the antioxidant enzymes that were studied, in order to improve the effectiveness of PDT.

3.1. SODs Inhibitors

3.1.1. 2-Methoxyestradiol (2-ME, SOD2 Inhibitor)

2-Methoxyestradiol, an estrogen metabolite, has been confirmed to be an enzymatic inhibitor of human and bovine SOD1 and *E.coli* SOD2 (Figure 8) [79,174]. Nonetheless, 2-ME was used as a selective SOD2 inhibitor in the study of antioxidant enzyme inhibitors against PDT [78,175]. 2-ME can enhance PDT-induced cell death in various human tumors. Corresponding to the report of Golab and co-workers, 2-ME showed a synergistic effect and enhanced the cytotoxic effect of Photofrin-based PDT in a dose-dependent manner in three murine cell lines (i.e., C-26, LLC, and MDC), five human cell lines (i.e., T47-D, PANC-1, HPAF-II, HPAC, and T24), and two xenograft tumor mice models (i.e., C-26 and LLC). Interestingly, C-26 adenocarcinoma-implanted Balb/c mice were cured by 60% after 14 days of 2-ME and Photofrin-based PDT treatment [79]. In the study of the cell cytoskeleton in human ovarian clear carcinoma OvBh-1 and breast adenocarcinoma MCF-7 cells, the 2-ME application, together with PDT, immediately induced cell shrinkage, disruption of actin filaments and microtubules architecture, followed by the reorganization of the cytoskeleton and nucleus [176]. 2-ME enhances PDT-induced apoptosis through an increase in caspase 3/7 and 12, with a lowering ratio of anti-apoptotic protein (Bcl-2) to pro-apoptotic protein (Bax). Kimáková et al. showed that SOD activity and its mRNA were significantly increased by hypericin-based PDT in breast adenocarcinoma MCF-7 cells, while this effect was not observed in MDA-MB-231 cells [177]. Treatment with 2-ME can prevent SOD mRNA expression using hypericin-based PDT, which further reduced the proliferative capability of MCF-7 cells with an increase in the caspase 3/7 activity and an enrichment of nucleosomes (DNA fragmentation). The 2-ME and PDT co-treatment further lowered the Bcl-2/Bax ratio from 0.19 to 0.5, compared with a single treatment of cells using hypericin-based PDT. It indicated that 2-ME can potentiate caspase 3/7 and apoptosis induction using hypericin-based PDT [177]. The enhancement of apoptosis due to 2-ME and cyanine IR-775-based PDT was observed in human breast (MDA-MB-231) and ovarian (SKOV-3) adenocarcinoma cells. Co-treatment with 2-ME and IR-775 significantly decreased MDA-MB-231 and SKOV-3 cell viability after 24 and 72 h, compared with treatment with 2-ME or IR-775 alone. Furthermore, the expression of SOD2 and caspase 12 were increased after cells' co-treatment with 2-ME and IR-775 in both cell lines [178].

3.1.2. Diethyldithiocarbamate (DDC, SOD1 Inhibitor)

Diethyldithiocarbamate, the primary metabolite of disulfiram, is a hydrophilic metal-chelating agent for Cu(II) and is well known as a SOD1 inhibitor (Figure 8) [175,179,180]. It is important to note that DDC can also decrease GSH levels [181,182]. DDC was investigated as a cytotoxicity enhancer for several photosensitizers [109]. The addition of DDC to zinc phthalocyanine-based PDT significantly enhanced the cytotoxicity of both free and liposome-encapsulated zinc phthalocyanine in mouse embryo fibroblast NIH3T3 and human breast cancer MDA-MB-231 cells, compared with zinc phthalocyanine treatment alone. The IC_{50} of zinc phthalocyanine-based PDT decreased from 64.9 to 32.43 and 6.78 to 3.39 μg/mL after co-treatment with DDC on mouse embryo fibroblast (NIH3T3) and MDA-MB 231 cell models, respectively. Co-encapsulation into liposomes of DDC and zinc phthalocyanine was confirmed to reduce SOD and GSH activities in MDA-MB 231 cells that resulted in sensitizing tumor cells to PDT [183]. The enhancement effect of DDC was also indicated in an in vivo study, in which DDC significantly potentiated an ear swelling response after Photofrin II-based PDT in female C3H mice, while the control group did not show any significant response [184]. Nevertheless, the enhancement effect of DDC in PDT was not shown in some tumors. Wright et al. investigated the effect of three antioxidant enzyme inhibitors delivered together with meta-tetrahydroxyphenyl chlorin (mTHPC)-based PDT in a murine dorsal root ganglion model composed of their neuron and associated satellite glia cells. The pretreatment of DDC at a dose of 50 μM significantly increased the sensitivity of neuron cells only, and an SOD2 inhibitor, 2-ME, at a dose of 1 μM, did not show any significant enhancing effects, whilst BSO pretreatment at a dose of 500 μM affected both neurons and satellite glia cells. Interestingly, a combinatory pretreatment of cells with DDC and BSO exhibited a near total loss of neuron and satellite glia cells after mTHPC-based PDT [185].

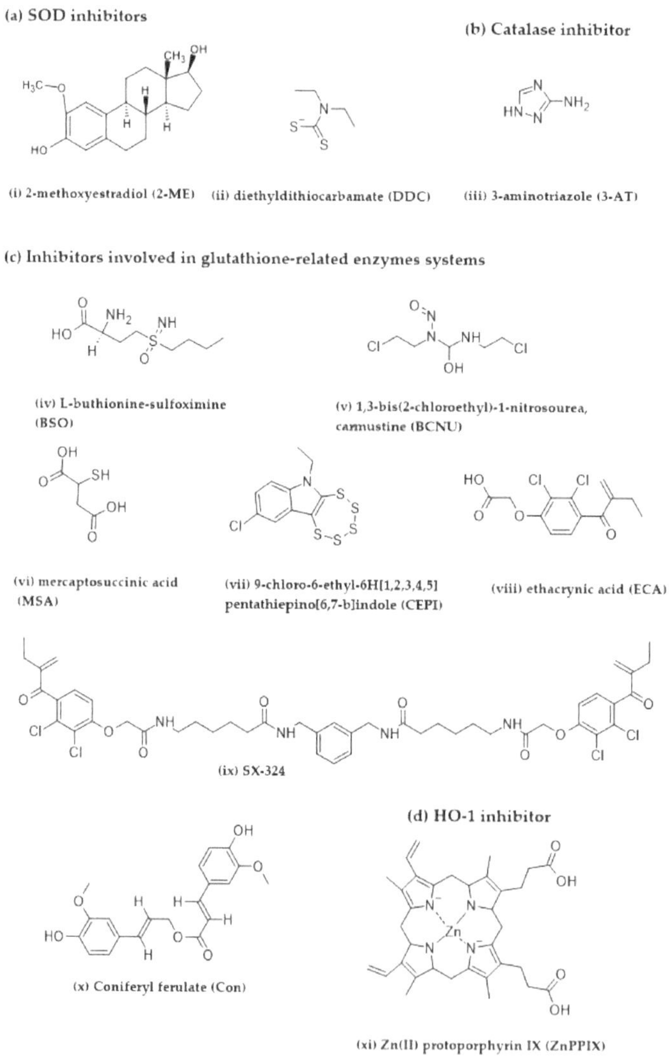

Figure 8. Inhibitors of antioxidant enzymes with potential applications in enhancing the effectiveness of photodynamic therapy.

3.2. *Catalase Inhibitors*

3-Aminotriazole (3-AT, Catalase Inhibitor)

3-aminotriazole is a triazole heterocycle derivative exhibiting several effects, including histamine H_2-receptor antagonistic, anti-asthmatic, and herbicidal (Figure 8) [186–188]. 3-AT is further used as a specific catalase inhibitor that can irreversibly inhibit catalase activity in the presence of a low and constant H_2O_2 level [189,190]. Many studies reported that concomitant treatment of 3-AT and PDT significantly improved PDT-induced cell death in various tumor cells [191,192]. Price and co-workers demonstrated the pro-apoptotic effect of H_2O_2 in benzoporphyrin derivative-based PDT [193]. Apoptosis-mediated PDT was enhanced due to 3-AT treatment by reducing the LD_{50} by 23.0% in a model murine leukemia P388 cell line. At the same time, the application of a catalase enzyme analogue, CAT^{-SKL}, and a ferrous iron chelating agent, 2,2-bipyridyl (BID), showed the opposite effect, protecting the cells from photokilling by increasing the LD_{50} of 18.0 and 8.2%, respectively. The conversion of procaspase-3 to active caspase-3 and the increase in H_2O_2 production were also confirmed in the cells after PDT treatment with 3-AT [193]. Soares' group reported that 3-AT can significantly enhance the cytotoxicity of redaporfin-based PDT in the low SOD and catalase activity cell line, A549. Whilst this effect did not occur in CT26 cells which showed higher SOD and catalase activity after PDT treatment [78]. Moreover, the effects of 3-AT were displayed in animal models. Catalase activity was significantly reduced by 3-AT pretreatment in EAC implanted mongrel mice. Pretreatment of 3-AT further enhanced the cytotoxicity of hematoporphyrin-based PDT by decreasing the LD_{50} of the PDT. The authors concluded that catalase potentially protects tumor cells against PDT [109]. The combination of Photofrin II-based PDT with a catalase inhibitor, 3-AT or hydroxyl amine, or with an SOD inhibitor, DDC, meaningfully promoted the potentiation of ear swelling response in female C3H mice. While the control group did not show any significant response. The authors suggested that superoxide anion and H_2O_2 were involved in Photofrin II-mediated cutaneous photosensitization [184].

3.3. *Inhibitors Involved in Glutathione-Related Enzyme Systems*

3.3.1. L-Buthionine Sulfoximine (BSO, GCS Inhibitor)

Guthionine sulfoximine was synthesized in 1979 as a specific enzymatic inhibitor of γ-glutamylcysteine synthetase (GCS) in the glutathione synthesis pathway (Figure 8) [194]. BSO caused GSH deficiency, sensitizing tumor cells to PDT-induced cell death [109,185,195]. Treatment with 0.002–10 mM BSO significantly depleted cellular GSH level in a dose-dependent manner in Chinese hamster ovary (CHO), Chinese hamster lung V-79, mouse-derived breast cancer EMT-6, and fibrosarcoma RIF cell lines. BSO further enhanced the cytotoxicity of Photofrin II-based PDT in all cell lines [196]. Likewise, the cytotoxicity of hematoporphyrin was enhanced when co-administered with BSO in murine leukemia L1210 cells [197]. BSO was employed in the microsphere system together with PDT agents to increase the cytotoxicity. BSO potentiated PDT cytotoxicity, mediated by Ce6 conjugated with an ethyldimethyl aminopropylcarbon diamide-activated polystyrene microsphere, in human bladder carcinoma MGH-U1 cells. It is important to note that the BSO's potentiation effect was not indicated after applying the Ce6-based PDT without conjugation to the microspheres [198]. In the study of the pro-oxidant and antioxidant effect of ascorbate performed by Soares et al., the inhibiting effects of 2-ME, 3-AT, and BSO were investigated [78]. 2-MT, 3-AT, and BSO significantly promoted the cytotoxic effect of superoxide anions and singlet oxygen produced by redaporfin-mediated PDT in A549 cells. Moreover, the application of the pro-oxidant molecule, ascorbate, can even further enhance this effect. Conversely, these inhibitors did not affect CT26 cells due to their high SOD2 activity and up-regulation of catalase after PDT treatment. In contrast to redaporfin, temoporfin that mainly generated singlet oxygen showed stronger cytotoxicity in CT26 than in A549 cells. It was suggested that the PS generated both superoxide anions and singlet oxygen, which offered better opportunities for cytotoxicity mediated by PDT in combination with antioxidant enzyme inhibitors and/or ascorbate. Interestingly, in the combination of PDT and ascorbate, ascorbate did not act only as a pro-oxidant molecule enhancing cytotoxic effects of superoxide anions and singlet oxygen, but also acted as an antioxidant, which quenched singlet oxygen, influencing the redox status of the cells [78]. However, the enhancement of the cytotoxic effect by BSO was not indicated after treatment of hypericin-based PDT in GPx4-expressing MCF-7 cells. Theodossiou and co-workers reported the cytotoxic effect of hypericin-based PDT in two phenotypically and genotypically different breast adenocarcinoma cell lines, MCF-7 and MDA-MB-231 [199]. High GSTP1-expressing MDA-MB-231 cells were more sensitive to hypericin than GPx4-expressing MCF-7 cells. Though co-treatment of BSO and hypericin-based PDT caused total GSH depletion in MCF-7 and MDA-MB-231 cells, the enhancement of the PDT cytotoxicity was exhibited only in MDA-MB-231 cells. Nevertheless, PDT cytotoxicity of MCF-7 cells can be enhanced in a combinatory treatment with BSO and BCNU, a GR inhibitor. The authors concluded that the GPx-4 enzyme could be used as a predictive marker for cell response to PDT, whilst GST corresponds to the chemoresistance of a cell line [199]. Kimani's group reported cytotoxicity enhancement after the application of four antioxidant enzyme inhibitors in PDT employing disulphonated aluminum phthalocyanine ($AlPcS_2$) as a photosensitizer [175]. BSO significantly reduced MCF-7 cell viability after 24 h of incubation with $AlPcS_2$, compared with $AlPcS_2$ treatment alone. Whilst cells' pretreatment with 2-ME, DDC, or 3-AT and $AlPcS_2$-based PDT did not result in any effect. The cytotoxicity of $AlPcS_2$-based PDT was further enhanced after a 24 hr preincubation with BSO plus 3-AT or 2-ME, or with a combination of four antioxidant enzyme inhibitors. The authors concluded that the most related antioxidant mechanism in protecting MCF-7 cells against PDT is a glutathione redox cycle, followed by SOD2, catalase, and SOD1 [175]. Lee et al. showed that BSO can enhance the effectiveness of PDT in tumors characterized by either a high or low GSH level [200]. Among ten tumor cell lines, colorectal HCT116 and ampulla vater carcinoma SNU478 cells exhibited the highest and lowest GSH level, respectively. The combination of BSO and Ce6-based PDT significantly reduced the total GSH level and increased ROS generation in both HCT116 and SNU478 cells, compared with Ce6 treatment alone. The addition of intracellular GSH levels using glutathione reduced ethyl ester displayed a cytoprotective effect against PDT, by providing higher HCT116 and SNU478 cell survival after co-treatment with BSO and Ce6-based PDT, compared with non-treated cells. Notably, BSO enhanced the cytotoxicity for a wider concentration range of Ce6 treatment in HCT116 than SNU478 cells. It suggests that BSO induced a less synergistic effect with Ce6-based PDT in cells that have a lower GSH level [200]. BSO with Photofrin significantly decreased the cell survival, colony-forming capacity, and invasion properties of two human glioma cell lines, U87 and U251n, in a dose-dependent manner, compared with Photofrin treatment alone. Therapy enhancement using BSO in combination with Photofrin was also confirmed in a xenograft rat model. Co-treatment of BSO with Photofrin-based PDT showed remarkable superficial tumor damage, necrosis, and focal hemorrhage in the brain of U87 glioma-implanted rats, while the tumor lesion after treatment with only Photofrin was not obvious. The lesion volume of xenografted U87 glioma in the rat brain after BSO and Photofrin treatment was meaningfully greater [201]. Moreover, co-treatment with BSO and Photofrin-based PDT significantly increased the lesion volume of tumor necrosis in the brain of male Fischer rats bearing an intracerebral 9L gliosarcoma, compared with Photofrin treatment alone. Interestingly, BSO did not increase lesion volume in the normal brain samples [202]. Additionally, both in vitro and in vivo studies of BSO application in nanospheres were performed. Chlorin e6-loaded poly(ethylene glycol)-block-poly(D,L lactide) nanoparticles (Ce6-PEG-PLA-NPs)-based PDT exhibited synergetic effects with BSO. The co-administration of BSO and Ce6-PEG-PLA-NPs significantly decreased cell viability compared with Ce6-PEG-PLA-NPs treatment alone in mouse squamous cell carcinoma SCC-7 cells. The results were confirmed in the SCC-7 xenografted mouse model. The co-treatment completely suppressed tumor growth after 14 days, while the treatment of Ce6-PEG-PLA-NPs alone showed a lower effect. Hematoxylin and eosin-staining showed increased apoptosis and tissue damage after the combinatory therapy. Additionally, the body weight and liver and kidney tissues of treated mice did not significantly change due to therapy, referring to a negligible systemic toxicity of the NPs and BSO [203]. Similarly, BSO co-encapsulated with indocyanine green in thermosensitive liposomes was employed [204]. This delivery system was named as an IR photothermal liposomal nanoantagonist (PLNA), due to it containing BSO, a GSH biosynthesis antagonist. The presence of BSO in this delivery system resulted in a significant depletion of intracellular GSH levels in murine breast cancer 4T1 cells, when compared to nanocarriers lacking BSO. The results revealed that PLNA application increased the intracellular ROS levels, PDT cytotoxicity, and the apoptosis rate of the cells. Furthermore, PLNA demonstrated interesting outcomes in murine breast cancer 4T1-implanted BALB/c mice. Notably, PLNA not only significantly reduced GSH levels, tumor growth, and weight after 16 days of treatment, but also exhibited in vivo biosafety. After 30 days of treatment, alterations were not evidenced in the histological morphology of vital organs, levels of biochemical indicators of liver and kidney function, and essential blood biochemistry parameters [204].

In addition to GSH depletion by BSO treatment, the inhibition of deubiquitinating enzymes substantially interferes with cancer cell survival upon oxidative stress [205]. Harris et al. indicated that the inhibition of deubiquitinating enzymes in combination with BSO treatment increased cell death by ferroptosis, a cell death pathway activated by excessive lipid peroxidation [206]. Therefore, the cytotoxicity of PDT-based therapy is feasibly enhanced by deubiquitinating enzyme inhibitors combined with BSO.

3.3.2. 1,3-Bis(2-chloroethyl)-1-nitrosourea or Carmustine (BCNU, GR Inhibitor)

Not only an alkylating agent, 1,3-bis(2-chloroethyl)-1-nitrosourea or carmustine is extensively used in the clinical treatment of malignant gliomas, but also as a selective inhibitor of GR in the glutathione redox cycle, which can further enhance PDT-induced cell death in several conditions (Figure 8) [207–210]. The study of fractionated light delivery in PDT found that BCNU increased ROS levels by diminishing the GSH detoxification that enhanced the PDT cytotoxicity. Although fractionated irradiation of aluminum (III) phthalocyanine tetrasulfonate ($AlPcS_4$)- and hypericin-based PDT decreased ROS production and PDT cytotoxicity in human epidermoid carcinoma A431 cells, BCNU could reverse these effects by enhancing the ROS production and cytotoxicity of both PDT types [211]. In the study of glucose deprivation on PDT efficacy, two antioxidant inhibitors, BCNU and BSO, significantly increased intracellular ROS generation and enhanced the cytotoxicity of $AlPcS_4$-based PDT, compared with $AlPcS_4$ alone, in human epidermoid carcinoma A431 cells. Moreover, co-treatment of $AlPcS_4$ with BCNU or BSO exhibited PDT-induced apoptosis via an increase in the caspase-3-like enzyme activity and nuclear fragmentation. It is important to note that BSO was more potent than BCNU, since BCNU did not decrease intracellular GSH levels, while BSO inhibited enzymes in approximately 90% [195]. Sun and co-workers showed that BCNU sensitized SOD2-overexpressing cells to Photofrin-based PDT [212]. Human breast carcinoma ZR-75-1 cells were transfected with an adenoviral construct containing the cDNA for *SOD2* (Ad*MnSOD*) to increase SOD2 expression. The cytotoxicity of Photofrin-based PDT did not change in ZR-75-1 cells together with Ad*MnSOD*, compared with ZR-75-15 cells alone, though a combination of Ad*MnSOD* with BCNU could significantly increase ROS accumulation and further enhanced the cytotoxicity of Photofrin. Authors hypothesized that an increase in the conversion of superoxide anions to H_2O_2 by elevating SOD2 levels with simultaneous inhibition of GR by BCNU could enhance the steady-state levels of superoxide and tumor cell killing [212]. BCNU enhanced PDT-induced cell death in a PDT-resistant cell line, MCF-7 cells, which highly expressed GPx4. Although BSO showed only a slight enhancing effect of the hypericin-based PDT in MCF-7 cells, a combination of BCNU and BSO significantly enhanced the cytotoxicity of the PDT [199]. In the study of the temperature effect on hematoporphyrin-based PDT efficacy, the pretreatment of BCNU in EAC-implanted mongrel mice remarkably reduced the GR activity and enhanced PDT-induced cell death via reducing the LD_{50} of the PDT. Likewise, pretreatment of the other three antioxidant enzyme inhibitors, DDC, BSO, and 3-AT, reduced the activity of antioxidant enzymes and lowered the LD_{50} of the PDT significantly [109,213]. Interestingly, these inhibitors could not only enhance PDT-induced cell death via reducing the activities of antioxidant enzymes, but also suppressed the photoinduced degradation of HPD [214].

3.3.3. Mercaptosuccinic Acid (MSA, GPx1 Inhibitor)

Mercaptosuccinic acid is a mercaptan derivative, which is generally employed as a GPx1 inhibitor due to competing with GSH to bind to the active site, active-site selenocysteine (Figure 8) [215,216]. Due to diminishing GPx activity, which is an antioxidant enzyme in the glutathione redox cycle, MSA could enhance PDT-induced cell death [217]. The study on the effectiveness of Rose Bengal-based PDT by Yao et al. indicated that primary human skin fibroblasts (FBs) grown in monolayers were more sensitive to the therapy than fibroblasts grown in collagen gels. However, the cytotoxicity of Rose Bengal-based PDT in fibroblasts grown in collagen gels was enhanced when combined with either an antioxidant enzyme inhibitor, MSA or 3-AT [192]. Lee and co-workers demonstrated the effect of combined treatment with MSA and Ce6-based PDT on cholangiocarcinoma cells. The authors used two different cell lines, intrahepatic HuCC-T1 and extrahepatic SNU1196. Both lines differed in GSH level, with SNU1196 cells having higher GSH basal levels, catalytic subunit GSC expression, and GPx and GR activity compared with HuCC-T1 cells. Nevertheless, co-treatment with MSA and Ce6 significantly decreased GPx activity, resulting in elevating ROS levels and cytotoxicity in SNU1196 cells [122].

3.3.4. 9-Chloro-6-ethyl-6H[1,2,3,4,5]pentathiepino[6,7-b]indole (CEPI, GPx1 Inhibitor)

9-chloro-6-ethyl-6H[1–5]pentathiepino[6,7-b]indole is a pentathiepin derivative that was recently developed as a potent GPx1 inhibitor (Figure 8). Among eight pentathiepin derivatives, CEPI showed the strongest inhibitory activity against bovine erythrocyte GPx activity, which was 15-fold higher than MSA [218]. Lange and Bednarski reported synergistic effects of mTHPC-based PDT with a GPx1 inhibitor, MSA or CEPI, in a few cell lines. Among the five human cell lines, co-treatment with CEPI and mTHPC showed a synergistic effect in esophageal carcinoma KYSE-70 and urinary bladder carcinoma RT-4 cells via increased cytotoxicity, ROS generation, and apoptosis. MSA synergized with mTHPC-based PDT in lung carcinoma A-427, oral carcinoma BHY, KYSE-70, and RT-4 cells. It is important to note that MSA or CEPI could also produce additive or antagonistic effects against mTHPC-based PDT depending on doses and types of tumor [217].

3.3.5. GST Inhibitors

Ethacrynic Acid (ECA, GSTP1-1 Inhibitor)

Ethacrynic acid is an FDA-approved GSTP1-1 inhibitor, which has been used as a diuretic and alkylating agent in cancer treatment that can reverse anticancer resistance by inhibiting GST activity (Figure 8) [219–221]. In addition, ECA has been extensively used as an inhibitor of GST in order to enhance the effectiveness of several tumor treatments, including PDT [222–224]. Won et al. showed new constructs of brominated BODIPY-based PDT conjugated with ethacrynic acid (EA-BPS) [225]. Not only does EA-BPS exhibit more potent cytotoxicity compared with free brominated BODIPY-based PDT in human breast adenocarcinoma MDA-MB-231 and MCF-7 cells, but it also showed higher ROS production and formation of singlet oxygen, superoxide anions, hydroxyl radicals, and peroxynitrite anions in MCF-7 cells. Furthermore, EA-BPS significantly reduced tumor volume in MDA-MB-231-implanted immunodeficient nude mice without alteration of body weights or levels of aspartate transaminase (AST), alanine aminotransferase (ALT), and creatinine activity [225].

SX-324 (GSTP1-1 Inhibitor)

A novel GSTP1-1 inhibitor, SX-324, was developed based on a previous GSTP1-1 inhibitor, ECA, on the principle of symmetric and bifunctional inhibition for occupying both GST active sites [226,227]. Dabrowski and co-workers indicated that the cytotoxic effect of hypericin-based PDT was lowered in human kidney 293 cells transfected with gene-encoding GSTP1–1. Co-treatment with SX-324 and hypericin reversed the protective effects of GSTP1-1 via the increased cytotoxicity of PDT. Nevertheless, SX-324 did not modify the cytotoxicity of hypericin-based PDT in 293 cells that did not overexpress *GSTP1-1* [117].

Coniferyl Ferulate (Con, GST Inhibitor)

Coniferyl ferulate is a natural substance isolated from the root of *Angelica sinensis* (Oliv.) Diels. Con, showing an over 15 times stronger inhibition (IC_{50} value of 0.3 μM) of GST activity than ECA (IC_{50} value of 4.89 μM) in a high-throughput screening model using GST from the human placenta (Figure 8) [228]. Li et al. developed a drug self-delivery system made of Ce6 and Con (CeCon) as the PS and PDT enhancer, respectively. CeCon self-assembled into a nanomedicine and generated singlet oxygen similarly to Ce6-based PDT. Compared with Ce6-based PDT or Con alone, CeCon significantly decreased GST expression and activity in the A549 cells, enhancing ROS production, PDT cytotoxicity, and cell apoptosis [229].

3.4. *HO-1 Inhibitor*

Zn(II) Protoporphyrin IX (ZnPPIX, HO-1 Inhibitor)

Zn(II) protoporphyrin IX is a metalloporphyrin complex well-known as a selective inhibitor of HO-1, a protective enzyme against various PDT-induced cell death [230–233]. Frank and co-workers showed that the diminishing of the HO-1 activity via *HO-1* gene silencing or using ZnPPIX remarkably enhanced the effectiveness of 5-ALA-based PDT [159]. Co-treatment of ALA with ZnPPIX or *HO-1* siRNA significantly increased 5- and 2-time melanoma cell death, respectively, compared with ALA-based PDT treatment alone. Particularly, the combination of ZnPPIX and *HO-1* siRNA with ALA additionally enhanced cell death by over 6.4 times [159]. The results were confirmed in metastatic human melanoma WM451Lu cells by Grimm and co-workers. Co-treatment with ZnPPIX and ALA-based PDT significantly enhanced the cytotoxicity. Interestingly, supplementation with vitamin C at a dose of 280 μM reduced the cytotoxicity of ALA-based PDT in this model [145]. The enhancement effect of ZnPPIX was observed in Photofrin- and Talaporfin sodium-based PDT. ZnPPIX significantly increased the cytotoxicity of Photofrin in human colon adenocarcinoma C-26 and ovarian carcinoma MDAH2774 cells [142]. The cell viability of rat meningioma KMY-J cells was significantly decreased in a dose-dependent manner, followed by an increase in morphological cell damage after co-treatment with ZnPPIX and Talaporfin sodium compared with the photosensitizer alone [143]. Zhong and co-workers investigated a versatile nanoparticle-based drug delivery system for protoporphyrin IX-based PDT, containing Zn^{2+} and BSO (PZB NP) [160]. Its application significantly increased ROS generation with a decrease in the GSH level and protein level of GCS and HO-1, compared with a control group in breast cancer 4T1 cells. PZB NPs showed dose-dependent cytotoxicity, reducing 4T1 cell viability from 87% to 5% after light exposure, whereas PZ NPs (without BSO) showed slightly lower cytotoxicity (90% to 18%). The results were consistent with the in vivo model of murine breast cancer using 4T1 cells implanted to BALB/c mice. Treatment with PZB NPs significantly reduced tumor volume and weight compared with PZ NPs or NPs (without Zn^{2+} and BSO) after 14 days. The authors concluded that the nanodrug possessed dual antioxidation defense suppression properties, enhancing efficient ROS-based therapies [160]. Interestingly, ZnPPIX was also employed as an enhancer in chemodynamic treatments (CDTs). A cupric ion (Cu^{2+}) was used as a CDT initiator in Cu–Zn Protoporphyrin nanoscale coordination polymers (NCPs) by converting endogenous H_2O_2 to a cytotoxic hydroxyl radical. ZnPPIX significantly inhibited HO-1 expression and activity in MDA-MB-231 cells. Moreover, it enhanced the cytotoxicity of the system by reducing the viability of murine breast cancer 4T1, human embryonic kidney HEK-293 T, A549 and MDA-MB-231 cells, and tumor growth in MDA-MB-231 tumor-bearing mice [234]. ZnPPIX not only acted as an HO-1 inhibitor to enhance the cytotoxicity of PDT and CDT, but could also be photoactivated and produced a cytotoxic hydroxyl radical, leading to PDT-induced cell death. Fang et al. studied the activity of polymeric ZnPPIX conjugated with the *N*-(2-hydroxypropyl)methacrylamide (pHPMA) copolymer in PDT application [235]. Polymer-conjugated Zinc Protoporphyrin showed cytotoxicity after being irradiated with 400 to 700 nm xenon light in murine sarcoma S180 model implanted into Sprague–Dawley rats and carcinogen-induced tumor models. No dark toxicity was observed in polymeric ZnPPIX-based PDT treatment [235].

4. Conclusions

PDT is a selective and minimal systemically toxic modality for tumor treatment that overcomes the problems generated by conventional chemotherapy in various aspects, particularly specificity and efficacy against tumor cells. Nevertheless, PDT can be limited by multiple factors, especially the alteration of the level of antioxidant molecules. At least four significant antioxidant enzymes, SOD, catalase, glutathione redox cycle, and HO-1, remarkably attenuated the effectiveness of PDT. In order to increase the sensitivity of PDT against cancer cells, antioxidant enzyme inhibitors can be employed to diminish their ROS detoxifying activity (Table 2). It is a challenge to study the use of antioxidant enzyme inhibitors to improve the efficiency of PDT in eliminating tumor cells. However, the effects of a combination of PDT with antioxidant enzyme inhibitors still needs to be studied to determine the appropriate conditions.

Table 2. Antioxidant enzyme inhibitors tested in PDT.

Enzyme Inhibitor		Dose of Enzyme Inhibitor	PDT Base	Test Condition		Incubation Time (hr.)	Effectiveness of enzyme inhibitor	Ref.
Name	Target			In Vitro	In Vivo			
2-methoxy estradiol (2-ME)	SOD2	50 mM	Photofrin	Human ovarian clear carcinoma OvBh-1 cells		18	- Cell shrinkage - Actin and microtubule disruption	[176]
				Human breast adenocarcinoma MCF-7 cells				
		10 μM	Hypericin	Human breast adenocarcinoma MCF-7 cells		16	- 87.5% clonogenic ability *	[177]
		50 μM	Cyanine IR-775	Human breast adenocarcinoma MDA-MB-231 cells		24	+ 350% PDT cytotoxicity after 24 hr of irradiation* + 73.3% PDT cytotoxicity after 72 hr of irradiation *	[178]
				Human ovary adenocarcinoma SKOV-3 cells			+ 300% PDT cytotoxicity after 24 hr of irradiation * + 57.1% PDT cytotoxicity after 72 hr of irradiation *	
		3 μM	Redaporfin	Human lung adenocarcinoma A549 cells		24	+ 45.4% PDT cytotoxicity *	[78]

Table 2. *Cont.*

Enzyme Inhibitor		Dose of Enzyme Inhibitor	PDT Base	Test Condition		Incubation Time (hr.)	Effectiveness of enzyme inhibitor	Ref.
Name	Target			In Vitro	In Vivo			
2-methoxy estra-diol (2-ME)	SOD2	0.25–10 μM	Photofrin	Murine colon adenocarcinoma C-26 cells		48	- 77.6% SOD activity after 48 hr incubation (0.5 μM) * - 87.4% SOD activity after 48 hr incubation (1 μM) * + 200% PDT cytotoxicity at 6 KJ/m^2 (0.5 μM) *	[79]
		0.25–10 μM		Murine Lewis lung carcinoma (LLC) cells			+ 500% PDT cytotoxicity at 6 KJ/m^2 (0.5 μM) *	
		0.06–10 μM		Murine macrophage-derived chemokine (MDC) cells			+ 1,000% PDT cytotoxicity at 5 KJ/m^2 (0.25 μM) *	
		0.06–10 μM		Human breast cancer T47-D cells			+ 250% PDT cytotoxicity at 5 KJ/m^2 (0.12 μM) *	
		0.25–10 μM		Human pancreatic cancer PANC-1 cells			+ 250% PDT cytotoxicity at 6 KJ/m^2 (0.5 μM) *	
		0.06–10 μM		Human pancreatic cancer HPAF-II cells			+ 200% PDT cytotoxicity at 6 KJ/m^2 (0.25 μM) *	
		0.25–10 μM		Human pancreatic cancer HPAC cells			+ 167% PDT cytotoxicity at 6 KJ/m^2 (0.5 μM) *	
		0.06–10 μM		Human bladder cancer T24 cells			+ 300% PDT cytotoxicity at 6 KJ/m^2 (0.25 μM) *	
		100 mg/Kg body weight			Murine lewis lung carcinoma (LLC) implanted into B6D2F1 mice	6 days	- 60.0% tumor volume * + Survival time	
					Murine C-26 adeno-carcinoma implanted into Balb/c mice		- >90.0% tumor volume * + Survival time (60.0% cure rate)	

Table 2. *Cont.*

Enzyme Inhibitor		Dose of Enzyme Inhibitor	PDT Base	Test Condition		Incubation Time (hr.)	Effectiveness of enzyme inhibitor	Ref.
Name	Target			In Vitro	In Vivo			
Diethyldithiocarbamate (DDC)	SOD1	2–16 μg/mL	Zinc phthalocyanine	Murine embryo fibroblast NIH3T3 cells		24	- 50.0% IC_{50} of the PDT	[183]
				Human breast adenocarcinoma MDA-MB-231 cells			- 50.0% IC_{50} of the PDT	
		50 μM	Meta-tetrahydroxyphenyl chlorin	Murine dorsal root ganglia; neuron cells		1.5	+ 318% PDT cytotoxicity *	[185]
		0.4 mM/Kg body weight	Photofrin II		C3H mice	2	+ 30% potentiation of ear swelling response *	[184]
		0.1 mM	Hematoporphyrin		Murine Ehrlich ascites carcinoma (EAC) implanted into mongrel mice	20mins	- 56.6% SOD1 activity - 25.5% LD_{50} of the PDT	[109]
3-amino triazole (3-AT)	Catalase	30 mM	Benzoporphyrin	Murine leukaemia P388 cells		0.5	- 83.3% catalase activity - 23.0% LD_{50} of the PDT	[193]
		10 mM	Redaporfin	Human lung adenocarcinoma A549 cells		24	+ 20.0% PDT cytotoxicity *	[78]
		10 mM	Rose Bengal	Primary human skin fibroblasts (FB) grown in collagen gels		2	+ 16.7% PDT cytotoxicity at 150 J/cm^2 *	[192]
		25 mM	Hematoporphyrin		Murine Ehrlich ascites carcinoma (EAC) implanted into mongrel mice	1	- 38.1% catalase activity - 21.8% LD_{50} of the PDT	[109]
		0.7 mM/Kgbody weight	Photofrin II		C3H mice	2	+ 50% potentiation of ear swelling response *	[184]

Table 2. *Cont.*

Enzyme Inhibitor		Dose of Enzyme Inhibitor	PDT Base	Test Condition		Incubation Time (hr.)	Effectiveness of enzyme inhibitor	Ref.
Name	Target			In Vitro	In Vivo			
L-buthionine-sulfoximine (BSO)	GCS	0.002–10 mM	Photofrin II	Chinese hamster ovary CHO cells		1–24	- 29.0% to undetected GSH level + PDT cytotoxicity	[196]
				Chinese hamster lung V-79 cells			- 13.0% to undetected GSH level + PDT cytotoxicity	
				Murine breast carcinoma EMT-6 cells			- 19.0% to undetected GSH level + PDT cytotoxicity	
				Murine fibrosarcoma RIF-1 cells			- 12.0% to undetected GSH level + PDT cytotoxicity	
		1 mM	Hemato porphyrin	Murine leukemia L1210 cells		12	+ 3-fold log kill at 0.75 μg/mL hematopor-phyrin	[197]
		1 mM	Chlorin e6 conjugated with polystyrene micro-sphere	Human bladder carcinoma MGH-U1 cells		18	+ 36.1% PDT cytotoxicity at 10 J/cm^2	[198]
		600 μM	Redaporfin	Human lung adenocarcinoma A549 cells		24	+ 18.0% PDT cytotoxicity *	[78]
		100 μM	Hypericin	Human breast adenocarcinoma MCF-7 cells		Overnight	- 80.0% total GSH level	[199]
				Human breast adenocarcinoma MDA-MB-231 cells			- 80.0% total GSH level + 38.5% PDT cytotoxicity *	
		300 μM	Disulphonated aluminum phthalocya-nine ($AlPcS_2$)	Human breast adenocarcinoma MCF-7 cells		24	+ 34.3% PDT cytotoxicity	[175]

Table 2. *Cont.*

Enzyme Inhibitor Name	Enzyme Inhibitor Target	Dose of Enzyme Inhibitor	PDT Base	Test Condition In Vitro	Test Condition In Vivo	Incubation Time (hr.)	Effectiveness of enzyme inhibitor	Ref.
L-buthionine-sulfoximine (BSO)	GCS	500 μM	Meta-tetrahydroxyphenyl chlorin	Murine dorsal root ganglia; neuron cells		24	+ 535% PDT cytotoxicity *	[185]
				Murine satellite glia cells			+ 30.0% PDT cytotoxicity	
		0.001–10 mM	Chlorin e6	Human colorectal carcinoma HCT116 cells		24	- 78.0% GSH level at 10 μM BSO * + 45.0% PDT cytotoxicity at 0.5 μg/mL Ce6 with 10 mM BSO *	[200]
				Human ampulla vater carcinoma SNU478 cells			- 66.7% GSH level (10 μM BSO) + 72.7% PDT cytotoxicity at 0.5 μg/mL Ce6 with 10 mM BSO *	
		3 mM	Aluminum (III) phthalocyanine tetrasulfonate ($AlPcS_4$)	Human epidermoid carcinoma A431 cells		18	- 83.3% GSH level + 144% PDT cytotoxicity at 2 J/cm^2 *	[195]
		0.5–1000 μg/mL	Photofrin	Human glioma U87 cells: and U251n cells		24	+ 70.0% PDT cytotoxicity at 5 μg/mL Photofrin with 0.5 μg/mL *	[201]
				Human glioma U251n cells			+ 60.0% PDT cytotoxicity at 5 μg/mL Photofrin with 0.5 μg/mL *	
		440 mg/Kg body weight			Human U87 glioblastoma implanted into rats		+ Superficial tumor damage + 114.3% lesion volume at 70 J/cm^2	
		440 mg/Kg body weight	Photofrin		Murine 9L gliosarcoma implanted into Fischer rats	24	- 67.1% GSH level + 111.1% lesion volume	[202]

Table 2. *Cont.*

Enzyme Inhibitor		Dose of Enzyme Inhibitor	PDT Base	Test Condition		Incubation Time (hr.)	Effectiveness of enzyme inhibitor	Ref.
Name	Target			In Vitro	In Vivo			
L-buthionine-sulfoximine (BSO)	GCS	10 mM	Chlorin e6-loaded poly(ethylene glycol)-block-poly(D,L lactide) nanoparticles	Murine carcinoma SCC-7 cells		28	- 75.6% GSH level + 50.0% PDT cytotoxicity at 2 μg/mL Ce6 *	[203]
		3 mmol/Kg body weight			Murine carcinoma SCC-7 into implanted mice	12	- 75% tumor size after 14 days * + Apoptosis and tissue damage	
		N/A	Indocyanine green in near-infrared (NIR) photothermal liposomal nanoantagonists	Murine breast cancer 4T1 cells		24	- 26.4% GSH level + 90.9% PDT cytotoxicity + 1.5-fold ROS level	[204]
					Murine breast cancer 4T1 implanted into BALB/c mice	18–24	- 2.9-fold GSH level - 2.0-fold tumor weight	
		4 mM/Kg body weight	Hematoporphyrin		Murine Ehrlich ascites carcinoma (EAC) implanted into mongrel mice	14	- 68.2% GSH level - 63.6% total glutathione level - 21.5% LD_{50} of the PDT	[109]
		0.2–4 μM	Protoporphyrin IX	Murine breast cancer 4T1 cells		8	- 28.0% GSH level at 4 μM BSO - GCS expression at 4 μM BSO + 50.0% PDT cytotoxicity at 0.8 μM BSO	[160]
		100 μL of 2 mM			Murine breast cancer 4T1 implanted into BALB/c mice	4	- 50.0% tumor volume after 12 days * - 62.5% tumor weight after 12 days *	

Table 2. *Cont.*

Enzyme Inhibitor		Dose of Enzyme Inhibitor	PDT Base	Test Condition		Incubation Time (hr.)	Effectiveness of enzyme inhibitor	Ref.
Name	Target			In Vitro	In Vivo			
1,3-bis(2-chloroethyl)-1-nitrosourea (BCNU)	GR	500 μM	Aluminum (III) phthalocyanine tetrasulfonate (AlPcS4)	Human epidermoid carcinoma A431 cells		1	+ 23.4% ROS level at 1.8 J/cm^2 continuous light * + 146% PDT cytotoxicity at 2.25 J/cm^2 continuous light *	[211]
			Hypericin				+ 23.5% ROS level at 0.162 J/cm^2 continuous light * + 38.5% PDT cytotoxicity at 0.2 J/cm^2 continuous light *	
		500 μM	Aluminum (III) phthalocyanine tetrasulfonate ($AlPcS_4$)	Human epidermoid carcinoma A431 cells		1	+ 35.3% PDT cytotoxicity at 2 J/cm^2 *	[195]
		50 μM	Photofrin	Ad*MnSOD* transfected human breast carcinoma ZR-75-1 cells		1	+ 120% PDT cytotoxicity	[212]
		100 μM	Hypericin	Human breast adenocarcinoma MCF-7 cells		Overnight	+ 100% PDT cytotoxicity in combination with 100 μM BSO *	[199]
		0.1 mM	Hematoporphyrin		Murine Ehrlich ascites carcinoma (EAC) implanted into mongrel mice	25 mins	- 64.2% GR activity - 21.8% LD_{50} of the PDT	[109]

Table 2. *Cont.*

Enzyme Inhibitor		Dose of Enzyme Inhibitor	PDT Base	Test Condition		Incubation Time (hr.)	Effectiveness of enzyme inhibitor	Ref.
Name	Target			In Vitro	In Vivo			
Mercapto succinic acid (MSA)	GPx1	1.5 mM	Rose Bengal	Primary human skin fibroblasts (FB) grown in collagen gels		2	+ 33.3% PDT cytotoxicity at 150 J/cm^2 *	[192]
		10 mM	Chlorin e6	Human extrahepatic cholangiocarcinoma SNU1196 cells		0.5	- 58.1% GPx activity * + 60.0% ROS level * + 60.0% PDT cytotoxicity *	[122]
		1–700 µmol/L	meta-tetrahydroxyphenyl chlorin	Human lung carcinoma A-427 cells		24	+ Synergistic effect (CI < 1)	[217]
				Human oral carcinoma BHY cells				
				Human esophageal carcinoma KYSE-70 cells				
				Human urinary bladder carcinoma RT-4 cells				
9-chloro-6-ethyl-6*H* [1,2,3,4,5] pentathiepino [6,7-b]indole (CEPI)	GPx1	0.01–50 µmol/L	meta-tetrahydroxyphenyl chlorin	Human esophageal carcinoma KYSE-70 cells		24	+ Synergistic effect (CI < 1)	[217]
		4.0–15.9 µmol/L		Human urinary bladder carcinoma RT-4 cells				
Ethacrynic acid (ECA)	GSTP1-1	5 µM	Ethacrynic acid-conjugated brominated BODIPY	Human breast adenocarcinoma MCF-7 cells		12	+ 50.0% PDT cytotoxicity *	[225]
				Human breast adenocarcinoma MDA-MB-231 cells			+ 133% PDT cytotoxicity* + 36.4% ROS level* + 7.14% Singlet oxygen level * + 13.1% Superoxide anion level * + 243% Hydroxyl radical and peroxynitrite anion level* - 15% GSH level without irradiation* - 730% GSH level with irradiation *	

Table 2. *Cont.*

Enzyme Inhibitor		Dose of Enzyme Inhibitor	PDT Base	Test Condition		Incubation Time (hr.)	Effectiveness of enzyme inhibitor	Ref.
Name	Target			In Vitro	In Vivo			
Ethacrynic acid (ECA)	GSTP1-1	5 mg/Kg body weight			Human breast adenocarcinoma MDA-MB-231 implanted into immunodeficient nude mice	6	- 56.9% tumor volume *	
SX-324	GSTP1-1	1 μM	Hypericin	GSTP1-1-overexpressed human kidney fibroblast K293 cells		1	+ 87.2% PDT cytotoxicity	[117]
Coniferyl ferulate (Con)	GST	0.2–2.7 mg/L	Drug self-delivery systems of chlorin e6 and coniferyl ferulate	Human lung adenocarcinoma A549 cells		20	+ 250% ROS level* + 200% PDT cytotoxicity at 2.7 mg/mL *	[229]
Zn(II) protoporphyrin IX (ZnPPIX)	HO-1	400 μM	5-aminolevulinic acid	Human melanoma WM451Lu cells		16	+ 499% PDT cytotoxicity + 641% PDT cytotoxicity (combined with HO-1 siRNA)	[159]
		5 μM	5-aminolevulinic acid	Human melanoma WM451Lu cells		16	+ 100% PDT cytotoxicity *	[145]
		1.25–2.5 μM	Photofrin	Murine colon adenocarcinoma C-26 cells		24	+ 77.5% PDT cytotoxicity at 4.5 KJ/m^2	[142]
				Human ovarian carcinoma MDAH2774 cells			+ >42.8% PDT cytotoxicity at 4.5 KJ/m^2	
		1 μM	Talaporfin sodium	Murine meningioma KMY-J cells		4	+ 900% PDT cytotoxicity at 19.2 μM talaporfin sodium * + Morphological cell damage	[143]

Table 2. *Cont.*

Enzyme Inhibitor		Dose of Enzyme Inhibitor	PDT Base	Test Condition		Incubation Time (hr.)	Effectiveness of enzyme inhibitor	Ref.
Name	Target			In Vitro	In Vivo			
Zn(II) protoporphyrin IX (ZnPPIX)	HO-1	2 μM	Protoporphyrin IX	Murine breast cancer 4T1 cells		8	- HO-1 expression	[160]
		2.81 mg/Kg body weight			Murine breast cancer 4T1 implanted into-BALB/c mice	4	- 70.0% tumor volume after 12 days * - 41.8% tumor weight after 12 days *	

Note. GCS, γ-glutamylcysteine synthetase; GPx, glutathione peroxidase; GR, glutathione reductase; GST, glutathione S-transferase; SOD, superoxide dismutase; *, estimated from the figure of references; N/A, no available data.

Author Contributions: Conceptualization, H.D.-K., M.K. and M.M.; writing—original draft preparation, W.U. and J.P.; writing—review and editing, H.D.-K., M.K., W.C. and M.M.; visualization, W.U. and M.K.; supervision, H.D.-K., M.K., W.C. and M.M.; project administration, H.D.-K. and M.M.; funding acquisition, M.K. and M.M. All authors have read and agreed to the published version of the manuscript.

Funding: This research was funded by the National Science Centre, Poland, grant number UMO-2021/43/B/NZ7/02476 (granted to M.M.).

Institutional Review Board Statement: Not applicable.

Informed Consent Statement: Not applicable.

Data Availability Statement: Not applicable.

Conflicts of Interest: The authors declare no conflicts of interest.

References

1. Dougherty, T.J. An Update on Photodynamic Therapy Applications. *J. Clin. Laser Med. Surg.* **2002**, *20*, 3–7. [CrossRef] [PubMed]
2. Kessel, D. Photodynamic Therapy: A Brief History. *J. Clin. Med.* **2019**, *8*, 1581. [CrossRef] [PubMed]
3. Michalak, M.; Mazurkiewicz, S.; Szymczyk, J.; Ziental, D.; Sobotta, Ł. Photodynamic Therapy Applications—Review. *J. Med. Sci.* **2023**, *92*, e865. [CrossRef]
4. Maharjan, P.S.; Bhattarai, H.K. Singlet Oxygen, Photodynamic Therapy, and Mechanisms of Cancer Cell Death. *J. Oncol.* **2022**, *2022*, 7211485. [CrossRef] [PubMed]
5. Mishchenko, T.; Balalaeva, I.; Gorokhova, A.; Vedunova, M.; Krysko, D.V. Which Cell Death Modality Wins the Contest for Photodynamic Therapy of Cancer? *Cell Death Dis.* **2022**, *13*, 455. [CrossRef]
6. Pola, M.; Kolarova, H.; Bajgar, R. Generation of Singlet Oxygen by Porphyrin and Phthalocyanine Derivatives Regarding the Oxygen Level. *J. Med. Sci.* **2022**, *91*, e752. [CrossRef]
7. Chen, D.; Xu, Q.; Wang, W.; Shao, J.; Huang, W.; Dong, X. Type I Photosensitizers Revitalizing Photodynamic Oncotherapy. *Small* **2021**, *17*, 2006742. [CrossRef]
8. Lucky, S.S.; Soo, K.C.; Zhang, Y. Nanoparticles in Photodynamic Therapy. *Chem. Rev.* **2015**, *115*, 1990–2042. [CrossRef]
9. Scherer, K.M.; Bisby, R.H.; Botchway, S.W.; Parker, A.W. New Approaches to Photodynamic Therapy from Types I, II and III to Type IV Using One or More Photons. *Anti-Cancer Agents Med. Chem.* **2017**, *17*, 171–189. [CrossRef]
10. Yao, Q.; Fan, J.; Long, S.; Zhao, X.; Li, H.; Du, J.; Shao, K.; Peng, X. The Concept and Examples of Type-III Photosensitizers for Cancer Photodynamic Therapy. *Chem* **2022**, *8*, 197–209. [CrossRef]
11. Almeida, R.D.; Manadas, B.J.; Carvalho, A.P.; Duarte, C.B. Intracellular Signaling Mechanisms in Photodynamic Therapy. *Biochim. Biophys. ActaBBA-Rev. Cancer* **2004**, *1704*, 59–86. [CrossRef] [PubMed]
12. Buytaert, E.; Dewaele, M.; Agostinis, P. Molecular Effectors of Multiple Cell Death Pathways Initiated by Photodynamic Therapy. *Biochim. Biophys. Acta BBA-Rev. Cancer* **2007**, *1776*, 86–107. [CrossRef] [PubMed]
13. Yoo, J.-O.; Ha, K.-S. New Insights into the Mechanisms for Photodynamic Therapy-Induced Cancer Cell Death. In *International Review of Cell and Molecular Biology*; Elsevier: Amsterdam, The Netherlands, 2012; Volume 295, pp. 139–174. ISBN 978-0-12-394306-4.

14. Tan, L.; Shen, X.; He, Z.; Lu, Y. The Role of Photodynamic Therapy in Triggering Cell Death and Facilitating Antitumor Immunology. *Front. Oncol.* **2022**, *12*, 863107. [CrossRef] [PubMed]
15. Mokoena, D.R.; George, B.P.; Abrahamse, H. Photodynamic Therapy Induced Cell Death Mechanisms in Breast Cancer. *Int. J. Mol. Sci.* **2021**, *22*, 10506. [CrossRef]
16. Evans, S.; Matthews, W.; Perry, R.; Fraker, D.; Norton, J.; Pass, H.I. Effect of Photodynamic Therapy on Tumqr Necrosis Factor Production by Murine Macrophages. *J. Natl. Cancer Inst.* **1990**, *82*, 34–39. [CrossRef]
17. Polo, L.; Valduga, G.; Jori, G.; Reddi, E. Low-Density Lipoprotein Receptors in the Uptake of Tumour Photosensitizers by Human and Rat Transformed Fibroblasts. *Int. J. Biochem. Cell Biol.* **2002**, *34*, 10–23. [CrossRef]
18. Casas, A.; Di Venosa, G.; Hasan, T.; Batlle, A. Mechanisms of Resistance to Photodynamic Therapy. *Curr. Med. Chem.* **2011**, *18*, 2486–2515. [CrossRef]
19. Agostinis, P.; Berg, K.; Cengel, K.A.; Foster, T.H.; Girotti, A.W.; Gollnick, S.O.; Hahn, S.M.; Hamblin, M.R.; Juzeniene, A.; Kessel, D.; et al. Photodynamic Therapy of Cancer: An Update. *CA A Cancer J. Clin.* **2011**, *61*, 250–281. [CrossRef]
20. Sai, D.L.; Lee, J.; Nguyen, D.L.; Kim, Y.-P. Tailoring Photosensitive ROS for Advanced Photodynamic Therapy. *Exp. Mol. Med.* **2021**, *53*, 495–504. [CrossRef]
21. Yang, Y.; Cui, W.; Zhao, J. Synergistic Treatment of Doxorubicin-Resistant Breast Cancer by the Combination of Chemotherapy and Photodynamic Therapy. *Colloids Surf. A Physicochem. Eng. Asp.* **2022**, *648*, 129167. [CrossRef]
22. Zuluaga, M.-F.; Lange, N. Combination of Photodynamic Therapy with Anti-Cancer Agents. *Curr. Med. Chem.* **2008**, *15*, 1655–1673. [CrossRef]
23. Dougherty, T.J.; Kaufman, J.E.; Goldfarb, A.; Weishaupt, K.R.; Boyle, D.; Mittleman, A. Photoradiation Therapy for the Treatment of Malignant Tumors. *Cancer Res.* **1978**, *38*, 2628–2635.
24. Brown, J.M.; Wilson, W.R. Exploiting Tumour Hypoxia in Cancer Treatment. *Nat. Rev. Cancer* **2004**, *4*, 437–447. [CrossRef]
25. Zhu, T.C.; Finlay, J.C. The Role of Photodynamic Therapy (PDT) Physics: PDT Physics. *Med. Phys.* **2008**, *35*, 3127–3136. [CrossRef]
26. Plaetzer, K.; Krammer, B.; Berlanda, J.; Berr, F.; Kiesslich, T. Photophysics and Photochemistry of Photodynamic Therapy: Fundamental Aspects. *Lasers Med. Sci.* **2009**, *24*, 259–268. [CrossRef]
27. Heckl, C.; Aumiller, M.; Rühm, A.; Sroka, R.; Stepp, H. Fluorescence and Treatment Light Monitoring for Interstitial Photodynamic Therapy. *Photochem. Photobiol.* **2020**, *96*, 388–396. [CrossRef] [PubMed]
28. de Andrade, C.T.; Nogueira, M.S.; Kanick, S.C.; Marra, K.; Gunn, J.; Andreozzi, J.; Samkoe, K.S.; Kurachi, C.; Pogue, B.W. Optical Spectroscopy of Radiotherapy and Photodynamic Therapy Responses in Normal Rat Skin Shows Vascular Breakdown Products. *SPIE Proceedings* **2016**, *9694*, 151–155. [CrossRef]
29. Larsen, E.L.P.; Randeberg, L.L.; Gederaas, O.A.; Arum, C.-J.; Hjelde, A.; Zhao, C.-M.; Chen, D.; Krokan, H.E.; Svaasand, L.O. Monitoring of Hexyl 5-Aminolevulinate-Induced Photodynamic Therapy in Rat Bladder Cancer by Optical Spectroscopy. *J. Biomed. Opt.* **2008**, *13*, 044031. [CrossRef] [PubMed]
30. Hamada, R.; Ogawa, E.; Arai, T. Continuous Optical Monitoring of Red Blood Cells During a Photosensitization Reaction. *Photobiomodul. Photomed. Laser Surg.* **2019**, *37*, 110–116. [CrossRef] [PubMed]
31. Allison, R.R.; Sibata, C.H. Oncologic Photodynamic Therapy Photosensitizers: A Clinical Review. *Photodiagn. Photodyn. Ther.* **2010**, *7*, 61–75. [CrossRef] [PubMed]
32. Henderson, B.W.; Busch, T.M.; Snyder, J.W. Fluence Rate as a Modulator of PDT Mechanisms. *Lasers Surg. Med.* **2006**, *38*, 489–493. [CrossRef] [PubMed]
33. Gunaydin, G.; Gedik, M.E.; Ayan, S. Photodynamic Therapy—Current Limitations and Novel Approaches. *Front. Chem.* **2021**, *9*, 691697. [CrossRef]
34. Jankun, J. A Thousand Words about the Challenges of Photodynamic Therapy: Challenges of Photodynamic Therapy. *J. Med. Sci.* **2019**, *88*, 195–199. [CrossRef]
35. Rapozzi, V.; Jori, G. (Eds.) *Resistance to Photodynamic Therapy in Cancer*; Resistance to Targeted Anti-Cancer Therapeutics; Springer International Publishing: Cham, Switzerland, 2015; Volume 5, ISBN 978-3-319-12729-3.
36. Wu, Y.; Li, Y.; Lv, G.; Bu, W. Redox Dyshomeostasis Strategy for Tumor Therapy Based on Nanomaterials Chemistry. *Chem. Sci.* **2022**, *13*, 2202–2217. [CrossRef]
37. Cheng, Q.; Yu, W.; Ye, J.; Liu, M.; Liu, W.; Zhang, C.; Zhang, C.; Feng, J.; Zhang, X.-Z. Nanotherapeutics Interfere with Cellular Redox Homeostasis for Highly Improved Photodynamic Therapy. *Biomaterials* **2019**, *224*, 119500. [CrossRef]
38. Liu, Y.; Li, Q.; Zhou, L.; Xie, N.; Nice, E.C.; Zhang, H.; Huang, C.; Lei, Y. Cancer Drug Resistance: Redox Resetting Renders a Way. *Oncotarget* **2016**, *7*, 42740–42761. [CrossRef] [PubMed]
39. Gorrini, C.; Harris, I.S.; Mak, T.W. Modulation of Oxidative Stress as an Anticancer Strategy. *Nat. Rev. Drug Discov.* **2013**, *12*, 931–947. [CrossRef] [PubMed]
40. Nakamura, H.; Takada, K. Reactive Oxygen Species in Cancer: Current Findings and Future Directions. *Cancer Sci.* **2021**, *112*, 3945–3952. [CrossRef]
41. Hamada, N.; Fujimichi, Y.; Iwasaki, T.; Fujii, N.; Furuhashi, M.; Kubo, E.; Minamino, T.; Nomura, T.; Sato, H. Emerging Issues in Radiogenic Cataracts and Cardiovascular Disease. *J. Radiat. Res.* **2014**, *55*, 831–846. [CrossRef]
42. Fukai, T.; Ushio-Fukai, M. Superoxide Dismutases: Role in Redox Signaling, Vascular Function, and Diseases. *Antioxid. Redox Signal.* **2011**, *15*, 1583–1606. [CrossRef]

43. Holmström, K.M.; Finkel, T. Cellular Mechanisms and Physiological Consequences of Redox-Dependent Signalling. *Nat. Rev. Mol. Cell Biol.* **2014**, *15*, 411–421. [CrossRef]
44. Andrés, C.M.C.; Pérez De La Lastra, J.M.; Andrés Juan, C.; Plou, F.J.; Pérez-Lebeña, E. Superoxide Anion Chemistry—Its Role at the Core of the Innate Immunity. *Int. J. Mol. Sci.* **2023**, *24*, 1841. [CrossRef]
45. Bielski, B.H.; Arudi, R.L.; Sutherland, M.W. A Study of the Reactivity of HO2/O2- with Unsaturated Fatty Acids. *J. Biol. Chem.* **1983**, *258*, 4759–4761. [CrossRef] [PubMed]
46. Fridovich, I. Superoxide Anion Radical (O_{2-}.), Superoxide Dismutases, and Related Matters. *J. Biol. Chem.* **1997**, *272*, 18515–18517. [CrossRef] [PubMed]
47. Guzik, T.J.; Harrison, D.G. Vascular NADPH Oxidases as Drug Targets for Novel Antioxidant Strategies. *Drug Discov. Today* **2006**, *11*, 524–533. [CrossRef] [PubMed]
48. Madamanchi, N.R.; Runge, M.S. Mitochondrial Dysfunction in Atherosclerosis. *Circ. Res.* **2007**, *100*, 460–473. [CrossRef] [PubMed]
49. Wang, Y.; Branicky, R.; Noë, A.; Hekimi, S. Superoxide Dismutases: Dual Roles in Controlling ROS Damage and Regulating ROS Signaling. *J. Cell Biol.* **2018**, *217*, 1915–1928. [CrossRef] [PubMed]
50. Abreu, I.A.; Cabelli, D.E. Superoxide Dismutases—A Review of the Metal-Associated Mechanistic Variations. *Biochim. Biophys. Acta BBA-Proteins Proteom.* **2010**, *1804*, 263–274. [CrossRef] [PubMed]
51. Mumbengegwi, D.R.; Li, Q.; Li, C.; Bear, C.E.; Engelhardt, J.F. Evidence for a Superoxide Permeability Pathway in Endosomal Membranes. *Mol. Cell Biol.* **2008**, *28*, 3700–3712. [CrossRef]
52. Tsang, C.K.; Liu, Y.; Thomas, J.; Zhang, Y.; Zheng, X.F.S. Superoxide Dismutase 1 Acts as a Nuclear Transcription Factor to Regulate Oxidative Stress Resistance. *Nat. Commun.* **2014**, *5*, 3446. [CrossRef]
53. Becuwe, P.; Ennen, M.; Klotz, R.; Barbieux, C.; Grandemange, S. Manganese Superoxide Dismutase in Breast Cancer: From Molecular Mechanisms of Gene Regulation to Biological and Clinical Significance. *Free Radic. Biol. Med.* **2014**, *77*, 139–151. [CrossRef] [PubMed]
54. Ushiofukai, M. Redox Signaling in Angiogenesis: Role of NADPH Oxidase. *Cardiovasc. Res.* **2006**, *71*, 226–235. [CrossRef]
55. Zelko, I.N.; Mariani, T.J.; Folz, R.J. Superoxide Dismutase Multigene Family: A Comparison of the CuZn-SOD (SOD1), Mn-SOD (SOD2), and EC-SOD (SOD3) Gene Structures, Evolution, and Expression. *Free Radic. Biol. Med.* **2002**, *33*, 337–349. [CrossRef]
56. Griess, B.; Tom, E.; Domann, F.; Teoh-Fitzgerald, M. Extracellular Superoxide Dismutase and Its Role in Cancer. *Free Radic. Biol. Med.* **2017**, *112*, 464–479. [CrossRef]
57. Bauer, G. Tumor Cell-Protective Catalase as a Novel Target for Rational Therapeutic Approaches Based on Specific Intercellular ROS Signaling. *Anticancer. Res.* **2012**, *32*, 2599–2624. [PubMed]
58. Behrend, L.; Henderson, G.; Zwacka, R.M. Reactive Oxygen Species in Oncogenic Transformation. *Biochem. Soc. Trans.* **2003**, *31*, 1441–1444. [CrossRef]
59. Weinberg, F.; Chandel, N.S. Reactive Oxygen Species-Dependent Signaling Regulates Cancer. *Cell. Mol. Life Sci.* **2009**, *66*, 3663–3673. [CrossRef] [PubMed]
60. Pottgiesser, S.J.; Heinzelmann, S.; Bauer, G. Intercellular HOCl-Mediated Apoptosis Induction in Malignant Cells: Interplay Between NOX1-Dependent Superoxide Anion Generation and DUOX-Related HOCl-Generating Peroxidase Activity. *Anticancer. Res.* **2015**, *35*, 5927–5943.
61. Bauer, G. HOCl and the Control of Oncogenesis. *J. Inorg. Biochem.* **2018**, *179*, 10–23. [CrossRef]
62. Bauer, G. HOCl-Dependent Singlet Oxygen and Hydroxyl Radical Generation Modulate and Induce Apoptosis of Malignant Cells. *Anticancer. Res.* **2013**, *33*, 3589–3602.
63. Bauer, G. Central Signaling Elements of Intercellular Reactive Oxygen/Nitrogen Species-Dependent Induction of Apoptosis in Malignant Cells. *Anticancer Res.* **2017**, *37*, 499–514. [CrossRef]
64. Heinzelmann, S.; Bauer, G. Multiple Protective Functions of Catalase against Intercellular Apoptosis-Inducing ROS Signaling of Human Tumor Cells. *Biol. Chem.* **2010**, *391*, 675–693. [CrossRef]
65. Lucena, S.R.; Zamarrón, A.; Carrasco, E.; Marigil, M.A.; Mascaraque, M.; Fernández-Guarino, M.; Gilaberte, Y.; González, S.; Juarranz, A. Characterisation of Resistance Mechanisms Developed by Basal Cell Carcinoma Cells in Response to Repeated Cycles of Photodynamic Therapy. *Sci. Rep.* **2019**, *9*, 4835. [CrossRef] [PubMed]
66. Scheit, K.; Bauer, G. Direct and Indirect Inactivation of Tumor Cell Protective Catalase by Salicylic Acid and Anthocyanidins Reactivates Intercellular ROS Signaling and Allows for Synergistic Effects. *Carcinogenesis* **2015**, *36*, 400–411. [CrossRef] [PubMed]
67. Clark, R.A.; Klebanoff, S.J. Role of the Myeloperoxidase-H2O2-Halide System in Concanavalin A-Induced Tumor Cell Killing by Human Neutrophils. *J. Immunol.* **1979**, *122*, 2605–2610. [CrossRef] [PubMed]
68. Schieven, G.L.; de Fex, H.; Stephenson, L. Hypochlorous Acid Activates Tyrosine Phosphorylation Signal Pathways Leading to Calcium Signaling and TNFα Production. *Antioxid. Redox Signal.* **2002**, *4*, 501–507. [CrossRef] [PubMed]
69. Levine, A.B.; Punihaole, D.; Levine, T.B. Characterization of the Role of Nitric Oxide and Its Clinical Applications. *Cardiology* **2012**, *122*, 55–68. [CrossRef] [PubMed]
70. Bauer, G. The Antitumor Effect of Singlet Oxygen. *Anticancer Res.* **2016**, *36*, 5649–5664. [CrossRef] [PubMed]
71. Bauer, G. Targeting Extracellular ROS Signaling of Tumor Cells. *Anticancer. Res.* **2014**, *34*, 1467–1482.
72. Sah, S.K.; Agrahari, G.; Kim, T.-Y. Insights into Superoxide Dismutase 3 in Regulating Biological and Functional Properties of Mesenchymal Stem Cells. *Cell Biosci.* **2020**, *10*, 22. [CrossRef]

73. Liu, X.; Wang, A.; Muzio, L.L.; Kolokythas, A.; Sheng, S.; Rubini, C.; Ye, H.; Shi, F.; Yu, T.; Crowe, D.L.; et al. Deregulation of Manganese Superoxide Dismutase (SOD2) Expression and Lymph Node Metastasis in Tongue Squamous Cell Carcinoma. *BMC Cancer* **2010**, *10*, 365. [CrossRef]
74. Ye, H.; Wang, A.; Lee, B.-S.; Yu, T.; Sheng, S.; Peng, T.; Hu, S.; Crowe, D.L.; Zhou, X. Proteomic Based Identification of Manganese Superoxide Dismutase 2 (SOD2) as a Metastasis Marker for Oral Squamous Cell Carcinoma. *Cancer Genom. Proteom.* **2008**, *5*, 85–94.
75. Liu, Z.; Li, S.; Cai, Y.; Wang, A.; He, Q.; Zheng, C.; Zhao, T.; Ding, X.; Zhou, X. Manganese Superoxide Dismutase Induces Migration and Invasion of Tongue Squamous Cell Carcinoma via H2O2-Dependent Snail Signaling. *Free Radic. Biol. Med.* **2012**, *53*, 44–50. [CrossRef] [PubMed]
76. Dolgachev, V.; Oberley, L.W.; Huang, T.-T.; Kraniak, J.M.; Tainsky, M.A.; Hanada, K.; Separovic, D. A Role for Manganese Superoxide Dismutase in Apoptosis after Photosensitization. *Biochem. Biophys. Res. Commun.* **2005**, *332*, 411–417. [CrossRef] [PubMed]
77. Korbelik, M.; Parkins, C.S.; Shibuya, H.; Cecic, I.; Stratford, M.R.L.; Chaplin, D.J. Nitric Oxide Production by Tumour Tissue: Impact on the Response to Photodynamic Therapy. *Br. J. Cancer* **2000**, *82*, 1835–1843. [CrossRef] [PubMed]
78. Soares, H.T.; Campos, J.R.S.; Gomes-da-Silva, L.C.; Schaberle, F.A.; Dabrowski, J.M.; Arnaut, L.G. Pro-Oxidant and Antioxidant Effects in Photodynamic Therapy: Cells Recognise That Not All Exogenous ROS Are Alike. *ChemBioChem* **2016**, *17*, 836–842. [CrossRef] [PubMed]
79. Golab, J.; Nowis, D.; Skrzycki, M.; Czeczot, H.; Barańczyk-Kuźma, A.; Wilczyński, G.M.; Makowski, M.; Mróz, P.; Kozar, K.; Kamiński, R.; et al. Antitumor Effects of Photodynamic Therapy Are Potentiated by 2-Methoxyestradiol. *J. Biol. Chem.* **2003**, *278*, 407–414. [CrossRef] [PubMed]
80. Zhang, Z.; Jayakumar, M.K.G.; Zheng, X.; Shikha, S.; Zhang, Y.; Bansal, A.; Poon, D.J.J.; Chu, P.L.; Yeo, E.L.L.; Chua, M.L.K.; et al. Upconversion Superballs for Programmable Photoactivation of Therapeutics. *Nat. Commun.* **2019**, *10*, 4586. [CrossRef] [PubMed]
81. Nandi, A.; Yan, L.-J.; Jana, C.K.; Das, N. Role of Catalase in Oxidative Stress- and Age-Associated Degenerative Diseases. *Oxidative Med. Cell. Longev.* **2019**, *2019*, 9613090. [CrossRef] [PubMed]
82. Lardinois, O.M. Reactions of Bovine Liver Catalase with Superoxide Radicals and Hydrogen Peroxide. *Free Radic. Res.* **1995**, *22*, 251–274. [CrossRef]
83. Deisseroth, A.; Dounce, A.L. Catalase: Physical and Chemical Properties, Mechanism of Catalysis, and Physiological Role. *Physiol. Rev.* **1970**, *50*, 319–375. [CrossRef]
84. Reimer, D.L.; Bailley, J.; Singh, S.M. Complete cDNA and 5′ Genomic Sequences and Multilevel Regulation of the Mouse Catalase Gene. *Genomics* **1994**, *21*, 325–336. [CrossRef]
85. Marín-García, J. Oxidative Stress and Cell Death in Cardiovascular Disease. In *Post-Genomic Cardiology*; Elsevier: Amsterdam, The Netherlands, 2014; pp. 471–498. ISBN 978-0-12-404599-6.
86. Li, G.; Chen, Y.; Saari, J.T.; Kang, Y.J. Catalase-Overexpressing Transgenic Mouse Heart Is Resistant to Ischemia-Reperfusion Injury. *Am. J. Physiol. Heart Circ. Physiol.* **1997**, *273*, H1090–H1095. [CrossRef]
87. Schriner, S.E.; Linford, N.J.; Martin, G.M.; Treuting, P.; Ogburn, C.E.; Emond, M.; Coskun, P.E.; Ladiges, W.; Wolf, N.; Van Remmen, H.; et al. Extension of Murine Life Span by Overexpression of Catalase Targeted to Mitochondria. *Science* **2005**, *308*, 1909–1911. [CrossRef]
88. Hyoudou, K.; Nishikawa, M.; Kobayashi, Y.; Umeyama, Y.; Yamashita, F.; Hashida, M. PEGylated Catalase Prevents Metastatic Tumor Growth Aggravated by Tumor Removal. *Free Radic. Biol. Med.* **2006**, *41*, 1449–1458. [CrossRef]
89. Goth, L.; Rass, P.; Pay, A. Catalase Enzyme Mutations and Their Association with Diseases. *Mol. Diagn.* **2004**, *8*, 141–149. [CrossRef]
90. Kodydková, J.; Vávrová, L.; Kocík, M.; Žák, A. Human Catalase, Its Polymorphisms, Regulation and Changes of Its Activity in Different Diseases. *Folia Biol.* **2014**, *60*, 153–167.
91. Goth, L.; Eaton, J.W. Hereditary Catalase Deficiencies and Increased Risk of Diabetes. *Lancet* **2000**, *356*, 1820–1821. [CrossRef] [PubMed]
92. Jiang, Z.; Akey, J.M.; Shi, J.; Xiong, M.; Wang, Y.; Shen, Y.; Xu, X.; Chen, H.; Wu, H.; Xiao, J.; et al. A Polymorphism in the Promoter Region of Catalase Is Associated with Blood Pressure Levels. *Hum. Genet.* **2001**, *109*, 95–98. [CrossRef] [PubMed]
93. Takahara, S. Progressive Oral Gangrene Probably Due to Lack of Catalase in the Blood (Acatalasaemia). *Lancet* **1952**, *260*, 1101–1104. [CrossRef] [PubMed]
94. Glorieux, C.; Zamocky, M.; Sandoval, J.M.; Verrax, J.; Calderon, P.B. Regulation of Catalase Expression in Healthy and Cancerous Cells. *Free Radic. Biol. Med.* **2015**, *87*, 84–97. [CrossRef]
95. Glorieux, C.; Calderon, P.B. Catalase, a Remarkable Enzyme: Targeting the Oldest Antioxidant Enzyme to Find a New Cancer Treatment Approach. *Biol. Chem.* **2017**, *398*, 1095–1108. [CrossRef]
96. Brunelli, L.; Yermilov, V.; Beckman, J.S. Modulation of Catalase Peroxidatic and Catalatic Activity by Nitric Oxide. *Free Radic. Biol. Med.* **2001**, *30*, 709–714. [CrossRef] [PubMed]
97. Bauer, G. Increasing the Endogenous NO Level Causes Catalase Inactivation and Reactivation of Intercellular Apoptosis Signaling Specifically in Tumor Cells. *Redox Biol.* **2015**, *6*, 353–371. [CrossRef] [PubMed]
98. Brown, G.C. Reversible Binding and Inhibition of Catalase by Nitric Oxide. *Eur. J. Biochem.* **1995**, *232*, 188–191. [CrossRef]

99. Wink, D.A.; Mitchell, J.B. Chemical Biology of Nitric Oxide: Insights into Regulatory, Cytotoxic, and Cytoprotective Mechanisms of Nitric Oxide. *Free Radic. Biol. Med.* **1998**, *25*, 434–456. [CrossRef] [PubMed]
100. Riethmüller, M.; Burger, N.; Bauer, G. Singlet Oxygen Treatment of Tumor Cells Triggers Extracellular Singlet Oxygen Generation, Catalase Inactivation and Reactivation of Intercellular Apoptosis-Inducing Signaling. *Redox Biol.* **2015**, *6*, 157–168. [CrossRef] [PubMed]
101. Di Mascio, P.; Bechara, E.J.H.; Medeiros, M.H.G.; Briviba, K.; Sies, H. Singlet Molecular Oxygen Production in the Reaction of Peroxynitrite with Hydrogen Peroxide. *FEBS Lett.* **1994**, *355*, 287–289. [CrossRef]
102. Glorieux, C.; Sandoval, J.M.; Dejeans, N.; Nonckreman, S.; Bahloula, K.; Poirel, H.A.; Calderon, P.B. Evaluation of Potential Mechanisms Controlling the Catalase Expression in Breast Cancer Cells. *Oxidative Med. Cell. Longev.* **2018**, *2018*, 5351967. [CrossRef]
103. Klingelhoeffer, C.; Kämmerer, U.; Koospal, M.; Mühling, B.; Schneider, M.; Kapp, M.; Kübler, A.; Germer, C.-T.; Otto, C. Natural Resistance to Ascorbic Acid Induced Oxidative Stress Is Mainly Mediated by Catalase Activity in Human Cancer Cells and Catalase-Silencing Sensitizes to Oxidative Stress. *BMC Complement. Altern. Med.* **2012**, *12*, 61. [CrossRef]
104. Smith, P.S.; Zhao, W.; Spitz, D.R.; Robbins, M.E. Inhibiting Catalase Activity Sensitizes 36B10 Rat Glioma Cells to Oxidative Stress. *Free Radic. Biol. Med.* **2007**, *42*, 787–797. [CrossRef] [PubMed]
105. Kang, M.Y.; Kim, H.-B.; Piao, C.; Lee, K.H.; Hyun, J.W.; Chang, I.-Y.; You, H.J. The Critical Role of Catalase in Prooxidant and Antioxidant Function of P53. *Cell Death Differ.* **2013**, *20*, 117–129. [CrossRef] [PubMed]
106. Zhao, M.-X.; Wen, J.-L.; Wang, L.; Wang, X.-P.; Chen, T.-S. Intracellular Catalase Activity Instead of Glutathione Level Dominates the Resistance of Cells to Reactive Oxygen Species. *Cell Stress Chaperones* **2019**, *24*, 609–619. [CrossRef] [PubMed]
107. Glorieux, C.; Dejeans, N.; Sid, B.; Beck, R.; Calderon, P.B.; Verrax, J. Catalase Overexpression in Mammary Cancer Cells Leads to a Less Aggressive Phenotype and an Altered Response to Chemotherapy. *Biochem. Pharmacol.* **2011**, *82*, 1384–1390. [CrossRef] [PubMed]
108. Kahlos, K.; Soini, Y.; Sormunen, R.; Kaarteenaho-Wiik, R.; Pääkkö, P.; Linnainmaa, K.; Kinnula, V.L. Expression and Prognostic Significance of Catalase in Malignant Mesothelioma. *Cancer* **2001**, *91*, 1349–1357. [CrossRef] [PubMed]
109. Chekulayeva, L.V.; Shevchuk, I.N.; Chekulayev, V.A. Influence of Temperature on the Efficiency of Photodestruction of Ehrlich Ascites Carcinoma Cells Sensitized by Hematoporphyrin Derivative. *Exp. Oncol.* **2004**, *26*, 125–139.
110. Flohé, L. The Impact of Thiol Peroxidases on Redox Regulation. *Free Radic. Res.* **2016**, *50*, 126–142. [CrossRef]
111. Flohé, L.; Toppo, S.; Cozza, G.; Ursini, F. A Comparison of Thiol Peroxidase Mechanisms. *Antioxid. Redox Signal.* **2011**, *15*, 763–780. [CrossRef]
112. Dickinson, D.A.; Forman, H.J. Cellular Glutathione and Thiols Metabolism. *Biochem. Pharmacol.* **2002**, *64*, 1019–1026. [CrossRef]
113. Franco, R.; Cidlowski, J.A. Apoptosis and Glutathione: Beyond an Antioxidant. *Cell Death Differ.* **2009**, *16*, 1303–1314. [CrossRef]
114. Sies, H.; Sharov, V.S.; Klotz, L.-O.; Briviba, K. Glutathione Peroxidase Protects against Peroxynitrite-Mediated Oxidations. *J. Biol. Chem.* **1997**, *272*, 27812–27817. [CrossRef]
115. Hayes, J.D.; Flanagan, J.U.; Jowsey, I.R. Glutathione Transferases. *Annu. Rev. Pharmacol. Toxicol.* **2005**, *45*, 51–88. [CrossRef]
116. Adler, V.; Yin, Z.; Fuchs, S.Y.; Benezra, M.; Rosario, L.; Tew, K.D.; Pincus, M.R.; Sardana, M.; Henderson, C.J.; Wolf, C.R.; et al. Regulation of JNK Signaling by GSTp. *EMBO J.* **1999**, *18*, 1321–1334. [CrossRef]
117. Dabrowski, M.J.; Maeda, D.; Zebala, J.; Lu, W.D.; Mahajan, S.; Kavanagh, T.J.; Atkins, W.M. Glutathione S-Transferase P1-1 Expression Modulates Sensitivity of Human Kidney 293 Cells to Photodynamic Therapy with Hypericin. *Arch. Biochem. Biophys.* **2006**, *449*, 94–103. [CrossRef] [PubMed]
118. Singhal, S.S.; Singh, S.P.; Singhal, P.; Horne, D.; Singhal, J.; Awasthi, S. Antioxidant Role of Glutathione S-Transferases: 4-Hydroxynonenal, a Key Molecule in Stress-Mediated Signaling. *Toxicol. Appl. Pharmacol.* **2015**, *289*, 361–370. [CrossRef] [PubMed]
119. Wang, L.; Ahn, Y.J.; Asmis, R. Sexual Dimorphism in Glutathione Metabolism and Glutathione-Dependent Responses. *Redox Biol.* **2020**, *31*, 101410. [CrossRef] [PubMed]
120. Cooper, A.J.L.; Hanigan, M.H. Metabolism of Glutathione S-Conjugates: Multiple Pathways. In *Comprehensive Toxicology*; Elsevier: Amsterdam, The Netherlands, 2018; pp. 363–406. ISBN 978-0-08-100601-6.
121. Townsend, D.M.; Tew, K.D. The Role of Glutathione-S-Transferase in Anti-Cancer Drug Resistance. *Oncogene* **2003**, *22*, 7369–7375. [CrossRef] [PubMed]
122. Lee, H.M.; Chung, C.-W.; Kim, C.H.; Kim, D.H.; Kwak, T.W.; Jeong, Y.-I.; Kang, D.H. Defensive Mechanism in Cholangiocarcinoma Cells against Oxidative Stress Induced by Chlorin E6-Based Photodynamic Therapy. *Drug Des. Dev. Ther.* **2014**, *8*, 1451–1462. [CrossRef]
123. Lin, S.; Lei, K.; Du, W.; Yang, L.; Shi, H.; Gao, Y.; Yin, P.; Liang, X.; Liu, J. Enhancement of Oxaliplatin Sensitivity in Human Colorectal Cancer by Hypericin Mediated Photodynamic Therapy via ROS-Related Mechanism. *Int. J. Biochem. Cell Biol.* **2016**, *71*, 24–34. [CrossRef] [PubMed]
124. Wang, H. Phospholipid Hydroperoxide Glutathione Peroxidase Protects against Singlet Oxygen-Induced Cell Damage of Photodynamic Therapy. *Free Radic. Biol. Med.* **2001**, *30*, 825–835. [CrossRef] [PubMed]
125. Lu, W.D.; Atkins, W.M. A Novel Antioxidant Role for Ligandin Behavior of Glutathione S-Transferases: Attenuation of the Photodynamic Effects of Hypericin. *Biochemistry* **2004**, *43*, 12761–12769. [CrossRef]

126. Spassov, S.G.; Donus, R.; Ihle, P.M.; Engelstaedter, H.; Hoetzel, A.; Faller, S. Hydrogen Sulfide Prevents Formation of Reactive Oxygen Species through PI3K/Akt Signaling and Limits Ventilator-Induced Lung Injury. *Oxidative Med. Cell. Longev.* **2017**, *2017*, 3715037. [CrossRef] [PubMed]
127. Calvo, G.; Céspedes, M.; Casas, A.; Di Venosa, G.; Sáenz, D. Hydrogen Sulfide Decreases Photodynamic Therapy Outcome through the Modulation of the Cellular Redox State. *Nitric Oxide* **2022**, *125–126*, 57–68. [CrossRef] [PubMed]
128. Wagener, F.A.D.T.G.; Volk, H.-D.; Willis, D.; Abraham, N.G.; Soares, M.P.; Adema, G.J.; Figdor, C.G. Different Faces of the Heme-Heme Oxygenase System in Inflammation. *Pharmacol. Rev.* **2003**, *55*, 551–571. [CrossRef] [PubMed]
129. Abraham, N.G.; Kappas, A. Pharmacological and Clinical Aspects of Heme Oxygenase. *Pharmacol. Rev.* **2008**, *60*, 79–127. [CrossRef] [PubMed]
130. Dunn, L.L.; Midwinter, R.G.; Ni, J.; Hamid, H.A.; Parish, C.R.; Stocker, R. New Insights into Intracellular Locations and Functions of Heme Oxygenase-1. *Antioxid. Redox Signal.* **2014**, *20*, 1723–1742. [CrossRef] [PubMed]
131. Linnenbaum, M.; Busker, M.; Kraehling, J.R.; Behrends, S. Heme Oxygenase Isoforms Differ in Their Subcellular Trafficking during Hypoxia and Are Differentially Modulated by Cytochrome P450 Reductase. *PLoS ONE* **2012**, *7*, e35483. [CrossRef] [PubMed]
132. Tenhunen, R.; Marver, H.S.; Schmid, R. Microsomal Heme Oxygenase. *J. Biol. Chem.* **1969**, *244*, 6388–6394. [CrossRef]
133. Hayashi, S.; Omata, Y.; Sakamoto, H.; Higashimoto, Y.; Hara, T.; Sagara, Y.; Noguchi, M. Characterization of Rat Heme Oxygenase-3 Gene. Implication of Processed Pseudogenes Derived from Heme Oxygenase-2 Gene. *Gene* **2004**, *336*, 241–250. [CrossRef]
134. Gene HMOX1—Heme Oxygenase 1 (Human). Available online: https://pubchem.ncbi.nlm.nih.gov/gene/HMOX1/human (accessed on 20 February 2023).
135. HMOX2 Heme Oxygenase 2 [Homo Sapiens (Human)]-Gene-NCBI. Available online: https://www.ncbi.nlm.nih.gov/gene/3163 (accessed on 26 September 2023).
136. Kutty, R.K.; Kutty, G.; Rodriguez, I.R.; Chader, G.J.; Wiggert, B. Chromosomal Localization of the Human Heme Oxygenase Genes: Heme Oxygenase-1 (HMOX1) Maps to Chromosome 22q12 and Heme Oxygenase-2 (HMOX2) Maps to Chromosome 16p13.3. *Genomics* **1994**, *20*, 513–516. [CrossRef]
137. UniProtKB HMOX1—Heme Oxygenase 1—Homo Sapiens (Human). Available online: https://www.uniprot.org/uniprotkb/P09601/entry#sequences (accessed on 20 February 2023).
138. Keyse, S.M.; Tyrrell, R.M. Heme Oxygenase Is the Major 32-kDa Stress Protein Induced in Human Skin Fibroblasts by UVA Radiation, Hydrogen Peroxide, and Sodium Arsenite. *Proc. Natl. Acad. Sci. USA* **1989**, *86*, 99–103. [CrossRef]
139. HMOX2—Heme Oxygenase 2—Homo Sapiens (Human) | UniProtKB | UniProt. Available online: https://www.uniprot.org/uniprotkb/P30519/entry (accessed on 26 September 2023).
140. Zakhary, R.; Gaine, S.P.; Dinerman, J.L.; Ruat, M.; Flavahan, N.A.; Snyder, S.H. Heme Oxygenase 2: Endothelial and Neuronal Localization and Role in Endothelium-Dependent Relaxation. *Proc. Natl. Acad. Sci. USA* **1996**, *93*, 795–798. [CrossRef]
141. Wu, M.-L.; Ho, Y.-C.; Lin, C.-Y.; Yet, S.-F. Heme Oxygenase-1 in Inflammation and Cardiovascular Disease. *Am. J. Cardiovasc. Dis.* **2011**, *1*, 150–158. [PubMed]
142. Nowis, D.; Legat, M.; Grzela, T.; Niderla, J.; Wilczek, E.; Wilczynski, G.M.; Głodkowska, E.; Mrówka, P.; Issat, T.; Dulak, J.; et al. Heme Oxygenase-1 Protects Tumor Cells against Photodynamic Therapy-Mediated Cytotoxicity. *Oncogene* **2006**, *25*, 3365–3374. [CrossRef] [PubMed]
143. Takahashi, T.; Suzuki, S.; Misawa, S.; Akimoto, J.; Shinoda, Y.; Fujiwara, Y. Photodynamic Therapy Using Talaporfin Sodium Induces Heme Oxygenase-1 Expression in Rat Malignant Meningioma KMY-J Cells. *J. Toxicol. Sci.* **2018**, *43*, 353–358. [CrossRef] [PubMed]
144. Takahashi, T.; Misawa, S.; Suzuki, S.; Saeki, N.; Shinoda, Y.; Tsuneoka, Y.; Akimoto, J.; Fujiwara, Y. Possible Mechanism of Heme Oxygenase-1 Expression in Rat Malignant Meningioma KMY-J Cells Subjected to Talaporfin Sodium-Mediated Photodynamic Therapy. *Photodiagn. Photodyn. Ther.* **2020**, *32*, 102009. [CrossRef] [PubMed]
145. Grimm, S.; Mvondo, D.; Grune, T.; Breusing, N. The Outcome of 5-ALA-Mediated Photodynamic Treatment in Melanoma Cells Is Influenced by Vitamin C and Heme Oxygenase-1. *BioFactors* **2011**, *37*, 17–24. [CrossRef] [PubMed]
146. Kocanova, S.; Buytaert, E.; Matroule, J.-Y.; Piette, J.; Golab, J.; de Witte, P.; Agostinis, P. Induction of Heme-Oxygenase 1 Requires the p38MAPK and PI3K Pathways and Suppresses Apoptotic Cell Death Following Hypericin-Mediated Photodynamic Therapy. *Apoptosis* **2007**, *12*, 731–741. [CrossRef] [PubMed]
147. Medina, M.V.; Sapochnik, D.; Garcia Solá, M.; Coso, O. Regulation of the Expression of Heme Oxygenase-1: Signal Transduction, Gene Promoter Activation, and Beyond. *Antioxid. Redox Signal.* **2020**, *32*, 1033–1044. [CrossRef]
148. Loboda, A.; Damulewicz, M.; Pyza, E.; Jozkowicz, A.; Dulak, J. Role of Nrf2/HO-1 System in Development, Oxidative Stress Response and Diseases: An Evolutionarily Conserved Mechanism. *Cell. Mol. Life Sci.* **2016**, *73*, 3221–3247. [CrossRef]
149. PubChem Carbon Monoxide. Available online: https://pubchem.ncbi.nlm.nih.gov/compound/281 (accessed on 20 February 2023).
150. Piantadosi, C.A.; Sylvia, A.L.; Saltzman, H.A.; Jobsis-Vandervliet, F.F. Carbon Monoxide-Cytochrome Interactions in the Brain of the Fluorocarbon-Perfused Rat. *J. Appl. Physiol.* **1985**, *58*, 665–672. [CrossRef] [PubMed]
151. Coceani, F.; Kelsey, L.; Seidlitz, E. Carbon Monoxide-Induced Relaxation of the Ductus Arteriosus in the Lamb: Evidence against the Prime Role of Guanylyl Cyclase. *Br. J. Pharmacol.* **1996**, *118*, 1689–1696. [CrossRef] [PubMed]

152. Lancel, S.; Hassoun, S.M.; Favory, R.; Decoster, B.; Motterlini, R.; Neviere, R. Carbon Monoxide Rescues Mice from Lethal Sepsis by Supporting Mitochondrial Energetic Metabolism and Activating Mitochondrial Biogenesis. *J. Pharmacol. Exp. Ther.* **2009**, *329*, 641–648. [CrossRef] [PubMed]
153. Ryter, S.W.; Otterbein, L.E. Carbon Monoxide in Biology and Medicine. *Bioessays* **2004**, *26*, 270–280. [CrossRef] [PubMed]
154. Jansen, T.; Hortmann, M.; Oelze, M.; Opitz, B.; Steven, S.; Schell, R.; Knorr, M.; Karbach, S.; Schuhmacher, S.; Wenzel, P.; et al. Conversion of Biliverdin to Bilirubin by Biliverdin Reductase Contributes to Endothelial Cell Protection by Heme Oxygenase-1—Evidence for Direct and Indirect Antioxidant Actions of Bilirubin. *J. Mol. Cell. Cardiol.* **2010**, *49*, 186–195. [CrossRef] [PubMed]
155. Jansen, T.; Daiber, A. Direct Antioxidant Properties of Bilirubin and Biliverdin. Is There a Role for Biliverdin Reductase? *Front. Pharmacol.* **2012**, *3*, 30. [CrossRef] [PubMed]
156. Stocker, R.; Yamamoto, Y.; McDonagh, A.F.; Glazer, A.N.; Ames, B.N. Bilirubin Is an Antioxidant of Possible Physiological Importance. *Science* **1987**, *235*, 1043–1046. [CrossRef]
157. Mancuso, C.; Barone, E.; Guido, P.; Miceli, F.; Di Domenico, F.; Perluigi, M.; Santangelo, R.; Preziosi, P. Inhibition of Lipid Peroxidation and Protein Oxidation by Endogenous and Exogenous Antioxidants in Rat Brain Microsomes in Vitro. *Neurosci. Lett.* **2012**, *518*, 101–105. [CrossRef]
158. Minetti, M.; Mallozzi, C.; Di Stasi, A.M.M.; Pietraforte, D. Bilirubin Is an Effective Antioxidant of Peroxynitrite-Mediated Protein Oxidation in Human Blood Plasma. *Arch. Biochem. Biophys.* **1998**, *352*, 165–174. [CrossRef]
159. Frank, J.; Lornejad-Schäfer, M.; Schöffl, H.; Flaccus, A.; Lambert, C.; Biesalski, H. Inhibition of Heme Oxygenase-1 Increases Responsiveness of Melanoma Cells to ALA-Based Photodynamic Therapy. *Int. J. Oncol.* **2007**, *31*, 1539–1545. [CrossRef]
160. Zhong, H.; Huang, P.; Yan, P.; Chen, P.; Shi, Q.; Zhao, Z.; Chen, J.; Shu, X.; Wang, P.; Yang, B.; et al. Versatile Nanodrugs Containing Glutathione and Heme Oxygenase 1 Inhibitors Enable Suppression of Antioxidant Defense System in a Two-Pronged Manner for Enhanced Photodynamic Therapy. *Adv. Healthc. Mater.* **2021**, *10*, 2100770. [CrossRef]
161. Cheng, P.-Y.; Lee, Y.-M.; Shih, N.-L.; Chen, Y.-C.; Yen, M.-H. Heme Oxygenase-1 Contributes to the Cytoprotection of Alpha-Lipoic Acid via Activation of P44/42 Mitogen-Activated Protein Kinase in Vascular Smooth Muscle Cells. *Free Radic. Biol. Med.* **2006**, *40*, 1313–1322. [CrossRef]
162. Sandland, J.; Malatesti, N.; Boyle, R. Porphyrins and Related Macrocycles: Combining Photosensitization with Radio- or Optical-Imaging for next Generation Theranostic Agents. *Photodiagnosis Photodyn. Ther.* **2018**, *23*, 281–294. [CrossRef]
163. Shan, Y.; Lambrecht, R.W.; Donohue, S.E.; Bonkovsky, H.L. Role of Bach1 and Nrf2 in Up-regulation of the Heme Oxygenase-1 Gene by Cobalt Protoporphyrin. *FASEB J.* **2006**, *20*, 2651–2653. [CrossRef]
164. Shi, L.; Fang, J. Implication of Heme Oxygenase-1 in the Sensitivity of Nasopharyngeal Carcinomas to Radiotherapy. *J. Exp. Clin. Cancer Res.* **2008**, *27*, 13. [CrossRef] [PubMed]
165. Marinissen, M.J.; Tanos, T.; Bolós, M.; de Sagarra, M.R.; Coso, O.A.; Cuadrado, A. Inhibition of Heme Oxygenase-1 Interferes with the Transforming Activity of the Kaposi Sarcoma Herpesvirusencoded G Protein-Coupled Receptor *♦. *J. Biol. Chem.* **2006**, *281*, 11332–11346. [CrossRef] [PubMed]
166. Tarhini, A.A.; Belani, C.P.; Luketich, J.D.; Argiris, A.; Ramalingam, S.S.; Gooding, W.; Pennathur, A.; Petro, D.; Kane, K.; Liggitt, D.; et al. A Phase I Study of Concurrent Chemotherapy (Paclitaxel and Carboplatin) and Thoracic Radiotherapy with Swallowed Manganese Superoxide Dismutase Plasmid Liposome Protection in Patients with Locally Advanced Stage III Non-Small-Cell Lung Cancer. *Hum. Gene Ther.* **2011**, *22*, 336–342. [CrossRef] [PubMed]
167. Ismy, J.; Sugandi, S.; Rachmadi, D.; Hardjowijoto, S.; Mustafa, A. The Effect of Exogenous Superoxide Dismutase (SOD) on Caspase-3 Activation and Apoptosis Induction in Pc-3 Prostate Cancer Cells. *Res. Rep. Urol.* **2020**, *12*, 503–508. [CrossRef] [PubMed]
168. Spitz, D.R.; Dornfeld, K.J.; Krishnan, K.; Gius, D. (Eds.) *Oxidative Stress in Cancer Biology and Therapy*; Humana Press: Totowa, NJ, USA, 2012; ISBN 978-1-61779-396-7.
169. Alexandre, J.; Nicco, C.; Chéreau, C.; Laurent, A.; Weill, B.; Goldwasser, F.; Batteux, F. Improvement of the Therapeutic Index of Anticancer Drugs by the Superoxide Dismutase Mimic Mangafodipir. *J. Natl. Cancer Inst.* **2006**, *98*, 236–244. [CrossRef] [PubMed]
170. Blanco, A.; Blanco, G. Chapter 16—Amino Acid Metabolism. In *Medical Biochemistry*, 2nd ed.; Blanco, A., Blanco, G., Eds.; Academic Press: Cambridge, MA, USA, 2022; pp. 401–435. ISBN 978-0-323-91599-1.
171. Villablanca, J.G.; Volchenboum, S.L.; Cho, H.; Kang, M.H.; Cohn, S.L.; Anderson, C.P.; Marachelian, A.; Groshen, S.; Tsao-Wei, D.; Matthay, K.K.; et al. A Phase I New Approaches to Neuroblastoma Therapy Study of Buthionine Sulfoximine and Melphalan With Autologous Stem Cells for Recurrent/Refractory High-Risk Neuroblastoma: Phase I BSO-Melphalan in Neuroblastoma. *Pediatr. Blood Cancer* **2016**, *63*, 1349–1356. [CrossRef] [PubMed]
172. Niu, B.; Liao, K.; Zhou, Y.; Wen, T.; Quan, G.; Pan, X.; Wu, C. Application of Glutathione Depletion in Cancer Therapy: Enhanced ROS-Based Therapy, Ferroptosis, and Chemotherapy. *Biomaterials* **2021**, *277*, 121110. [CrossRef] [PubMed]
173. Yuan, J.-L.; Zheng, W.-X.; Yan, F.; Xue, Q.; Wu, G.-J.; Qin, W.-J.; Wang, F.-L.; Qin, J.; Tian, C.-J. Heme Oxygenase-1 Is a Predictive Biomarker for Therapeutic Targeting of Advanced Clear Cell Renal Cell Carcinoma Treated with Sorafenib or Sunitinib. *OncoTargets Ther.* **2015**, *8*, 2081–2088. [CrossRef] [PubMed]
174. Huang, P.; Feng, L.; Oldham, E.A.; Keating, M.J.; Plunkett, W. Superoxide Dismutase as a Target for the Selective Killing of Cancer Cells. *Nature* **2000**, *407*, 390–395. [CrossRef] [PubMed]

175. Kimani, S.G.; Phillips, J.B.; Bruce, J.I.; MacRobert, A.J.; Golding, J.P. Antioxidant Inhibitors Potentiate the Cytotoxicity of Photodynamic Therapy. *Photochem. Photobiol.* **2012**, *88*, 175–187. [CrossRef] [PubMed]
176. Saczko, J.; Choromańska, A.; Rembiałkowska, N.; Dubińska-Magiera, M.; Bednarz-Misa, I.; Bar, J.; Marcinkowska, A.; Kulbacka, J. Oxidative Modification Induced by Photodynamic Therapy with Photofrin®II and 2-Methoxyestradiol in Human Ovarian Clear Carcinoma (OvBH-1) and Human Breast Adenocarcinoma (MCF-7) Cells. *Biomed. Pharmacother.* **2015**, *71*, 30–36. [CrossRef] [PubMed]
177. Kimáková, P.; Solár, P.; Fecková, B.; Sačková, V.; Solárová, Z.; Ilkovičová, L.; Kello, M. Photoactivated Hypericin Increases the Expression of SOD-2 and Makes MCF-7 Cells Resistant to Photodynamic Therapy. *Biomed. Pharmacother.* **2017**, *85*, 749–755. [CrossRef]
178. Waszkiewicz, M.; Choromanska, A.; Kulbacka, J.; Saczko, J. The Photodynamic Reaction with IR-775 Cyanine Combined with 2-Methoxyestradiol in Ovarian (SKOV-3) and Human Breast Adenocarcinoma (MDA MB-231) Cell Lines. *Photodiagn. Photodyn. Ther.* **2022**, *38*, 102766. [CrossRef]
179. Cocco, D.; Calabrese, L.; Rigo, A.; Argese, E.; Rotilio, G. Re-Examination of the Reaction of Diethyldithiocarbamate with the Copper of Superoxide Dismutase. *J. Biol. Chem.* **1981**, *256*, 8983–8986. [CrossRef]
180. Misra, H.P. Reaction of Copper-Zinc Superoxide Dismutase with Diethyldithiocarbamate. *J. Biol. Chem.* **1979**, *254*, 11623–11628. [CrossRef] [PubMed]
181. Kanno, S.; Matsukawa, E.; Miura, A.; Shouji, A.; Asou, K.; Ishikawa, M. Diethyldithiocarbamate-Induced Cytotoxicity and Apoptosis in Leukemia Cell Lines. *Biol. Pharm. Bull.* **2003**, *26*, 964–968. [CrossRef] [PubMed]
182. Skrott, Z.; Cvek, B. Diethyldithiocarbamate Complex with Copper: The Mechanism of Action in Cancer Cells. *Mini-Rev. Med. Chem.* **2012**, *12*, 1184–1192. [CrossRef] [PubMed]
183. Feuser, P.E.; Cordeiro, A.P.; de Bem Silveira, G.; Borges Corrêa, M.E.A.; Lock Silveira, P.C.; Sayer, C.; de Araújo, P.H.H.; Machado-de-Ávila, R.A.; Dal Bó, A.G. Co-Encapsulation of Sodium Diethyldithiocarbamate (DETC) and Zinc Phthalocyanine (ZnPc) in Liposomes Promotes Increases Phototoxic Activity against (MDA-MB 231) Human Breast Cancer Cells. *Colloids Surf. B Biointerfaces* **2021**, *197*, 111434. [CrossRef] [PubMed]
184. Athar, M.; Mukhtar, H.; Elmets, C.A.; Tarif Zaim, M.; Lloyd, J.R.; Bickers, D.R. In Situ Evidence for the Involvement of Superoxide Anions in Cutaneous Porphyrin Photosensitization. *Biochem. Biophys. Res. Commun.* **1988**, *151*, 1054–1059. [CrossRef]
185. Wright, K.E.; MacRobert, A.J.; Phillips, J.B. Inhibition of Specific Cellular Antioxidant Pathways Increases the Sensitivity of Neurons to Meta-Tetrahydroxyphenyl Chlorin-Mediated Photodynamic Therapy in a 3D Co-Culture Model. *Photochem. Photobiol.* **2012**, *88*, 1539–1545. [CrossRef] [PubMed]
186. Noël, R.; Song, X.; Jiang, R.; Chalmers, M.J.; Griffin, P.R.; Kamenecka, T.M. Efficient Methodology for the Synthesis of 3-Amino-1,2,4-Triazoles. *J. Org. Chem.* **2009**, *74*, 7595–7597. [CrossRef] [PubMed]
187. Naito, Y.; Akahoshi, F.; Takeda, S.; Okada, T.; Kajii, M.; Nishimura, H.; Sugiura, M.; Fukaya, C.; Kagitani, Y. Synthesis and Pharmacological Activity of Triazole Derivatives Inhibiting Eosinophilia. *J. Med. Chem.* **1996**, *39*, 3019–3029. [CrossRef] [PubMed]
188. Hartmann, M.; Bauer, H.-J.; Wermann, K. Biocide Polymers. *Polym. Bull.* **1985**, *13*, 195–200. [CrossRef]
189. Margoliash, E.; Novogrodsky, A.; Schejter, A. Irreversible Reaction of 3-Amino-1:2:4-Triazole and Related Inhibitors with the Protein of Catalase. *Biochem. J.* **1960**, *74*, 339–348. [CrossRef]
190. Darr, D.; Fridovich, I. Irreversible Inactivation of Catalase by 3-Amino-1,2,4-Triazole. *Biochem. Pharmacol.* **1986**, *35*, 3642. [CrossRef]
191. Mariño-Ocampo, N.; Dibona-Villanueva, L.; Escobar-Álvarez, E.; Guerra-Díaz, D.; Zúñiga-Núñez, D.; Fuentealba, D.; Robinson-Duggon, J. Recent Photosensitizer Developments, Delivery Strategies and Combination-based Approaches for Photodynamic Therapy. *Photochem. Photobiol.* **2023**, *99*, 469–497. [CrossRef]
192. Yao, M.; Gu, C.; Doyle, F.J.; Zhu, H.; Redmond, R.W.; Kochevar, I.E. Why Is Rose Bengal More Phototoxic to Fibroblasts In Vitro Than In Vivo? *Photochem. Photobiol.* **2014**, *90*, 297–305. [CrossRef] [PubMed]
193. Price, M.; Terlecky, S.R.; Kessel, D. A Role for Hydrogen Peroxide in the Pro-Apoptotic Effects of Photodynamic Therapy. *Photochem. Photobiol.* **2009**, *85*, 1491–1496. [CrossRef]
194. Griffith, O.W.; Meister, A. Potent and Specific Inhibition of Glutathione Synthesis by Buthionine Sulfoximine (S-n-Butyl Homocysteine Sulfoximine). *J. Biol. Chem.* **1979**, *254*, 7558–7560. [CrossRef]
195. Kiesslich, T.; Plaetzer, K.; Oberdanner, C.B.; Berlanda, J.; Obermair, F.J.; Krammer, B. Differential Effects of Glucose Deprivation on the Cellular Sensitivity towards Photodynamic Treatment-Based Production of Reactive Oxygen Species and Apoptosis-Induction. *FEBS Lett.* **2005**, *579*, 185–190. [CrossRef] [PubMed]
196. Miller, A.C.; Henderson, B.W. The Influence of Cellular Glutathione Content on Cell Survival Following Photodynamic Treatment in Vitro. *Radiat. Res.* **1986**, *107*, 83. [CrossRef] [PubMed]
197. Thomas, J.P.; Girotti, A.W. Role of Lipid Peroxidation in Hematoporphyrin Derivative-Sensitized Photokilling of Tumor Cells: Protective Effects of Glutathione Peroxidase. *Cancer Res.* **1989**, *49*, 1682–1686.
198. Bachor, R.; Scholz, M.; Shea, C.R. Mechanism of Photosensitization by Microsphere-Bound Chlorin e 6 in Human Bladder Carcinoma Cells. *Cancer Res.* **1991**, *51*, 4410–4414.
199. Theodossiou, T.A.; Olsen, C.E.; Jonsson, M.; Kubin, A.; Hothersall, J.S.; Berg, K. The Diverse Roles of Glutathione-Associated Cell Resistance against Hypericin Photodynamic Therapy. *Redox Biol.* **2017**, *12*, 191–197. [CrossRef]

200. Lee, H.M.; Kim, D.H.; Lee, H.L.; Cha, B.; Kang, D.H.; Jeong, Y.-I. Synergistic Effect of Buthionine Sulfoximine on the Chlorin E6-Based Photodynamic Treatment of Cancer Cells. *Arch. Pharm. Res.* **2019**, *42*, 990–999. [CrossRef]
201. Jiang, F.; Robin, A.M.; Katakowski, M.; Tong, L.; Espiritu, M.; Singh, G.; Chopp, M. Photodynamic Therapy with Photofrin in Combination with Buthionine Sulfoximine (BSO) of Human Glioma in the Nude Rat. *Lasers Med. Sci.* **2003**, *18*, 128–133. [CrossRef]
202. Jiang, F.; Lilge, L.; Belcuig, M.; Singh, G.; Grenier, J.; Li, Y.; Chopp, M. Photodynamic Therapy Using Photofrin in Combination with Buthionine Sulfoximine (BSO) to Treat 9L Gliosarcoma in Rat Brain. *Lasers Surg. Med.* **1998**, *23*, 161–166. [CrossRef]
203. Yoo, J.; Jang, S.; Park, C.; Lee, D.; Kwon, S.; Koo, H. Lowering Glutathione Level by Buthionine Sulfoximine Enhances in Vivo Photodynamic Therapy Using Chlorin E6-Loaded Nanoparticles. *Dye. Pigment.* **2020**, *176*, 108207. [CrossRef]
204. Sun, H.; Feng, M.; Chen, S.; Wang, R.; Luo, Y.; Yin, B.; Li, J.; Wang, X. Near-Infrared Photothermal Liposomal Nanoantagonists for Amplified Cancer Photodynamic Therapy. *J. Mater. Chem. B* **2020**, *8*, 7149–7159. [CrossRef]
205. Snyder, N.A.; Silva, G.M. Deubiquitinating Enzymes (DUBs): Regulation, Homeostasis, and Oxidative Stress Response. *J. Biol. Chem.* **2021**, *297*, 101077. [CrossRef] [PubMed]
206. Harris, I.S.; Endress, J.E.; Coloff, J.L.; Selfors, L.M.; McBrayer, S.K.; Rosenbluth, J.M.; Takahashi, N.; Dhakal, S.; Koduri, V.; Oser, M.G.; et al. Deubiquitinases Maintain Protein Homeostasis and Survival of Cancer Cells upon Glutathione Depletion. *Cell Metab.* **2019**, *29*, 1166–1181.e6. [CrossRef] [PubMed]
207. Puppa, A.D.; Lombardi, G.; Rossetto, M.; Rustemi, O.; Berti, F.; Cecchin, D.; Gardiman, M.P.; Rolma, G.; Persano, L.; Zagonel, V.; et al. Outcome of Patients Affected by Newly Diagnosed Glioblastoma Undergoing Surgery Assisted by 5-Aminolevulinic Acid Guided Resection Followed by BCNU Wafers Implantation: A 3-Year Follow-Up. *J. Neurooncol.* **2017**, *131*, 331–340. [CrossRef] [PubMed]
208. Nathan, C.; Arrick, B.; Murray, H.; DeSantis, N.; Cohm, Z. Tumor Cell Anti-Oxidant Defenses. Inhibition of the Glutathione Redox Cycle Enhances Macrophage-Mediated Cytolysis. *J. Exp. Med.* **1981**, *153*, 766–782. [CrossRef]
209. Watts, C.; Ashkan, K.; Jenkinson, M.D.; Price, S.J.; Santarius, T.; Matys, T.; Zhang, T.T.; Finch, A.; Collins, P.; Allinson, K.; et al. An Evaluation of the Tolerability and Feasibility of Combining 5-Amino-Levulinic Acid (5-ALA) with BCNU Wafers in the Surgical Management of Primary Glioblastoma. *Cancers* **2021**, *13*, 3241. [CrossRef] [PubMed]
210. Westphal, M.; Hilt, D.C.; Bortey, E.; Delavault, P.; Olivares, R.; Warnke, P.C.; Whittle, I.R.; Jääskeläinen, J.; Ram, Z. A Phase 3 Trial of Local Chemotherapy with Biodegradable Carmustine (BCNU) Wafers (Gliadel Wafers) in Patients with Primary Malignant Glioma1,2. *Neuro Oncol.* **2003**, *5*, 79–88. [CrossRef]
211. Oberdanner, C.B.; Plaetzer, K.; Kiesslich, T.; Krammer, B. Photodynamic Treatment with Fractionated Light Decreases Production of Reactive Oxygen Species and Cytotoxicity In Vitro via Regeneration of Glutathione. *Photochem. Photobiol.* **2005**, *81*, 609–613. [CrossRef]
212. Sun, W.G.; Weydert, C.J.; Zhang, Y.; Yu, L.; Liu, J.; Spitz, D.R.; Cullen, J.J.; Oberley, L.W. Superoxide Enhances the Antitumor Combination of AdMnSOD Plus BCNU in Breast Cancer. *Cancers* **2010**, *2*, 68–87. [CrossRef]
213. Chekulayeva, L.; Chekulayeva, I.; Chekulayev, V. On the Mechanism of the Phototoxic Action of Haematoporphyrin Derivative towards Tumour Cells. *Proc. Est. Acad. Sci. Biology. Ecol.* **2005**, *54*, 83. [CrossRef]
214. Chekulayeva, L.V.; Chekulayev, V.A.; Shevchuk, I.N. Active Oxygen Intermediates in the Degradation of Hematoporphyrin Derivative in Tumor Cells Subjected to Photodynamic Therapy. *J. Photochem. Photobiol. B Biol.* **2008**, *93*, 94–107. [CrossRef]
215. Chaudiere, J.; Wilhelmsen, E.C.; Tappel, A.L. Mechanism of Selenium-Glutathione Peroxidase and Its Inhibition by Mercaptocarboxylic Acids and Other Mercaptans. *J. Biol. Chem.* **1984**, *259*, 1043–1050. [CrossRef]
216. Lubos, E.; Loscalzo, J.; Handy, D.E. Glutathione Peroxidase-1 in Health and Disease: From Molecular Mechanisms to Therapeutic Opportunities. *Antioxid. Redox Signal.* **2011**, *15*, 1957–1997. [CrossRef]
217. Lange, C.; Bednarski, P.J. In Vitro Assessment of Synergistic Effects in Combinations of a Temoporfin-Based Photodynamic Therapy with Glutathione Peroxidase 1 Inhibitors. *Photodiagn. Photodyn. Ther.* **2021**, *36*, 102478. [CrossRef]
218. Behnisch-Cornwell, S.; Bandaru, S.S.M.; Napierkowski, M.; Wolff, L.; Zubair, M.; Urbainsky, C.; Lillig, C.; Schulzke, C.; Bednarski, P.J. Pentathiepins: A Novel Class of Glutathione Peroxidase 1 Inhibitors That Induce Oxidative Stress, Loss of Mitochondrial Membrane Potential and Apoptosis in Human Cancer Cells. *ChemMedChem* **2020**, *15*, 1515–1528. [CrossRef] [PubMed]
219. Musdal, Y.; Hegazy, U.M.; Aksoy, Y.; Mannervik, B. FDA-Approved Drugs and Other Compounds Tested as Inhibitors of Human Glutathione Transferase P1-1. *Chem.-Biol. Interact.* **2013**, *205*, 53–62. [CrossRef] [PubMed]
220. Wang, J.; Seebacher, N.; Shi, H.; Kan, Q.; Duan, Z. Novel Strategies to Prevent the Development of Multidrug Resistance (MDR) in Cancer. *Oncotarget* **2017**, *8*, 84559–84571. [CrossRef] [PubMed]
221. Khil, M.S.; Kim, S.H.; Pinto, J.T.; Kim, J.H. Ethacrynic Acid: A Novel Radiation Enhancer in Human Carcinoma Cells. *Int. J. Radiat. Oncol. *Biol. *Phys.* **1996**, *34*, 375–380. [CrossRef] [PubMed]
222. Awasthi, S.; Srivastava, S.K.; Ahmad, F.; Ahmad, H.; Ansari, G.A.S. Interactions of Glutathione S-Transferase-π with Ethacrynic Acid and Its Glutathione Conjugate. *Biochim. Biophys. Acta BBA-Protein Struct. Mol. Enzymol.* **1993**, *1164*, 173–178. [CrossRef]
223. Yu, L.; Lee, H.; Rho, S.B.; Park, M.K.; Lee, C.H. Ethacrynic Acid: A Promising Candidate for Drug Repurposing as an Anticancer Agent. *Int. J. Mol. Sci.* **2023**, *24*, 6712. [CrossRef]
224. Yutaka, S.; Shinya, F.; Yasuhiko, F.; Toshio, K. Antiproliferative Effects of Glutathione S -Transferase Inhibitors on the K562 Cell Line. *Biochem. Pharmacol.* **1990**, *39*, 1263–1266. [CrossRef]

225. Won, M.; Koo, S.; Li, H.; Sessler, J.L.; Lee, J.Y.; Sharma, A.; Kim, J.S. An Ethacrynic Acid-Brominated BODIPY Photosensitizer (EA-BPS) Construct Enhances the Lethality of Reactive Oxygen Species in Hypoxic Tumor-Targeted Photodynamic Therapy. *Angew. Chem. Int. Ed.* **2021**, *60*, 3196–3204. [CrossRef]
226. Lyon, R.P.; Hill, J.J.; Atkins, W.M. Novel Class of Bivalent Glutathione *S* -Transferase Inhibitors. *Biochemistry* **2003**, *42*, 10418–10428. [CrossRef] [PubMed]
227. Oakley, A.J.; Bello, M.L.; Battistoni, A.; Ricci, G.; Rossjohn, J.; Villar, H.O.; Parker, M.W. The Structures of Human Glutathione Transferase P1-1 in Complex with Glutathione and Various Inhibitors at High Resolution. *J. Mol. Biol.* **1997**, *274*, 84–100. [CrossRef]
228. Chen, C.; Wu, C.; Lu, X.; Yan, Z.; Gao, J.; Zhao, H.; Li, S. Coniferyl Ferulate, a Strong Inhibitor of Glutathione S-Transferase Isolated from Radix *Angelicae Sinensis*, Reverses Multidrug Resistance and Downregulates P-Glycoprotein. *Evid.-Based Complement. Altern. Med.* **2013**, *2013*, 639083. [CrossRef]
229. Li, X.; Kong, R.; Li, Y.; Huang, J.; Zhou, X.; Li, S.; Cheng, H. Carrier-Free Nanomedicine for Enhanced Photodynamic Tumor Therapy through Glutathione S-Transferase Inhibition. *Chem. Commun.* **2022**, *58*, 3917–3920. [CrossRef] [PubMed]
230. Drummond, G.S.; Kappas, A. Prevention of Neonatal Hyperbilirubinemia by Tin Protoporphyrin IX, a Potent Competitive Inhibitor of Heme Oxidation. *Proc. Natl. Acad. Sci. USA* **1981**, *78*, 6466–6470. [CrossRef]
231. Fang, J.; Sawa, T.; Akaike, T.; Akuta, T.; Sahoo, S.K.; Khaled, G.; Hamada, A.; Maeda, H. In Vivo Antitumor Activity of Pegylated Zinc Protoporphyrin: Targeted Inhibition of Heme Oxygenase in Solid Tumor. *Cancer Res.* **2003**, *63*, 3567–3574. [PubMed]
232. Maines, M.D. Zinc · Protoporphyrin Is a Selective Inhibitor of Heme Oxygenase Activity in the Neonatal Rat. *Biochim. Biophys. Acta BBA-Gen. Subj.* **1981**, *673*, 339–350. [CrossRef] [PubMed]
233. Nowis, D.; Bugajski, M.; Winiarska, M.; Bil, J.; Szokalska, A.; Salwa, P.; Issat, T.; Was, H.; Jozkowicz, A.; Dulak, J.; et al. Zinc Protoporphyrin IX, a Heme Oxygenase-1 Inhibitor, Demonstrates Potent Antitumor Effects but Is Unable to Potentiate Antitumor Effects of Chemotherapeutics in Mice. *BMC Cancer* **2008**, *8*, 197. [CrossRef] [PubMed]
234. Zhang, Y.; Wang, F.; Shi, L.; Lu, M.; Lee, K.-J.; Ditty, M.M.; Xing, Y.; He, H.-Z.; Ren, X.; Zheng, S.-Y. Nanoscale Coordination Polymers Enabling Antioxidants Inhibition for Enhanced Chemodynamic Therapy. *J. Control. Release* **2023**, *354*, 196–206. [CrossRef] [PubMed]
235. Fang, J.; Liao, L.; Yin, H.; Nakamura, H.; Subr, V.; Ulbrich, K.; Maeda, H. Photodynamic Therapy and Imaging Based on Tumor-Targeted Nanoprobe, Polymer-Conjugated Zinc Protoporphyrin. *Future Sci. OA* **2015**, *1*, fso.15.2. [CrossRef]

International Journal of
Molecular Sciences

MDPI

Review

Oxidative Mechanisms and Cardiovascular Abnormalities of Cirrhosis and Portal Hypertension

Hongqun Liu, Henry H. Nguyen, Sang Youn Hwang † and Samuel S. Lee *

Liver Unit, University of Calgary Cumming School of Medicine, Calgary, AB T2N 4N1, Canada;
hhnguye@ucalgary.ca (H.H.N.); mongmani@daum.net (S.Y.H.)
* Correspondence: samlee@ucalgary.ca
† Current address: Department of Internal Medicine, Dongnam Institute of Radiological & Medical Sciences, Busan 46033, Republic of Korea.

Abstract: In patients with portal hypertension, there are many complications including cardiovascular abnormalities, hepatorenal syndrome, ascites, variceal bleeding, and hepatic encephalopathy. The underlying mechanisms are not yet completely clarified. It is well known that portal hypertension causes mesenteric congestion which produces reactive oxygen species (ROS). ROS has been associated with intestinal mucosal injury, increased intestinal permeability, enhanced gut bacterial overgrowth, and translocation; all these changes result in increased endotoxin and inflammation. Portal hypertension also results in the development of collateral circulation and reduces liver mass resulting in an overall increase in endotoxin/bacteria bypassing detoxication and immune clearance in the liver. Endotoxemia can in turn aggravate oxidative stress and inflammation, leading to a cycle of gut barrier dysfunction → endotoxemia → organ injury. The phenotype of cardiovascular abnormalities includes hyperdynamic circulation and cirrhotic cardiomyopathy. Oxidative stress is often accompanied by inflammation; thus, blocking oxidative stress can minimize the systemic inflammatory response and alleviate the severity of cardiovascular diseases. The present review aims to elucidate the role of oxidative stress in cirrhosis-associated cardiovascular abnormalities and discusses possible therapeutic effects of antioxidants on cardiovascular complications of cirrhosis including hyperdynamic circulation, cirrhotic cardiomyopathy, and hepatorenal syndrome.

Keywords: oxidative stress; cardiovascular; cirrhosis; liver; portal hypertension

1. Introduction

Oxidative stress is an imbalance between the production of reactive oxygen species (ROS) and the antioxidant system reducing its capability to detoxify ROS or repair the resulting damage, i.e., ROS overwhelms antioxidants. Oxidative stress is a key pathogenic factor in chronic liver injury of various etiologies, such as alcoholic liver disease [1], nonalcoholic fatty liver diseases (NAFLD) [2], chronic viral hepatitis, and cholestatic diseases. This damage will ultimately lead to cirrhosis (defined as hepatic architectural damage characterized by nodular regeneration and diffuse fibrosis) [3]. Furthermore, oxidative stress also plays an important pathogenic role in portal hypertension (defined as a portal venous pressure of greater than 12 mm Hg) [4], cirrhotic cardiomyopathy (CCM) [5], hepatorenal syndrome (HRS) [6], cirrhosis-related pulmonary complications [7], and hepatic encephalopathy [8]. The present review aims to summarize the role of oxidative stress in cirrhosis-related cardiovascular changes including hyperdynamic circulation, CCM, cardiac arrhythmias, acute kidney injury (AKI), and hepatorenal syndrome (HRS). We will also review a potential therapeutic role of antioxidants in cardiovascular anomalies of cirrhosis.

2. Pathogenic Mechanisms of Oxidative Stress

Oxidative stress plays a crucial role in the progression of chronic liver diseases to cirrhosis and the development of associated complications. The liver plays a central role in the detoxification of endogenous and exogenous toxins, and harbors a high antioxidant function [3]. In cirrhosis, liver function is significantly impaired and therefore antioxidant function is also jeopardized. This is coupled with excess oxidative stress resulting from portal hypertension driven by gastrointestinal congestion and bacterial translocation [9]. The overactivated ROS can damage the intestine structurally and functionally, as increased lipid peroxidation and protein oxidation have been found in the intestinal mucosa of cirrhotic rats [10] and decompensated cirrhotic patients [11]. Using a carbon tetrachloride (CCl_4) model of cirrhosis, Ramachandran and coworkers [10] evaluated oxidative stress status in the gastrointestinal tract. In comparison with controls, xanthine oxidase (XO) activity (an index of oxidative stress) was significantly increased, and xanthine dehydrogenase activity (a parameter of antioxidant status) was significantly decreased in the intestine of cirrhotic rats. This alteration of oxidative stress was associated with a significant reduction in villus fraction, increased enterocyte necrosis, loss of tight junctions, and abnormal intestinal brush border. The damaged intestinal mucosa is thought to enhance intestinal permeability and bacterial translocation that in combination with collateral circulation and an impaired liver results in endotoxemia. Endotoxemia can then further increase oxidative stress, intestinal barrier dysfunction, and organ injury, leading to a 'vicious cycle': gut barrier dysfunction $\rightarrow$ endotoxemia $\rightarrow$ organ injury. Endotoxemia in cirrhotic subjects plays critical role in cirrhotic complications such as CCM [11], and AKI/HRS [12].

3. Overview of Cardiovascular Abnormalities of Cirrhosis and Portal Hypertension

The cardiovascular system in cirrhotic patients is abnormal, and is characterized by portal hypertension, systemic hyperdynamic circulation (increased cardiac output and decreased peripheral vascular resistance), and arterial pressure [13]. The decrease in peripheral vascular resistance is thought to be due to an imbalance between vasoconstrictive and vasodilatory factors. The former is mainly driven by the sympathetic system [14], renin–angiotensin system (RAS) [15], endothelin-1 [16], and thromboxane [17]; the latter by glucagon [18], prostaglandins [19], bile acids, nitric oxide (NO) [20], carbon monoxide (CO) [21], and hydrogen sulfate (H_2S) [22]. Although the vasoconstrictors such as the sympathetic system [23,24] and RAS [25,26] are increased in subjects with cirrhosis, the response of cirrhotic subjects to vasoconstrictors as a whole is impaired [27]. Vasodilators play a dominant role in cirrhotic patients and therefore the cardiovascular system in patients with cirrhosis is characterized by peripheral vascular dilation, decreased systemic vascular resistance (SVR), and mean arterial pressure (MAP). The cardiac output is increased at rest with cirrhotic patients having been described to have hyperdynamic circulation [22]. Under stress, the cardiac functional reserve is insufficient in cirrhosis, with decreased left ventricular responsiveness having been described [28]. Moreover, cardiac diastolic dysfunction has also been reported and can lead to significantly smaller increases in stroke volume when challenged [28]. This collection of cardiac functional abnormalities in patients with cirrhosis is called cirrhotic cardiomyopathy. The diagnosis of cirrhotic cardiomyopathy is based on advanced imaging examination at rest [29].

The pathophysiology of cardiovascular changes in cirrhosis is multifaceted, with inflammation (evidenced by increases of proinflammatory cytokines) [30] and oxidative stress as significant contributors to these changes [5]. There is evidence that oxidative stress also plays an essential role in non-cirrhotic cardiovascular diseases [31]. However, the role of oxidative stress in the pathophysiology of cardiovascular changes in cirrhosis remains incompletely clarified.

4. Oxidative Stress in Pathogenesis of Hyperdynamic Circulation

Cirrhosis and portal hypertension cause hyperdynamic circulation. There are two theories explaining hyperdynamic circulation in subjects with cirrhosis and portal hypertension: the humoral theory and central neural dysregulation [9].

5. Oxidative Stress in the Humoral Theory

The humoral hypothesis suggests that in cirrhosis, mesenteric congestion causes endotoxemia. Endotoxin stimulates the generation of vasodilators such as glucagon [18], prostaglandins [19], NO [32], CO [33], and H_2S [34]. All these vasodilators additively/synergically dilate peripheral vasculature which results in hyperdynamic circulation.

Oxidative stress also plays an important role in hyperdynamic circulation. In bile duct ligation (BDL)-induced cirrhosis in rats, Lee et al. [35] found that mesenteric markers of oxidative stress, such as thiobarbituric acid reactive substances (TBARS, an index of lipoperoxidation), and malondialdehyde (MDA), are significantly increased. Congruent with these data, our group has also shown that mesenteric myeloperoxidase (MPO) is significantly increased in portal hypertensive rats [9]. Furthermore, the levels of oxidative stress in the mesentery are closely related to circulating proinflammatory cytokines, such as TNF-α, IL-1β, and IL-6. Lee's study suggests that oxidative stress may have an additive/synergic effect on systemic inflammation on hyperdynamic circulation in cirrhotic animal models [35]. Now it is clear that cellular enzymes called nicotinamide adenine dinucleotide phosphate (NADPH) oxidases produce a considerable amount of ROS in humans [36] and a rat model of partial portal vein ligation (PPVL) [37]. Deng and coworkers [37] demonstrated that H_2O_2 is significantly increased in mesenteric tissues and in parallel, phosphorylated eNOS (p-eNOS) is elevated. NADPH oxidase inhibitor, GKT137831, significantly reduces mesenteric H_2O_2 and p-eNOS, linking oxidative stress and the vasodilator, NO [37]. Interestingly, GKT137831 also reduces cardiac index, portal vein pressure, portal vein blood flow, and portal–systemic shunting in PPVL rats. GKT137831 reverses the decreased mesenteric artery contractile response to norepinephrine in PPVL rats. The final effect of NADPH oxidase inhibition is ameliorating hyperdynamic circulation [37].

In 1998, the Moore lab [38] demonstrated that PPVL rats develop hyperdynamic circulation; this was reversed when these rats were treated with N-acetylcysteine (NAC) (Figure 1). Licks et al. [39] later found that in PPVL rats, in parallel with hyperdynamic circulation, the levels of gastric TBARS, nitrates, and nitrites are increased. In their four groups of rats (Sham, Sham + NAC, PPVL, and PPVL + NAC), the levels of oxidative stress markers paralleled that of nitrates and nitrites. The antioxidant parameters, such as superoxide dismutase (SOD) and glutathione peroxidase (GPx), were significantly decreased in PPVL rats. Histology showed that the vessels in the gastric mucosa in the PPVL group were dilated. NAC treatment significantly reversed these changes and resulted in a circulation that resembled what was observed in sham operated control rats. With these results, they concluded that oxidative stress contributes to portal hypertension and hyperdynamic circulation via the regulation of nitrates and nitrites, and antioxidant reverses these changes in the rat PPVL model.

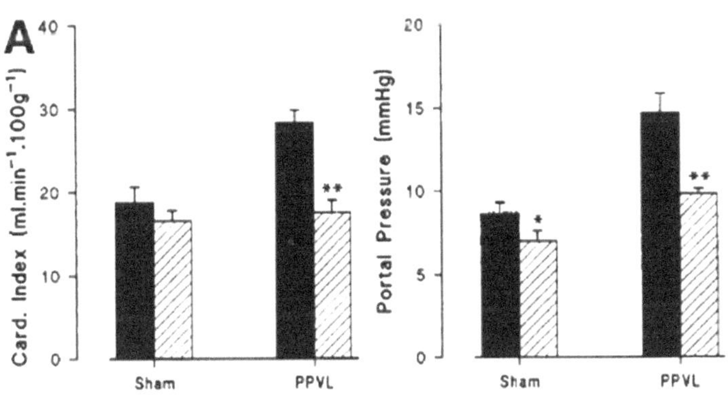

Figure 1. *Cont.*

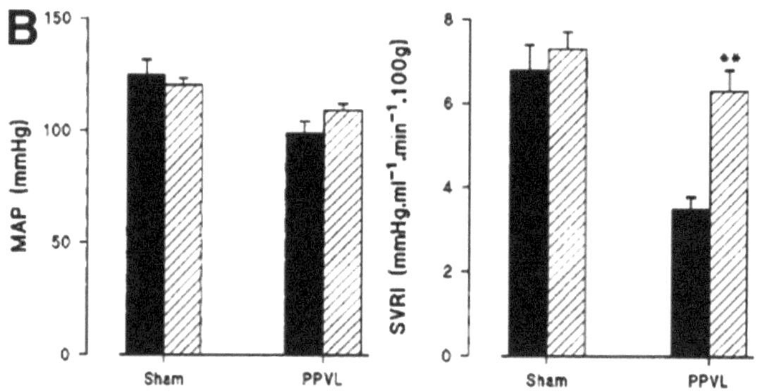

Figure 1. Hemodynamic studies in placebo-treated (■) and NAC-treated (▨) rats. Following PPVL and administration of placebo (n = 6), there was an increased cardiac output, portal pressure (**A**) and a reduction of MAP and systemic vascular resistance (**B**) compared with placebo-treated sham animals (n = 8). These hemodynamic changes were prevented by the twice-daily administration of NAC (PPVL + NAC) (n = 6). Values represent means ± SEM. PPVL + NAC vs. PPVL + placebo: ** $p < 0.0005$. Sham + placebo vs. sham + NAC: * $p < 0.05$. (Reproduced from reference [38]).

Interestingly, Iwakiri et al. [40] used a double knockout (iNOS, eNOS) mice in a PPVL model and observed that these mice still develop hyperdynamic circulation. This suggests that other variables in addition to the humoral theory may be at play in this complex condition.

6. Oxidative Stress in Central Neural Dysregulation

Hyperdynamic circulation due to the dysregulation of the central neural system [41] has also been described in subjects with cirrhosis and portal hypertension. This theory proposes that there is a reflex arc which regulates the cardiovascular system. The reflex arc includes the receptors in mesentery, afferent nerves, cardiovascular nuclei, and efferent nerves. The signals originating from receptors in mesentery are relayed via afferent nerves to the central neural system which then dispatches signals to the cardiovascular system via efferent nerves. The integrity of the reflex arc is essential for the regulation of the cardiovascular system [9,41,42]. Portal hypertension causes congestion in the mesentery which activates chemoreceptors and/or baroreceptors in the splanchnic area. Our study found that 10 days after PPVL, the MAP and SVR are significantly decreased and cardiac output significantly increased, indicating a hyperdynamic circulation [42]. We examined different interventions to test the role of this reflex arc in hyperdynamic circulation. We first tested the role of capsaicin-sensitive nerves in hyperdynamic circulation. Capsaicin was used to denervate the afferent nerves in rat pups. These rats were subjected to PPVL or BDL-induced cirrhosis when they reached adulthood [43]. We showed that capsaicin-treated PPVL or cirrhotic rats had similar cardiac output and systemic vascular resistance compared to the sham-operated group. In comparison, the PPVL or cirrhotic rats treated with vehicle (DMSO + ethanol) demonstrated hyperdynamic circulation. These data confirmed that capsaicin-treated rats have no capacity to develop hyperdynamic circulation when subjected to PPVL or cirrhosis. Capsaicin had no hemodynamic effect on sham-operated rats. These results showed that capsaicin treatment blocks the development of vasodilation in cirrhotic and portal hypertensive rats. Thus, primary afferent innervation is important in the pathogenesis of hyperdynamic circulation in portal hypertension and cirrhosis.

We then tested the central neural system in the regulation of hyperdynamic circulation in PPVL rats [42]. *c-fos* is an immediate-early gene and has important roles in cellular signal transduction. The *c-fos* protein product Fos is significantly increased in central cardiovascular nuclei such as the nucleus tractus solitarius (NTS) and paraventricular nucleus (PVN). Fos is an activation marker in the central neural system. We found that Fos expression is the prerequisite of hyperdynamic circulation in PPVL rats. Fos is detectable at day 1 after PPVL with immunohistochemistry and persistently increased when examined daily in the PPVL rats. However, the hyperdynamic circulation developed on day 3 and remained thereafter. When Fos expression in the NTS was blocked by local microinjection of *c-fos* antisense oligonucleotides, the increased cardiac output decreased SVR and MAP were reversed in PPVL rats. *c-fos* antisense oligonucleotides had no effect on circulation in sham-control rats. This experiment indicated that cardiovascular nuclei are crucial to the regulation of hyperdynamic circulation in PPVL rats [42].

We then tried to clarify the afferent nervous pathway. An inflatable cuff around the portal vein was used to acutely increase the portal pressure, then the vagal nerve electrical activity in the cervical area was recorded [41]. The acute increase in portal pressure immediately increased the vagal nerve electrical activity. In another experiment, the cervical vagus nerve was ablated by capsaicin. Three weeks after vagal ablation, the rats were subjected to PPVL. Our results showed that vagal nerve ablation significantly decreased Fos expression in the PVN of PPVL rats. Furthermore, vagal nerve blocked the development of hyperdynamic circulation in PPVL rats. This implied that an intact vagal nerve is a sine qua non in the pathogenesis of hyperdynamic circulation in PPVL rats [41].

The initial signal that triggers the hyperdynamic circulation in PPVL rats is thought to be mesenteric congestion. The congestion impacts two types of receptors, baroreceptors and chemoreceptors, as congestion not only increases the mesenteric venous pressure, but also causes ischemia. Chen et al. [44] induced cirrhosis in rats by CCl_4, and reported that H_2O_2 content in the mesenteric arterial wall was significantly increased in comparison to control animals. Several studies demonstrated that an antioxidant such as NAC significantly reverses hyperdynamic circulation in portal hypertensive animal models.

One of these studies from the Moore Lab demonstrated that NAC alleviates oxidative stress and prevents hyperdynamic circulation in the PPVL rats. They showed that the portal pressure remains significantly higher in the PPVL + NAC animals compared with sham + NAC rats [38]. However, that study did not further investigate the mechanism of NAC on the attenuation of hyperdynamic circulation.

We therefore performed a study to investigate the role of oxidative stress in the pathogenesis of hyperdynamic circulation, specifically aiming to evaluate whether oxidative stress is the initiating signal in the gut. We also used the PPVL model in rats because prehepatic portal hypertension creates mesenteric congestion and ischemia without significant liver parenchymal injury. Our study also reconfirmed the effect of NAC on hyperdynamic circulation in PPVL rats [10] (Figure 2). Furthermore, we found that jejunal MPO, an index of intestinal oxidative stress, is significantly increased in the PPVL model in rats; NAC treatment significantly decreased the activity of jejunal MPO (Figure 3). Interestingly, NAC also significantly decreased cardiac output, increased MAP and SVR, and reversed the hyperdynamic circulation in PPVL rats (Figure 2). To confirm that it is the oxidative stress that inaugurates hyperdynamic circulation, H_2O_2 was applied directly to the mesenteric area. We confirmed that H_2O_2 stimulates Fos expression in PVN (Figure 4), and decreased MAP, a direct index of hyperdynamic circulation. All these data indicate that it is the oxidative stress that triggers the hyperdynamic circulation in portal hypertension [9].

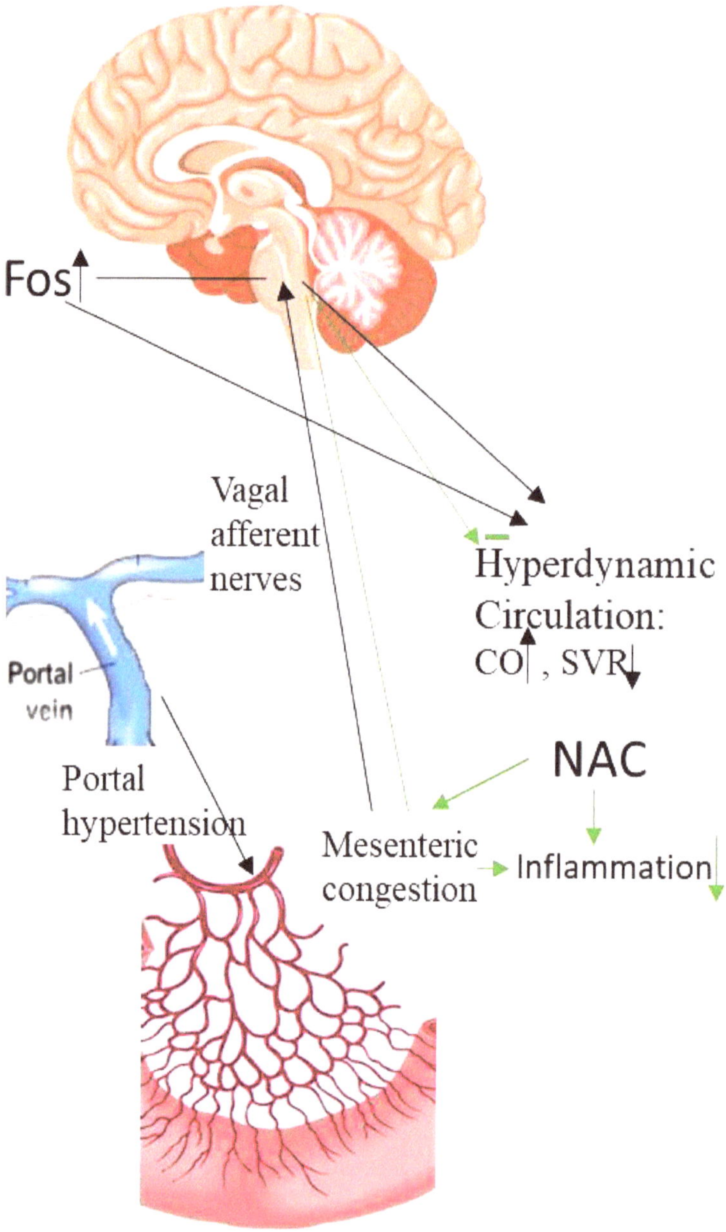

Figure 2. Changes in circulation indices. Schematic diagram to show the correlation among portal hypertension, mesenteric congestion, central neural activation and hyperdynamic circulation. CO: Cardiac output; MAP: mean arterial pressure; SVR: systemic vascular resistant; NAC: N-acetylcysteine. (Reproduced from reference [9]: Liu H et al., Hepatol Int 2023;17:689–697).

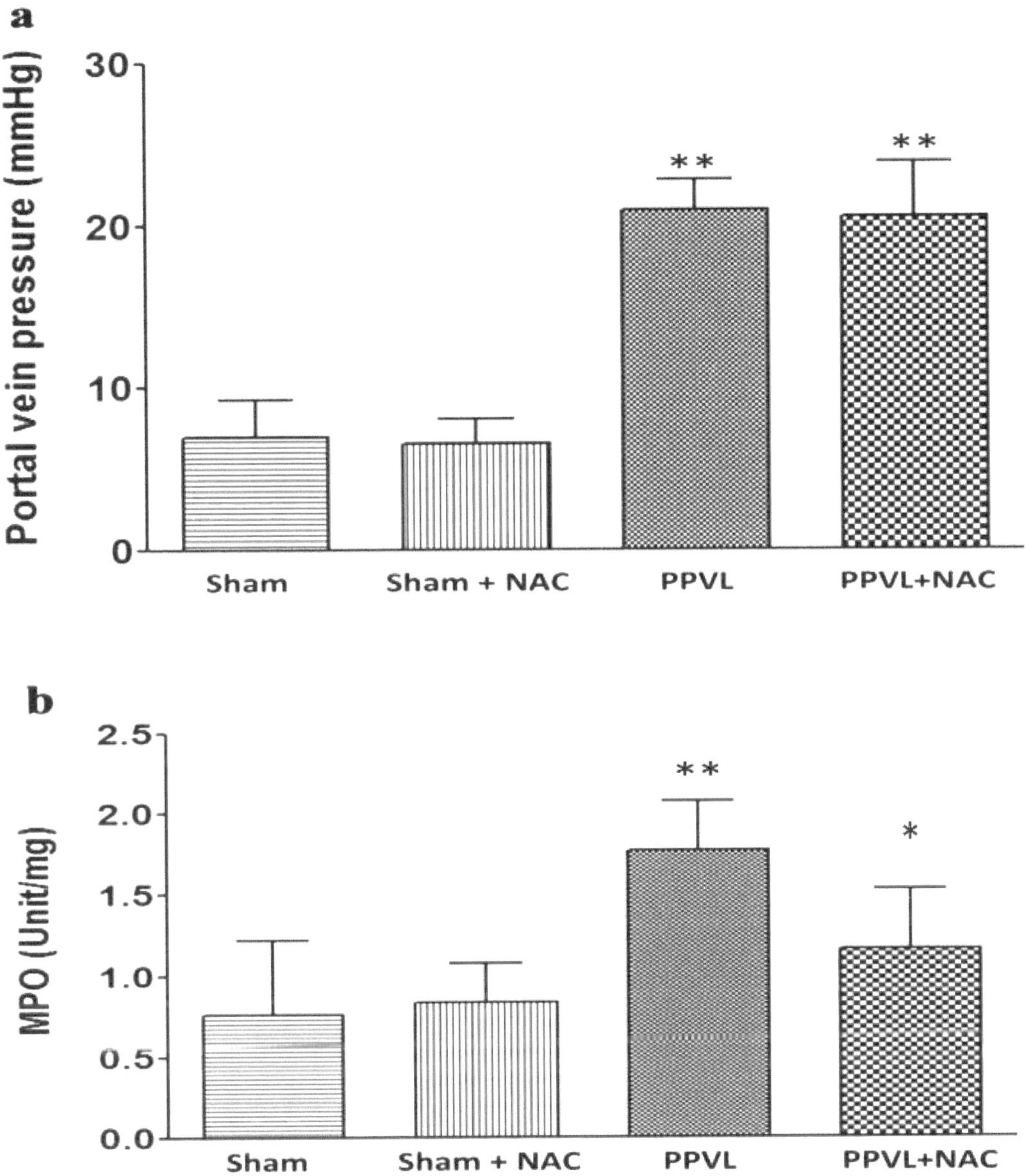

Figure 3. The effect of NAC on portal vein pressure and oxidative stress in mesentery area. (**a**) NAC has no effect on portal vein pressure either in Sham or BDL rats. (**b**) The effect of NAC on myeloperoxidase (MPO) status in the jejunum (** $p < 0.01$ compared with sham controls, * $p < 0.05$ compared eith PPVL group) NAC: N-acetylcysteine; PPVL: partial portal vein ligation. [Reproduced from reference [9]: Liu H et al., Hepatol Int 2023;17:689–697].

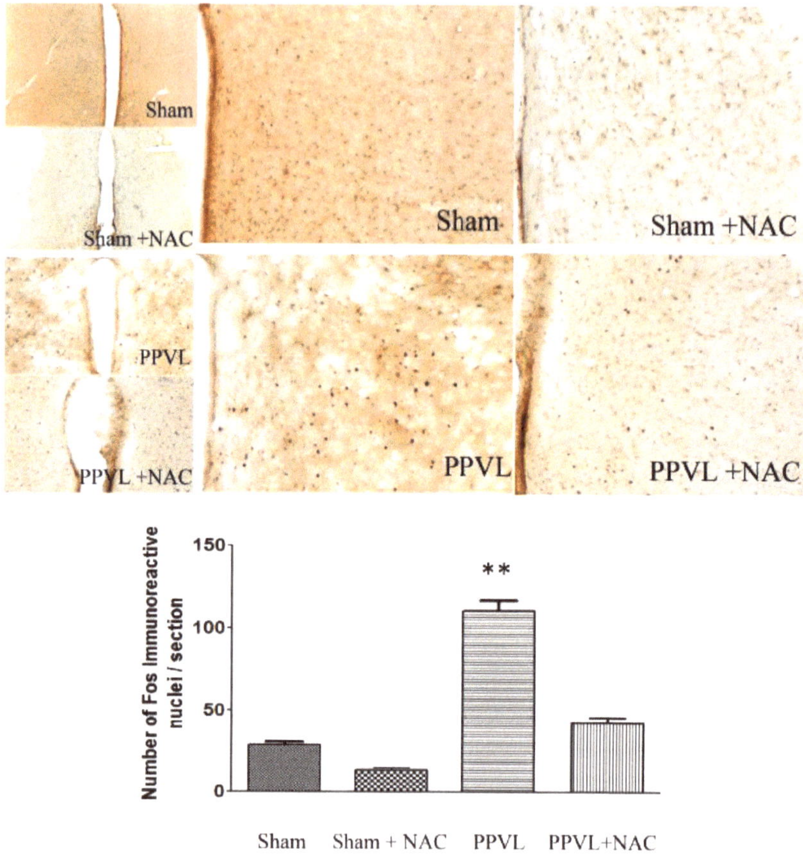

Figure 4. Fos density in the paraventricular nucleus (PVN) of the hypothalamus. Partial portal vein ligation (PPVL) significantly increased the density of Fos in PVN in PPVL rats. *N*-acetyl-cysteine (NAC) significantly decreased the density of Fos in PVN in PPVL rats, but did not change Fos density in PVN in sham-operated rats (** $p < 0.01$ compared with sham controls). (Reproduced from reference [9]: Liu H et al., Hepatol Int 2023; 17: 689–697).

7. Cirrhotic Cardiomyopathy

Cardiac dysfunction underlying cirrhosis in the absence of pre-existing heart disease is known as CCM [29]. The diagnostic criteria of CCM include systolic and diastolic dysfunction (Table 1). The mechanisms of CCM include endotoxemia, increased proinflammatory cytokines such as TNFα and IL-1β [45], apoptosis [46], changes in cardiac myofilament proteins [47], and oxidative stress [48].

ROS were previously thought to be produced almost exclusively from mitochondrial metabolism. Now it is clear that cellular enzymes called NADPH oxidases produce a considerable amount of ROS in humans [36] and animal models of PPVL in rats [37]. NADPH is located predominantly in the cytosolic compartment while NADH is localized predominantly to mitochondria and therefore, mitochondria are a main site of ROS production [49]. The first three cellular sources of ROS are neutrophils, monocytes, and cardiomyocytes. ROS is overproduced in subjects with cirrhosis [50].

Table 1. Diagnostic criteria proposed by Cirrhotic Cardiomyopathy Consortium.

Systolic Dysfunction	Advanced Diastolic Dysfunction	Areas for Future Research
Any of the following: • LV ejection fraction ≤ 50% • Absolute * GLS < 18%	≥3 of the following: • Septal e′ velocity < 7 cm/s • E/e′ ratio ≥ 15 • LAVI > 34 mL/m^2 TR velocity > 2.8 m/s	• Abnormal chronotropic or inotropic response • Electrocardiographic changes • Electromechanical uncoupling • Myocardial mass change • Serum biomarkers • Chamber enlargement • CMRI

* GLS (global longitudinal strain) is reported as a negative value in echocardiography reports. Changes in GLS should be described as changes in the absolute value. LV, left ventricle; e′, early diastolic mitral annular velocity; E/e′, ratio of mitral peak velocity of early filling to early diastolic mitral annular velocity; LAVI, left atrial (LA) volume index; TR, tricuspid regurgitation; CMRI, cardiac magnetic resonance imaging.

It is well known that the heart is an energy-consuming organ and around one-third of the cardiomyocyte is mitochondria in adults [49]. Ninety-five percent of energy supplied to the cardiomyocyte is derived from mitochondria (ref) [51]. Our study demonstrated that monocytes are increased in the hearts of cirrhotic animals [52] and highlights the innate immune response as a contributing source of ROS. Mousavi and colleagues [5] evaluated oxidative stress in cirrhotic hearts induced by BDL in rats and found that the ROS level, lipid peroxidation, and protein carbonylation were significantly increased in cirrhotic hearts compared with those in control hearts. Glutathione (GSH) in the cirrhotic heart was significantly depleted and oxidized glutathione (GSSG) was significantly increased, and the GSH/GSSG ratio was significantly decreased. The total antioxidant capacity was significantly reduced. Moreover, Mousavi's study revealed that the content of ATP, a marker of myocardial mitochondrial function, was significantly decreased (less than 50% of controls) in cirrhotic animals [5]. When mitochondria cannot meet the demands of a cell for ATP, ROS will be produced [49]. Mitochondria generate many types of ROS, including superoxide anion (O_2^-), H_2O_2, and hydroxyl radical (HO). Although the reactivity is different in each individual ROS, they all cause cardiomyocyte dysfunction. Mitochondrial homeostasis is therefore vital for preserving cardiac function [53]. The dysfunction of mitochondria causes a cellular energy crisis which plays an essential role in CCM (Figure 5). Our previous study also demonstrated that in the cirrhotic rat heart, 2,4-dinitrophenylhydazone, an indicator of oxidative stress, is significantly increased, and Nrf2, an antioxidant protein, is significantly decreased. Erythropoietin, an antioxidant, significantly reduced oxidative stress and augmented antioxidant proteins. Furthermore, erythropoietin significantly improved cardiac function in a rat cirrhotic model. These data imply that oxidative stress plays an important pathogenic role in the cirrhotic heart [48]

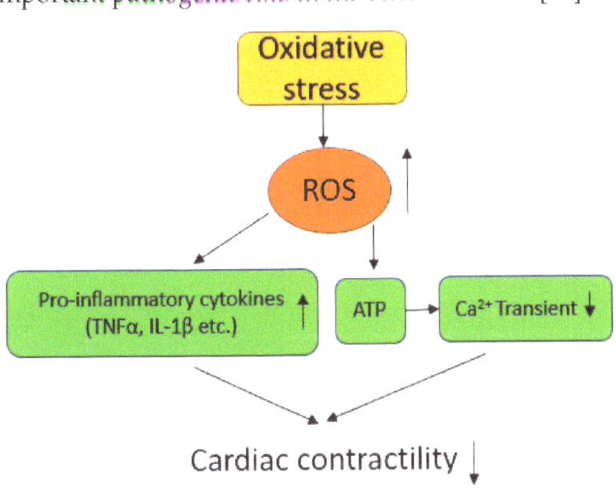

Figure 5. Pathogenic mechanism of oxidative stress on cardiac function.

8. Role of Oxidative Mechanisms in Cardiac Arrhythmias

In patients with cirrhosis, atrial fibrillation is the most common arrhythmia [54]. Oxidative stress is significantly increased and antioxidants are significantly decreased in noncirrhotic patients with atrial fibrillation [55,56]. Corradi and colleagues [55] reported that molecular markers of oxidative stress such as heme oxygenase-1 and 3-nitrotyrosine were significantly elevated and antioxidant biomarkers such as SOD-2 were significantly reduced in patients with atrial fibrillation. Bezna et al. [56] studied 80 patients with supraventricular cardiac arrhythmias and 40 healthy volunteers, and reported that specific antioxidant biomarkers such as SOD and glutathione peroxidase were significantly decreased in all patients with arrhythmias. Is there a direct *causal effect* of increased oxidative stress in cardiac arrhythmias? Morita et al. [57] directly exposed isolated hearts to H_2O_2 (0.1 mM) in a Langendorff setup and demonstrated that H_2O_2 directly induces ventricular fibrillation. Ranolazine, which inhibits late inward sodium current and has an antioxidant effect, prevents/terminates H_2O_2-induced ventricular fibrillation. Morita's study provides solid evidence that oxidative stress causes arrhythmias.

9. Acute Kidney Injury (AKI) and Hepatorenal Syndrome

HRS is defined as renal failure developing in patients with pre-existing chronic liver failure (acute or chronic) in the absence of any other identifiable cause of renal disease [58].

HRS is a serious and life-threatening complication of decompensated cirrhosis. HRS is not a purely 'functional' renal failure due to hemodynamic perturbation, as oxidative stress and inflammation are also thought to play a significant role in the pathogenesis of this condition. Local/systemic oxidative stress and inflammation cause structural changes [59]. The International Club of Ascites in 2007 classified HRS as types 1 and 2 (HRS-1 and HRS-2) [60]. HRS-1 is defined as a rapid deterioration of renal function due to precipitating factors, such as bacterial infection, large volume paracentesis, and gastrointestinal hemorrhage [61]. HRS-2 is a relatively slow process of progressive renal dysfunction. HRS-2 usually has no obvious precipitating factors. HRS-1 therefore manifests as acute renal failure and HRS-2 is mainly characterized by refractory ascites.

The pathogenesis of HRS is the underfilling of the arterial circulation due to arterial vasodilation combined with inadequate renal perfusion due to the ventricular dysfunction of CCM [62]. The causal connection between oxidative stress and HRS/AKI is whether oxidative stress contributes to arterial vasodilation and CCM. The pathogenic role of oxidative stress in CCM has been reviewed above. As for arterial vasodilatation, accumulating evidence indicates that oxidative stress contributes to the structural and functional derangement of the intestinal mucosa which results in the disruption of gut barrier integrity and increases permeability. The increased permeability, mesenteric congestion due to portal hypertension, and decreased hepatic detoxication capacity due to cirrhosis result in bacterial overgrowth, translocation, and increased lipopolysaccharides (LPS) which escape the liver via collateral circulation; the final result is endotoxemia. Endotoxin causes kidney damage in multifaceted ways [63] including vasodilation via TNFα, nitric oxide, and carbon monoxide. Therefore, oxidative stress is an Important factor in the pathogenesis of HRS.

10. Antioxidants as Potential Treatment Options in Cardiovascular Anomalies of Cirrhosis

There is no accepted specific treatment for the management of cardiovascular anomalies of cirrhosis. Traditional therapeutic strategies for non-cirrhotic heart diseases, such as vasodilators, are not suitable for heart dysfunction in cirrhosis because cirrhotic patients often have vasodilation and hypotension. As such, vasodilators may worsen a cirrhotic patient's clinical status [64]. Therefore, angiotensin-converting enzyme (ACE) inhibitors or angiotensin receptor blockers are not applicable in advanced cirrhosis and are contraindicated in HRS [64]. Liver transplantation is the definitive 'cure' for cardiovascular anomalies of cirrhosis. However, the shortage of donor organs may limit its application, and transplantation is not widely available in all global regions. Moreover, it is an expensive, complex procedure which is not feasible for many medical centers. Finally, long term immunosuppression is associated with adverse effects, including risk of infections and malignancy. Thus, the search for medical therapies for the cardiovascular complications of cirrhosis must continue. Accordingly, any study that finds a link between cardiovascular anomalies and certain molecules may lead to a potential therapeutic strategy. Oxidative stress-related molecules may thus be targets for this purpose.

11. Nonspecific Beta-Adrenergic Blockers (NSBBs)

Taprantzia et al. [65] investigated the status of oxidative stress in cirrhotic patients and demonstrated that oxidative indicators such as lipid hydroperoxides and malondialdehyde were significantly increased in cirrhotic patients compared with healthy controls. Propranolol treatment for one month significantly reduced oxidative stress by decreasing portal pressure in cirrhotic patients [66], improving mesenteric venous congestion, and decreasing intestinal permeability [67]. These effects indirectly alleviated endotoxemia and systemic inflammation [65].

Improvement in systemic inflammation benefits the cardiovascular system. Another potential benefit is that NSBBs shorten the prolonged QTc interval and decrease the risk of ventricular arrhythmias [68]. However, Silvestre et al. [69], in a randomized controlled trial, treated CCM patients with metoprolol and did not find significant improvement of cardiac function after 6 months in the metoprolol-treated group compared to a placebo. A lack of significant response was thought to reflect heterogeneity of the patient population and sympathetic neural response relative to severity of cirrhosis [70].

12. Taurine

Taurine has pleiotropic functions including anti-oxidation, anti-inflammation, and anti-apoptosis. It impacts many organs including retina, skeletal muscle, liver, platelets, and leukocytes [71]. Taurine is also thought to be essential for cardiovascular function as studies evaluating taurine transporter knockout mice note cardiac dysfunction as a phenotype [72]. Taurine has been shown to have a protective effect on oxidative stress-induced vascular dysfunction [73]. The role of taurine in CCM needs to be further investigated and characterized. The biosynthesis of taurine occurs primarily in the liver [71]. Cirrhosis decreases the functional liver mass and consequently the synthesis of taurine [64]. Low taurine serum levels have been closely associated with many oxidative stress-mediated pathologies, including hepatic disorders and cardiomyopathy [74].

Given that the antioxidant capacity in patients with cirrhosis is decreased, supplementation of taurine may be potentially beneficial. Taurine has been shown to reduce lipid peroxidation and protects cells from damage [75]. Using a model of transverse aortic constriction-induced heart failure in mice, Liu et al. [76] demonstrated that taurine has a protective effect on cardiac function. The mechanisms are thought to be secondary to reducing myocyte oxidative stress, apoptosis, hypertrophy, and cardiac fibrosis. These protective effects of taurine on non-cirrhotic heart failure may also apply to CCM. Mousavi and colleagues [5] showed that taurine significantly reduced tissue oxidative stress which includes lipid peroxidation, ROS, protein carbonylation, and the GSH/GSSG ratio in a bile duct ligation model of cirrhosis. Overall, taurine increased total antioxidant capacity and mitochondrial ATP content in this study. In summary, taurine decreases oxidative stress and improves mitochondrial function in the cirrhotic rat heart. Furthermore, taurine also decreases the level of creatine kinase MB (CK-MB), a marker of heart injury. Taurine is a valuable candidate worth further investigation in cirrhotic patients with cardiovascular complications.

13. Spermidine

Similar to taurine, spermidine also possesses antioxidant, anti-inflammatory, and anti-apoptotic properties [77,78]. Omar et al. [79] evaluated the effects of spermidine on isoproterenol-induced acute myocardial infarction and reported that it significantly increased electrocardiographic RR and QRS intervals to normal values, and decreased QT intervals and ST segment height to normal ranges, compared to the untreated group. Spermidine also significantly reduced serum CK-MB and lactate dehydrogenase (LDH), both parameters of serum cardiac injury. In parallel, the reduced antioxidant capacity in the untreated AMI group was rescued with spermidine treatment, indicating that the protective effect of spermidine is at least partially mediated via inhibition of oxidative stress [79].

Furthermore, Sheibani et al. [78] investigated the effects of spermidine in BDL-cirrhotic rats and demonstrated that spermidine significantly reduced the cardiac oxidative stress and inflammation. Moreover, spermidine significantly decreased the QTc interval in the BDL group (204 vs. 170 ms, $p < 0.001$). The cardiac contractility of spermidine-treated cirrhotic rats was also significantly increased in comparison with that from untreated BDL rats. These studies raise the possibility of the clinical application of spermidine in cirrhotic patients with cardiovascular diseases.

14. Direct Antioxidants

A meta-analysis [80] demonstrated that NAC not only significantly decreased oxidative markers, such as MDA and homocysteine, but also inflammatory markers, such as TNF-α and IL-6. Subjects with cirrhosis have both oxidative stress and inflammation, and this raises the question whether agents such as NAC can be used in this clinical setting. Using the BDL model of cirrhosis in rats, Lee and coworkers [35] reported that TBARS and MDA markers of oxidative stress were significantly increased in BDL vs. control rats. In parallel with this, inflammatory markers such as TNF-α, IL-1β, and IL-6 were also significantly increased in BDL rats. NAC significantly decreased both oxidative and inflammatory markers. Interestingly, one month treatment of NAC significantly attenuated systemic and splanchnic hyperdynamic circulation, improved hepatic endothelial dysfunction, and reduced intrahepatic resistance [27].

Another direct antioxidant is hydrogen. Because of the small size of the hydrogen molecule, it easily penetrates the cell membrane to the cytosol. Another advantage is that there are no side effects because it can be metabolized without residue [81]. Hydrogen exerts antioxidant [82], anti-inflammatory, and antiapoptotic effects [83,84], which has cardioprotective benefits. Hydrogen might be a novel treatment in various cardiovascular conditions such as ischemia–reperfusion injury [85] and cardiac transplantation because hydrogen protects cardiac allografts and reduces intimal hyperplasia of aortic allografts [86]. Lee et al. [35] revealed that hydrogen-rich saline significantly decreased TBARS and MDA, markers of oxidative stress, and increased SOD, GSH, markers of antioxidant in BDL rats compared with BDL + vehicle. Furthermore, hydrogen-rich saline decreased inflammatory markers such as TNF-α, IL-1β, and IL-6. The final results were the improvement of hepatic endothelial function, intrahepatic resistance, and systemic and splanchnic hyperdynamic circulation [35]. The studies on hydrogen at present are limited to animals, but there is potential for clinical application.

Other antioxidants, such as resveratrol [87], melatonin [88], and albumin [89] also have protective/therapeutic effects on cardiovascular diseases; these antioxidants may thus be applicable to treat cardiovascular complications in cirrhosis.

In conclusion, in subjects with cirrhosis and portal hypertension, oxidative stress plays an essential role in the pathogenesis of several complications. These complications include hyperdynamic circulation, cirrhotic cardiomyopathy, and acute kidney injury/hepatorenal syndrome. Oxidative stress stimulates inflammation and impacts the production of cardiac energy, which result in cardiac and vascular dysfunction. Antioxidants can reverse or mitigate these processes and thus may have potential therapeutic effects on cardiovascular and renal abnormalities in cirrhosis.

Author Contributions: Conceptualization, S.S.L.; writing—original draft preparation, H.L., H.H.N. and S.Y.H. All authors have read and agreed to the published version of the manuscript.

Funding: This research received no external funding.

Institutional Review Board Statement: Not applicable.

Informed Consent Statement: Not applicable.

Conflicts of Interest: The authors declare no conflict of interest.

References

1. Salete-Granado, D.; Carbonell, C.; Puertas-Miranda, D.; Vega-Rodriguez, V.J.; Garcia-Macia, M.; Herrero, A.B.; Marcos, M. Autophagy, Oxidative Stress, and Alcoholic Liver Disease: A Systematic Review and Potential Clinical Applications. *Antioxidants* **2023**, *12*, 1425. [CrossRef] [PubMed]
2. Barrea, L.; Verde, L.; Savastano, S.; Colao, A.; Muscogiuri, G. Adherence to Mediterranean Diet: Any Association with NAFLD? *Antioxidants* **2023**, *12*, 1318. [CrossRef]
3. Tanikawa, K.; Torimura, T. Studies on oxidative stress in liver diseases: Important future trends in liver research. *Med. Mol. Morphol.* **2006**, *39*, 22–27. [CrossRef]
4. Boyer-Diaz, Z.; Morata, P.; Aristu-Zabalza, P.; Gibert-Ramos, A.; Bosch, J.; Gracia-Sancho, J. Oxidative Stress in Chronic Liver Disease and Portal Hypertension: Potential of DHA as Nutraceutical. *Nutrients* **2020**, *12*, 2627. [CrossRef]
5. Mousavi, K.; Niknahad, H.; Ghalamfarsa, A.; Mohammadi, H.; Azarpira, N.; Ommati, M.M.; Heidari, R. Taurine mitigates cirrhosis-associated heart injury through mitochondrial-dependent and antioxidative mechanisms. *Clin. Exp. Hepatol.* **2020**, *6*, 207–219. [CrossRef]
6. Nickovic, V.P.; Miric, D.; Kisic, B.; Kocic, H.; Stojanovic, M.; Buttice, S.; Kocic, G. Oxidative stress, NOx/l-arginine ratio and glutathione/glutathione S-transferase ratio as predictors of 'sterile inflammation' in patients with alcoholic cirrhosis and hepatorenal syndrome type II. *Ren. Fail.* **2018**, *40*, 340–349. [CrossRef] [PubMed]
7. Ommati, M.M.; Mobasheri, A.; Ma, Y.; Xu, D.; Tang, Z.; Manthari, R.K.; Abdoli, N.; Azarpira, N.; Lu, Y.; Sadeghian, I.; et al. Taurine mitigates the development of pulmonary inflammation, oxidative stress, and histopathological alterations in a rat model of bile duct ligation. *Naunyn Schmiedebergs Arch. Pharmacol.* **2022**, *395*, 1557–1572. [CrossRef]
8. Bai, Y.; Li, K.; Li, X.; Chen, X.; Zheng, J.; Wu, F.; Chen, J.; Li, Z.; Zhang, S.; Wu, K.; et al. Effects of oxidative stress on hepatic encephalopathy pathogenesis in mice. *Nat. Commun.* **2023**, *14*, 4456. [CrossRef]
9. Liu, H.; Alhassan, N.; Yoon, K.T.; Almutlaq, L.; Lee, S.S. Oxidative stress triggers hyperdynamic circulation via central neural activation in portal hypertensive rats. *Hepatol. Int.* **2023**, *17*, 689–697. [CrossRef]
10. Ramachandran, A.; Prabhu, R.; Thomas, S.; Reddy, J.B.; Pulimood, A.; Balasubramanian, K.A. Intestinal mucosal alterations in experimental cirrhosis in the rat: Role of oxygen free radicals. *Hepatology* **2002**, *35*, 622–629. [CrossRef]
11. Assimakopoulos, S.F.; Tsamandas, A.C.; Tsiaoussis, G.I.; Karatza, E.; Zisimopoulos, D.; Maroulis, I.; Kontogeorgou, E.; Georgiou, C.D.; Scopa, C.D.; Thomopoulos, K.C. Intestinal mucosal proliferation, apoptosis and oxidative stress in patients with liver cirrhosis. *Ann. Hepatol.* **2013**, *12*, 301–307. [CrossRef]
12. Gilchrist, I.C. Dorsal Radial Access: Is the Back Door to the Arterial System Ready to Be the Workhorse Entry? *Cardiovasc. Revasc. Med.* **2019**, *20*, 735–736. [CrossRef]
13. Danielsen, K.V.; Wiese, S.; Busk, T.; Nabilou, P.; Kronborg, T.M.; Petersen, C.L.; Hove, J.D.; Moller, S.; Bendtsen, F. Cardiovascular Mapping in Cirrhosis From the Compensated Stage to Hepatorenal Syndrome: A Magnetic Resonance Study. *Am. J. Gastroenterol.* **2022**, *117*, 1269–1278. [CrossRef]
14. Dietrich, P.; Moleda, L.; Kees, F.; Muller, M.; Straub, R.H.; Hellerbrand, C.; Wiest, R. Dysbalance in sympathetic neurotransmitter release and action in cirrhotic rats: Impact of exogenous neuropeptide Y. *J. Hepatol.* **2013**, *58*, 254–261. [CrossRef]
15. Fialla, A.D.; Thiesson, H.C.; Bie, P.; Schaffalitzky de Muckadell, O.B.; Krag, A. Internal dysregulation of the renin system in patients with stable liver cirrhosis. *Scand. J. Clin. Lab. Investig.* **2017**, *77*, 298–309. [CrossRef]
16. Hsu, S.J.; Lin, T.Y.; Wang, S.S.; Chuang, C.L.; Lee, F.Y.; Huang, H.C.; Hsin, I.F.; Lee, J.Y.; Lin, H.C.; Lee, S.D. Endothelin receptor blockers reduce shunting and angiogenesis in cirrhotic rats. *Eur. J. Clin. Investig.* **2016**, *46*, 572–580. [CrossRef] [PubMed]
17. Sola, E.; Gines, P. Challenges and Management of Liver Cirrhosis: Pathophysiology of Renal Dysfunction in Cirrhosis. *Dig. Dis.* **2015**, *33*, 534–538. [CrossRef] [PubMed]
18. Ohara, N.; Jaspan, J.; Chang, S.W. Hyperglucagonemia and hyperdynamic circulation in rats with biliary cirrhosis. *J. Lab. Clin. Med.* **1993**, *121*, 142–147. [PubMed]
19. Oberti, F.; Sogni, P.; Cailmail, S.; Moreau, R.; Pipy, B.; Lebrec, D. Role of prostacyclin in hemodynamic alterations in conscious rats with extrahepatic or intrahepatic portal hypertension. *Hepatology* **1993**, *18*, 621–627. [CrossRef] [PubMed]
20. Papagiouvanni, I.; Sarafidis, P.; Theodorakopoulou, M.P.; Sinakos, E.; Goulis, I. Endothelial and microvascular function in liver cirrhosis: An old concept that needs re-evaluation? *Ann. Gastroenterol.* **2022**, *35*, 471–482. [CrossRef] [PubMed]
21. Liu, H.; Song, D.; Lee, S.S. Role of heme oxygenase-carbon monoxide pathway in pathogenesis of cirrhotic cardiomyopathy in the rat. *Am. J. Physiol. Gastrointest. Liver Physiol.* **2001**, *280*, G68–G74. [CrossRef] [PubMed]

22. Moller, S.; Bendtsen, F. The pathophysiology of arterial vasodilatation and hyperdynamic circulation in cirrhosis. *Liver Int.* **2018**, *38*, 570–580. [CrossRef] [PubMed]
23. Henriksen, J.H.; Ring-Larsen, H.; Christensen, N.J. Sympathetic nervous activity in cirrhosis. A survey of plasma catecholamine studies. *J. Hepatol.* **1985**, *1*, 55–65. [CrossRef]
24. Vidal Gonzalez, D.; Perez Lopez, K.P.; Vera Nungaray, S.A.; Moreno Madrigal, L.G. Treatment of refractory ascites: Current strategies and new landscape of non-selective beta-blockers. *Gastroenterol. Hepatol.* **2022**, *45*, 715–723. [CrossRef]
25. Gunarathne, L.S.; Rajapaksha, H.; Shackel, N.; Angus, P.W.; Herath, C.B. Cirrhotic portal hypertension: From pathophysiology to novel therapeutics. *World J. Gastroenterol.* **2020**, *26*, 6111–6140. [CrossRef] [PubMed]
26. Hartl, L.; Rumpf, B.; Domenig, O.; Simbrunner, B.; Paternostro, R.; Jachs, M.; Poglitsch, M.; Marculescu, R.; Trauner, M.; Reindl-Schwaighofer, R.; et al. The systemic and hepatic alternative renin-angiotensin system is activated in liver cirrhosis, linked to endothelial dysfunction and inflammation. *Sci. Rep.* **2023**, *13*, 953. [CrossRef]
27. Jimenez, W.; Rodes, J. Impaired responsiveness to endogenous vasoconstrictors and endothelium-derived vasoactive factors in cirrhosis. *Gastroenterology* **1994**, *107*, 1201–1203. [CrossRef]
28. Wong, F.; Girgrah, N.; Graba, J.; Allidina, Y.; Liu, P.; Blendis, L. The cardiac response to exercise in cirrhosis. *Gut* **2001**, *49*, 268–275. [CrossRef]
29. Izzy, M.; VanWagner, L.B.; Lin, G.; Altieri, M.; Findlay, J.Y.; Oh, J.K.; Watt, K.D.; Lee, S.S.; Cirrhotic Cardiomyopathy Consortium. Redefining Cirrhotic Cardiomyopathy for the Modern Era. *Hepatology* **2020**, *71*, 334–345. [CrossRef]
30. Yang, Y.Y.; Liu, H.; Nam, S.W.; Kunos, G.; Lee, S.S. Mechanisms of TNFalpha-induced cardiac dysfunction in cholestatic bile duct-ligated mice: Interaction between TNFalpha and endocannabinoids. *J. Hepatol.* **2010**, *53*, 298–306. [CrossRef]
31. Teuber, J.P.; Essandoh, K.; Hummel, S.L.; Madamanchi, N.R.; Brody, M.J. NADPH Oxidases in Diastolic Dysfunction and Heart Failure with Preserved Ejection Fraction. *Antioxidants* **2022**, *11*, 1822. [CrossRef]
32. Groszmann, R.J. Hyperdynamic state in chronic liver diseases. *J. Hepatol.* **1993**, *17* (Suppl. 2), S38–S40. [CrossRef]
33. Bolognesi, M.; Di Pascoli, M.; Verardo, A.; Gatta, A. Splanchnic vasodilation and hyperdynamic circulatory syndrome in cirrhosis. *World J. Gastroenterol.* **2014**, *20*, 2555–2563. [CrossRef]
34. Ebrahimkhani, M.R.; Mani, A.R.; Moore, K. Hydrogen sulphide and the hyperdynamic circulation in cirrhosis: A hypothesis. *Gut* **2005**, *54*, 1668–1671. [CrossRef]
35. Lee, P.C.; Yang, Y.Y.; Huang, C.S.; Hsieh, S.L.; Lee, K.C.; Hsieh, Y.C.; Lee, T.Y.; Lin, H.C. Concomitant inhibition of oxidative stress and angiogenesis by chronic hydrogen-rich saline and N-acetylcysteine treatments improves systemic, splanchnic and hepatic hemodynamics of cirrhotic rats. *Hepatol. Res.* **2015**, *45*, 578–588. [CrossRef] [PubMed]
36. Bardaweel, S.K.; Gul, M.; Alzweiri, M.; Ishaqat, A.; ALSalamat, H.A.; Bashatwah, R.M. Reactive Oxygen Species: The Dual Role in Physiological and Pathological Conditions of the Human Body. *Eurasian J. Med.* **2018**, *50*, 193–201. [CrossRef]
37. Deng, W.; Duan, M.; Qian, B.; Zhu, Y.; Lin, J.; Zheng, L.; Zhang, C.; Qi, X.; Luo, M. NADPH oxidase 1/4 inhibition attenuates the portal hypertensive syndrome via modulation of mesenteric angiogenesis and arterial hyporeactivity in rats. *Clin. Res. Hepatol. Gastroenterol.* **2019**, *43*, 255–265. [CrossRef]
38. Fernando, B.; Marley, R.; Holt, S.; Anand, R.; Harry, D.; Sanderson, P.; Smith, R.; Hamilton, G.; Moore, K. N-acetylcysteine prevents development of the hyperdynamic circulation in the portal hypertensive rat. *Hepatology* **1998**, *28*, 689–694. [CrossRef]
39. Licks, F.; Marques, C.; Zetler, C.; Martins, M.I.; Marroni, C.A.; Marroni, N.P. Antioxidant effect of N-acetylcysteine on prehepatic portal hypertensive gastropathy in rats. *Ann. Hepatol.* **2014**, *13*, 370–377. [CrossRef]
40. Iwakiri, Y.; Cadelina, G.; Sessa, W.C.; Groszmann, R.J. Mice with targeted deletion of eNOS develop hyperdynamic circulation associated with portal hypertension. *Am. J. Physiol. Gastrointest. Liver Physiol.* **2002**, *283*, G1074–G1081. [CrossRef]
41. Liu, H.; Schuelert, N.; McDougall, J.J.; Lee, S.S. Central neural activation of hyperdynamic circulation in portal hypertensive rats depends on vagal afferent nerves. *Gut* **2008**, *57*, 966–973. [CrossRef]
42. Song, D.; Liu, H.; Sharkey, K.A.; Lee, S.S. Hyperdynamic circulation in portal-hypertensive rats is dependent on central c-fos gene expression. *Hepatology* **2002**, *35*, 159–166. [CrossRef]
43. Lee, S.S.; Sharkey, K.A. Capsaicin treatment blocks development of hyperkinetic circulation in portal hypertensive and cirrhotic rats. *Am. J. Physiol.* **1993**, *264 Pt 1*, G868–G873. [CrossRef]
44. Chen, W.; Liu, D.J.; Huo, Y.M.; Wu, Z.Y.; Sun, Y.W. Reactive oxygen species are involved in regulating hypocontractility of mesenteric artery to norepinephrine in cirrhotic rats with portal hypertension. *Int. J. Biol. Sci.* **2014**, *10*, 386–395. [CrossRef]
45. Liu, H.; Ma, Z.; Lee, S.S. Contribution of nitric oxide to the pathogenesis of cirrhotic cardiomyopathy in bile duct-ligated rats. *Gastroenterology* **2000**, *118*, 937–944. [CrossRef]
46. Nam, S.W.; Liu, H.; Wong, J.Z.; Feng, A.Y.; Chu, G.; Merchant, N.; Lee, S.S. Cardiomyocyte apoptosis contributes to pathogenesis of cirrhotic cardiomyopathy in bile duct-ligated mice. *Clin. Sci.* **2014**, *127*, 519–526. [CrossRef]
47. Glenn, T.K.; Honar, H.; Liu, H.; ter Keurs, H.E.; Lee, S.S. Role of cardiac myofilament proteins titin and collagen in the pathogenesis of diastolic dysfunction in cirrhotic rats. *J. Hepatol.* **2011**, *55*, 1249–1255. [CrossRef]
48. Liu, L.; Liu, H.; Nam, S.W.; Lee, S.S. Protective effects of erythropoietin on cirrhotic cardiomyopathy in rats. *Dig. Liver Dis.* **2012**, *44*, 1012–1017. [CrossRef]
49. Manolis, A.S.; Manolis, A.A.; Manolis, T.A.; Apostolaki, N.E.; Apostolopoulos, E.J.; Melita, H.; Katsiki, N. Mitochondrial dysfunction in cardiovascular disease: Current status of translational research/clinical and therapeutic implications. *Med. Res. Rev.* **2021**, *41*, 275–313. [CrossRef]

50. Banerjee, P.; Gaddam, N.; Chandler, V.; Chakraborty, S. Oxidative Stress-Induced Liver Damage and Remodeling of the Liver Vasculature. *Am. J. Pathol.* **2023**, *193*, 1400–1414. [CrossRef]
51. Szyller, J.; Jagielski, D.; Bil-Lula, I. Antioxidants in Arrhythmia Treatment-Still a Controversy? A Review of Selected Clinical and Laboratory Research. *Antioxidants* **2022**, *11*, 1109. [CrossRef]
52. Gaskari, S.A.; Liu, H.; D'Mello, C.; Kunos, G.; Lee, S.S. Blunted cardiac response to hemorrhage in cirrhotic rats is mediated by local macrophage-released endocannabinoids. *J. Hepatol.* **2015**, *62*, 1272–1277. [CrossRef]
53. Goracy, A.; Rosik, J.; Szostak, J.; Szostak, B.; Retfinski, S.; Machaj, F.; Pawlik, A. Improving mitochondrial function in preclinical models of heart failure: Therapeutic targets for future clinical therapies? *Expert Opin. Ther. Targets* **2023**, *27*, 593–608. [CrossRef]
54. Vandenberk, B.; Altieri, M.H.; Liu, H.; Raj, S.R.; Lee, S.S. Review article: Diagnosis, pathophysiology and management of atrial fibrillation in cirrhosis and portal hypertension. *Aliment. Pharmacol. Ther.* **2023**, *57*, 290–303. [CrossRef]
55. Corradi, D.; Callegari, S.; Manotti, L.; Ferrara, D.; Goldoni, M.; Alinovi, R.; Pinelli, S.; Mozzoni, P.; Andreoli, R.; Asimaki, A.; et al. Persistent lone atrial fibrillation: Clinicopathologic study of 19 cases. *Heart Rhythm* **2014**, *11*, 1250–1258. [CrossRef]
56. Bezna, M.C.; Danoiu, S.; Bezna, M.; Voisneanu, I.A.; Genunche-Dumitrescu, A.; Istratoaie, O. The Importance of Oxidative Stress Biomarkers and the Need of Antioxidant Therapy in the Control of Cardiac Arrhythmias. *Eur. Cardiol.* **2023**, *18*, e32. [CrossRef]
57. Morita, N.; Lee, J.H.; Xie, Y.; Sovari, A.; Qu, Z.; Weiss, J.N.; Karagueuzian, H.S. Suppression of re-entrant and multifocal ventricular fibrillation by the late sodium current blocker ranolazine. *J. Am. Coll. Cardiol.* **2011**, *57*, 366–375. [CrossRef]
58. Arroyo, V.; Gines, P.; Gerbes, A.L.; Dudley, F.J.; Gentilini, P.; Laffi, G.; Reynolds, T.B.; Ring-Larsen, H.; Scholmerich, J. Definition and diagnostic criteria of refractory ascites and hepatorenal syndrome in cirrhosis. International Ascites Club. *Hepatology* **1996**, *23*, 164–176. [CrossRef]
59. Angeli, P.; Garcia-Tsao, G.; Nadim, M.K.; Parikh, C.R. News in pathophysiology, definition and classification of hepatorenal syndrome: A step beyond the International Club of Ascites (ICA) consensus document. *J. Hepatol.* **2019**, *71*, 811–822. [CrossRef]
60. Salerno, F.; Gerbes, A.; Gines, P.; Wong, F.; Arroyo, V. Diagnosis, prevention and treatment of hepatorenal syndrome in cirrhosis. *Gut* **2007**, *56*, 1310–1318. [CrossRef]
61. Chinnasamy, V.; Dhande, S.K.; Kumar, K.M.; M, J. Precipitating Factors and Outcome of Hepatorenal Syndrome in Liver Cirrhosis. *J. Assoc. Physicians India* **2023**, *71*, 1.
62. Gines, P.; Sola, E.; Angeli, P.; Wong, F.; Nadim, M.K.; Kamath, P.S. Hepatorenal syndrome. *Nat. Rev. Dis. Primers* **2018**, *4*, 23. [CrossRef]
63. Peng, J.L.; Techasatian, W.; Hato, T.; Liangpunsakul, S. Role of endotoxemia in causing renal dysfunction in cirrhosis. *J. Investig. Med.* **2020**, *68*, 26–29. [CrossRef]
64. Yoon, K.T.; Liu, H.; Lee, S.S. Cirrhotic Cardiomyopathy. *Curr. Gastroenterol. Rep.* **2020**, *22*, 45. [CrossRef]
65. Taprantzi, D.; Zisimopoulos, D.; Thomopoulos, K.C.; Spiliopoulou, I.; Georgiou, C.D.; Tsiaoussis, G.; Triantos, C.; Gogos, C.A.; Labropoulou-Karatza, C.; Assimakopoulos, S.F. Propranolol reduces systemic oxidative stress and endotoxemia in cirrhotic patients with esophageal varices. *Ann. Gastroenterol.* **2018**, *31*, 224–230. [CrossRef]
66. Iwakiri, Y.; Trebicka, J. Portal hypertension in cirrhosis: Pathophysiological mechanisms and therapy. *JHEP Rep.* **2021**, *3*, 100316. [CrossRef]
67. Reiberger, T.; Ferlitsch, A.; Payer, B.A.; Mandorfer, M.; Heinisch, B.B.; Hayden, H.; Lammert, F.; Trauner, M.; Peck-Radosavljevic, M.; Vogelsang, H.; et al. Non-selective betablocker therapy decreases intestinal permeability and serum levels of LBP and IL-6 in patients with cirrhosis. *J. Hepatol.* **2013**, *58*, 911–921. [CrossRef]
68. Lee, W.; Vandenberk, B.; Raj, S.R.; Lee, S.S. Prolonged QT Interval in Cirrhosis: Twisting Time? *Gut Liver* **2022**, *16*, 849–860. [CrossRef]
69. Silvestre, O.M.; Farias, A.Q.; Ramos, D.S.; Furtado, M.S.; Rodrigues, A.C.; Ximenes, R.O.; de Campos Mazo, D.F.; Yoshimura Zitelli, P.M.; Diniz, M.A.; Andrade, J.L.; et al. beta-Blocker therapy for cirrhotic cardiomyopathy: A randomized-controlled trial. *Eur. J. Gastroenterol. Hepatol.* **2018**, *30*, 930–937. [CrossRef]
70. Krag, A.; Wiest, R.; Albillos, A.; Gluud, L.L. The window hypothesis: Haemodynamic and non-haemodynamic effects of beta-blockers improve survival of patients with cirrhosis during a window in the disease. *Gut* **2012**, *61*, 967–969. [CrossRef]
71. Baliou, S.; Adamaki, M.; Ioannou, P.; Pappa, A.; Panayiotidis, M.I.; Spandidos, D.A.; Christodoulou, I.; Kyriakopoulos, A.M.; Zoumpourlis, V. Protective role of taurine against oxidative stress (Review). *Mol. Med. Rep.* **2021**, *24*, 605. [CrossRef]
72. Ito, T.; Oishi, S.; Takai, M.; Kimura, Y.; Uozumi, Y.; Fujio, Y.; Schaffer, S.W.; Azuma, J. Cardiac and skeletal muscle abnormality in taurine transporter-knockout mice. *J. Biomed. Sci.* **2010**, *17* (Suppl. 1), S20. [CrossRef]
73. Ozsarlak-Sozer, G.; Sevin, G.; Ozgur, H.H.; Yetik-Anacak, G.; Kerry, Z. Diverse effects of taurine on vascular response and inflammation in GSH depletion model in rabbits. *Eur. Rev. Med. Pharmacol. Sci.* **2016**, *20*, 1360–1372.
74. Schaffer, S.W.; Jong, C.J.; Ramila, K.C.; Azuma, J. Physiological roles of taurine in heart and muscle. *J. Biomed. Sci.* **2010**, *17* (Suppl. 1), S2. [CrossRef]
75. Goodman, C.A.; Horvath, D.; Stathis, C.; Mori, T.; Croft, K.; Murphy, R.M.; Hayes, A. Taurine supplementation increases skeletal muscle force production and protects muscle function during and after high-frequency in vitro stimulation. *J. Appl. Physiol. (1985)* **2009**, *107*, 144–154. [CrossRef]
76. Liu, J.; Ai, Y.; Niu, X.; Shang, F.; Li, Z.; Liu, H.; Li, W.; Ma, W.; Chen, R.; Wei, T.; et al. Taurine protects against cardiac dysfunction induced by pressure overload through SIRT1-p53 activation. *Chem. Biol. Interact.* **2020**, *317*, 108972. [CrossRef]

77. Jiang, D.; Wang, X.; Zhou, X.; Wang, Z.; Li, S.; Sun, Q.; Jiang, Y.; Ji, C.; Ling, W.; An, X.; et al. Spermidine alleviating oxidative stress and apoptosis by inducing autophagy of granulosa cells in Sichuan white geese. *Poult. Sci.* **2023**, *102*, 102879. [CrossRef]
78. Sheibani, M.; Nezamoleslami, S.; Mousavi, S.E.; Faghir-Ghanesefat, H.; Yousefi-Manesh, H.; Rezayat, S.M.; Dehpour, A. Protective Effects of Spermidine Against Cirrhotic Cardiomyopathy in Bile Duct-Ligated Rats. *J. Cardiovasc. Pharmacol.* **2020**, *76*, 286–295. [CrossRef]
79. Omar, E.M.; Omar, R.S.; Shoela, M.S.; El Sayed, N.S. A study of the cardioprotective effect of spermidine: A novel inducer of autophagy. *Chin. J. Physiol.* **2021**, *64*, 281–288. [CrossRef]
80. Faghfouri, A.H.; Zarezadeh, M.; Tavakoli-Rouzbehani, O.M.; Radkhah, N.; Faghfuri, E.; Kord-Varkaneh, H.; Tan, S.C.; Ostadrahimi, A. The effects of N-acetylcysteine on inflammatory and oxidative stress biomarkers: A systematic review and meta-analysis of controlled clinical trials. *Eur. J. Pharmacol.* **2020**, *884*, 173368. [CrossRef]
81. Saengsin, K.; Sittiwangkul, R.; Chattipakorn, S.C.; Chattipakorn, N. Hydrogen therapy as a potential therapeutic intervention in heart disease: From the past evidence to future application. *Cell. Mol. Life Sci.* **2023**, *80*, 174. [CrossRef]
82. Graves, J.; Mason, M.; Laws, D. A case of orthodeoxia platypnoea in a patient with adult polycystic kidney and liver disease with a patent foramen ovale. *Acute Med.* **2007**, *6*, 126–127. [CrossRef]
83. Ohta, S. Molecular hydrogen as a preventive and therapeutic medical gas: Initiation, development and potential of hydrogen medicine. *Pharmacol. Ther.* **2014**, *144*, 1–11. [CrossRef]
84. Yao, L.; Chen, H.; Wu, Q.; Xie, K. Hydrogen-rich saline alleviates inflammation and apoptosis in myocardial I/R injury via PINK-mediated autophagy. *Int. J. Mol. Med.* **2019**, *44*, 1048–1062. [CrossRef]
85. Sun, Q.; Kang, Z.; Cai, J.; Liu, W.; Liu, Y.; Zhang, J.H.; Denoble, P.J.; Tao, H.; Sun, X. Hydrogen-rich saline protects myocardium against ischemia/reperfusion injury in rats. *Exp. Biol. Med.* **2009**, *234*, 1212–1219. [CrossRef]
86. Noda, K.; Tanaka, Y.; Shigemura, N.; Kawamura, T.; Wang, Y.; Masutani, K.; Sun, X.; Toyoda, Y.; Bermudez, C.A.; Nakao, A. Hydrogen-supplemented drinking water protects cardiac allografts from inflammation-associated deterioration. *Transpl. Int.* **2012**, *25*, 1213–1222. [CrossRef]
87. Breuss, J.M.; Atanasov, A.G.; Uhrin, P. Resveratrol and Its Effects on the Vascular System. *Int. J. Mol. Sci.* **2019**, *20*, 1523. [CrossRef]
88. Ma, X.; Wang, S.; Cheng, H.; Ouyang, H.; Ma, X. Melatonin Attenuates Ischemia/Reperfusion-Induced Oxidative Stress by Activating Mitochondrial Fusion in Cardiomyocytes. *Oxid. Med. Cell. Longev.* **2022**, *2022*, 7105181. [CrossRef]
89. Bortoluzzi, A.; Ceolotto, G.; Gola, E.; Sticca, A.; Bova, S.; Morando, F.; Piano, S.; Fasolato, S.; Rosi, S.; Gatta, A.; et al. Positive cardiac inotropic effect of albumin infusion in rodents with cirrhosis and ascites: Molecular mechanisms. *Hepatology* **2013**, *57*, 266–276. [CrossRef]

MDPI AG
Grosspeteranlage 5
4052 Basel
Switzerland
Tel.: +41 61 683 77 34

International Journal of Molecular Sciences Editorial Office
E-mail: ijms@mdpi.com
www.mdpi.com/journal/ijms

www.ingramcontent.com/pod-product-compliance
Lightning Source LLC
Chambersburg PA
CBHW041102270926
51850CB00025B/3309
9783725843237